Building Blocks in Paediatrics

Building Blocks in Paediatrics

EDITED BY

Alfred Nicholson, FRCPI, FRCPCH

Head of School
Royal College of Surgeons in Ireland (RCSI)
Bahrain, Kingdom of Bahrain

Kevin Dunne, FRCPCH, DCH

Professor of Paediatrics and Child Health
Royal College of Surgeons in Ireland (RCSI)
Bahrain, Kingdom of Bahrain

ELSEVIER

Notices

Practitioners and researchers must always rely on their own experience and knowledge in evaluating and using any information, methods, compounds or experiments described herein. Because of rapid advances in the medical sciences in particular, independent verification of diagnoses and drug dosages should be made. To the fullest extent of the law, no responsibility is assumed by Elsevier, authors, editors or contributors for any injury and/or damage to persons or property as a matter of products liability, negligence or otherwise, or from any use or operation of any methods, products, instructions, or ideas contained in the material herein.

ISBN: 978-0-3238-3421-6

Content Strategist: Alexandra Mortimer
Content Project Manager: Shubham Dixit
Design: Bridget Hoette
Illustration Manager: Narayanan Ramakrishnan
Marketing Manager: Deborah Watkins

Printed in Scotland

Last digit is the print number: 9 8 7 6 5 4 3 2 1

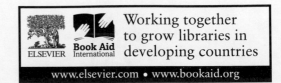

Contents

Foreword

In calling this gem of a textbook 'Building blocks', Alf Nicholson and Kevin Dunne have set themselves a difficult task. Fortunately, its one they succeed at with great aplomb. The book indeed provides the reader with the building blocks of knowledge of clinical child health and makes a good fist of going beyond knowledge to influencing attitudes and imparting basic skills.

There are many textbooks of paediatrics and child health, but this will, I am sure, become one of 'the' textbooks for students and even senior doctors alike. It very much gives the lie to the suggestion that textbooks have been superseded by online sources. In our age where the endless availability of information is overwhelming, a concise pragmatic summary is a huge asset and will be very much valued by medical students, generalists such as GPs and paediatric trainees.

Reading through it I remembered a great deal that I had forgotten, as well as learning much that I never knew (or had forgotten I ever knew).

Everything the medical student and trainee doctor needs is here, from the basics of taking a history and examination of children and teenagers through to core specialist knowledge (such as congenital heart disease) through to ethics and prevention. Each condition is described by an expert yet in an uncomplicated and pragmatic way, providing a brief summary of the key conditions, common findings and diagnostic dilemmas, and practical management. This is as true of the most specialised chapters as for general chapters on toddlers and adolescents.

I suspect the most useful may be the excellent chapters based around problems or symptoms. The series of 'The Child with' chapters on cough, diarrhoea, fever, frequent infections and so on will be particularly useful for GPs I imagine, and also provide paediatricians with sensible approaches to these common clinical presentations. I was particularly gratified to see obesity, mental health and adolescent medicine given so much space, recognising the importance of each of these in modern clinical child health.

I loved the many practical examples, showing the humanity and years of experience of the writers. The chapter entitled 'Frequent Flyers in the Toddler Years' is full of this wisdom, and I can imagine many general practitioners (which I briefly once was) and paediatric trainees keeping this section particularly to hand for ready reference. My favourite section was 'A Toddler Who Just Will Not Sleep'.

I thoroughly recommend this book and believe it will give readers continuing value through their undergraduate and post-graduate years.

Russell Viner

Preface

In modern medical and nursing practice, great emphasis is placed on lifelong learning and continuing professional development. In writing this book, we sought to produce a comprehensive textbook that would have broad appeal and take the reader from the basic principles of child health right through the complex and difficult decisions required of an experienced consultant.

This book satisfies the needs of the medical or nursing student, the GP or paediatric trainee, and other child health professionals and the experienced paediatrician or general practitioner. It has been written to reflect requirements for both the undergraduate student encountering paediatrics for the first time, for international postgraduate training curricula in paediatrics and to prepare trainees for postgraduate examinations.

It is supported by summary key points and case scenarios to enable a greater understanding of various clinical presentations. Short podcasts by subject matter experts reflect key principles and clinical vignettes.

The book is aptly named, we believe, in that it equips the reader with the core knowledge and understanding to deal with the varied presentations in paediatrics and apply these building blocks to their interactions with children. It is divided into four sections:

Section one is designed for the undergraduate as it goes through the key concepts of paediatrics, not least how to take a history, conduct a system-based examination and the key concepts of growth and development unique to paediatrics. We have devoted a chapter to the modern worldwide problem of childhood obesity with a contemporary contribution by Professor Sir Stephen O'Rahilly on the genetics of obesity.

Section two is symptom-based and we have had excellent input from all our chapter editors from the United Kingdom, the United States of America and Ireland. This section covers the core theoretical curriculum required in paediatric training.

Section three is unique and reflects the common presentations across the various age groups ranging from infancy, through toddlerhood, school aged children and, finally, adolescence. We know that first responders in general practice, child health professionals and trainees will find these chapters particularly helpful in managing the very common presentations across these age groups. We are indebted to Dr Sarah Taaffe for her input into this section. So often 'the forgotten tribe', Dr Orla Walsh deals with common issues in adolescence in a comprehensive way.

Section four will appeal in particular to trainees in paediatrics and specialist paediatricians and explores the issues of the consultation, illness without disease, dealing with errors and complex ethical decisions and the interpretation of ECGs and laboratory investigations. As a bonus there are unique chapters looking at critical appraisal of the literature and both neonatal and paediatric practical procedures.

This is a textbook to use throughout a full career and is packed with clinical vignettes and high-quality clinical images.

We thank all of the chapter editors for their expertise and patience and both Ms Alexandra Mortimer and Mr Shubham Dixit from Elsevier for their highly professional approach throughout.

This is a book written in initial draft form during the global pandemic and I thank Professor Kevin Dunne, co-editor, for his unshakeable enthusiasm and commitment and Ms Bincy Mathew for all her help and expertise with the typing of the drafts of the book. We are indebted to an array of sub-specialist chapter editors who have generously given their time and contributed handsomely to each of the chapters. We also thank Mr Killian Holmes, Mr Emiliano Grimaldi and Dr Joy Tan from the Royal College of Surgeons in Ireland for their professional production of the podcasts available in the e-version of the book. We thank all the subject matter experts who contributed to these podcasts.

Finally, we wish to sincerely thank Professor Russell Viner, Past President of the Royal College of Paediatrics and Child Health in the United Kingdom, for agreeing to write the foreword for this book.

We hope you enjoy this book and that it remains a companion textbook throughout your career.

Alf Nicholson

Kevin Dunne

Contributors

Stephen Atkin, FRCP, PhD
Head of Research and Postgraduate Studies
Royal College of Surgeons in Ireland (RCSI)
Bahrain, Kingdom of Bahrain

Louise Baker, MB, Bch, BAO, MRCPI(CH), FRACP(CH), FRCPI
General paediatrician with special interest in Neurodisability
Children's Health Ireland at Temple Street
Dublin, Ireland

Cormac Breatnach, MRCPI, FJFICMI
Paediatric Intensivist
Children's Health Ireland at Crumlin
Dublin, Ireland

Fiona Browne, MB, BCh, BAO, MSc, MRCPI
Consultant Dermatologist
Children's Health Ireland at Crumlin and Temple Street
Dublin, Ireland

Karina Butler, MB, BCh, FRCPI, FFPHMI (Hon.)
UCD Clinical Professor of Paediatrics
Paediatrician with a special interest in infectious diseases
Children's Health Ireland at Crumlin and Temple Street
Dublin, Ireland

Michael Cosgrove, FRCPCH
Paediatric Gastroenterologist
Singleton Hospital
Swansea, Wales, UK

Ellen Crushell, FRCPI, FRCPCH
Paediatrician with special interest in metabolic disorders
Children's Health Ireland at Temple Street and Crumlin
Dublin, Ireland

Wayne Cunningham, MBChB, MGP, MD, FRNZCGP
General Practitioner
Wellington, New Zealand

Eugene Dempsey, MD, MSc, MA, FRCPI
Horgan Chair in Neonatology
University College Cork
Cork, Ireland

William Evans, MD
Professor of Clinical Paediatrics
Children's Heart Center
Las Vegas, Nevada, USA

Aisling Flinn, MB, BAO, BCh, MRCPCH, PhD
Academic Clinical Lecturer in Paediatric Immunology
Great North Children's Hospital
Newcastle upon Tyne, UK

Fionnuala Gough, MB, BCh, BAO, MMedSc (Pharm), LLB, PhD
Lecturer in Healthcare Ethics
Royal College of Surgeons in Ireland (RCSI)
Bahrain, Kingdom of Bahrain

Conor Hensey, MB, BCh, BAO, PDipHSc, FRCPI
General Paediatrician
Children's Health Ireland at Temple Street
Dublin, Ireland

Jonathan Hourihane, FRCPCH, FRCPI
Professor of Paediatrics and Child Health
Royal College of Surgeons in Ireland (RCSI)
Dublin, Ireland

Kris Hughes, MB, BCh, BAO, MRCSI, BSc
Surgical Fellow
Children's Health Ireland at Crumlin
Dublin, Ireland

Louise Kyne, MB, Bch, BAO, MRCPI(CH), FRACP(CH), FRCPI
General Paediatrician
Children's Health Ireland at Temple Street
Dublin, Ireland

Ronan Leahy, MB, BCh, PhD, FRCPI
Paediatric Immunologist
Children's Health Ireland at Crumlin and Temple Street
Dublin, Ireland

Clodagh Lowry, MB, BCh, BAO, MRCPI
Paediatric Rheumatologist
Children's Health Ireland at Temple Street
Dublin, Ireland

Bryan Lynch, FRCPI
Paediatric Neurologist
Children's Health Ireland at Temple Street
Dublin, Ireland

Sabine Maguire, MBE, MBBCh, MRCPI, FRCPCH
Honorary Research Fellow
Cardiff University
Wales, UK

Naomi McCallion, FRCPI, MD, PG Dip, TLHE
Professor of Neonatology
Royal College of Surgeons in Ireland (RCSI)
Rotunda Hospital
Dublin, Ireland

Niamh McGrath, MD, MRCPI
Paediatrician with a special interest in endocrinology
University College Hospital
Galway, Ireland

David Misselbrook, MSc, MA, FRCGP
Past Associate Professor of Family Medicine
Royal College of Surgeons in Ireland (RCSI)
Bahrain, Kingdom of Bahrain

Alan Mortell, MB, BCH, BAO, FRCSI, MD, FEBPS, FRCS (Paed Surg)
Associate Professor of Paediatric Surgery
Royal College of Surgeons in Ireland (RCSI)
Consultant Paediatric Surgeon
Children's Health Ireland at Crumlin
Dublin, Ireland

Nuala Murphy, MD, FRCPI, DCH
Paediatric Endocrinologist
Children's Health Ireland at Temple Street
Dublin, Ireland

Sinead Murphy, MD, FRCPI
Director of Paediatric Education
University College Dublin School of Medicine
Consultant Paediatrician
Children's Health Ireland at Temple Street
Dublin, Ireland

John Murphy, FRCPI
RCSI Associate Professor of Neonatology
National Maternity Hospital
Holles Street, Dublin, Ireland

Aengus O'Marcaigh, MD, FRCPI, FFPaed, FAAP
Consultant Paediatric Haematologist
Children's Health Ireland at Crumlin
Dublin, Ireland

James O'Byrne, PhD, MRCPI
Professor (Assoc.) in Genetics
Mater Hospital
Dublin, Ireland

Susan O'Connell, MD, FRACP, FRCPI
Paediatric Endocrinologist
Children's Health Ireland at Crumlin
Dublin, Ireland

Ikechukwu Okafor, MBBS, PGDip, MSc, MRCPI, FRCPI
Consultant in Paediatric Emergency Medicine
Children's Health Ireland at Temple Street
Dublin, Ireland

Terence Prendiville, MD, FRCPI
Professor of Paediatric Cardiology
Children's Health Ireland at Crumlin
Dublin, Ireland

Michael Riordan, MD, FRCPCH
Paediatric Nephrologist
Children's Health Ireland at Temple Street and Crumlin
Dublin, Ireland

Shaista Salman, FRCR2A, Cert, Dip, MMedEd
Lecturer in Professionalism
Royal College of Surgeons in Ireland (RCSI)
Bahrain, Kingdom of Bahrain

Amre Shahwan, MD, MRCPCH
Consultant Clinical Neurophysiologist & Epileptologist
Royal College of Surgeons in Ireland (RCSI)
Children's Health Ireland at Temple Street
Dublin, Ireland

Orla Walsh, MB, MSc Ed, FRCPCH
General Paediatrician with an interest in adolescent health
Children's Health Ireland at Temple Street
Dublin, Ireland

Martin White, MD, FRCPI
Professor of Neonatology
Coombe Women and Infants Hospital
Children's Health Ireland at Crumlin
Dublin, Ireland

Michael Williamson, MB, FRCPI
Paediatric Respirologist
Children's Health Ireland at Temple Street
Dublin, Ireland

'To my wife Helen, children Katie, Mark, Marie Louise and Alfie for all their love and support in writing this book'
– Alfred Nicholson

'To my wife Denise and children Patrick, Kevin and Aisling for their unwavering belief in me and support in editing this book.'
– Kevin Dunne

The Core Essentials

1

The Big Picture in Child Health

ALF NICHOLSON

All of us do not have equal talent, but all of us should have equal opportunity to develop those talents.

JOHN F. KENNEDY (1963)

Paediatrics is a fascinating area, and there have been staggering advances over the past 40 years to ensure that our children and young people have never been healthier. Unfortunately, despite dramatic improvements in survival, nutrition and education in childhood, issues such as climate change, conflict with consequent migration, persistent inequalities and predatory commercial practices threaten the health and future of children in every country. Even in rich countries, children live in conditions of relative poverty, especially those belonging to ethnic minorities or indigenous populations.

The adolescent period, debatably extending from 10 to 24 years of age, is another window of opportunity in terms of both identity and vulnerability. Patterns can be laid for a lifetime of poor nutrition, poor mental health, reduced exercise, interpersonal violence and alcohol and tobacco use.

Interventions to improve child health and wellbeing have long-term intergenerational benefits, and the investment in child health and education is highly cost-effective.

Children differ from adults in that they are subject to developmental change, dependent on their parents, have different illnesses and disabilities and are highly influenced by socioeconomic factors. Children use health services differently, with short stay observation units often replacing overnight hospitalisation.

High-quality care requires a combination of different elements of the system to most effectively meet the needs of the child and family. In Ireland and the UK, children and young people most often receive care in primary care, with most specialist expertise residing in hospitals. Pathways for both acute care and the care of chronic long-term conditions must be flexible and need to cross institutional borders, often on multiple occasions. A higher level of integration improves outcomes and the child and family experience and may also lower costs by reducing unnecessary hospital and emergency department attendances.

Better integration of paediatric specialist expertise with primary care could potentially reduce the burden on hard-pressed emergency departments by over 30 per cent. The future care of children and adolescents should be integrated across the health system and is an essential element of planned changes in primary and urgent care delivery.

Research in Paediatrics

There is no doubt about the importance of research as today's research is tomorrow's standard of care.

The **_seven_** great achievements in paediatric research over the past 40 years were highlighted by Cheng, et al. in 2016 and include:

- preventing infections via vaccinations (a stunning success)
- reducing SIDS via the 'back to sleep' campaign with a dramatic fall death rate
- acute lymphoblastic leukaemia survival (now over 90 per cent cure rate) with personalised treatment
- significantly increased survival of markedly preterm infants (hats off to neonatal staff worldwide in both developed and developing countries)
- preventing HIV transmission from mother to baby (important worldwide)
- increased life expectancy of cystic fibrosis (CF) patients (gets better and better with newborn screening and new treatments with additional benefits)
- saving lives with seatbelts and car seats (again a major success in countries with an emphasis on road safety measures such as car seats and traffic calming).

However, the great influencers of child health and wellbeing continue to be parenting, prevention and poverty. Measures to support positive parenting, reduce income inequality (thereby reducing poverty, still as high as 25 per cent in some EU countries), and a focus on prevention will always bring success and improve child health.

Primary Prevention and Health Promotion

The foundations of future health and wellbeing are laid down during pregnancy and the first years of life. There is growing evidence linking adverse childhood experiences to the subsequent development of unhealthy lifestyles, poor overall health and persistent socioeconomic inequalities. On the other hand, nurturing care provides a stable environment sensitive to the growing child's health, nutrition, sense of security and safety and fosters early learning. Successful child health programmes worldwide establish a primary screening and prevention service for all children with additional 'proportionate universalism' to ensure additional services for vulnerable groups.

Organised, scheduled visits by healthcare professionals or trained volunteers help women breast-feed their babies for longer. Maternal postnatal depression can significantly impact a mother's ability to develop a stable, responsive relationship with her baby. Home visiting (usually by a public health nurse or health visitor) is the intervention of choice as it allows earlier identification and a more accurate assessment of family need.

PROMOTING INFANT AND CHILD DEVELOPMENT

From birth to 2 years of age, the brain goes through a period of rapid development and growth. During this time, the brain displays a remarkable capacity to absorb information and adapt to its surroundings. At 3 years of age, a child's brain is twice as active as an adult brain. Parenting plays a key role in developing the capacity for emotional regulation in young children.

PROMOTING HEALTHY NUTRITION

Apart from providing excellent nutrition, breast milk confers passive immunity via immunoglobulin A, macrophages, T cells and stem cells. Alpha-lactalbumin in breast milk has both antibacterial and immunostimulatory properties. Oligosaccharides in breast milk encourage the growth of beneficial microbes in the infant's gut. While breast milk cannot guarantee perfect health, breast-fed infants enjoy better health than their bottle-fed counterparts.

Mothers living in relative poverty are less likely to initiate breast-feeding or to continue exclusive breast-feeding until the infant is at least 6 months. Skin to skin contact between mother and baby immediately after birth is vital for initiating lactation, as is keeping the mother and infant together to allow unrestricted, frequent feeds. Good positioning is essential to ensure effective breast-feeding and prevent painful sucking and nipple trauma.

The transition from milk feeding to supplementary solid foods (weaning) begins at around 4 to 6 months old. Once established, solid feeds should be offered two or three times per day, initially rising to three meals and two nutritious snacks per day by 12 to 24 months of age. A wide variety of solid foods are recommended, and meat, fish or eggs should be given daily if possible. Recent evidence has suggested that infants at risk of allergy are protected by exposure in the first year. Therefore, allergenic foods should be introduced one by one with weaning solids after the age of 6 months. Traditionally feeding starts with thin purees with the consistency gradually increased to stimulate oromotor development. At around 6 months of age, most infants can reach out for and attempt to feed themselves finger food.

Iron-containing solid foods become important by 6 months of age. Iron bound into haem from red meat and oil-rich fish is the most easily absorbed source of iron. In practice, the most common sources of iron for children are breakfast cereals and formula milk fortified with non-haem iron. Unmodified cow's milk is an inferior source of iron, and toddlers who drink a lot of milk to the exclusion of solid foods are at high risk of iron deficiency.

Mothers are advised to include meat, eggs, beans and dried fruit from 6 months of age to prevent iron deficiency. For most children, there is no need to continue formula milk beyond 12 months of age, but unmodified cow's milk should be restricted to no more than 500 mL/day.

Vitamin D is essential for the growth and maturation of the skeleton and is predominantly synthesised in the skin by the action of sunlight. Where there is little sunlight exposure, dietary sources then become important.

Vitamin D supplementation until 1 year of age has been recommended for some time, but uptake is less than ideal. Vitamin D supplementation is particularly important in children born prematurely, those with low exposure to sunlight, children with dark skin and those with limited diets.

PROMOTING A HEALTHY DIET

Young toddlers should have three meals and two nutritious snacks per day. Grazing on sweet snacks and drinks between meals places them at risk of dental caries, becoming overweight, spoiling their appetite and causing food refusal at mealtimes (Fig. 1.1). Eating behaviour can be challenging at times; parents should limit meal duration (20 to 30 minutes), reduce serving size and enable the child to self-feed. For instance, eating together with other children (at creche or nursery) may help model appropriate eating behaviour. Parents of overweight children should receive specific advice to prevent further weight gain, such as limiting portion sizes, reducing intake of high energy foods and promoting physical activity.

PROMOTING PHYSICAL ACTIVITY

Physical activity should be encouraged from birth through tummy time, crawling, rolling and pushing or pulling up against furniture in the home. Preschool children capable of walking unaided should be physically active for 3 hours spread throughout the day and should minimise the amount of time being sedentary for extended periods.

All school-going children and young people should engage in moderate to vigorous physical activity for at least 1 hour and up to several hours per day. Vigorously intense activities (such as skipping, gymnastics, jumping, aerobics and most sports) should happen at least 3 days/week. Children should minimise the amount of time spent watching television, playing computer games or on a computer. It is important to provide safe, attractive and accessible outdoor

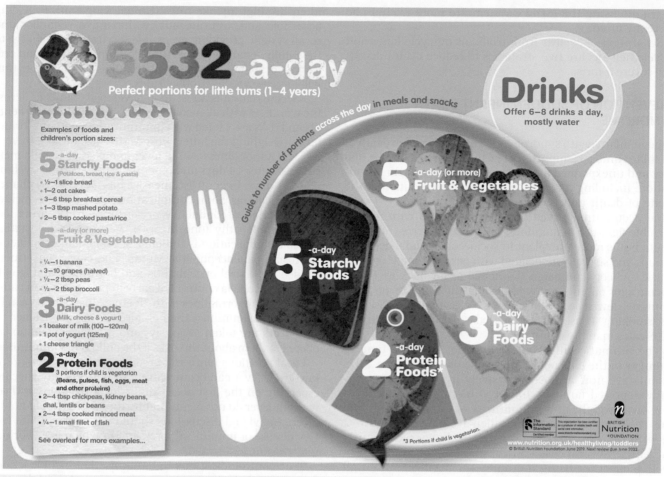

Figure 1.1   5532-a-day. (Image courtesy of British Nutrition Foundation www.nutrition.org.uk.)

play facilities in local communities to facilitate physical activity for all children.

PROMOTION OF GOOD DENTAL HEALTH

Tooth decay occurs when a child consumes food or drink containing free sugars from which cariogenic bacteria in the mouth over a period of time produce acid, which affects a susceptible tooth surface. Risk factors for dental caries include sugar-sweetened drinks, lack of access to fluoride and social disadvantage.

In preventing dental caries up to 6 years of age, effective interventions include breast-feeding, parents brushing their child's teeth or supervising their child's brushing twice daily with fluoridated toothpaste and reducing the number of sugary drinks. Fluoridated toothpaste should contain at least 1000 ppm fluoride. Water fluoridation provides a universal programme to prevent dental caries in young children and is very effective.

UNINTENTIONAL INJURIES AND THEIR PREVENTION

Most deaths and hospitalisations due to injuries in the under 5-year-old age group occur in or around the home. Deaths relate to high falls, smoke inhalation due to house fires, drowning, choking and accidental suffocation or strangulation.

Risk factors for increased injury risk include gender (risk for boys is far higher across all age groups), socioeconomic deprivation, a history of epilepsy or attention hyperactivity disorder, overcrowding and maternal depression.

Intensive home visiting programmes significantly reduce injury risk in young children, especially if the programme is targeted towards more vulnerable groups.

Home safety education and the provision of safety equipment helps families make homes safer. Safety education includes increasing possession of functional smoke alarms, safety gate use on stairs, secure storage of poisons, fireguard use and a fire escape plan, reducing baby walker use and having a safe hot tap water temperature.

On the roads, reducing vehicle speed is of paramount importance. Therefore, it is essential to reduce speed to 30 km per hour in streets that are primarily residential or with high volumes of pedestrians and cyclists and traffic-calming speed bumps. The most important factor in cars is age-appropriate child restraints or car seats, as these measures significantly reduce death and serious injury in a road collision. Properly fitted and used rearward-facing child car restraints are most effective in children under 2 years. Child restraints are only effective if they are correctly fitted and used. There is some evidence that restraints using the ISOFIX system are more likely to be correctly fitted.

Separation of cyclists from traffic using cycle lanes and bicycle helmets are two strategies to reduce cyclist deaths and severe injuries.

PREVENTION OF SUDDEN INFANT DEATH SYNDROME

Sudden infant death syndrome (SIDS) is the sudden death of an infant under 12 months of age that is unexpected by history and unexplained after a thorough postmortem examination, including a complete autopsy, investigation at the scene of death and review of the medical history. Death often occurs unobserved during infant sleep with no discernible signs of a major illness. SIDS occurs across all social strata but is more prevalent in socioeconomically deprived groups and strongly associated with parental smoking. The 'Back to Sleep' campaign (launched as far back as 1991) encourages parents to avoid placing their infants on their front, use fewer bedclothes, avoid co-sleeping and discourage smoking. These precautions led to a dramatic decline in SIDS rates in many countries.

The dramatic fall in SIDS rates has led over time to changes in the characteristic profile of SIDS deaths. SIDS infants are now almost exclusively from socioeconomically deprived families. Infant vulnerability in terms of low birth weight and prematurity is more marked, and the peak age of death has fallen from 3 months to 2 months of age. Co-sleeping deaths have significantly increased. Several case-control studies have found a protective effect for using a dummy (or pacifier), although the mechanism for protection is unclear. Key advice to reduce the risk of SIDS includes consistently placing an infant on their back to sleep, avoiding cigarette smoke (keeping the infant smoke-free during pregnancy and after birth), breast-feeding and keeping infants in a separate cot (or Moses's basket) in the same room as the parents for the first 6 months. Likewise, one should never sleep on a sofa or in an armchair with a young infant and avoid co-sleeping at night.

IMMUNISATION

The evidence for the effectiveness of immunisation is powerful, and vaccine uptake rates are acceptable (above 90 per cent) in most developed countries. Despite this, outbreaks of measles, mumps and pertussis continue to occur.

A small but vocal group of the population (up to 5 per cent) declines immunisation for their children because they consider vaccines to be unsafe or unnecessary. Outbreaks can then occur, as these unvaccinated children may cluster in a given population. The level of vaccine hesitancy has risen in recent years in both Europe and the USA. Advice from a trusted healthcare professional is a pivotal factor to enable a parent to change their mind over immunisations they have previously delayed or declined.

Different strategies are used in different countries to promote high vaccine uptake. Examples include 'no jabs no school' (USA), immunisation status tagged to child welfare allowances (France) or providing incentives to providers to ensure high uptake rates (United Kingdom). Providing accessible and accurate advice, having a reminder and recall system, providing accessible services free of charge to the family, enabling opportunistic immunisation and collecting local and national data are all essential factors that will increase vaccine uptake rates.

Vaccine refusal is an issue in developed countries across the world. As with all medical interventions, there are benefits and risks associated with immunisation, with the former far outweighing the latter. Post-MMR vaccination, there is a risk of minor illness with a fever and possibly a mild measles rash after 14 days and potentially mild parotid swelling after 21 days. In contrast, measles has a one in 10 chance of complications. Some complications can be severe, including pneumonia, conductive or sensorineural hearing loss or encephalopathy (one in 500). A rare but devastating possible complication is the later development of subacute sclerosing panencephalitis. Mumps can cause sensorineural deafness, viral encephalitis and both male and female infertility. Rubella contracted early in pregnancy can cause congenital abnormalities in the foetus. Most parents can be persuaded to immunise their children if they are listened to, their fears are taken seriously, and a clear explanation is offered to them about the risks if the child is not immunised.

Local reactions (with mild reddening and swelling) and low-grade fever can occur within 24 hours of any vaccine, especially on the first dose. Minor local reactions with or without fever do not mean that further doses should not be given. Individual discussions should occur if an infant has HIV disease or immunosuppression, in which live vaccines may be contraindicated.

True contraindications to immunisation include a confirmed anaphylactic reaction to a previous dose of the vaccine, acute illness with fever or systemic upset.

Live vaccines such as BCG and MMR are contraindicated in children being treated for malignant disease with chemotherapy or radiotherapy, post-transplantation until 12 months post-cessation of immunosuppressive therapy, high-dose steroids within the previous 3 months and those with primary immunodeficiency (such as severe combined immunodeficiency). Children with HIV should not receive BCG, oral polio, yellow fever or oral typhoid vaccines.

Over the coming years, immunisation programmes may include the prevention of neonatal group B streptococcal infection and respiratory syncytial virus (RSV) bronchiolitis.

Immunisation schedules may change in response to emerging evidence on optimal approaches to maximise protection through herd immunity, with the perceived crowding of schedules and new vaccines driving change. (Figs. 1.2 and 1.3).

Monitoring Growth and the Use of Growth Charts

Growth charts allow us to compare a child's measurements to the normal range of measurements in children of the same age and sex. The 50th centile represents the average (median) for the population, while the second and 98th centiles are two standard deviations above and below the median. In addition, there are 0.4th and 99.6th centiles below or above which only one in 250 growing

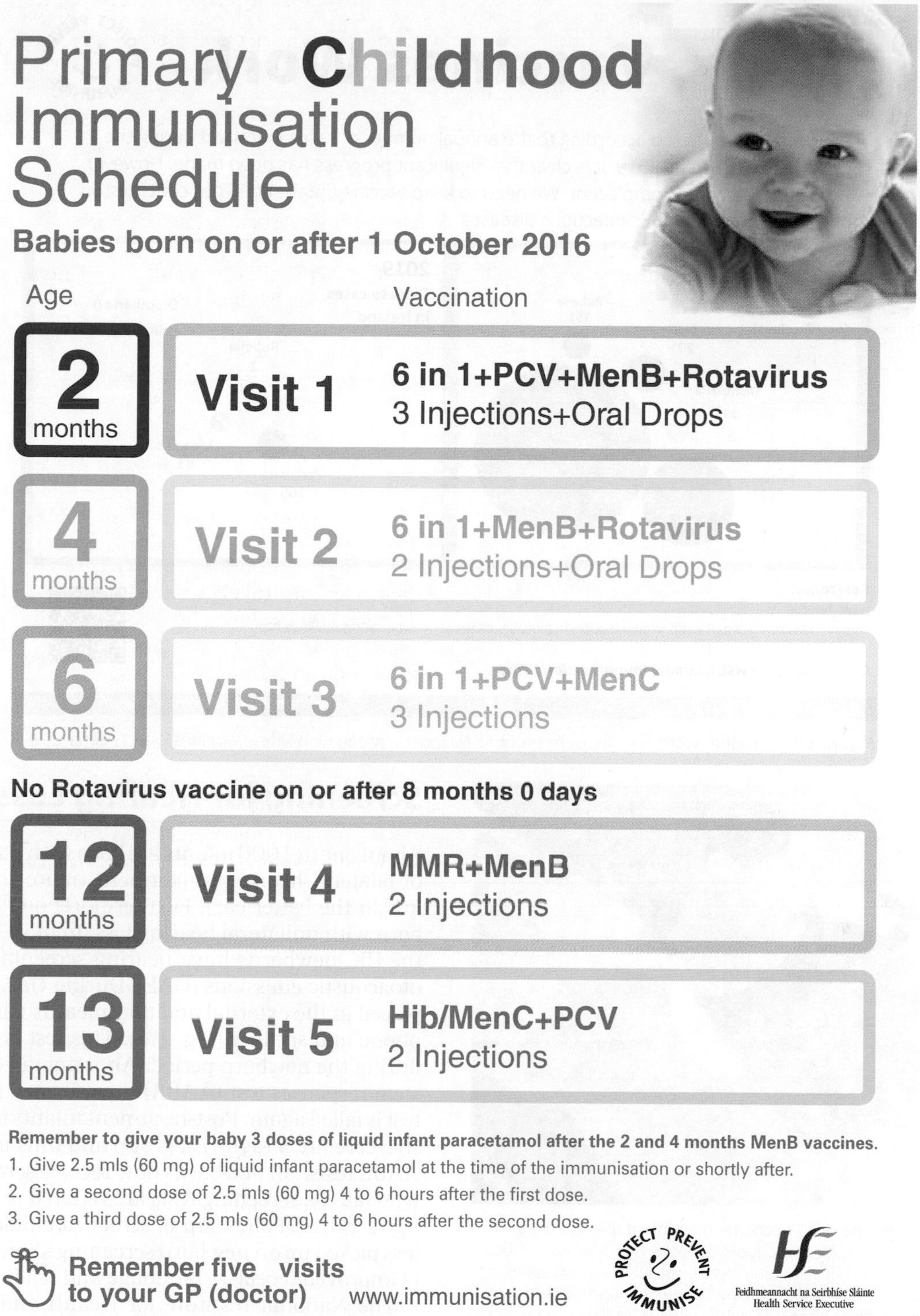

Primary **Childhood** Immunisation Schedule

Babies born on or after 1 October 2016

Age	Vaccination

2 months — **Visit 1** — **6 in 1+PCV+MenB+Rotavirus** 3 Injections+Oral Drops

4 months — **Visit 2** — **6 in 1+MenB+Rotavirus** 2 Injections+Oral Drops

6 months — **Visit 3** — **6 in 1+PCV+MenC** 3 Injections

No Rotavirus vaccine on or after 8 months 0 days

12 months — **Visit 4** — **MMR+MenB** 2 Injections

13 months — **Visit 5** — **Hib/MenC+PCV** 2 Injections

Remember to give your baby 3 doses of liquid infant paracetamol after the 2 and 4 months MenB vaccines.
1. Give 2.5 mls (60 mg) of liquid infant paracetamol at the time of the immunisation or shortly after.
2. Give a second dose of 2.5 mls (60 mg) 4 to 6 hours after the first dose.
3. Give a third dose of 2.5 mls (60 mg) 4 to 6 hours after the second dose.

 Remember five   visits to your GP (doctor)   www.immunisation.ie

Feidhmeannacht na Seirbhíse Sláinte
Health Service Executive

Figure 1.2 Primary childhood immunisation schedule. (Image courtesy of HSE National Immunisation Office, Primary Childhood Immunisation Schedule 2020.)

children will fall. The World Health Organisation (WHO) Child Growth Standards for infants and children up to the age of 5 years were published in 2006 and are based on the growth of healthy, breast-fed, non-deprived children from six different countries (Brazil, Ghana, India, Norway, Oman and the USA). The UK 1990 growth charts are based on measurements from a large cohort of British children collected in the late 1980s and describe typical children in the United Kingdom from 1980 to 1990.

Vaccines Work

These bubbles are sized according to the annual number of cases in Ireland during the pre-vaccine era versus 2019. It is clear that significant progress has been made. However, we must not become complacent. We need to keep vaccine uptake at 95 per cent to stop outbreaks of these serious infectious diseases.

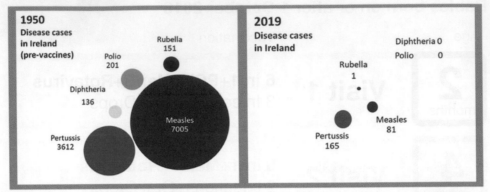

1950
Disease cases in Ireland (pre-vaccines)

Rubella 151
Polio 201
Diphtheria 136
Measles 7005
Pertussis 3612

2019
Disease cases in Ireland

Diphtheria 0
Polio 0
Rubella 1
Measles 81
Pertussis 165

Reference:
www.hpsc.ie
https://www.hse.ie/eng/health/immunisation/hcpinfo/guidelines/immunisationguidelines.html

Developed by the **HSE National Immunisation Office**

www.immunisation.ie   @hseimm #VaccinesWork #KeepVaccinating

Figure 1.3   Vaccines work. (Image courtesy of HSE National Immunisation Office, Vaccines Work Graphic 2020.)

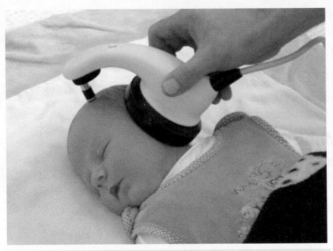

Figure 1.4   BERAphone MB 11 screening an infant. (Reproduced with permission from van Dyk, M., Swanepoel de, W., & Hall, J. W. (2015). Outcomes with OAE and AABR screening in the first 48 h – Implications for newborn hearing screening in developing countries. *International Journal of Pediatric Otorhinolaryngology, 79*(7), 1034–1040.)

Body Mass Index (BMI)

Body mass index tells you how heavy a child is relative to their height and is the most practical measure of being overweight or obese from 2 years of age. Most children will have a BMI between the 25th and 75th centiles, whatever their height centile. The higher the BMI, the more indicative it is of excess fat.

Learning materials are available from the Royal College of Paediatrics and Child Health UK for further information on growth monitoring charts.

Screening for Hearing Loss

About one in 1000 infants are born with a significant degree of bilateral hearing impairment (more than a 40-decibel loss in the better ear). Furthermore, one in 500 infants is born with unilateral hearing loss. In most EU countries and the UK, newborns have hearing screening via automated otoacoustic emissions (OAE). During OAE, a small probe is placed in the external auditory meatus with a small microphone and speaker (Fig. 1.4). This test is repeated if failed during the newborn period. An automated auditory brainstem responses test (AABR) is performed if the repeat OAE test is failed again. Post-treatment infants in neonatal intensive care are a high-risk group and thus undergo OAE and AABR tests. All newborns now receive screening, and those who fail the screening tests are referred promptly to audiology services. Follow up of screened children with hearing loss picked up on newborn screening shows ample evidence of improved receptive language and reading ability.

The National Institute for Health and Care Excellence lists several features in *older children* which should raise the suspicion of hearing loss:

- hearing issues requiring instructions to be repeated, especially at school
- delayed language development
- repeated ear infections
- poor educational progress or attention problems
- intolerance of loud sounds

Concerning serous otitis media or glue ear, the balance between watchful waiting and surgical intervention (insertion of grommets) is still hotly debated. Children with persistent bilateral serous otitis media documented over 3 months with a hearing level in the better ear of 25 to 30 dBHL should be considered for grommet insertion.

PICKING UP VISUAL IMPAIRMENT

Many causes of blindness are treatable if diagnosed early (particularly cataracts, retinopathy of prematurity and glaucoma).

One should suspect a significant impairment of visual acuity if:

- an infant does not fix, follow or smile by 6 to 8 weeks of age
- obvious strabismus at a young age
- nystagmus or 'roving' eye movements

Strabismus is relatively common in children and requires assessment and referral in children over 6 months of age. Clinical assessment involves firstly shining a light beyond accommodation distance to see if it lands symmetrically on both pupils. A cover-uncover test is performed to test eye movements. Finally, the red reflex is tested to out rule conditions such as retinoblastoma. Strabismus requires referral to an ophthalmologist with treatments including patching the non-squinting eye, orthoptic exercises and use of glasses. Very rarely is a corrective operation required for strabismus. Amblyopia of the squinting eye may occur if strabismus is not picked up. It is recommended that children should have vision screening soon after school entry.

(Box 1.1)

Box 1.1   Key Points

The great influencers of child health and wellbeing continue to be poverty, prevention and parenting.

Foundations of future health and wellbeing are laid down during pregnancy and the first years of life.

There is growing evidence linking adverse childhood experiences to the subsequent development of unhealthy lifestyles (poor eating and exercise habits and substance abuse), poor overall health and persistent socioeconomic inequalities.

Mothers living in relative poverty are less likely to initiate breast-feeding or to continue exclusive breast-feeding until the infant is at least 6 months.

The transition from milk feeding to supplementary solid foods (weaning) begins at around 4 to 6 months.

All school-going children and young people should engage in moderate to vigorous physical activity for at least 1 hour and up to several hours per day.

The most effective way to prevent injury or death in children travelling in cars is to use an appropriate restraint in the rear of the vehicle.

The 'Back to Sleep' campaign has led to a dramatic decline in SIDS rates in many countries.

Advice from a trusted healthcare professional is a pivotal factor to enable a parent to change their mind over immunisations they have previously delayed or declined.

Follow up of screened children with hearing loss picked up on newborn screening shows good evidence of improved receptive language and reading ability.

Many causes of blindness are treatable if diagnosed early (particularly cataracts, retinopathy of prematurity and glaucoma).

Key References

Cheng, T. L., Monteiro, N., DiMeglio, L. A., Chien, A. T., Peeples, E. S., Raetz, E., et al. (2016). Seven great achievements in pediatric research in the past 40 y. *Pediatric Research*, 80(3), 330–337. https://doi.org/10.1038/pr.2016.95.

Cheung, R. (2018, March 15). *International comparisons of health and wellbeing in early childhood.* Nuffield Trust. https://www.nuffieldtrust.org.uk/research/international-comparisons-of-health-and-wellbeing-in-early-childhood.

Clark, H., Coll-Seck, A. M., Banerjee, A., Peterson, S., Dalglish, S. L., Ameratunga, S., et al. (2020). A future for the world's children? A WHO-UNICEF-Lancet Commission. *Lancet (London, England)*, 395(10224), 605–658. https://doi.org/10.1016/S0140-6736(19)32540-1.

Devakumar, D., Edwards, E., & Kossarova, L. (2016, August 2). Nuffield Trust. *The future of child health services: New models of care.* https://www.nuffieldtrust.org.uk/research/the-future-of-child-health-services-new-models-of-care.

Emond, A. (Ed.), (2019). *Health for all children* (5th ed.). Oxford University Press.

Lang, S., Loving, S., McCarthy, N. D., Ramsay, M. E., Salisbury, D., & Pollard, A. J. (2020). Two centuries of immunisation in the UK (part II). *Archives of Disease in Childhood*, 105(3), 216–222.

National Immunisation Office in Ireland (n.d.). National Immunisation Office. http://www.immunisation.ie

Royal College of Paediatrics and Child Health. (n.d.). Growth charts. http://www.rcpch.ac.uk/growthcharts

Royal College of Paediatrics and Child Health. (2009). *UK-WHO Growth Charts – Face Sheet 3: Measuring and Plotting.* https://www.rcpch.ac.uk/sites/default/files/Measuring_and_plotting_advice.pdf.

Viner, R. M., & Hargreaves, D. S. (2018). A forward view for child health: integrating across the system to improve health and reduce hospital attendances for children and young people. *Archives of Disease in Childhood*, 103(2), 117–118.

2 Taking a History

ALF NICHOLSON, KEVIN DUNNE, and ORLA WALSH

Listen to the patient. He is telling you the diagnosis.

SIR WILLIAM OSLER

Introduction

An essential skill for any student (undergraduate or postgraduate) is the ability to take a detailed and comprehensive history, usually from the child's parents. Taking a history from a third party does pose additional challenges. The history may be taken directly in adolescence but is given added detail and context by input from one or both parents.

Thus, taking a paediatric history poses unique but surmountable challenges. The first priority is establishing good rapport with the parent providing the history, and listening attentively to their concerns.

Answers are remarkably consistent when parents are asked to identify the most important qualities they seek in their family doctor or paediatrician. Answers include 'a doctor who gives us enough time', 'a doctor who is an attentive listener', and perhaps most importantly, 'a doctor who explains things to me in words I can understand'. Good listening skills and a clear explanation are thus two essential elements in a successful paediatric or adolescent consultation. Always show empathy and understanding with an appreciation of the family's concerns. Reassurance is of the utmost importance to relieve parental anxiety. (Box 2.1).

The presenting symptoms are key to the paediatric history and should first be itemised and then filled in with additional detail. The ability to accurately elucidate the presenting symptoms is critical in generating an appropriate differential diagnosis.

A few pointers are key to effective history taking in paediatrics:

- Parents are not perfect historians but have an innate sense of whether or not their child is sick; this innate concern should be harnessed.
- Do not attempt to 'lead the witness', as it were. In other words, do not ask direct questions where the parent might be tempted to give the answer they think you want. Suppose you are taking a history in the winter season, for instance. In that case, you may see many children with lower respiratory infections or infants with bronchiolitis, and it may be tempting to frame the history with an expectation that you already know the diagnosis. Favouring one possible diagnosis is not advisable, and the student should always take a history with an open mind about the diagnosis.
- When taking a history, the presenting symptoms are critically important and should be the focal point of your overall picture of the child. A good analogy to keep in mind is the central importance of the bride and groom in a wedding photo.
- Aim to obtain at least three presenting symptoms and details for each (abdominal pain, fever and vomiting may be present in a case of suspected acute appendicitis).
- Always focus on the presenting symptoms and not on parental observations about interactions with healthcare professionals over the previous 48 hours. Always go back to the presenting symptoms.
- When practising giving a history, it is essential that you accurately clarify the presenting symptoms. Over time, you will find that clear, descriptive patterns will emerge.
- Practice makes perfect. The more histories you take and present, the better you become, and the easier it is to

Box 2.1   Key Components of a Successful Consultation or History Taking

Introduce yourself and call the child by name
Greet the family and identify who is present
Try to eliminate distractions or interruptions
Listen attentively
Sustain eye contact throughout the consultation as much as possible
Go through a logical sequence with a clear focus on the presenting symptoms
Be aware of important nonverbal cues
Show empathy and support throughout the interview

navigate your way to a differential diagnosis that considers all the likely possibilities.

■ The remainder of the history provides context and scaffolding around the presenting symptoms to enable a robust set of differential diagnoses to be considered.

■ During your period in paediatrics, you should take histories on the most common presenting scenarios to ensure that you are at ease with the common presenting symptoms of illness.

■ Develop a strong rapport with the parent giving the history and always keep an open mind about rare diagnoses during the illness. The adage that 'not all that wheezes is asthma' rings true.

■ In clinical practice, always revisit the paediatric history and refocus on the presenting complaints if the child is not improving. An important detail in the history may have been left out in initial discussions. This is a key point in clinical practice: revisit the working diagnosis if the child is not getting better. An example of this might be an infant who presents with vomiting and diarrhoea with a presumptive diagnosis of acute gastroenteritis, goes markedly pale and has blood PR hours later. On further investigation, this infant transpired to have intussusception. The lesson is that differential diagnoses may have to be revised if the infant or child is not improving.

■ It is rare for parents to fabricate symptoms (called Factitious or Fabricated Induced Illness or FII). Over the course of a near lifetime in paediatrics, we have come across FII only a handful of times.

PREPARATION

Before you see the child, you should review any pre-existing information available. Be aware of ambulance or nursing triage notes and prior attendances or admissions. Handover from colleagues is vital once you are qualified, and robust handover is essential to ensure accurate transfer of information. Be aware that parents are often highly anxious and stressed, impairing their ability to give an accurate history in an emergency situation. Parents will often be exhausted, thus requiring an understanding and compassionate approach on your part (sometimes tricky to do in a busy emergency department).

Start by greeting the parent or caregiver and child and by introducing yourself, including your title. Be confident and empathetic with good eye contact. Try to put the family at ease as much as possible. Give parents time to speak, and explore their concerns about their child. Avoid medical jargon, and explain unfamiliar words and concepts in a way the parents can fully understand.

Presenting Symptoms

As mentioned above, the presenting symptoms are the centrepiece of the history and enable a proper differential diagnosis. Always begin with open questions and allow the parent to itemise their concerns. Once itemised, then tackle each of these key symptoms individually, enabling a detailed history of each. Resist the temptation to ask questions too quickly. Three to four key presenting symptoms are often sufficient for an accurate reflection of the presenting complaint. Detail the presenting symptoms to give a greater sense of severity (e.g. detail the nature and frequency of vomiting and the volume of vomitus, thus enabling a more accurate reflection of severity).

The true test of accurately taken presenting symptoms is your ability to develop a reliable and sensible differential diagnosis. The importance of the accurate elucidation of presenting symptoms cannot be overemphasised.

Recent developments include an artificial intelligence (AI) classification of cough sounds using the unique sound signatures of a child's cough recorded by a smartphone. Parent-reported symptoms can later enhance this information. This form of AI holds promise for the future.

HISTORY OF PRESENTING COMPLAINT

Vital questions to be answered include when the various symptoms started, in what sequence they appeared and how they were managed. As in the pointers above, avoid simply a series of parental observations about healthcare professional interactions over the previous 48 hours. Is the child improving or deteriorating?

FOCUSED SYSTEMATIC REVIEW

In addition to the presenting symptoms, seek detail from a **focused** review of symptoms to find additional symptoms that will help make a diagnosis or relevant negatives to generate a robust differential diagnosis.

PAST MEDICAL HISTORY

Enquire about any prior emergency presentations or admissions to the hospital and any previous surgical procedures. Ask if this has ever happened before. If the child has a chronic illness such as asthma, enquire about the age at initial presentation, diagnosis, treatment given, duration of hospital stays, subsequent follow-up and current medications.

DRUG HISTORY/ALLERGIES/IMMUNISATIONS

One needs an accurate drug history regarding current medications (proper name – not brand name) regarding dosage and frequency (and a sense of whether the patient is compliant with therapy), and any previous allergies or drug reactions. Ask about any over-the-counter or complementary drugs the child may be taking.

A detailed immunisation history is essential and reasons for not immunising need to be explored with sensitivity.

PERINATAL/BIRTH HISTORY

Enquire about the pregnancy, gestation, complications of pregnancy, birth weight, and neonatal complications, if any. Enquire about the mode of delivery and indications for instrumental or caesarian section delivery, if not spontaneous vertex delivery. Details of admission in the neonatal unit are also necessary, as are any complications or procedures in the neonatal period. The Apgar score and need for resuscitation should also be clarified.

FEEDING HISTORY

Feeding history is most relevant in infancy and should reflect whether the child is breast- or bottle-fed, any feeding issues or prior interventions for faltering growth. Also ask about age of weaning to solids.

FAMILY HISTORY

Family history is significant as many conditions have a genetic basis. Enquire about siblings and their health issues. Ask about a family history of diabetes, congenital heart disease or deaths in infancy, making it relevant to the presenting symptoms explained above. Ask about pertinent genetic conditions, depending on where the child was born and raised. Examples include G6PD, sickle cell, thalassemia or diabetes in a family from the Middle East, and cystic fibrosis or coeliac disease in a northern European family. Construct a family tree and ask (with sensitivity) about consanguinity.

SOCIAL AND TRAVEL HISTORY

Again, these questions require sensitivity. Never be judgmental or discriminatory. Key issues relate to who looks after the child on a daily basis, what social and family supports are available and parent employment status. Housing conditions (e.g. house or apartment, direct provision, refugee accommodation or even homelessness) are directly relevant to a child's physical and mental wellbeing at all ages. Issues such as domestic or intimate partner violence are rare but highly relevant. Passive smoking in households is also worth ascertaining, especially if the child presents chronic respiratory symptoms. Questions about alcohol intake also require sensitivity. Any pets may be relevant as a source of disease or allergy. The ability to take an accurate and comprehensive social history is a key discriminator of student ability.

DEVELOPMENTAL HISTORY

A detailed developmental history is critical and should focus on the key domains (gross motor development, fine motor development and vision, hearing and language development, and social and play development). Key questions relate to whether the parents or healthcare professionals have concerns about their child's developmental progress across the above domains. Enquire about academic performance in a school-age child. Developmental history and assessment are necessary for every paediatric history.

Foreign travel (especially to exotic locations) is also relevant, especially if there is an unexplained prolonged fever (malaria or dengue fever).

SYSTEMS REVIEW

For those symptoms not already covered in questions relating to the presenting symptoms, the remainder of the systems review is required and likely to be non-contributory or negative, unlike in adult medicine. One should consider somatisation symptoms if numerous symptoms span many systems in which the answer to almost all questions is yes. In general, these symptoms are more relevant in adolescence but are not exclusive to this age group.

PRESENTING YOUR FINDINGS

Over the years, we have become struck by the importance of handover, especially between healthcare professionals. Therefore, we believe the best approach to present your findings is to use the **ISBAR** technique.

- **I** is for you to identify yourself (your name and perhaps that you are the senior house officer on call).
- **S** as in the military analogy for Situation but with S standing for Symptoms at presentation. Give a concise summary of the presenting symptoms (one or two sentences).
- **B** is for background, including a tight summary of prior attendances, diagnosis and overall context.
- **A** is for your assessment, which requires examining the child and assessing their illness severity, and whether or not they are stable.
- **R** is essential and calls for your recommendation, which might be to admit to a hospital or high dependency or intensive care, start treatment, or embark on appropriate urgent investigations.

Interprofessional robust communication requires all involved to hand over efficiently ill or unstable patients in particular and, especially when seeking senior advice, allows a more precise picture to emerge.

PRACTICE MAKES PERFECT (THE TOP 25)

Take histories during your time in paediatrics on a broad range of presenting symptoms, including:
- the child with faltering growth (failure to thrive)
- the child with acute abdominal pain
- the child with constipation
- the child with recurrent abdominal pain
- the infant or child with a fever (with or without a rash)
- the infant or child with a rash (acute or chronic)
- the infant or child with a cough, wheeze or respiratory distress
- the child with headaches
- the child with a suspected seizure

- the child with a heart murmur, syncope or chest pain
- the child with joint pain or a limp
- the crying or distressed infant
- the vomiting infant
- the infant or child with a suspected urinary tract infection
- the pale child
- the child with bruising
- the child with an inguinoscrotal issue
- the infant or child with suspected delayed developmental milestones
- the infant or child with a physical disability (e.g. cerebral palsy or a neural tube defect)
- the child with type 1 diabetes mellitus
- the child with a chronic condition (e.g. cerebral palsy, cystic fibrosis, sickle cell anaemia, beta thalassemia)
- the infant or child with Trisomy 21
- the child with short stature
- the infant with a large head
- the child with early or delayed puberty

Thus, taking history is a key element of a paediatric consultation and presenting symptoms are fundamental to unlocking the diagnosis. Take as many histories on varied presentations as you can – just like crosswords, you will get much better at accurately taking and giving histories with practice. An observed history is an essential component of undergraduate paediatric examinations, the significance of which cannot be overstated.

The Adolescent History

Interviewing adolescents in clinical practice is extremely rewarding, provided you follow a few straightforward guidelines. You must spend part of the interview speaking to the adolescent alone – this is an important step in teaching adolescents to manage their own health care and provides them with an opportunity to discuss sensitive issues.

Parents play a central role in supporting the developmental steps of the adolescent while maintaining safety, clear limits and reasonable expectations. These issues are important to clarify and emphasise when speaking with them.

Some parents may initially question why you want to speak with the adolescent alone. However, with an explanation of its importance, most parents respect that this private conversation is vital for the interview.

Adolescents will occasionally offer information that they do not want their parents to know. Therefore, it is critical that you explain to the adolescent and their parents what can and cannot be kept confidential at the start of the interview.

Young people have a right to confidentiality, even if they are not yet competent. However, if the safety of the adolescent or others is of concern, confidentiality should not be maintained (referred to as conditional confidentiality). Examples of this include disclosure of sexual abuse or significant suicidal thoughts.

The following are key factors when communicating with adolescents:

- See the young person with their parents at the start of the consultation.
- Conditional confidentiality should be discussed with both the parents and young person to ensure trust.
- The young person should be central in the communication process, making it necessary for you to spend some time with the young person alone.
- Many young people can be initially ambivalent, but this can be overcome with skill and patience.
- A psychosocial history is key and should focus on factors of risk and resilience.

HEEADSSS SCREENING TOOL

HEEADSSS is a psychosocial screening tool first described by Goldenring. Clinicians use it to identify psychosocial risks and resilience factors contributing to adolescent mortality (injury, suicide) and morbidity (mental health problems, STIs).

HEEADSSS is a structured interview with a series of domains:

- Home and relationships
- Education and employment
- Eating
- Activities
- Drugs, alcohol and tobacco
- Sex and relationships
- Self-harm, suicidality and depression
- Safety

It is not easy to comprehensively cover all these topics in an interview, and basic screening questions may be required to target risk areas. Always start with general questions before leading into more sensitive questions.

The following questions are suggestions based on the answers to the opening questions. Not all need to be asked.

HOME AND RELATIONSHIPS

The home environment should ideally provide adolescents with stability and meet their basic needs, including love, acceptance and discipline. However, home can be very stressful for some, especially if drug or alcohol use or physical violence is present.

Opening questions: *Who lives with you? Where do you live? What are relationships like at home? Who can you talk to at home when you feel stressed? Has anyone moved in or out of your home recently?*

Follow-ups: *Have you moved recently? Have you ever lived away from home? Does your home feel safe? Have you ever run away from home?*

Resilience factors: connected with careers or other family members; undertakes appropriate chores and responsibilities within the home, including care for other relatives.

EDUCATION AND EMPLOYMENT

The academic environment at school may be positive, negative or neutral and may involve significant peer issues such as bullying (in-person or online) that should be explored.

Opening questions: *Can you tell me about school? Do you feel connected at school/feel like you belong there? How are your grades? Do you need any extra help at school? What are your plans for the future? Do you have a job? Where? How many hours do you work?*

Follow-ups: *How much school time have you missed? Have you ever been suspended or expelled? How do you get on with people at school? Tell me about your friends at school.*

Resilience factors: better than average school performance; feeling connected with school; limited employment (under 20 hours/week); strong participation in school-related extra-curricular activities.

EATING

Eating disorders often present in adolescence. Questions to screen for a possible eating disorder may include the following.

Opening questions: *Do you have any concerns about your body weight or shape? Have there been any recent changes in your weight? Have you dieted in the last year?*

Follow-ups: *What do you like/dislike about your body? What else have you done to control your weight? Tell me about the exercise you do each week. Does it ever seem like your eating is out of control? Have you ever taken diet pills?*

ACTIVITIES

Ask about any activities (sporting or otherwise) outside of home and school to get a sense as to whether healthy or unhealthy lifestyle choices are being made.

Opening questions: *What do you do after school/work in your spare time? What do you like to do for fun/to relax? How many hours a day do you spend using a screen?*

Follow-ups: *Do you do any sports/exercise? Do you regularly attend religious/spiritual activities? How do you spend your time online? Can you think of a friend who has been harmed online?*

Resilience factors: participation in peer activities supervised by adults; leadership amongst peer groups; religious affiliation.

DRUGS, ALCOHOL AND TOBACCO

Substance and alcohol use can occur in adolescence and may be associated with significant morbidity. It can also be a gateway into crime and more addictive drugs for some.

Opening questions: *Do any of your friends/family smoke/drink/do drugs? Do you vape or use an e-cigarette? Have you ever tried smoking/alcohol/drugs? Have you carried on using? Have you used any medications that weren't prescribed to you? Do you use steroids/energy drinks?*

Follow-ups: *Is there any history of alcohol/drug problems in your family? Do you ever drink/use drugs alone? (Assess frequency, pattern of use/abuse, and how they obtain/pay for it.)*

Resilience factors: non-use or limited use (of alcohol only); non-use or limited use (of alcohol only) amongst family and friends; refusal skills.

SEX AND RELATIONSHIPS

The subject of sex and relationships is significant due to the risk of sexually transmitted infections (STIs) and unwanted pregnancy. Some adolescents have issues related to their sexuality. These are sensitive questions, the answers to which adolescents will want to remain confidential.

Opening questions: *How do you identify your gender? Are you interested in boys/girls/both/not sure yet? Have you ever been in a relationship? Have any of your relationships been sexual (involving kissing/touching)?*

Follow-ups: *Have any of your relationships been violent? Have you been involved in sexting? Have you ever been made to do something sexual you didn't want to? How many sexual partners have you had? Are you using contraception? Do you use condoms every time you have sex? Have you ever been pregnant/had an STI or been worried about being pregnant/having an STI?*

Resilience factors: abstinence; consistent use of contraception including condoms to prevent STIs; supportive intimate relationship with a peer; participates in sexual health screening and prevention programmes.

SELF-HARM, SUICIDALITY AND DEPRESSION

Depression in adolescents may present as irritability, withdrawal, poor sleep, poor hygiene, or deterioration in school performance. Suicide is one of the leading causes of death; risk factors include prior deliberate self-harm, substance abuse and a family history of suicide.

Opening questions: *Do you ever feel depressed, anxious or stressed? Are you bored much of the time? Have you been struggling to sleep? Have you ever thought about hurting yourself or someone else?*

Follow-ups: *Does it seem like you have lost interest in things you used to enjoy? Do you find yourself spending less time with your friends? Have you ever hurt yourself/used alcohol or drugs to calm down or feel better? Have you ever tried to kill yourself?*

Resilience factors: no personal or family history of self-harm, suicidality or depression; access to support from family, friends or professionals; no substance misuse; successful coping skills.

SAFETY

Injuries and homicide are significant causes of morbidity and mortality in adolescents. Safety threats may include school violence and guns in some settings and risks related to motor vehicles in others.

Opening questions: *Do you feel safe at home/school/in your neighbourhood? Have you ever been seriously injured? Has anyone picked on you or made you feel uncomfortable online? Have you ever been in a car with a driver who was drunk or high on drugs?*

Follow-ups: *Do you use safety equipment for sports and activities? Have you ever been in a road traffic accident? Do you get into fights? Have you ever felt that you need to carry a weapon to protect yourself? Have you ever been in trouble with the police?*

Resilience factors: seatbelt and helmet use; conflict resolution skills; no substance misuse; no weapon carrying; avoids unsafe situations (such as sharing a car with an intoxicated driver).

(Box 2.2)

Box 2.2   **Key Points**

The ability to accurately elucidate the <u>presenting symptoms</u> is critical to generating an appropriate differential diagnosis. Three to four main presenting symptoms are most often sufficient to accurately reflect the presenting complaint.

<u>Practice makes perfect</u> – the more histories you take and present, the better you become and the easier it is for you to navigate your way to a differential diagnosis that considers all likely possibilities.

The remainder of the history provides both context and scaffolding around the presenting symptoms to enable a robust set of differential diagnoses to be examined.

<u>If the child is not getting better, revisit the working diagnosis</u>. Revisit the presenting symptoms to ensure no vital information is missing.

The ability to take an <u>accurate and comprehensive social history</u> is a key discriminator of student ability.

Take as many histories on varied presentations as you can. With practice, you will significantly improve at taking and giving accurate histories (just like crosswords).

HEEADSSS is a psychosocial screening tool used by clinicians to identify psychosocial risks and resilience factors contributing to adolescent mortality and morbidity.

Key References

Chan, J., Raju, S. C., & Topol, E. (2019). Towards a tricorder for diagnosing paediatric conditions. *Lancet (London, England)*, 394(10202), 907. https://doi.org/10.1016/S0140-6736(19)32087-2.

Doukrou, M., & Segal, T. Y. (2018). Fifteen-minute consultation: Communicating with young people–how to use HEEADSSS, a psychosocial interview for adolescents. *Archives of Disease in Childhood. Education and Practice Edition, 103*(1), 15–19. https://doi.org/10.1136/archdischild-2016-311553.

Goldenring, J. M., & Cohen, E. (1988). Getting into adolescent heads. *Contemporary Pediatrics, 5*, 75–90.

Goldenring, J. M., & Rosen, D. S. (2004, January). Getting into adolescent heads: An essential update. *Contemporary Pediatrics, 21*(64), 64–90. https://peds.arizona.edu/sites/default/files/curriculumfiles/headss.pdf.

Kneebone, R. L. (2017). Performing magic, performing medicine. *Lancet, 389*(10065), 148–149.

Liang, H., Tsui, B. Y., Ni, H., Valentim, C., Baxter, S. L., Liu, G., et al. (2019). Evaluation and accurate diagnoses of pediatric diseases using artificial intelligence. *Nature Medicine, 25*(3), 433–438. https://doi.org/10.1038/s41591-018-0335-9.

Royal College of Paediatrics and Child Health. (n.d.). *The YPHSIG App.* Young People's Health Special Interest Group. https://www.yphsig.org.uk/resources-1/app.

Smith, G. L., & McGuinness, T. M. (2017). Adolescent Psychosocial Assessment: The HEEADSSS. *Journal of Psychosocial Nursing and Mental Health Services, 55*(5), 24–27. https://doi.org/10.3928/02793695-20170420-03.

Thompson, J. E., Collett, L. W., Langbart, M. J., Purcell, N. J., Boyd, S. M., Yuminaga, Y., et al. (2011). Using the ISBAR handover tool in junior medical officer handover: A study in an Australian tertiary hospital. *Postgraduate Medical Journal, 87*(1027), 340–344. https://doi.org/10.1136/pgmj.2010.105569.

Western Australian Clinical Training Network. (2016, August). *Simulation Scenario – Adolescent Health (HEADSS) Screen* [Video]. YouTube. https://www.youtube.com/watch?v=IaXq43U1t3I&ab_channel=WesternAustralianClinicalTrainingNetwork.

3 | *The Paediatric Examination*

ALF NICHOLSON, KEVIN DUNNE, and CONOR HENSEY

It's a funny thing, the more I practice the luckier I get.

ARNOLD PALMER

A Different Approach

When considering the differences between an adult and paediatric examination, you will find that many of your skills are transferable and apply equally. The critical difference is in the approach. Carefully observe senior paediatricians – watch how they approach the examination and try to emulate their approach – after getting consent from the parent to examine their child.

As a general rule, introduce yourself to the parents and child after washing your hands and immediately begin the examination.

The Power of Observation

Experience has taught us the necessary power of observation, especially when examining sick infants with respiratory distress.

General observation and the <u>six Os</u>:
- **Observe** whether the child is ill or well. Respiratory distress is a common cause of illness in paediatrics.

Observe the colour of the child's skin, assessing whether it is pink or cyanosed, pale (which may be an ill child as well as anaemia) or yellow (jaundiced).

Observe if the child shows signs of dehydration, particularly dry mucous membranes or sunken eyes.

Observe for apparent growth and nutrition issues, such as a child who is clearly under or overweight. Always cross-check your observations by plotting on the growth charts.

Observe for any dysmorphic features, such as those of Trisomy 21.

Finally, **observe** for bedside clues such as oxygen via a nasal cannula, a pulse oximeter or a nebuliser in a respiratory case.

Leave potentially unpleasant elements until the end of the examination, one example being evaluation of the ears. Children, especially toddlers, are best examined in their preferred position of comfort (often on their mother's knee). Always explain what you are about to do and provide reassurance.

You should practise the timing and technique of individual system-based examinations and develop the ability to summarise your findings accurately.

Growth and development are the additional central elements in paediatric examination. You must become proficient in assessing growth parameters (weight, length or height, and head circumference) and accurately plotting these measurements on an age-appropriate centile chart.

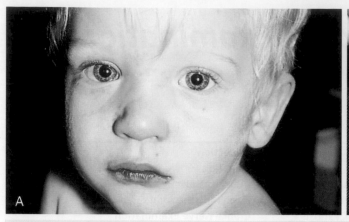

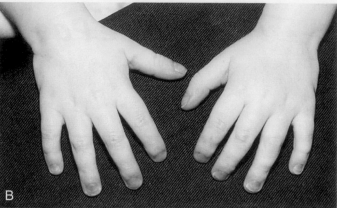

Figure 3.1   Moderate cyanosis. This child demonstrates moderate cyanosis of the lips (A) and nails (B). Note also the reddish discoloration of the eyes resulting from conjunctival suffusion (Reproduced with permission from Zitelli, B. J., McIntire, S.C., Nowalk, A.J. and Garrison, J. (Eds.), (2018). *Zitelli and Davis' Atlas of Pediatric Physical Diagnosis*. Elsevier Inc.)

You must also be able to perform a complete neurodevelopmental examination, which requires considerable practice over time.

The Cardiovascular Examination

Examining the cardiovascular system – especially listening for murmurs – can be daunting for many students and some postgraduate students. It may seem unfair for a medical student with little paediatric experience to accurately interpret various murmurs. A murmur is defined as an audible turbulent flow within the heart or great vessels. Up to 40 per cent of healthy schoolchildren have innocent murmurs. Approximately 1 per cent of children have a structural heart defect.

Observe from the end of the bed for evidence of central cyanosis, dysmorphic features, signs of respiratory distress, sternotomy or thoracotomy scars, intravenous lines, a saturation monitor or nasogastric tube placement.

There are several essential elements in a cardiovascular examination.

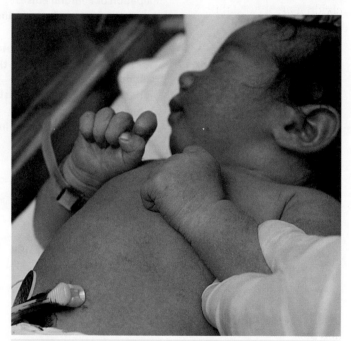

Figure 3.2   Acrocyanosis of hands of a newborn. (Reproduced with permission from Ball, J. W., et al. (Eds.), (2018). *Seidel's guide to physical examination* (chap. 9). Elsevier.)

ASCERTAIN IF EVIDENCE OF DYSMORPHIC FEATURES

One should look for dysmorphic features, particularly those of known syndromes associated with congenital heart disease (Trisomy 21, Trisomy 18, Noonan's syndrome and Turner's syndrome). Trisomy 21 has a very strong association with congenital heart disease (40 per cent), with A-V canal defects being the most common. An infant with a cleft palate has a 20 per cent chance of having a congenital heart lesion.

ASSESS FOR EVIDENCE OF CENTRAL CYANOSIS

Parents are often concerned about blueness of the hands and feet or around the lips. These symptoms often represent peripheral cyanosis or acrocyanosis. Central cyanosis of the lips and tongue (Fig. 3.1) is always abnormal but may be difficult to recognise. Acrocyanosis in an otherwise well

child should be considered benign (Fig. 3.2). These difficulties have led to the successful introduction of pulse oximetry screening in newborns to detect central cyanosis.

Clubbing is first evident from six months onwards in those with cyanotic congenital heart disease and is first apparent in the thumbs or toes. Clubbing takes a few years to disappear after corrective surgery for cyanotic congenital heart disease.

ASSESS FOR EVIDENCE OF CONGESTIVE HEART FAILURE (CCF)

The main features of CCF include tachypnoea with associated subcostal recession, fatigue and poor weight gain with excessive perspiration. Always consider CCF if an infant cannot take the same number of feeds as usual, especially if there is associated rapid breathing or sweating of the head.

Heart failure that develops in the first week of life (especially the first three days) is usually due to an obstructive lesion (critical aortic stenosis, hypoplastic left heart syndrome or pre-ductal coarctation of the aorta).

Examination findings in CCF include tachypnoea, tachycardia, a left parasternal heave and hepatomegaly.

Auscultation

Auscultation of the heart can be challenging for students, as crying and breath sounds may interfere with interpreting heart sounds and picking up a murmur. Establishing whether you consider a murmur to be innocent or significant is critical. The great majority of murmurs heard in well children are innocent in type.

PALPATION OF FEMORAL PULSES

Palpation of the femoral pulses is challenging and requires gentleness, good technique, persistence, patience and warm hands. Always check the lower limb pulses – one must consider the possibility of coarctation of the aorta if the femoral pulses are weak or impalpable.

EXAMINATION OF THE PRAECORDIUM

Inspect the chest thoroughly, looking for evidence of use of accessory muscles of respiration with tracheal tug, intercostal and subcostal recession, midline sternotomy scars lateral thoracotomy or pacemaker scars.

Palpate for the apex beat, which is defined as the most downward and lateral position where the heart's impulse lifts the index finger. Do not forget to place one hand on each side of the chest to ensure that the apex beat is on the left side to exclude dextrocardia. Palpate also for heaves and thrills at the apex, the left sternal border (LSB), the aortic and pulmonary areas, and the suprasternal notch.

During auscultation, try to determine the heart sounds and their character, any additional sounds (30 per cent of children have a third heart sound) and murmurs (their character and where they are heard).

The first heart sound (HS 1) is due to closure of the mitral and tricuspid valves. The HS 1 should be auscultated at the apex and the lower LSB. The second heart sound (HS 2) is due to closure of first the aortic and then the pulmonary valve. The HS 2 is auscultated at the aortic and pulmonary areas. It is important to determine whether the HS 2 is loud (pulmonary hypertension) or split. Usually, with inspiration, the sounds of HS 2 separate and come together on expiration (physiological splitting) (Fig. 3.3). In atrial septal defect (ASD), you will hear fixed splitting of HS 2 (Fig. 3.4). To hear a split HS 2, ask the child to sit up and listen at the mid-lower LSB with the bell during expiration. If the HS 2 is found to be split at that time, then it can be fixed and split.

Physiological splitting of the HS 2 occurs in healthy children and children with a minor ventricular septal defect.

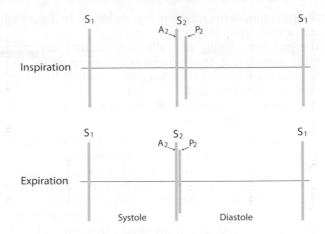

Normal Heart Sounds. Inspiration accentuates S2 split.

Figure 3.3 Normal heart sounds. (Courtesy Dr W Evans.)

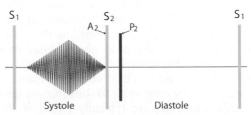

ASD. Ejection murmur, fixed wide S2 split

Figure 3.4 Atrial septal defect. Ejection systolic murmur with fixed wide split S2. (Courtesy Dr W Evans.)

I	Barely audible
II	Easily audible but not loud
III	Moderately loud but no thrill
IV	Loud with palpable thrill from high velocity turbulent flow
V	Loud with thrill and heard with stethoscope's chest piece in contact with the praecordium but slightly tilted
VI	Very loud with thrill and still audible with the stethoscope just off the chest

Figure 3.5 Grades of systolic murmurs. (Courtesy Dr W Evans.)

Exaggerated splitting is typical of pulmonary valve stenosis, while fixed splitting is a cardinal feature of an atrial septal defect.

ASSESSING HEART MURMURS

Key issues include the following:

- the <u>timing</u> of the murmur (either systolic, diastolic or continuous);
- its <u>intensity</u> (ranging from grade 1 to 6) (Fig. 3.5);
- the <u>site of maximum intensity</u> (if ejection systolic in the second intercostal space on the right favours aortic valve stenosis and the left favours pulmonary valve stenosis);

- the radiation of the murmur (e.g. radiation to the neck if aortic valve stenosis);
- the murmur quality and whether the murmur varies with posture (e.g. the murmur of aortic regurgitation is best heard with the child leaning forward with breath held in expiration); and
- respiration (the murmur of tricuspid regurgitation increases with inspiration).

Innocent murmurs are always systolic, soft, localised and may vary with either respiration or posture. A venous hum is heard in the sitting position but disappears by laying the child supine. Conversely, a vibratory Still's murmur is maximally heard in the supine position and may disappear on standing. A mid-systolic click is a clinical marker for mitral valve prolapse in the supine position and, if the child stands up, the click moves earlier in systole, and a late systolic murmur is heard.

Ejection systolic murmurs are typically found at the upper LSB above the nipple line and imply outflow tract obstruction. In mild pulmonary stenosis, the murmur peaks in the first half of systole and, as the obstruction becomes more severe, the peak occurs later in systole, and the murmur becomes longer in duration. Try to determine whether an ejection click is present – this is recognised as a very crisp start to the ejection murmur.

Pansystolic murmurs are typically found at the lower LSB below the nipple line or the apex. The most common pansystolic murmur at the lower LSB and apex is one associated with a Ventriculo-septal defect (VSD).

Continuous murmurs are characteristically heard in the left infraclavicular area, indicating flow across a patent ductus arteriosus (PDA). The classical continuous murmur of a PDA begins in systole and extends into diastole.

Diastolic murmurs are unusual in children and are never innocent. A diastolic murmur that is best heard at the LSB with a diaphragm and on expiration is typical of aortic regurgitation and may be associated with a collapsing pulse. This murmur is heard immediately after the HS 2.

Suppose a posterolateral thoracotomy scar is found after lifting the arms and inspecting the back. In that case, either an operative PDA repair, placement of a Blalock-Taussig (BT) shunt, repair of coarctation of the aorta or pulmonary artery banding is implied. Any child with a BT shunt who is cyanosed is likely to have a diagnosis of Fallot's Tetralogy.

A median sternotomy scar signifies a repair of intracardiac pathology with open-heart surgery.

The Respiratory Examination

A complete examination of the respiratory system in an infant or young child is best done with the child sitting on the parent's knee. Regular respiratory rates are faster in infancy and early childhood, with the average respiratory rate between 25 and 40 breaths per minute in infancy.

Observation is a critical element of the respiratory examination, especially in infants. Observe the respiratory rate and for signs of respiratory distress and whether there is excessive use of the accessory muscles of respiration such as the sternocleidomastoids.

- Check for the presence of finger clubbing (a cardinal feature of bronchiectasis).
- Look for nasal polyposis (typical of Cystic fibrosis (CF)) and check for nasal obstruction using the *sniff test*.
- Check if the trachea is central and whether or not tracheal tug is evident.

The Three Key Questions in the Respiratory Examination

SIGNS OF ACUTE RESPIRATORY DISTRESS

Signs include tachypnoea, grunting, stridor and use of the accessory muscles of respiration. Subcostal and intercostal recession may progress to a tracheal tug if respiratory distress increases. The tracheal tug will then progress to a supraclavicular recession and, lastly, sternal recession in severe cases (a worrying sign that may indicate impending respiratory failure). Flaring of the alae nasi with grunting may also be present.

Stridor, classically inspiratory, implies an upper airway pathology (commonly croup).

Wheeze, classically expiratory, implies a lower airway pathology (commonly asthma).

EVIDENCE OF CLUBBING

Clubbing is a significant finding in a child with respiratory symptoms and points to evidence of bronchiectasis (most commonly associated with cystic fibrosis but may also relate to other causes).

SIGNS OF CHRONIC CHEST HYPERINFLATION

Chest hyperinflation or air trapping features include a fixed chest wall deformity (pectus carinatum or excavatum), Harrison's sulcus, reduced chest expansion, hyperresonance to percussion and depressed liver dullness on the right side. Common causes of hyperinflation are poorly controlled asthma and cystic fibrosis in Caucasian children.

Check chest expansion in an older, cooperative child. Percussion can demonstrate hyperresonance or areas of dullness and may be useful. Tactile or vocal fremitus are rarely of value. Remember to auscultate over the intercostal spaces, and do not forget the axillae. Normal vesicular breath sounds in a child are high-pitched, but because chest compliance is far higher in young children, transmitted sounds are commonly heard. Signs of infection may include crepitations, decreased air entry and bronchial breathing.

Abdominal Examination

Attempts to perform an abdominal examination in an upset or uncooperative child are futile.

Firstly, try to gain the child's cooperation. The abdomen should be fully exposed, and you should examine the inguinal regions and the external genitalia.

The child should be lying flat and supine, arms by their side, and feet together – the abdominal muscles are most relaxed in this position. In older children, flexion at the knees may also help. Infants and toddlers may resist lying down and may be best examined while sitting on the parent's lap.

INSPECTION

Check to see whether the abdomen is flat, distended or scaphoid. Healthy toddlers (due to lumbar lordosis) can have a somewhat protuberant abdomen. Abdominal distension is an important sign of intestinal obstruction. Umbilical hernias are common in infancy and are almost universal in some ethnic groups. Separation of the rectus abdominis muscle (diastasis recti) is normal in young children. Scars on the abdominal wall will confirm previous surgery. Check for masses.

PALPATION

A relaxed abdomen is essential for palpation. Your hands should be warm and your touch gentle. Have the child lie flat with arms by their sides and knees flexed to encourage relaxation. Palpate all around the abdomen to detect tenderness and check for guarding and rebound tenderness in any tender areas.

For the palpation of the liver and spleen, always begin your palpation in the right iliac fossa. Gently rest your fingertips on the abdomen and depress them intermittently. As the child breathes in and out, the liver will come down to make contact with your fingers on inspiration. Advance your fingers upwards on expiration towards the right costal margin in increments of one to two cm. The liver edge is usually palpable one to two cm below the costal margin in the midclavicular line, especially in young infants. Measure the liver span by percussion of the lower and upper liver margins and the distance between them. The liver span is six to 12 cm in children six to 12 years of age.

Hepatomegaly may relate to acute infection (hepatitis A or EBV infection), autoimmune hepatitis, CHF, malignancy (such as neuroblastoma, leukaemia or hepatoblastoma), mucopolysaccharidoses or storage disorders.

The spleen tip is palpable in 10 per cent of healthy children and is often palpable in newborns. In infants, the spleen enlarges downwards towards the left lower quadrant, whereas in older children, enlargement is towards the right lower quadrant. An enlarged spleen's characteristic findings are that it moves with respiration, is dull to percussion, a notch may be felt, and one cannot get above it.

Splenomegaly is found in portal hypertension and chronic haemolytic anaemias such as hereditary spherocytosis.

The kidneys are retroperitoneal, ballotable, and are best palpated bimanually. Bilateral renal enlargement suggests either polycystic kidneys or bilateral obstructive uropathy.

Check for ascites by demonstrating shifting dullness or, rarely, a fluid thrill.

In toddlers, testes are best examined in the standing position or lying flat on the couch. Place a finger first on both external inguinal rings and then palpate the scrotum for testicular descent. This ensures that the testis does not retract into the inguinal canal as most young boys have a very strong cremasteric reflex. This bimanual approach is essential to rule out retractile testes.

Auscultation

Listen for bowel sounds, which are essential in several acute scenarios such as abdominal trauma, suspected peritonitis and a post-laparotomy child. Listen for renal artery bruits, especially if the child is hypertensive.

EXAMINING THE JOINTS

Watch the child closely, observing any noticeable abnormalities while the child is walking or playing. Observe the child's gait during walking and running over a reasonable distance with the child sufficiently undressed to give you a good view of the legs and pelvis. If a child spends a shorter time bearing weight on the painful leg, the gait is described as antalgic.

Examine the back for scoliosis by observing the child standing from behind with the shoulders level. Ask the child to bend forward at the waist while keeping the knees straight and allowing the arms to hang down freely.

Ask some pGALS screening questions regarding any difficulties or pain during movement of the arms, legs, neck or back, whether or not the child can dress without help, and whether or not the child can walk up or down stairs without assistance. A formal pGALS assessment of gait, arms, leg and spine movements should follow to assess movements of individual joints (Fig. 3.6).

For individual joints, check for swelling, redness of overlying skin and evidence of muscle wasting.

Always check active movements first and only check passive movements if active movements are incomplete.

CRANIAL NERVE EXAMINATION

Examining a child's cranial nerves is far less daunting than you might think and is very similar to cranial nerve examination in adults. Observation is critical; look for evident strabismus, ptosis or facial nerve palsy. Examine the cranial nerves in sequence.

I. Test sense of smell separately in each nostril, the other being occluded by finger pressure (coffee/almonds/cocoa).

II. Visual acuity via Snellen charts (distant vision) and Jaeger chart (near vision). Visual fields are tested using a finger equidistant from examiner and patient.

III, IV, VI: Inspect eyelids and pupils, check the direct and consensual response to light and eye movements in an H–distribution. A third nerve palsy is associated with a dilated pupil and ptosis on the affected side. An isolated sixth nerve palsy may be due to raised intracranial pressure (Fig. 3.7).

V: The sensory part comprises the ophthalmic, maxillary, and mandibular divisions and the corneal reflex. Check also the jaw jerk and muscles of mastication.

VII: Inspect for facial droop and involvement of the frontalis muscle as an upper motor neuron lesion of the facial nerve spares frontalis muscle. Test muscles of

Questions

- Do you (or does your child) have any pain or stiffness in your (their) joints, muscles or back?
- Do you (or does your child) have any difficulty getting yourself (him/ herself) dressed without any help? Or lifting an object above shoulder level?
- Do you (or does your child) have any problem going up and down steps ? Or being able to squat?

Figure	Manoeuvres	What is being assessed ?
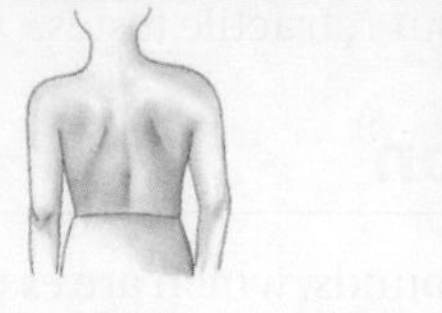	Observe the child standing (from front, back and sides)	Posture, habitus, skin rashes, Deformity (leg length inequality, alignment, scoliosis, joint swelling, muscle wasting, flat feet)
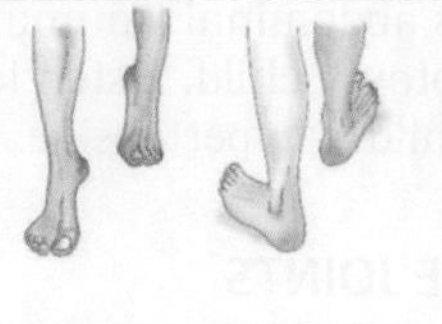	Observe the child walking, turning and returning then "Walk on your tip-toes" then "Walk on your heels"	Feet, ankles, subtalar, midtarsal and small joints of feet and toes Foot posture (check medial longitudinal arch when on tip toes)
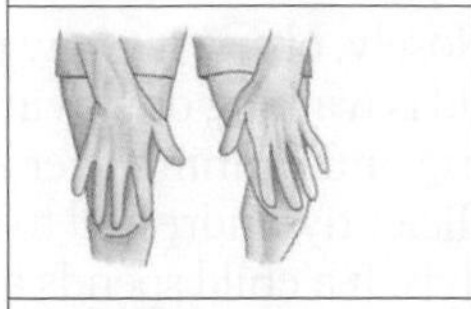	"Hold your hands out straight in front of you"	Forward flexion of shoulders Elbow extension, wrist extension, extension of small joints of fingers
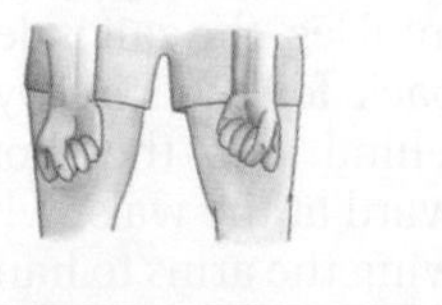	"Turn your hands over & make a fist"	Wrist supination, Elbow supination, Flexion of small joints of fingers
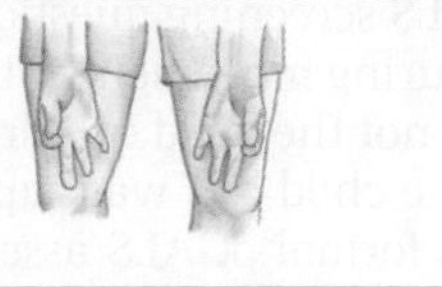	"Pinch your index finger & thumb together"	Manual dexterity Co-ordination of small joints of fingers

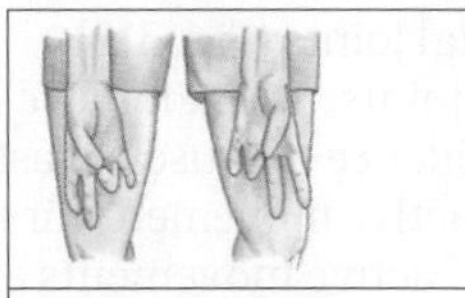	"Touch the tips of your fingers"	Manual dexterity Co-ordination of small joints of fingers
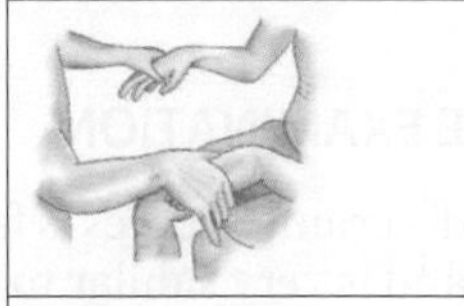	Squeeze the metacarpophalangeal joints	Metacarpophalangeal joints (for tenderness)
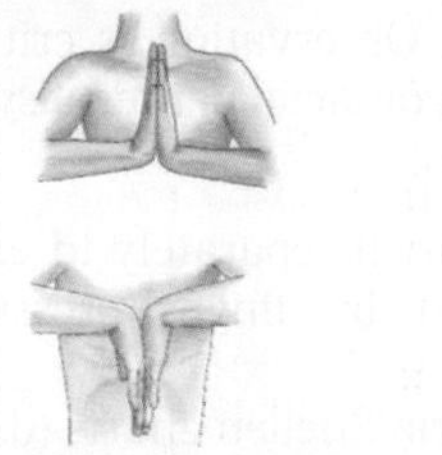	"Put your hands together palm to palms and "Put your hands together back to back"	Extension of small joints of fingers, Wrist extension / flexion, Elbow flexion
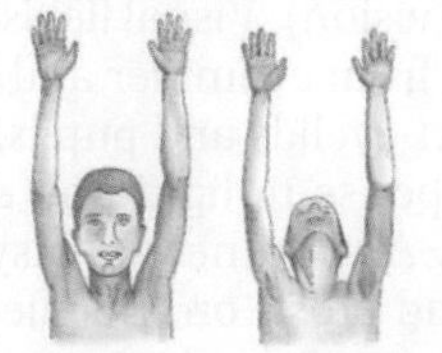	"Reach up, 'touch the sky', and "Look at the ceiling"	Neck extension, Shoulder abduction, Elbow extension, Wrist extension
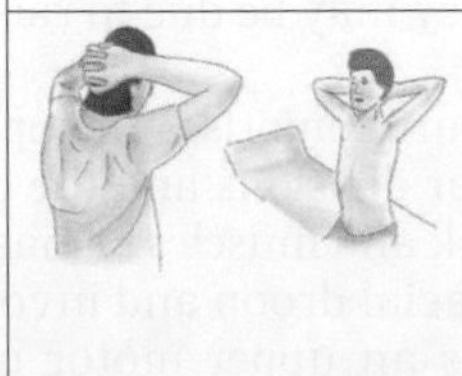	"Put your hands behind your neck"	Shoulder abduction, External rotation of shoulders, Elbow flexion

Figure 3.6 The pGALS musculoskeletal screen. (Reproduced from Reports on the Rheumatic Diseases Series 5, Hands on No. 15 (June 2008) – by kind permission from Arthritis Research UK www.arthritisresearchuk.org.)

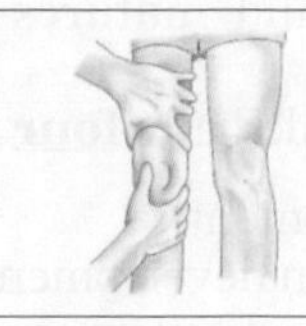 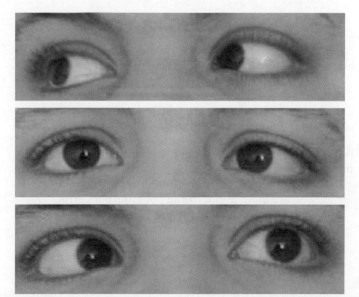 Feel for effusion at the knee (patellar tap or cross fluctuation)	Knee effusion (small effusion may be missed by patellar tap alone)
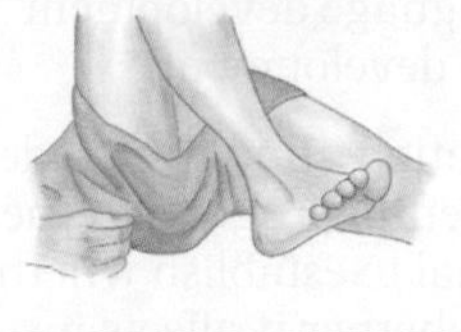 Active movement of knees & feel for crepitus (passive flexion)	Knee flexion / extension
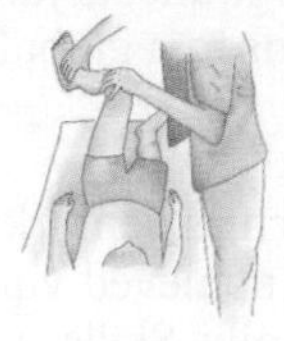 Passive movement (full flexion, internal rotation of hip	Hip flexion and internal rotation
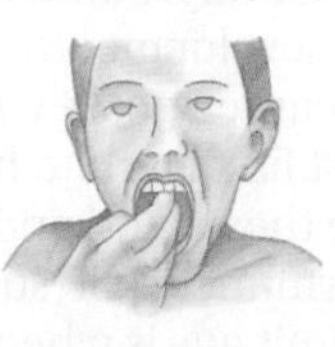 "Open wide and put 3 (child's own) fingers in your mouth"	Temporomandibular joints (check deviation of jaw movement)
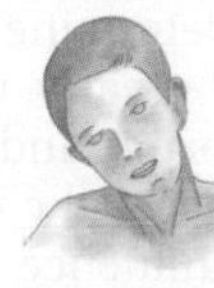 "Try and touch your shoulder with your ear"	Cervical spine lateral flexion
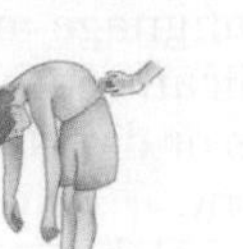 "Bend forwards & touch your toes"	Thoraco-lumbar spine forward flexion (check for scoliosis)

Figure 3.6   *Continued*

Figure 3.7   Left sixth nerve palsy. (Reproduced with permission from Poropat, F., Ventura, G., Murru, F. M., Orzan, F., & Maschio, M. (2012). A boy with acute strabismus. *The Journal of Pediatrics*. 161(6), 1178.e1, Fig. 1, © 2012.)

facial expression by asking the child to look up and raise their eyebrows, screw their eyes up tight and bury their eyelashes, keep them shut (tests orbicularis oculi), show their teeth (look for asymmetry of naso-labial folds), and puff out their cheeks (Fig. 3.8). Also, check the external auditory canal to look for herpetic vesicles).

VIII: For the Rinne test, the tuning fork is first placed on the mastoid process. When the sound can no longer be heard, the tuning fork is placed in front of the external auditory meatus. Air conduction is typically better than bone conduction. For the Weber test, the tuning fork is held in the midline of the forehead, and the sound should be heard in the centre without lateralisation to either ear. With conductive hearing loss, the sound is heard on the side of the conductive loss; likewise, the sound is better heard on the opposite (unaffected) side with sensorineural hearing loss.

IX/X: Both the gag response and movement of the uvula are tested.

XI: Check both the sternomastoid and trapezius muscles.

XII: Inspect the tongue on protrusion and ask the child to push their tongue against both cheeks.

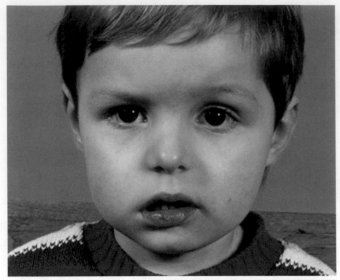

Figure 3.8 Right-sided facial nerve palsy. (Reproduced with permission from Andreassen, C. S., & Therese, O. (2015) Multiple recurrences of ipsilateral facial palsy in a patient with widening of the facial canal. *International Journal of Pediatric Otorhinolaryngology*, 79(2), 274–277. Fig. 2 Persistent right-sided facial nerve palsy (House-Brackmann grade 3) in the patient at 41 months of age following 15 incidents of recurrent right-sided facial nerve palsy since the age of 13 months. © 2014.)

ASSESSMENT OF A POTENTIAL SQUINT

Strabismus is a deviation of the eyes which may appear at the time of examination (manifest squint) or may be detected only when the two eyes are dissociated by testing (latent squint). Latent squints may become evident under conditions of stress, fatigue or acute illness.

Strabismus (or squint) is the leading cause of amblyopia in children and can be convergent or divergent. It is a widespread problem in young children (affecting up to ten per cent) and early detection is vital.

Convergent strabismus is most common and is usually evident by six to nine months of age. Early correction may result in near full restoration of normal binocular vision.

Clinical Assessment

Check first the light reflex. Perform the cover/uncover test (the squint will disappear when the non-squinting eye is covered and reappear when uncovered). Check the eye movements (possible sixth nerve palsy or lateral rectus paresis), the red reflex (looking for absent red reflex or leukocoria) and, finally, the visual acuity in both eyes.

Management of Strabismus

If over six months of age, refer to a paediatric ophthalmologist. Treatment consists of both occlusion of the non-squinting eye, glasses, orthoptic exercises and, rarely, an operation for cosmetic purposes.

DEVELOPMENTAL EXAMINATION

Performing a developmental examination is a core skill for undergraduate and postgraduate trainees and unique to paediatrics. The child's skills are assessed and compared to infants and children of a similar age. With development, the child matures into an independent adult.

Development is divided into **four** main domains:

- gross motor development
- fine motor and vision development
- speech and language development
- social and play development

Every consultation should include questions about the child's developmental progress. If there is delayed development, it is essential to establish whether the delay is mild or significant and whether it affects just one domain (isolated delay) or all four domains in a global delay.

Normal Development

The development pattern is remarkably constant, but the rate at which goals are achieved varies from child to child, even within the same family. Skills are acquired sequentially. Acquisition of later developmental goals often depends on the achievement of earlier goals within the same field. For instance, a child must first learn to have head control and sit independently before they stand and then walk. The acquisition of a critical performance skill (such as walking) is referred to as a milestone. A limit age is when a skill should have been achieved and is two standard deviations above the mean.

Genetic factors may determine a child's potential, but their environment may greatly influence their developmental progress. A supportive and nurturing environment in infancy and early childhood can enhance the development of the brain and influence development, especially in the domains of language and social skills. Conversely, children with significant early challenges, such as those living in orphanages or direct provision centres, may have impaired development.

Global developmental delay affects 1 to 3 per cent of children. Just over 1 per cent of children have autism spectrum disorder, and 1 to 2 per cent have a mild learning disability.

Early identification and early intervention improve the outcomes in children with developmental delay.

TAKING A DEVELOPMENTAL HISTORY

Parents, especially those with previous children, are excellent observers, and any concern they have about their child's development must be taken seriously as they are usually correct. They are often more knowledgeable about the pattern of normal motor skills development than perhaps speech development, but all concerns must be noted. Any history of regression (a loss of previously acquired skills) is a major red flag, and the child should immediately be referred for specialist paediatric assessment (Table 3.1). Developmental screening questionnaires are popular worldwide and are quite useful to flag potential concerns.

Specific questions should relate to gestation in weeks as developmental issues are more frequently seen if neonatal complications are related to prematurity. Also, if premature, the child should be assessed for their corrected age rather than their chronological age for at least the first two years of life.

Complications during pregnancy or birth may include maternal infections in early pregnancy, antenatal complications, perinatal asphyxia, abnormal neurological behaviour in the neonatal period and evident congenital malformations.

Table 3.1 Normal Developmental Milestones and Red Flags

Age	Gross Motor	Fine Motor and Vision	Hearing and Language	Social and Play	Red Flags
6–8 weeks	Raises head to 45 degrees in prone Head in line with body on ventral suspension	Fixes and follows the parents' faces to 90 degrees	Responds to loud noises	Social smile	No responses to visual or auditory stimuli Poor head control with significant head lag
3–4 months	Raises head to 90 degrees in ventral suspension Rolls front to back (4 months)	Holds object placed in hand Reaches out for object (4 months)	Coos and Aah sounds	Early hand regard and laughs	Not fixing No social responses or sounds
6–7 months	Sits without support with round back No head lag on pulling to sit Lifts up on forearms if prone and turns head to both sides	Evident crude palmar grasp Objects transferred from hand to mouth, and hand to hand (7 months)	Tuneful babbling	Finger feeding started Stranger anxiety begins	Head lag still present or excessive floppiness Not reaching for objects
9–10 months	Sits without support with straight back Pulls to a standing position and attempts to crawl	Index finger approach with the development of a scissors grip Brings two blocks together	Babbles in two syllables with use of 'baba', 'dada' or 'mama'	Plays 'peek a boo' and waves bye-bye Understands objects still exist even if out of view (termed object permanence)	Not able to sit without support No babbling
12 months	Cruises around furniture (termed 'coastal navigation') Stands independently Walks if 2 hands held	Mature pincer grasp Throws objects to floor (Casts) Puts blocks into a cup or container	Has 4–5 single words and constantly trying to imitate sounds uses mama and dada appropriately for parents	Points to indicate needs and initiates activities Is able to drink from a cup with 2 hands	Not able to stand with support Not pointing to objects No stranger anxiety
18 months	Walks well even if carrying a toy Runs	Begins to show hand preference Builds a tower of three 1-inch blocks Marks the page with crayon	Has 6–10 words Points to 2 parts of the body without prompting	Uses a spoon without spills and engages in symbolic play 'feeds' doll	Not walk independently Lack of words with meaning
24 months	Climbs upstairs two feet per step, kicks a ball and throws overhead	Scribbles and copies a line. Builds a tower of 6 blocks	Joins 2 or 3 words in short phrases, e.g. Daddy car Identifies animals in pictures	Is able to remove some clothes	Not able to run No symbolic play or to join two words into a phrase
36 months	Climbs upstairs alternating feet and is able to stand briefly on 1 foot	Draws a circle and matches five geometric shapes in a puzzle Builds a tower of 9 blocks	Talks in 3–4 word clear sentences	Uses a fork and spoon to eat Attempts to put on clothes May be dry by day	Not able to climb stairs Not able to communicate with words
48 months	Is able to balance on one foot for 5 seconds Hops on 1 foot	Builds a bridge from a model, tower of 12 blocks Draws a cross Traces a diamond shape Picks the longer of two lines	Asks lots of questions and engages in full conversation Gives opposites Points to colours on request	Dresses with supervision Goes to the toilet without prompting Plays interactive games such as hide and seek Takes turns	Not able to hop or climb upstairs Does not participate in interactive games with siblings or peers Not able to complete sentences or be understood

Adapted from Bellman M et al

History of early childhood illness should focus on neonatal infections such as meningitis, abusive or accidental head trauma or significant hyperbilirubinemia or hypoglycaemia in the newborn period.

Gross Motor Development

Ask whether the child can sit with or without support, crawl, stand or cruise, and assess the ability to walk unaided. Forward parachute reflexes are evident from 12 to 15 months of age.

Walking up and down stairs starts with two feet per step at two years of age, one foot per step going up and two feet per step going down at three years of age, and one foot per step both up and downstairs at four years of age.

Fine Motor and Vision

Ask the parents about any concerns about the child's vision. Assess grasp as to whether palmar, crude pincer or fine pincer. At six months, the child should reach

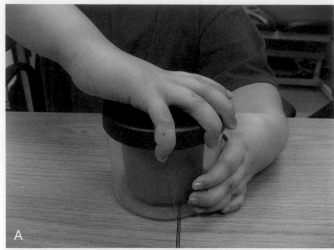

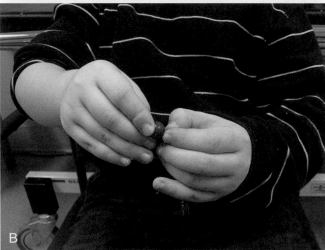

Figure 3.9 Palmar and pincer grasp. (Reproduced with permission from Ho, E. S., Curtis, C. G., & Clarke, H. M. (2012). The brachial plexus outcome measure: Development, internal consistency, and construct validity. *Journal of Hand Therapy*, 25(4), 406–417. © 2012.)

Table 3.2   **Red flags** requiring referral to paediatric services
■ regression of developmental skills at any age ■ head circumference above 97th centile or below 0.4th centile ■ persistently low tone or increased muscle tone
GROSS MOTOR ABILITIES: ■ if an infant cannot sit unsupported by 12 months ■ if a child cannot walk by 18 months in boys (always consider Duchenne muscular dystrophy) or 24 months in girls ■ persistent toe walking (consider spastic diplegia) ■ if a child cannot run by two years and six months
FINE MOTOR AND VISION ABILITIES: ■ parental concerns about vision require prompt ophthalmological review ■ if an infant cannot hold an object placed in their hand by five months or reach out for objects by six months ■ definite hand preference under 18 months (may indicate hemiplegia)
HEARING AND SPEECH ABILITIES: ■ no speech by 18 months ■ significant hearing loss
SOCIAL ABILITIES: ■ if a child cannot point at objects to express interest to others by two years of age

Adapted from Bellman M, et al

potty trained (dry during the day, usually by two years, and dry during the night, usually by three years).

Normal variants include bottom shuffling and rolling. Advanced motor skills are more likely in Black and Indian infants. Language development may be delayed in bilingual households.

Correctable causes of developmental issues include severe iron deficiency, severe failure to thrive or undiagnosed coeliac disease, maternal depression or significant social isolation.

CONCERNS ABOUT DEVELOPMENT

One of the key learning outcomes for an undergraduate paediatric student is to understand normal development and its variation. Normal variants such as bottom shufflers and rollers are not a source of concern in general terms, and parents can be rightly reassured. Likewise, isolated expressive speech delay, particularly in multilingual families, is very common.

The following tables 3.2 and 3.3 are important signals of abnormality.

Assessment and investigation of delayed development are necessary to enable a diagnosis, appropriate early intervention, and make predictions for the future. When delayed development is suspected, a detailed clinical assessment is required. Always bear in mind that you are looking for strengths as well as weaknesses.

NEURODEVELOPMENTAL EXAMINATION

A neurodevelopmental examination combines a neurological examination of the infant or child with a developmental examination across the four domains. The examination should initially focus on height, weight, head circumference and prior recordings to assess trends. Look for dysmorphic features and neurocutaneous

out and bring objects to the midline, have hand-to-hand transfer, and have a palmar grasp with no hand preference (Fig. 3.9).

A fine pincer grasp should be seen at 10 months. At 12 months, the child should cast objects away, point and look for a fallen toy or object (object permanence).

Hearing, Speech and Language

Ask about any parental concerns about hearing, speech or communication. Ask if more than one language is spoken at home.

Ask whether the child responds to their name, can talk, and ask how many words they can say. Ask whether the child can speak in sentences and express their wishes.

Social and Play Development

Ask about the onset of a social smile, whether a fear of strangers and whether the child feeds with a spoon.

Enquire whether the child's play is either symbolic (18 months) or make-believe (three years), whether or not they interact with other children, and whether or not they are

Table 3.3   Red flags for salient groups of disorders

METABOLIC DISORDERS
- loss of skills
- parental consanguinity
- family history of unexplained developmental delay especially if severe
- a symptom-free interval in the neonatal period
- slowing of developmental skills acquisition
- evidence of encephalopathy
- coarse facial features
- organomegaly

NEUROMUSCULAR DISORDERS
- reduced foetal movements
- early feeding difficulties
- marked truncal and limb hypotonia as an infant
- delayed motor milestones (not walking by 18 months)
- inability to jump by three years or hop by five years
- depressed or absent deep tendon reflexes
- a positive Gower's sign

Adapted from Horrridge KA

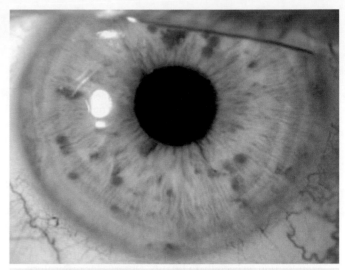

Figure 3.11   Lisch nodules. (Reproduced with permission from Lambert, S. E. (2017). *Taylor and Hoyt's pediatric ophthalmology and strabismus* (5th ed.). Elsevier.)

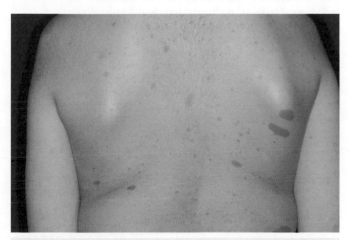

Figure 3.10   Neurofibromatosis type 1 (NF1). The presence of six or more café-au-lait (CAL) spots larger than 0.5cm in diameter in children and 1.5cm in adolescents suggests the possibility of NF1, although having CAL spots alone does not allow for definitive diagnosis. (Reproduced with permission from Mancini, A. J., & Paller, A. S. (Eds.), (2016). Hurwitz clinical pediatric dermatology: *A textbook of skin disorders of childhood and adolescence* (5th ed.). Elsevier Inc.)

lesions. Although café au lait spots are commonly seen, the presence of **six** or more spots (over 0.5 cm in pre-pubertal children and over 1.5 cm in post-pubertal children) fulfils one of the diagnostic criteria for neurofibromatosis type 1 (NF1) (Fig. 3.10). Other diagnostic criteria include axillary freckling, Lisch nodules of the iris (Fig. 3.11), and neurofibromas.

Start the neurological examination by checking tone, power and reflexes, and look for features of spasticity or hypotonia. Truncal tone is assessed by looking for head lag and evaluating the infant in both ventral and vertical suspension. Peripheral tone is assessed by measuring passive movement of the limbs. Deep tendon reflexes are easy to elicit in infancy, and plantar responses are often upgoing in the first year of life.

Check for preserved primitive reflexes (in particular the Moro and Asymmetrical Tonic Neck Reflex) as both should have disappeared by four months of age. Formal ophthalmology and hearing assessments should be performed.

Begin with careful observation of their posture and their play skills. Young children and those with significant delay should be examined where they feel comfortable, usually on a parent's knee. Start by assessing their gross motor abilities – can the child sit unsupported with a straight back? Rather than upsetting the child by moving them to a standing or sitting position, move on to vision and fine motor abilities. To examine a pincer grip, use small safe objects like a crumpled ball of paper. Assess their grasp of a pencil or crayon and their ability to draw, place shapes or build a tower of one-inch wooden cubes.

Note any vocalisations heard and their understanding. Can they follow simple commands? Do they know body parts? How many words, phrases or sentences are heard?

Social skills in this age group can be assessed by questioning the parents about their ability to feed themselves, dress and undress, and play. Note their interaction with you and their parents. Now that the child should be cooperative, their gross motor skills can be observed with them standing, walking or running. Also, ask about their ability to manage stairs.

Older children should be able to sit at a desk at a suitable height. Warm them up with simple tasks before assessing fine motor abilities through copying or imitating shapes with a pencil/crayon and paper, or ability to draw a person. Test their vision and ability to recognise letters and colours. Assess their speech output and use of grammar. Enquire about their social skills and observe them dressing and undressing. Finally, check their gross motor skills and ability to run and kick or catch a ball.

SPECIALIST ASSESSMENT

A specialist multidisciplinary team should assess any child presenting with significant developmental concern, often in a child development centre. Members of this team may include a paediatrician, occupational therapist, physiotherapist, psychologist, social worker or other family support,

Box 3.1   Key Points

Children – especially toddlers – are best examined in their preferred position of comfort (often on their mother's knee). Always explain what you are about to do and be as reassuring as possible. Observation is a major skill in paediatrics. The additional key elements of paediatric examination are growth and development.

During the cardiovascular examination, look for dysmorphic features, assess for central cyanosis or features of congestive heart failure and check peripheral pulses before auscultation of the heart.

Murmur variations with posture are important. A venous hum is heard in the sitting position but disappears by laying the child supine. Conversely, a Still's murmur is maximally heard in the supine position and may disappear on standing.

Observation is a critical element of the respiratory examination, especially in infants. Observe for respiratory distress and whether or not there is excessive use of the accessory muscles of respiration.

Relevant questions in the respiratory examination include enquiring about the presence of respiratory distress, clubbing and features of significant chest hyperinflation.

A relaxed abdomen is essential for palpation. Your hands should be warm and your touch gentle. Palpate all around the abdomen to detect tenderness and, if an area of tenderness is discovered, check for guarding and rebound tenderness.

Always begin your palpation in the right iliac fossa for the palpation of the liver and spleen. The bimanual approach is essential to rule out retractile testes.

For individual joints, check for swelling, redness of overlying skin, and evidence of muscle wasting. Always check active joint movements first and only check passive movements if active movements are incomplete.

Performing a developmental examination is a core skill for undergraduate and postgraduate trainees and unique to paediatrics. The child's skills are assessed and compared to infants and children of a similar age.

The acquisition of an essential performance skill (such as walking) is referred to as a milestone. A limit age is when a skill should have been achieved and is two standard deviations above the mean.

The neurodevelopmental examination combines a full developmental assessment with head circumference measurement, assessment for dysmorphic features, evaluation of both truncal tone and peripheral tone and deep tendon reflexes in both upper and lower limbs, and examination looking for preserved primitive reflexes.

Observation is key in examining the cranial nerves and looking for obvious strabismus, ptosis or facial nerve palsy.

Strabismus (or squint) is the leading cause of amblyopia in children and may be convergent or divergent. Refer to a paediatric ophthalmologist if a squint is detected in an infant over six months of age.

---

and a speech and language therapist. Developmental assessments used in secondary care include the Griffith mental development scales, the Bayley scales and the Weschler pre-school and primary scale of intelligence. Specific tests such as ADOS-2 are also available to diagnose autism.

The key benefits of specialist developmental assessment are early diagnosis and intervention to reassure parents if the infant or child has developmental milestones within the normal range or if a developmental delay is detected.

 Video on the topic developmental delay is available online at Elsevier eBooks+.

Key References

Bellman, M., Byrne, O., & Sege, R. (2013). Developmental assessment of children. *BMJ, 346,* e8687. https://doi.org/10.1136/bmj.e8687.

Clerihew, L., Rowney, D., & Ker, J. (2016). Simulation in paediatric training. *Archives of Disease in Childhood. Education and Practice Edition, 101*(1), 8–14.

Cohen, H. (2018). Syncope and dizziness. In R. M. Kliegman, P. S. Lye, B. Bordini, H. Toth, & D. Basel (Eds.), *Nelson pediatric symptom-based diagnosis* (1st ed., pp. 83–103). Elsevier – Health Sciences Division.

Craze, J., & Hope, T. (2006). Teaching medical students to examine children. *Archives of Disease in Childhood, 91*(12), 966–968.

Horridge, K. A. (2011). Assessment and investigation of the child with disordered development. *Archives of Disease in Childhood: Education and Practice Edition, 96*(1), 9–20.

Lang, B. A. (2010, August 2). Musculoskeletal Examination. In R. B. Goldbloom (Ed.), *Pediatric clinical skills* (4th ed., pp. 215–235). Elsevier.

Rashid, M. (2010, August 2). Evaluating gastrointestinal symptoms. In R. B. Goldbloom (Ed.), *Pediatric clinical skills* (4th ed., pp. 215–235). Elsevier.

Online References

unicyclemedic. (2016, October 11). *Poop demons.* Unicyclemedic.com. https://unicyclemedic.com/2016/10/11/poop-demons/.

Warren, A. E., & Roy, D. L. (2015, October 6). Cardiovascular assessments of infants and children. https://clinicalgate.com/cardiovascular-assessment-of-infants-and-children/

4

The Newborn and the Six-Week Examination

NAOMI MCCALLION and JOHN MURPHY

A core skill for both undergraduate and postgraduate students is the performance of a newborn examination and subsequent six-week check. A comprehensive examination ideally takes place within 24 hours of birth (but certainly by 72 hours) in order to:

- detect congenital abnormalities (affecting 1 to 2 per cent of newborns)
- confirm and manage abnormalities detected antenatally
- identify common problems such as jaundice, pallor or plethora, cyanosis, respiratory distress, or minor skin disorders
- ensure adequate infant feeding, discuss neonatal screening and vaccination

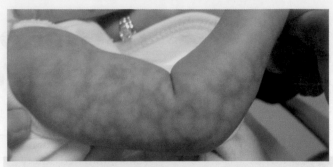

Figure 4.1 Cutis marmorata telangiectasia congenita on the right arm of a neonate. (Reproduced with permission from Weston, W., Morelli, J. (2017). *Pediatric dermatology DDX deck* (2nd ed.). Elsevier Inc.)

Newborn Examination

The core purpose of the newborn examination is to identify significant, important anomalies that might impact on the health of the child. It also presents an opportunity to assess and reassure parents about minor anomalies or normal variants. It is a critical examination and sufficient time must be set aside to undertake it thoroughly.

Although comprehensive, <u>particular attention</u> is focussed on specific conditions as part of the newborn examination:

- Eyes – screening for congenital cataract
- Heart – screening for congenital heart disease by both examination and pulse oximetry
- Hips – screening for developmental dysplasia of the hip
- Testes – screening for undescended testes

One or both parents should be present for the examination of the infant. Most infants are examined ideally on an examination table or in their cot.

A SHORT, TARGETED HISTORY

Try to ascertain any concerns the parents have about their newborn infant. It is important to inform parents that certain conditions may not be evident at birth and these conditions may require subsequent examinations to be identified. An example of this is a ventricular septal defect where there is often no murmur evident at birth.

Enquire from both the mother and the obstetric case notes about the history of labour, the birth weight and APGAR scores of the infant, whether any issues were identified during the pregnancy, and whether a fetal anomaly scan was performed and if any abnormalities were identified therein. Ask about a family history of developmental dysplasia of the hip (DDH) in a first-degree relative (mother, father, brother or sister).

Clinical Examination

Begin the clinical examination by noting the infant's general appearance and state of alertness. The normal term newborn sleeps for up to 20 hours per day, but when awake is alert and responsive. The infant generally lies with their limbs in a semi-flexed position. From a neurological examination perspective, the examination should ideally take place 30 to 60 minutes prior to the next feed – however, this may not always be practical.

Observing the Appearance of the Skin

JAUNDICE

Jaundice is very common in term infants and is most often physiological. It may be difficult to detect in dark-skinned children; in these infants, one must carefully check for yellow discolouration of the sclera of the eye. It is seen more commonly in breast-fed infants. Jaundice at less than 24 hours of age is invariably of concern and indicates acute haemolysis (Rhesus isoimmunisation, ABO incompatibility, and Glucose 6 phosphate dehydrogenase deficiency) or other important underlying conditions. It must be investigated promptly. If a jaundiced newborn appears ill, always consider either sepsis or the rare metabolic condition galactosemia as potential causes.

CYANOSIS

It is quite common to see peripheral cyanosis of both the hands and feet in the first 48 hours after birth. Central cyanosis, on the other hand, is always abnormal and requires urgent investigation. It is important to look under the tongue to detect central cyanosis. If in any doubt about cyanosis, check with pulse oximetry. All newborns should have pulse oximetry prior to discharge to detect subtle cyanosis and to rule out cyanotic congenital heart disease.

MOTTLING

Skin mottling is associated with a blue lacy appearance of the baby's skin and generally disappears once the infant warms up. Cutis marmorata is more persistent and does not disappear on warming the infant (Fig. 4.1). Occasionally cutis marmorata may indicate poor perfusion in infants developing sepsis or may be associated with syndromes.

MILIA

These are very frequent and are seen as small white spots on the infant's nose, chin, or cheeks, and resolve within a few weeks.

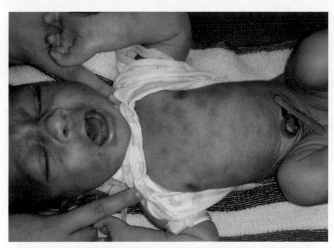

Figure 4.2 Erythema toxicum neonatorum. (Reproduced with permission from Thirunavukkarasu, A. B. (2017). *Pediatrics for medical graduates.* Elsevier, a division of RELX India Pvt. Ltd.)

SALMON PATCHES

These pink, flat, irregular shaped patches are most often seen between the eyebrows, on one of the eyelids, or over the back of the neck and are present in up to 70 per cent of infants. They fade by one to two years, but those on the back of the neck may persist longer.

ERYTHEMA TOXICUM

This is very common and has a 'nettle sting' appearance with areas of erythema with white papules (Fig 4.2). It often begins on the face and spreads to the trunk and limbs with both the palms and soles being spared.

PORT-WINE STAINS

These are typically found on the face, neck, scalp, arms, or legs. Port-wine stains are flat, permanent birthmarks that have cosmetic implications. If on the face around the eye, they may indicate Sturge-Weber syndrome.

CONGENITAL DERMAL MELANOCYTOSIS

Congenital dermal melanocytosis (previously known mongolian blue spots) are very frequently seen on the buttocks of African (90 per cent) and Asian (80 per cent) infants and less so in fair-haired infants (under 10 per cent). They are blue-black in colour and may be confused with bruising (Fig. 4.3). They do not change in colour and tend to fade by two years and disappear by five years.

INFANTILE HAEMANGIOMA

This is a benign vascular growth that generally first presents as a blanching or red macule of varying size. The natural history of an infant haemangioma is to first increase in size and then to involute slowly over months or years. Dermatology referral is indicated if the haemangioma is extensive, interfering with feeding or situated close to the eyes. Treatment with propranolol is rarely required.

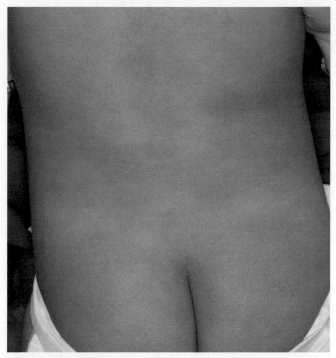

Figure 4.3 Mongolian spots. Large blue-grey patches over the lumbosacral area and buttocks of an African American baby. These spots often fade or clear within the first few years of life. (Reproduced with permission from Paller, A. S., & Mancini, A. J. (2016). *Hurwitz clinical pediatric dermatology: A textbook of skin disorders of childhood and adolescence* (5th ed.). Elsevier Inc.)

EXAMINATION OF THE HEAD

Examine the head for size, shape, and evidence of any swellings, then palpate the cranial sutures (sagittal, coronal, and lambdoid).

The occipitofrontal circumference (OFC), from the frontal area to the occipital protuberance, should be measured at its largest diameter. If over 38 cm, consider the possibility of hydrocephalus, and if under 32 cm in a term infant, consider primary microcephaly.

HEAD SHAPE

Following a normal cephalic vaginal delivery, the head is often moulded into an oblong shape. Pronounced moulding is also seen after a breech delivery but corrects quickly over the first few days after birth.

Marked head shape asymmetry may be due to craniosynostosis. In sagittal craniosynostosis, the sagittal suture is ridged, and the infant has an elongated head shape. In coronal craniosynostosis early marked plagiocephaly is seen in the first few months of life.

FONTANELLES

Always palpate both the anterior and posterior fontanelles and ensure they are open. Both fontanelles should be soft, firm, and flat. Infants with Down syndrome may have a third fontanelle. Even at birth, the diameter of the anterior fontanelle varies greatly.

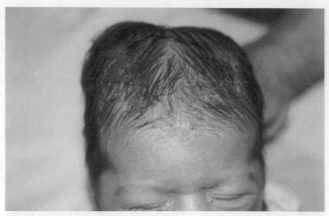

Figure 4.4 Bilateral cephalhaematoma in a three-day-old infant. (Reproduced with permission from Pai, M. V., & Hebbar, S. (Eds.), (2016). *Obstetrics & gynaecology: prep manual for undergraduates.* Elsevier Inc.)

Head Swellings

CAPUT SUCCEDANEUM

The key characteristic of this relatively common swelling is that it is **not** limited by suture lines and tends to resolve within 48 to 72 hours.

CEPHALHAEMATOMA

A cephalhaematoma is a swelling usually confined within the suture lines. No drainage is required, and it may take several weeks to settle fully. Jaundice may occur as the swelling resolves. (Fig. 4.4).

CHIGNON

A mark or bump occurring after a ventouse delivery resolving within 48 to 72 hours.

SUBGALEAL HAEMORRHAGE

A subgaleal haemorrhage is suggested by a boggy swelling without clear margins and can cross suture lines. It may lead to acute blood loss which may occasionally be life-threatening – close infant monitoring is required.

Examination of the Face

Cleft lip and palate requires prompt referral to a specialist cleft lip and palate service coordinator and careful assessment of infant feeding to ensure adequate intake (Fig. 4.5). Check for dysmorphic features and see if micrognathia is present. Micrognathia can be a sign of Pierre-Robin sequence, which may interfere with the baby's feeding and breathing.

Examination of the Nose

Mild nasal compression may relate to reduced amniotic fluid and tends to correct spontaneously within several days.

CHOANAL ATRESIA

Suspect choanal atresia if there is respiratory difficulty relieved by crying. Most cases are unilateral but in bilateral choanal atresia, the infant rapidly becomes cyanosed when the mouth is closed or obstructed but goes pink when the mouth reopens.

To test for choanal atresia, either assess movement of a wisp of cotton wool under the nostril, demonstrate an absence of fogging of a mirror placed under the nostril or try to pass a size 6 Fr catheter down the nostril.

Examination of the Eyes

CONJUNCTIVAL HAEMORRHAGE

This is very common and of no significance.

PTOSIS

Ptosis is a significant finding and requires referral to paediatric ophthalmology if the upper eyelid margin obscures the pupil.

LARGE EYE

A large eye may indicate congenital glaucoma (buphthalmos) and should prompt urgent paediatric ophthalmology referral (Fig. 4.6).

ANIRIDIA

Aniridia is characterised by an excessively large pupil due to the absence of the iris. In some cases, it is associated with the development of a Wilm's tumour, particularly when there is WT 1 deletion present.

EYE DISCHARGE

Eye discharge with excess watering may be due to a blocked nasolacrimal duct and may be associated with a bluish swelling (a dacrocystocoele). If eye discharge is purulent or blood-stained, *Chlamydia trachomatis* and *Neisseria gonorrhoea* should be suspected, and special swabs sent.

RED REFLEX

This should be elicited for both eyes to exclude the presence of a congenital cataract or retinoblastoma. An absent red reflex should be urgently referred to an ophthalmologist and seen within one week.

Examination of the Mouth

CLEFT LIP ± PALATE

Use a tongue depressor and light to check for a cleft palate. Ensure that the gum margin and the hard and soft palate

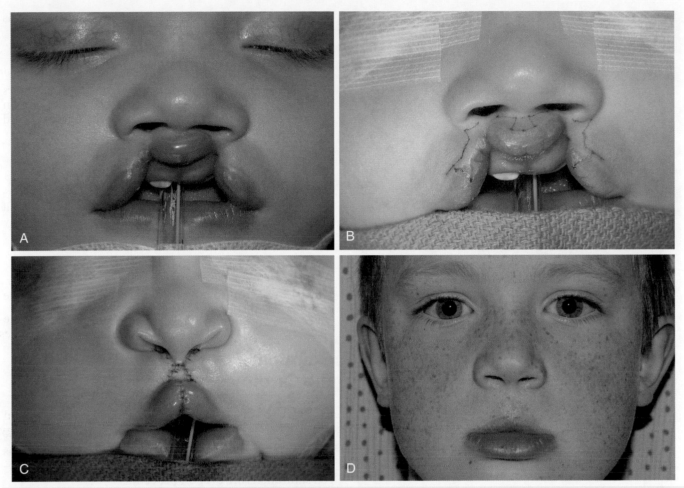

Figure 4.5 Incomplete bilateral cleft lip and palate. (A) preoperative view at five months of age; (B) intraoperative markings for the Fisher bilateral technique; (C) immediate postoperative view; and (D) appearance at 10 years of age. (Reproduced with permission from Farhadieh, R., Bulstrode, N., Mehrara, B. J., & Cugno, S. (Eds.), (2022). *Plastic surgery – principles and practice.* Elsevier Inc.)

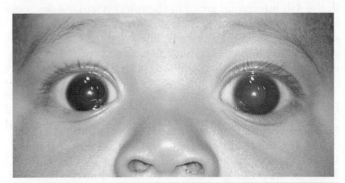

Figure 4.6 Congenital glaucoma: left eye larger than the right eye with greyish discolouration secondary to corneal oedema in the left eye. (Reproduced with permission from Martin, R. J., Fanaroff, A. A., & Walsh, M. C. (2020). *Fanaroff and Martin's neonatal-perinatal medicine, 2-volume set: diseases of the fetus and infant* (11th ed.). Elsevier Inc.)

are intact and that the uvula is present. A cleft lip should be easy to detect. An isolated cleft palate can be missed unless one examines the entire palate, particularly the soft palate. If the uvula is bifid, it can be a marker for a submucous cleft. Milk regurgitating through the nostrils can point to a cleft palate.

FACIAL NERVE PALSY

Features include incomplete eyelid closure and asymmetry of the lower face obvious mainly when crying (Fig. 4.7). The most common cause in newborns is post-instrumental delivery. Lubricating eye drops may be required to protect the cornea.

TONGUE-TIE

The frenulum is short and the tongue is more adherent to the floor of the mouth. It is only of importance if it significantly interferes with breast-feeding.

Examination of the Ears

The ears should be examined for placement, shape, and symmetry. Examine the auditory meatus for patency. Check that newborn hearing screening has been performed.

LOW SET EARS

For ears to be considered low set, the root of the helix (the top of the ear) is found to be below a horizontal line drawn from the corner of the orbit to the occipital protuberance.

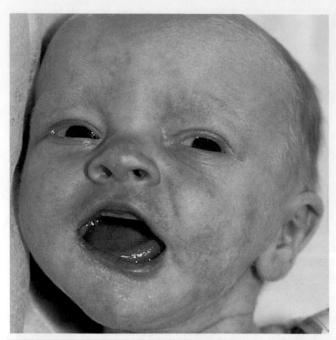

Figure 4.7   Facial nerve palsy. This infant incurred injury to the right facial nerve, resulting in loss of the nasolabial fold on the affected side and asymmetrical movement of the mouth. The side of the mouth that appears to droop is the normal side. (Reproduced with permission from Zitelli, B. J., McIntire, S. C., & Nowalk, A. J. (Eds.), (2018). *Zitelli and Davis' atlas of pediatric physical diagnosis* (7th ed.). Elsevier Inc.)

Low set ears are a feature of numerous syndromes including Down and Noonan.

PREAURICULAR SKIN LESIONS

These occur on the face anterior to the ear. They may be fleshy papules (tags) or superficial dimples (pits). Renal ultrasound examination is <u>not</u> recommended unless they are multiple or other anomalies are present.

MICROTIA

The external ear is underdeveloped in microtia, and in most cases the external auditory canal is absent. It is encountered in several syndromes including Treacher-Collins. A hearing deficit will invariably be present.

HEMIFACIAL MICROSOMIA

This is where the lower half of one side of the face is underdeveloped. It varies in severity, but it always includes maldevelopment of the mandible and the ear. The mouth is also involved. Referral to plastic surgery is advised.

Examination of the Neck

A very short neck may be indicative of Klippel-Feil syndrome. Those with Klippel-Feil syndrome have a low hairline and limited neck movements. The syndrome is caused by cervical vertebral fusion.

FRACTURED CLAVICLE

These can be injured during birth if shoulder dystocia occurs with a fractured clavicle being felt as crepitus. It requires an x-ray for confirmation and tends to heal rapidly. One should also examine for possible Erb's palsy.

BRANCHIAL CYSTS

These are small cysts on the side of the neck that may intermittently discharge. Surgical intervention is warranted if the cysts are causing repeated infections or if cosmetically unappealing.

CYSTIC HYGROMA

This is a soft, transilluminable, fluctuant swelling in the posterior triangle.

Examination of the Cardiovascular System

INSPECTION

Examine the mucous membranes. Ensure that the mucous membranes are pink. Check that routine pulse oximetry is performed predischarge and confirm the post-ductal oxygen saturations are over 94 per cent.

PALPATION

Locate the apex beat and determine its position. It is usually in the 4th intercostal space in the midclavicular line. Look for a left parasternal heave by placing two fingers immediately to the left of the sternum. The presence of a left parasternal heave indicates right ventricular hypertrophy and is encountered in cardiac conditions with a left to right shunt.

PERIPHERAL PULSES

Palpate for presence and volume of the brachial and femoral pulses. Brachial pulses are best felt with forearms extended. Weak brachial pulses may indicate poor cardiac output. Then identify and palpate the femoral pulses. Weak or absent femoral pulses suggest coarctation which requires a prompt cardiology referral.

AUSCULTATION

Auscultate over the precordium. The normal heart rate is 100 to 160 per minute in a term newborn. If a murmur is heard, note where it is maximal – murmurs are loudest along the left sternal border. Note if the murmur is soft or harsh. Harsh or loud murmurs are more likely to be clinically significant.

Examination of the Respiratory System

INSPECTION

Note the rate and pattern of respiration. The normal respiratory rate in a newborn is 30 to 60 breaths per minute. The presence of intercostal recession, subcostal recession, flared nostrils, head bobbing, stridor and grunting all point to respiratory distress. Observe chest wall symmetry during respiration. Examine the mucous membranes to ensure that they are pink.

Pectus excavatum is a depression seen over the sternum. It is most often an incidental finding and is not clinically important. Although rare, it may be one of the presenting features of Marfan's syndrome.

AUSCULTATION

In terms of surface anatomy for auscultation, the apices correspond to the upper lobes the right axilla corresponds to the right middle lobe, and the back corresponds to the lower lobes. Ensure air entry is equal on both sides during auscultation.

Examination of the Abdomen

INSPECTION

Inspect for distension and for masses. Diastasis recti is a normal finding that reflects a gap in the rectus abdominis muscle.

PALPATION

Palpate the liver and spleen for organomegaly. In newborns, a one to two cm liver edge below the costal margin is normally felt. A newborn's spleen enlarges down towards the left iliac fossa, whereas it enlarges across the abdomen in adults.

Check the umbilical stump to ensure there are no signs of infection. Check the number of umbilical vessels with normally three vessels evident (two umbilical arteries and one vein). The umbilical cord involutes over the first seven days and separates at the umbilical stump. Cord separation is defined as being delayed if still attached beyond 14 days. A delayed umbilical cord separation may be an indication of an underlying immunodeficiency, particularly if it becomes infected.

Umbilical hernias are especially common in infants of colour. They do not strangulate or incarcerate and will resolve spontaneously within a few months.

Inguinal hernias pose a higher risk of incarceration or strangulation than they do in adults. These occur more commonly in preterm infants and require early surgical referral.

Separate the buttocks and check for position and for anorectal patency. Anal atresia can easily be overlooked (Fig. 4.8). The presence of meconium on the nappy does not exclude anal atresia because it may have been

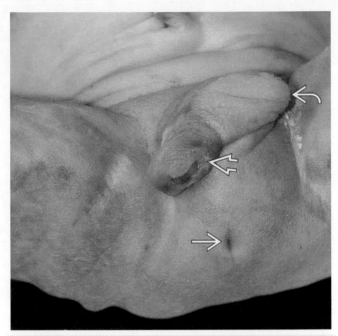

Figure 4.8 Clinical photograph shows a tiny perineal opening indicating low anal atresia. Note the undescended testes and hypospadias. (Reproduced with permission from Woodward, P. J., Kennedy, A., Sohaey, R. (2021). *Diagnostic imaging: Obstetrics* (4th ed.). Elsevier Inc.)

passed through a perineal, rectovaginal or rectovesical fistula.

Examination of the Genitalia

AMBIGUOUS GENITALIA

Ambiguous genitalia is an emergency requiring an early ultrasound to check for the presence of a uterus, investigation of endocrine anomalies including 17-hydroxyprogesterone levels and karyotyping for gender. The female infant with congenital adrenal hyperplasia will have an enlarged clitoris and normal internal female sexual organs. An infant with an XY karyotype may have ambiguous genitalia due to 5-alpha reductase deficiency preventing the conversion of testosterone to dihydrotestosterone. This deficiency leads to a small phallus, bifid scrotum, a urogenital sinus with perineal hypospadias, and a blind vaginal pouch. Early endocrine assessment is advised.

In females, inspect the vulva for anatomical anomalies. Note the normal structures, the labia majora and labia minora. Note if the clitoris is enlarged and hypertrophied. Blood-stained vaginal discharge is common, and no action is required.

In males, check the position of the urethral meatus for hypospadias or epispadias. In a typical case of hypospadias, the urethral meatus is on the ventral surface of the glans, the foreskin is hood-shaped and there is a ventral curvature of the penis called a chordee.

Check for scrotal swellings such as hydrocoele. Hydrocoeles are common in the newborn. The testis appears swollen. It may be unilateral or bilateral, the examiner can get above the swelling, and it readily transilluminates.

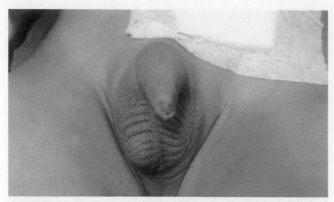

Figure 4.9 Unilateral (left) undescended testes (empty left scrotum). (Reproduced with permission from Swearingen, P.L., & Bhargavi, C.N. (Eds.), *Nursing care planning resource, volume III: Child and neonatal health,* (1st South Asia Edition). Elsevier Inc.)

Palpate the scrotum and note whether each testis is present and palpable in the scrotal sac.

UNDESCENDED TESTES

Undescended testes are relatively common (3 to 5 per cent of term male infants and 30 per cent of preterm infants) with 15 per cent being bilateral. Testes tend not to descend after one year of age and there is little, if any, benefit in delaying an orchidopexy procedure much beyond that age (Fig. 4.9).

Examination of the Spine

INSPECTION

Inspect for curvature, intact spine and any midline abnormality including midline birthmarks that could indicate an underlying problem.

A non-intact spine suggests a neural tube defect such as a lumbar myelomeningocele.

SACRAL DIMPLES

Sacral dimples are common and not of significance if they are below the level of the coccyx.

PALPATION

Palpate for spinal abnormalities such as lipomas or dermoid cysts.

Examination of the Upper Limbs

Examine arms for length, proportion and symmetry. Lack of active movements is noteworthy. Erb's palsy can result from brachial plexus injury and causes asymmetric posture and movements of the arm (Fig. 4.10). A brachial plexus injury may also affect an infant's grasp (Klumpke's palsy).

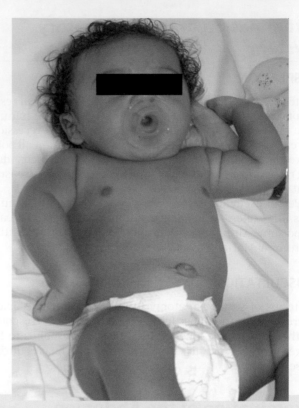

Figure 4.10 Right-sided brachial plexus injury (Erb-Duchenne palsy) in newborn infant. The Moro reflex was absent in the right upper extremity. Recovery was complete. (Reproduced with permission from Chung, K., Yang, L. J., & McGillicuddy, J. E. (Eds.), (2011). *Practical management of pediatric and adult brachial plexus palsies.* Philadelphia: Saunders.)

Lack of active movements and pain on passive movements (if acute) suggests a fracture or infection.

HANDS

Note the structure and number of digits. Preaxial polydactyly is where the extra digit is outside the thumb; this type is less common and warrants urgent assessment by a plastic surgeon and further investigation for underlying conditions.

Postaxial polydactyly is where the extra digit is outside the little finger. This is also called ulnar polydactyly. This finding is usually isolated and more common than preaxial polydactyly. It is often familial and is particularly common in babies of African descent. More than one extra digit on any hand should warrant investigation. Clinodactyly and abnormal palmar crease patterns can be familial, but look carefully for other dysmorphic features.

Examination of the Lower Limbs

LEGS

Examine legs for length, proportion, and spontaneous movement.

FEET

Note the structure and number of digits. Overriding toes tend to resolve spontaneously. Syndactyly is often familial and needs no treatment. Deformities of the feet are common in the neonate, particularly talipes, and may be positional or structural.

The most common of these are positional talipes where the affected foot is the same size as the normal foot. There is good dorsiflexion on stroking the skin on the dorsum of the foot. There is a full range of passive movement around the ankle joint. The calf muscles are similar in size to the other leg.

On the other hand, the foot is smaller in structural talipes equinovarus (TEV), there is no dorsiflexion on stroking the dorsum of the foot, the ankle is 'fixed', and the calf muscle is thinner on the affected side. There is an increased risk of hip problems. Structural talipes requires a prompt orthopaedic referral.

Examination of the Hips

DEVELOPMENTAL DYSPLASIA OF THE HIP (DDH)

Risk factors include a first-degree family history of DDH, whether the baby has been a breech presentation after 36 weeks of gestation, even if cephalic at birth and female sex. In multiple births, both infants should be screened if one had a breech presentation. Risk factors require a screening hip ultrasound to be performed within six weeks.

The Ortolani test is one of the tests recommended to screen for DDH. With the infant on their back, flex the knees and grasp the legs with the thumbs along the inner side of the thighs and the middle finger over the greater trochanter. Abduct the leg while the middle finger presses upwards on the greater trochanter. A 'clunk' will be felt if the hip is dislocated.

The Barlow Test is the other test recommended to screen for DDH. Hold the legs as previously described for the Ortolani test. Adduct the hip and apply light downward pressure on the knee. If the hip is unstable, it will pop out of the acetabulum.

Simple ligamentous clicks in a stable hip joint reflect newborn ligamentous laxity and are not significant. A positive Ortolani or Barlow test or an unstable hip joint require early investigation and treatment.

Examination of the Central Nervous System

MUSCLE TONE

Assessment of the infant's tone is important. Tone is defined as the passive resistance to movement about a joint. Abnormal tone may reflect systemic illness or a neurological (or neuromuscular) condition. The examination of central tone consists of eliciting head lag, ventral suspension and vertical suspension. The examination of peripheral tone

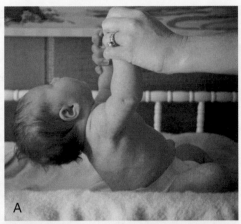

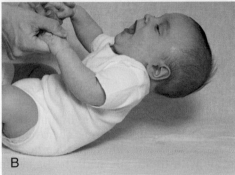

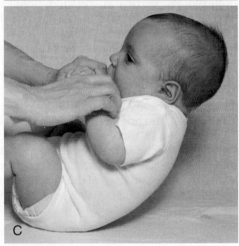

Figure 4.11   Head control while pulled to sitting position. (A) Complete head lag at one month; (B) partial head lag at two months; and (C) almost no head lag at four months. (Reproduced with permission from Hockenberry, M. J., Wilson, D., & Rodgers, C.C. (2018). *Wong's nursing care of infants and children* (11th ed.). Mosby.)

involves the passive assessment of tone in the upper and lower limbs.

EXAMINATION OF CENTRAL TONE

For head lag, begin by gently holding the infant by the forearms and pulling them upright (Fig. 4.11). There is an initial head lag over the first 30 degrees; the infant should then lift their head and hold it upright momentarily, while rounding the back.

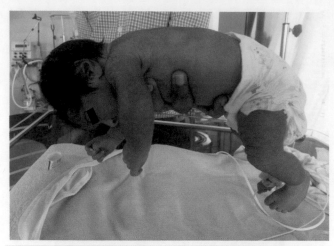

Figure 4.12 Full-term newborn baby, ventral suspension. Note flexion of elbows and knees with some extension of hips. (Reproduced with permission from Illingworth, R. S. (2021). In N. Jain, M. K. C. Nair, & P. Russell (Eds.), *Illingworth's the development of the infant and the young child: Normal and abnormal* (11th ed.). Elsevier Inc.)

For ventral suspension, turn the infant prone and lift them off the couch, placing a hand under their chest (Fig. 4.12). The normal newborn lifts both their head and pelvis almost in line with the trunk, with the upper and lower limbs semi-flexed. For vertical suspension, hold the infant under the armpits and lift them in an upright position with the legs dangling. Scissoring or hyperextension of the legs is abnormal and may suggest hypertonia or spasticity.

EXAMINATION OF PERIPHERAL TONE

Tone in the upper limbs involves testing the passive range of movement around the shoulders, elbows, wrists, and pronation and supination of the forearms. Check flexion and extension at the shoulder and the elbow and pronation and supination at the wrist. In the lower limbs, examine the tone by flexing the hips and then abducting the hips. Next, flex and extend the knees and dorsiflex and plantarflex the ankles.

Examination for Normal Newborn Reflexes

SUCKING AND SWALLOWING

Sucking and swallowing reflexes are present in all term infants and preterm infants over 35 weeks of gestation.

ROOTING REFLEX

When the corner of the infant's mouth is touched, the lower lip on that side and the tongue moves towards the point of stimulation.

GRASP REFLEX

When the infant's palm is stimulated, the hand closes. It disappears by two to three months.

THE MORO REFLEX

Explain to the parents that their baby may cry during this assessment. Lift the infant placing one hand behind their head and the other hand behind their back. Allow the head to drop a few degrees. There is a rapid abduction and extension of the arms with opening of the hands. The arms then come together. The Moro reflex is a very useful clinical test when assessing an infant for Erb's palsy, wherein asymmetry is readily obvious. It disappears by four to six months of age.

THE ASYMMETRIC TONIC NECK RESPONSE

When the infant turns their head to one side, the arm extends to the same side and the contralateral arm flexes in a so-called 'fencer position'. It disappears by two to three months of age.

THE PLACING AND WALKING REFLEXES

The placing reflex is elicited by bringing the anterior aspect of the tibia against the edge of the table. The infant will lift the leg up to step onto the table. The walking reflex is obtained by holding the infant upright so that the sole of the foot presses against the table. This initiates reciprocal flexion and extension of the legs, simulating walking. These reflexes disappear by six weeks of age.

Baseline Measurements

WEIGHT

A baby's birth weight is an important indicator of their health. Newborn babies may often lose up to 10 per cent of their birth weight but will regain it within one to two weeks. The weight should be recorded and plotted on the UK WHO growth chart if applicable.

LENGTH

The baby's length should be measured from the top of the head to the heel of one foot.

HEAD CIRCUMFERENCE

This involves measurement of the occipitofrontal circumference – accurate measurement is essential. It is also important to plot and if applicable, to act if outside normal range. It is important to use consistent technique (disposal paper 'Lassoo' tapes at the correct position on the head) and to measure three times and plot the largest of the three measurements.

The Six-Week Check

The six-week check is largely carried out in a family practice and is an excellent opportunity to rescreen for any conditions not evident on examination during the newborn period.

Key developmental milestones include improved head control and the ability to fix and follow and the development of a social smile. It is a period of considerable adjustment for the parents and the infant during which it is vital to assess both infant and parental wellbeing (particularly that of the mother). Feeding is a key issue – parents should be questioned about the frequency of feeds (if breast-fed), the length of time taken to feed, and if the infant is satisfied post-feed. Breast-feeding issues may prompt further support by a lactation consultant or public health nurse (health visitor). Mild regurgitation or gastroesophageal reflux occurs in 50 per cent of young infants and requires simple reassurance and positioning, with the possible addition of feed thickeners. Significant infant distress requires a comprehensive and compassionate approach and a more detailed assessment. Colic peaks at six to eight weeks of age and predominantly occur in the evening. Stool habit varies greatly and may occur after each feed or once every few days. Breast milk jaundice is common and tends to clinically resolve by six weeks of age. Always enquire about hearing concerns and reassure the parents that all newborns undergo hearing screening.

The six-week examination is identical to the examination in the newborn period in structure but with several conditions to look out for:

PROLONGED JAUNDICE (ASK ABOUT PALE STOOLS AND DARK URINE)

Although biliary atresia is very rare (one in 17,000 births), the success of the Kasai procedure directly relates to the time of diagnosis (ideally under 40 days of age). Always ask about stool and urine colour. If possible, observe that the stool is pigmented in an infant with prolonged jaundice and seek a measurement of the conjugated bilirubin.

POOR WEIGHT GAIN

During the first three months of life, infants tend to have an initial weight loss over the first two weeks and regain back to their birth weight by the end of week two. Thereafter, weight gain is usually between 180 and 200 grams per week but may be less for exclusively breast-fed infants (see section on faltering growth).

SIGNIFICANT INFANT DISTRESS

Infant colic affects 30 per cent of infants and is defined as paroxysmal uncontrollable crying in otherwise healthy infants less than three months of age with more than three hours crying per day (usually during the evening) for more than three days per week. Colic causes great distress and anxiety to parents and grandparents, and requires careful and compassionate assessment and a detailed assessment to exclude other differentials. Cow's milk protein intolerance may be considered, especially if no evening predominance, and responds well and quickly to exclusion of milk protein. If parents are at their wits' end, paediatric referral and possible hospitalisation is recommended for extreme infant colic.

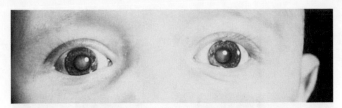

Figure 4.13   Congenital cataracts in an infant. (Reproduced with permission from Phillips, A. J., & Speedwell, L. (2019). *Contact lenses* (6th ed.). Elsevier Inc.)

RAPID HEAD GROWTH

The importance of accurate measurement of the infant's head circumference both at birth and again at six weeks cannot be overemphasised. The measurement is the occipitofrontal circumference and the newborn head circumference is 32 to 37 cms. Repeated measurements are critical to diagnosis.

Familial macrocephaly is common; a head circumference growing along the 90th to 97th centile is reassuring, whereas a head circumference crossing upwards across centiles is concerning. In this instance, it is important to look for other features of hydrocephalus such as dilated scalp veins, splayed sutures, a full anterior fontanelle and, as a late sign, 'sunsetting' of the eyes.

ABSENT FEMORAL PULSES

Coarctation of the aorta is the most commonly overlooked congenital heart disease. It is difficult to detect on antenatal scanning, and the normal neonatal circulatory changes over the first few days of life may mask the clinical findings. Every newborn examination should specifically check for coarctation of the aorta, which occurs in one per 2000 live births. Early detection and treatment reduce morbidity and mortality. Specific physical signs include weak or absent femoral pulses. Infants may be asymptomatic until closure of the ductus arteriosus. Weak or absent femoral pulses are found in over 90 per cent of cases of coarctation but may not be as obvious until the ductus arteriosus closes so may not be appreciated in the initial newborn examination. Severe symptoms of heart failure (tachypnoea, tachycardia and hepatomegaly) and cardiogenic shock (delayed capillary refill and grey discolouration of the skin of the peripheries) may develop acutely, or infants may present with poor weight gain due to poor feeding. Confirmation is by urgent echocardiography – the finding of weak or absent femoral pulses should prompt immediate paediatric cardiology referral.

UNDESCENDED TESTES (UDT)

The six-week check is another golden opportunity to check for UDT. Diagnosis involves a bimanual examination approach and should prompt routine referral to a paediatric surgical service, as correction via orchidopexy should

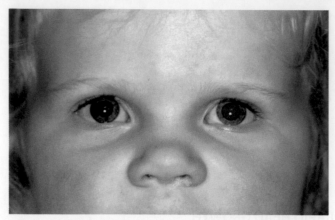

Figure 4.14   Absent red reflex in right eye. (Courtesy Childhood Eye Cancer Trust.)

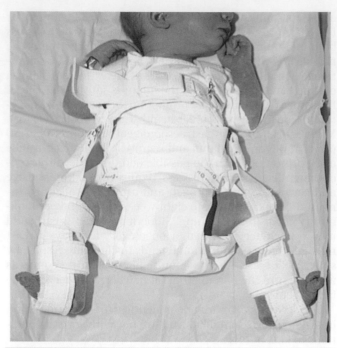

Figure 4.15   An infant in a Pavlik harness to treat developmental dysplasia of the hip. (Reproduced with permission from McKinney, E. S., Murray, S. S., Mau, K., James, S. R., Nelson, K., Ashwill, C., & Ashwill, J. (2022). *Maternal-child nursing* (6th ed.). Elsevier Inc.)

take place before 12 months of age. Six per cent of male infants have one or both testes undescended at birth, with a far higher rate in those born preterm. A high proportion of UDT will descend normally by three months of age, and so the prevalence of UDT at three months has dropped to 2 per cent.

PARENTAL CONCERNS ABOUT VISION (CATARACT)

A congenital cataract is an uncommon but important cause of preventable blindness wherein surgical correction is needed by three months of age for an optimal visual outcome (Fig. 4.13). The six-week check is an important opportunity for diagnosis. The red reflex examination can be difficult to perform in the newborn period as eyelid swelling at birth may make eye opening difficult. Infant upright positioning or suckling may help with spontaneous eye opening. Urgent paediatric ophthalmology referral is warranted if the red reflex is absent or if a white pupillary reflex (leukocoria) is identified. (Fig. 4.14). Leukocoria raises concerns about retinoblastoma, which are rare but potentially treatable. Visually significant congenital cataracts are managed by prompt cataract surgery to preserve vision.

DEVELOPMENTAL DYSPLASIA OF THE HIP (DDH)

Developmental dysplasia of the hip is a spectrum of hip joint instability ranging from mild acetabular dysplasia with a stable hip to a frankly dislocated hip. Early identification of DDH improves outcome, as the early use of simple dynamic abduction splints such the Pavlik harness (Fig. 4.15) may stabilise the hip whereas delayed diagnosis requires more complex interventional treatment and is less likely to have a successful outcome. The older the child is at presentation, the more likely it is that open reduction will be required, with femoral or acetabular osteotomies to stabilise the reduction. Traditional screening for DDH involves newborn examination of the hips at birth and then at six weeks, including both Barlow and Ortolani manoeuvres. At the six-week check, the presence of limited hip abduction may be the most sensitive sign for detecting a dislocated hip. In addition to universal examination at birth and six weeks, screening for DDH involves selective 'at risk' hip ultrasound for those infants with a breech presentation at birth or those that have a first-degree relative with DDH.

CLEFT PALATE

A cleft lip and/or palate is a common congenital malformation with a birth prevalence of one in 700. A cleft lip is obvious at birth, but an isolated cleft palate may be more difficult to recognise and up to 30 per cent of isolated cleft palate may be missed on examination during the newborn period. Infants, if not picked up, may have symptoms of milk regurgitation through the nose during feeds.

TONGUE-TIE

Ankyloglossia or tongue-tie is characterized by a short, thickened, or abnormally tight lingual frenulum and is present in 2 to 5 per cent of newborn infants. It may cause difficulty with breast-feeding in some infants. If identified during the neonatal examination, a detailed feeding history should be taken with referral to a lactation specialist to support the infant during latching and feeding. A recent Cochrane review (O'Shea et al., 2017) reported that frenotomy results in short-term improvement in self-reported breast-feeding efficacy and maternal pain but no difference in breast-feeding rates overall.

[Box 4.1]

Box 4.1 **Key Points**

A core element of both undergraduate and postgraduate teaching in paediatrics is the performance of the newborn check and the six-week check.

The core purpose of the newborn and six-week examinations is to identify significant anomalies that might impact the child's health.

Central cyanosis is always abnormal and needs urgent investigation.

The head should be examined for size, shape, and swellings and the cranial sutures (sagittal, coronal and lambdoid) should be palpated.

An absent red reflex should be referred to an ophthalmologist and seen within one week.

An isolated cleft palate can be missed unless one examines the entire palate, particularly the soft palate.

Palpate for presence and volume of the brachial and femoral pulses.

In newborns, a one to two cm liver edge can be normally felt below the costal margin.

Structural talipes requires a prompt orthopaedic referral. A positive Ortolani or Barlow test, or an unstable hip joint, require early investigation and treatment.

The Moro reflex is a very useful clinical test when assessing an infant for Erb's palsy, in which asymmetry is apparent.

At six weeks of age, key developmental milestones include improved head control and the ability to fix and follow and the development of a social smile.

Familial macrocephaly is common and a head circumference growing along the 90th to 97th centile is reassuring, whereas a head circumference moving upwards across centiles is concerning.

A high proportion of undescended testes will descend normally by three months of age, causing the prevalence of UDT at three months to drop to 2 per cent.

Visually significant congenital cataracts are managed by prompt cataract surgery to preserve vision.

At the six-week check, the presence of limited hip abduction may be the most sensitive sign for detecting a dislocated hip.

Key References

O'Shea, J. E., Foster, J. P., O'Donnell, C. P., Breathnach, D., Jacobs, S. E., Todd, D. A., et al. (2017). Frenotomy for tongue-tie in newborn infants. *Cochrane Database of Systematic Reviews, 3*(3), CD011065.

Reidy, M., Collins, C., MacLean, J. G. B., & Campbell, D. (2019). Examining the effectiveness of examination at 6–8 weeks for developmental dysplasia: testing the safety net. *Archives of Disease in Childhood, 104*(10), 953–955.

Online References

Health Service Executive. (n.d.). Growth Monitoring Resources. http://www.hse.ie/eng/health/child/growthmonitoring/

The National Healthy Childhood Programme. (n.d.). The Newborn Clinical Examination Handbook. https://www.hse.ie/eng/about/who/healthwellbeing/our-priority-programmes/child-health-and-wellbeing/newborn-%20exam.pdf

5 Feeding Issues and Faltering Growth

ALF NICHOLSON and KEVIN DUNNE

Breast-Feeding Issues

Breast milk is the sole food required for the first 6 months of life, and it confers passive immunity via immunoglobulin A, macrophages, T cells, stem cells and lymphocytes. Alpha-lactalbumin in breast milk has antibacterial properties; lactoferrin binds iron; and oligosaccharides selectively encourage the growth of beneficial bacteria in the infant's gut. Breast milk plays a role in gut maturation (especially if born preterm), brain development, and preventing dental caries.

While breast-feeding is perfectly natural, it is still a skill that both the mother and infant need to learn. Skin-to-skin contact between mother and infant immediately after birth plays a key role. Thereafter advice and support from a midwife, lactation consultant, public health nurse or health visitor or an experienced friend can make all the difference.

The *World Health Organisation* recommends breast-feeding for up to 2 years with the introduction of solids at 6 months of age. Problems most frequently encountered amongst breast-feeding mothers are nipple pain and poor milk supply.

NIPPLE AND BREAST PAIN

Nipple pain may be due to poor infant attachment and referral to a lactation consultant may be required. If the infant is attached correctly, there should be no friction of the tongue or gums on the nipple and no movement of the breast tissue in and out of the infant's mouth. The nipple and most of the areola should be inside the infant's mouth. When mothers are taking their infant off the breast post-feed, they should insert their fifth finger into the corner of the mouth to break the suction. Rarely, tongue-tie may restrict tongue movement, which can be associated with problems relating to latching on leading to sore nipples and poor feeding. A diagnosis of tongue-tie should be considered if breast-feeding problems persist despite a review of attachment and positioning by an experienced midwife or lactation consultant.

Mastitis is clinically characterised by a fever and a red, firm, tender area of the breast. It usually starts with breast engorgement and a blocked duct that progresses to mastitis infection and, rarely, a breast abscess. Treatment is by improving milk drainage by either increased feed frequency or a breast pump and improving infant attachment. Using a warm compress to gently massage the breast can also help increase the flow of milk. Although *Staphylococcus aureus* is the most common pathogen found in the milk of women with mastitis, antibiotics such as flucloxacillin are only indicated if problems persist after 24 hours of improved drainage. Fungal and herpes simplex infections are rare causes of severe pain and discomfort of the nipple area.

LOW MILK SUPPLY

Not producing enough milk is the most common reason women give for stopping breast-feeding but this may simply reflect a lack of confidence in the mother to successfully breast-feed. Early skin-to-skin contact between mother and infant is critical in the immediate period after birth to establish milk supply. It will also increase the duration of breast-feeding. Strategies to increase milk supply include offering both breasts at each feed, increasing the frequency of feeds, or expressing milk after feeds.

SUCCESSFUL BREAST-FEEDING

Evidence for successful breast-feeding includes the infant being satisfied after most feeds, proper latching on to the breast, satisfactory weight gain, at least six wet nappies per day, at least three soft stools per day, and no evidence of sore nipples or breast pain.

BREAST-FEEDING PROBLEMS

Breast-feeding is demanding as it initially requires the mother to be close to their infant 24 hours/day, making support for new mothers essential in the first few weeks after birth. Weight gain will be slow at first, and supplementary formula feeds may allay short term anxiety but at a much greater long-term cost. In practice, the key presenting features will relate to infants not being satisfied and gaining weight poorly with consequent referral to healthcare professionals. Sadly, breast-feeding rates are lowest in families of low socioeconomic status and mothers who are young or obese.

FORMULA FEEDING

Formula milks have improved dramatically over the past 30 years but still do not match the unique properties of breast milk. First milks are whey-dominant and milks for hungrier infants are casein dominant. Whey-dominant or first milks (70 per cent whey content) contrast with second milks (80 per cent casein). Follow-on milks (casein dominant) are used when the infant is over 6 months and has higher levels of iron, protein, calcium and phosphorus. Try to advise avoidance of 'milk roulette', or the constant switching from one formula to another, as it is very unsettling for infants.

Flow rates of teats are broadly categorised as slow, medium, or fast. All bottle-feeding equipment (bottles, teats and lids) should be sterilised until the infant reaches 12 months of age, with steam sterilising being the best method. Advise parents to use freshly boiled then cooled tap water to make infant formula.

For the first 2 weeks, advise the parents to feed the infant two to three hourly (60 mL/feed). From two to 12 weeks of age, advise three to four hourly feeds (90 to 210 mL/feed). At six months of age, offer four formula feeds hourly (210 to 240 mL/feed), and start weaning at around six months of age.

Goat's milk should not be used in an infant with an allergy to cow's milk, as it is very likely a cross-reaction will occur; infants allergic to cow's milk protein are also very likely to be allergic to goat's milk protein. Fresh goat's milk and unmodified soya milk are both unsuitable for infants under 12 months.

All infants should start solids from around six months of age. Parents should be advised to start with solids delivered as a smooth puree with no lumps and foods such as baby rice, stewed apple and pear, root vegetables in puree form and natural yoghurt. Breast milk or formula milk can be mixed into the solids. Potentially allergenic foods (eggs, fish, nuts, soya and citrus fruits) should be introduced one by one during the first year of life to reduce the risk of food allergic reactions. Advise avoidance of honey, added sugar, added salt, undercooked eggs and soft and unpasteurised cheeses until at least 12 months of age.

Avoidance of tea and coffee, carbonated drinks, natural mineral water (high sodium content) and cola in infants under one year old should be advised.

Vomiting in Early Infancy

OVERVIEW

Gastro-oesophageal reflux or regurgitation of milk is prevalent, affecting over 50 per cent of young infants. It is usually self-limiting and mild, with resolution in most cases by 12 months of age. No specific treatment is required in infants who are thriving, apart from feed thickeners and positioning post-feed. Likewise, no investigations are needed. These infants are sometimes referred to as 'happy spitters'. Tips to reduce reflux include proper winding of infants post-feed, ensuring teat flow is not too rapid, avoiding large volumes of feed, keeping the infant upright for 30 minutes post-feed if possible, and avoiding placing the infant in a car seat soon after a feed.

A common cause of reflux is over-feeding, so a thorough history of the amount and timing of feeds must be obtained. The prevalence of reflux is similar in bottle-fed and breast-fed infants.

THICKENING OF MILK

Systematic reviews of thickening of feeds with carob bean gum, corn starch, rice starch or cereal have been shown to reduce reflux and increase weight gain, so feed thickeners are moderately effective in managing reflux in healthy infants. Pre-thickened formula milks are an available alternative to feed thickeners added to milk.

INFANT POSITIONING

Based on a recent systematic review, elevating the head of the cot so that the infant's head is uppermost when lying supine is not justifiable. The prone position is not recommended as it may increase the risk of Sudden Infant Death Syndrome (SIDS).

ALGINATE COMBINATIONS

Alginate preparations increase the viscosity of gastric contents and form a protective coating over the lower end of the oesophagus. Gaviscon infant contains both sodium and magnesium alginate and has been found to reduce vomiting episodes in infants who reflux. Gaviscon is not recommended if intestinal obstruction or renal impairment is suspected.

GASTRO-OESOPHAGEAL REFLUX DISEASE

When reflux is associated with poor weight gain, marked distress with crying or oesophagitis, it is then termed gastro-oesophageal reflux disease (GORD). Oesophagitis may present with marked irritability, distress after feeds, faltering growth and possibly haematemesis or melaena. Oesophageal pH monitoring is generally accepted as the gold standard investigation for GORD.

Drugs for GORD include ranitidine (an H2 receptor antagonist) and omeprazole or lansoprazole (both proton pump inhibitors).

Faltering Growth

Faltering growth (formerly referred to as failure to thrive) is defined in its broadest sense as failure to gain weight at the expected rate and implies that weight will drop down two major centile lines over time. It is relatively common with a myriad of potential causes, but most cases are non-organic, and investigations are likely to be normal.

NORMAL GROWTH

Growth is an important measure of health and wellbeing in infants and children. While it is normal for infants to lose weight in the first few days of life, this will usually stop after 3 to 4 days, and most will have returned to their birth weight by 3 weeks.

Measuring and plotting weight and length/height on the appropriate growth chart helps to evaluate growth patterns over time.

Epidemiological data suggest that healthy children usually progress relatively consistently along a growth centile.

MEASUREMENT OF WEIGHT AND LENGTH/HEIGHT

Under 2 years of age:

Measure weight on a digital infant scale if available. Ideally, infants should be weighed without clothes (Fig. 5.1).

Measure length by lying the child on a length mat, with one person holding the child in position so that their head, back and legs are straight; heels are against the footboard; shoulders are touching the baseboard; and the crown of the head is touching the headboard (Fig. 5.2).

Over 2 years of age:

Remove shoes and ensure the child is wearing light clothing only. Measure weight on a calibrated digital scale and measure standing height using a calibrated stadiometer (Fig. 5.3), ensuring that the back and legs are straight, heels, buttocks, shoulders and back of the head are touching the measurement board, and that the child is looking straight ahead.

PLOTTING ON GROWTH CHARTS

Growth charts provide a visual representation of growth over time and indicate where a child's weight or length/height sits in relation to population norms for that age.

The World Health Organisation (WHO) has developed standards for growth based on healthy breast-fed infants from six countries, which should be used to represent

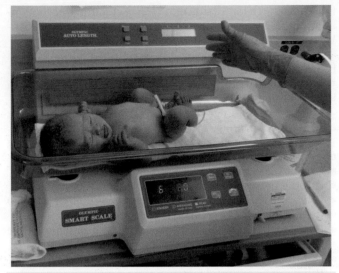

Figure 5.1   Weighing the Infant. Note the barrier placed under the infant and the nurse's hand, held above the infant for safety and protection. The scale used may be a balance scale or digital scale that locks in and displays the weight in kilograms. Some scales enable conversion of kilograms to pounds when the parents request to know the birth weight in pounds. Gloves should be worn when handling a nude infant. (Reproduced with permission from Leifer, G. (2019). *Introduction to maternity and pediatric nursing* (8th ed.). Saunders.)

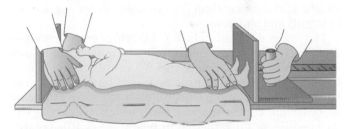

Figure 5.2   Measurement of the length of an infant. Crown-to-heel length of children 3 years and younger should be measured as follows: (1) Lay the child on a ruled board that has an attached piece of wood at one end and a movable piece at the other. (2) Stretch the child out on the board for the most accurate measurement. (3) Place the movable end flat against the bottom of the child's foot and read the length from the side of the board. (Reproduced with permission from Mahan, L. K., Escott-Stump, S., & Raymond, J. L. (2014). *Krause's food & the nutrition care process – Middle Eastern edition* (13th ed.). W.B. Saunders.)

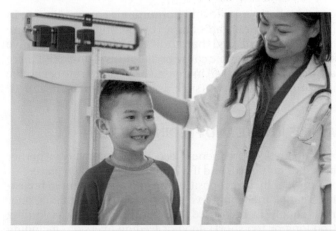

Figure 5.3   A medical professional measures the height of a child using a measurement scale. (Reproduced with permission from McKinney, E. S., James, S. R., Murray, S. S., Nelson, K., & Ashwill, J. (2022). *Maternal-child nursing* (6th ed.). Elsevier Inc.)

healthy growth for infants and young children internationally. These standards have been incorporated into the UK-WHO growth charts used in Ireland and the UK.

Gestational correction will be required for infants born before 37 weeks, and corrected age should be used up to 2 years of age. No gestational correction is required for term infants born at 37 to 42 weeks.

When plotting on growth charts, the child's age must be calculated accurately.

The charts should be examined to answer the following questions:

- Are the measurements of length and weight proportionate?
- Has the head grown proportionately?
- When did the problem start and progress (does it relate to the introduction of solids)?
- How severe are the deficits of each measurement relative to what is expected?
- Is the problem acute or chronic?
- What environmental factors are present?
- Has correction for degree of prematurity taken place if born under 37 weeks' gestation?

INTERPRETING GROWTH AND IDENTIFYING FALTERING GROWTH

Faltering growth refers to a pattern of growth in which weight gain is slower than the expected rate for age and sex in infants and children.

The agreed thresholds for faltering growth (NICE, 2017) are a fall across one or more weight centile spaces if birth weight was below the 9th centile, a fall across two or more weight centile spaces if birth weight was between the 9th and 91st centiles, a fall across three or more weight centile spaces if birth weight was above the 91st centile, or current weight below 2nd centile regardless of birth weight.

A weight that is more than two centiles below length/height centile is also considered a concern for faltering growth.

Only 5 per cent of children with faltering growth will have an underlying medical condition.

TAKING A HISTORY

Consider both organic and non-organic causes, bearing in mind that major organic causes of faltering growth are rare (under 5 per cent) and that studies on faltering growth have shown that an organic cause or diagnosis is unlikely if there are no signs (such as an increased respiratory rate or cardiac murmur) or symptoms (such as vomiting or diarrhoea).

ASSESS INTAKE AND FEEDING PATTERN

Ask about feed frequency feed during the day, whether breast or bottle-fed, and if weaning has yet taken place.

Consider incorrect positioning and attachment in breast-fed infants, inadequate volumes in bottle-fed infants, poor milk supply in breast-fed infants, the duration of feeding (too long or too short), food or feeding aversion, including aversion to solids, the presence of physical impairments that may affect feeding (e.g. cleft lip and/or palate), mealtime routine and eating behaviours and whether the infant or child is irritable or crying after feeds

ASSESS OUTPUT – URINARY OUTPUT, STOOL FREQUENCY AND CONSISTENCY, VOMITING

Ask about the frequency of wet nappies per day, whether vomiting is present, and the frequency and consistency of stools passed. Tachypnoea or dyspnoea during feeding may relate to chronic respiratory illness or congestive heart failure.

ASSESS OVERALL DEVELOPMENT

Enquire about developmental concerns and look for dysmorphic features as many syndromes are associated with faltering growth.

EXPLORE FAMILY DYNAMICS AND SOCIAL SUPPORTS

Seek information in a sensitive manner about the family composition, parental employment and living conditions.

PHYSICAL EXAMINATION

Look for any dysmorphic features (*Trisomy 21, Turner Syndrome, Russell–Silver Syndrome, 22q11 deletion*).

Assess whether tachypnoeic or if features of respiratory distress.

Look for any signs of discolouration (e.g. jaundice, cyanosis, pallor) and if any signs of undernutrition such as muscle wasting, poor skinfold thickness (subcutaneous fat stores Fig. 5.4) or thin hair.

Abdominal examination should rule out hepatosplenomegaly.

Observe behaviour throughout examination, direct observation of feeding may also be required (especially in breast-feeding so that positioning, attachment and behaviours during feeds can be assessed).

RED FLAGS

- If an infant has lost more than 10 per cent of their birth weight in the early days of life, or they have not returned to their birth weight by 3 weeks
- If infant is not feeding regularly from breast, or not draining breast, or if feeding frequently but for long periods
- If infant is feeding for very short periods <u>or</u> very long periods
- If not gaining appropriate weekly weight on two consecutive occasions
- If infant has fewer than five to six wet nappies in 24 hours or nappies do not feel heavy
- Recurrent infections
- Recurrent vomiting
- Tachypnoea or dyspnoea during feeds

FURTHER INVESTIGATIONS

Investigations may be required **only** if the initial assessment identifies relevant signs or symptoms:

(Table 5.1)

Table 5.1 Further Investigations of Faltering Growth

Investigations	Organic Diagnosis Being Considered
Full blood count, ferritin	Iron deficiency anaemia or low lymphocyte count in Severe combined immunodeficiency (SCID)
Urea, electrolytes, creatinine	Chronic renal failure, posterior urethral valves, nephrogenic diabetes insipidus
Thyroid function tests	Transient hyperthyroidism
Coeliac screen (tTG and IgA Endomysial antibody (EMA))	Coeliac disease (if faltering growth occurs post-weaning)
Sweat test	Cystic fibrosis
Vitamin D	Rickets (consider ethnicity)
Karyotype	Down, Edwards, or Turner syndrome
Chest x-ray	Congenital lobar emphysema or cystic adenomatoid malformation
Urinalysis	Urinary tract infection
Stool analysis + faecal elastase	Giardiasis or malabsorption

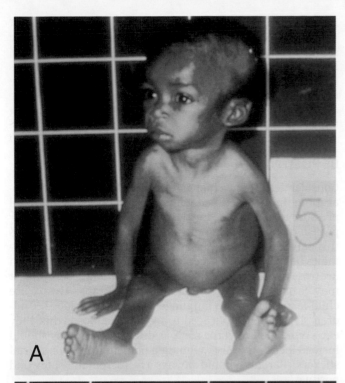

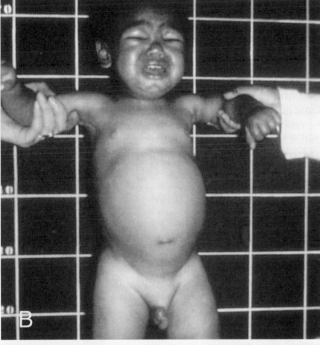

Figure 5.4 (A) Failure to thrive is a general nutritional calorie deficiency. Note the profound wasting found in malnutrition or starvation. (B) Kwashiorkor caused by a protein deficiency. The infant has generalised oedema with a white streak in the hair. (Reproduced with permission from Leifer, G. (2018). *Introduction to maternity and pediatric nursing* (8th ed.). Saunders.)

MANAGEMENT OF FALTERING GROWTH

In the first instance, community-based management of faltering growth is preferred. This will require the expertise of the public health nurse or health visitor and community dietitian.

The public health nurse (or health visitor) will usually monitor weight and length and refer to the General Practitioner (GP) and/or dietitian for further assessment if concerns.

Where possible, weight should be monitored at the same time of day and using the same weighing scales.

If faltering growth is confirmed, the dietitian will assess nutritional intake and compare to growth standards and calculated nutritional requirements. An increase in energy beyond the estimated average requirement (EAR) for age may be required.

Advice from the dietitian on management will be individualised and may include guidance on optimum feeding practices. This may include positioning and attachment in breast-fed infants, frequency of feeding, appropriate preparation of feeds, progression of weaning and perhaps advising increased energy intake through increased volumes (quantities), fortification, introduction of high energy formula or oral nutritional supplements.

Breast-feeding mothers should be supported to continue breast-feeding with advice on positioning and attachment and expressing breastmilk if appropriate to promote supply and provide as top-up to breast-feeds. Breast milk should be given first before any infant formula top-up. Information on local peer support groups should also be provided.

Hospital admission may be required if there is no improvement with community-based interventions or if the child is acutely unwell. Enteral tube feeding should only be considered when there are severe concerns about weight gain, and other interventions have been tried without improvement.

Involvement of a social worker may be required if there are social issues identified, or if there are any child protection concerns.

Clinical psychology, speech and language therapy, and occupational therapy may play a role in the management of food aversion.

Depending on the cause(s) identified, management of faltering growth may involve treatment by a range of healthcare professionals, including a paediatric dietitian. Management should be individualise and may include strategies to increase energy intake and improve feeding practices.

Information provided should be specific to the parents and child, and clearly explained and understood. Infants and children with faltering growth should be followed up by the appropriate healthcare professionals to ensure resolution of the problem.

Food Refusal

Feeding and nurturing their children is instinctive in parents – therefore, considerable anxiety and distress are caused when a child (typically a toddler) refuses to eat. This anxiety can affect the whole family.

Fussy or selective feeding is the rejection by the toddler or young child of a large proportion of familiar foods resulting in a diet with a very low variety of foods. A newer term, avoidant/restrictive food intake disorder (ARFID), is defined as a feeding practice resulting in persistent failure to meet appropriate nutritional or energy needs in the child.

Most of the issues surrounding food refusal arise due to excessive parental concern and attention on a child who is not eating. Distractions at mealtimes, a poor routine, excessive intake of juices, a limited variety of foods, manipulative behaviour in the child and parent anxiety can all contribute to food refusal.

It is normal for toddlers to eat well on some days and poorly on others, and that their intake will drop during intercurrent illness.

The prevalence of food refusal or faddy eating in preschool children is 10 to 30 per cent. For some, faddy eating may relate to a prior history of choking, vomiting or reflux with vomiting. Children with autism spectrum disorder often have selective eating patterns. Constipation is more common in selective eaters.

When taking a history, find out what the child is eating daily and enquire about past conditions that may contribute such as food allergies, severe gastro-oesophageal reflux, or marked prematurity with prolonged nasogastric feeds.

A complete examination, including weight and height measurement, will establish whether the child is well-grown and thriving. Look for features of iron deficiency anaemia.

Some key strategies are helpful for parents to tackle the issue:

DRINKS

Excessive intake of fluids (especially milk or juices) is probably the most typical cause of food refusal. The approach limits milk and juice intake (if deemed excessive) to no more than 600 mL of milk or one to two small glasses of juice per day. Try to avoid fizzy drinks altogether and ensure no drinks in the 30 minutes before meals.

REGULAR FAMILY MEALTIMES

Setting out a clear structure of meals and one or two snacks per day is key and helps avoid constant snacking.

A practical tip is to serve vegetables first and be aware that young children tend to eat better when others (especially siblings) are also eating with positive facial expressions. Parents eating target food and commenting positively is also an effective strategy. A key aim should be to make the meal table a relaxed and positive environment free of family conflict, tensions, and distractions, including television.

BE POSITIVE

Consider getting the child involved in gardening, food preparation, and food-related games. Avoid excessive parental pressure to eat, reduce meal times to 30 minutes and never punish a child for food refusal. Do not hide target foods, as this may lead to increased anxiety and a loss of trust. Vegetables have increased acceptance when initially paired with dextrose and calories and, once the vegetable is accepted, it may be offered in plainer non-sweetened forms. Always use child-focused positive language in describing foods. Children should be encouraged to taste but choose what they eat. Avoid food rewards such as desserts – rewards should instead focus on praise, reading a book together, or special stickers. Parents should always try to remain calm and positive.

SET REALISTIC EXPECTATIONS

In introducing new foods, select one target food at a time and begin with food close in flavour to an already accepted food. Continue to offer new foods with novel tastes to the child. Some effective approaches to introducing new foods include the child purchasing a vegetable or fruit in the shop, playing games with the vegetable or fruit, and exploring the texture and smell before being encouraged to lick, bite or chew.

FOCUS ON THE LONG TERM

Positive reassurance that young children will not be harmed by short periods of low intake is helpful as a consistent approach by both parents and grandparents of the child. Advise that no alternative meals or calorie-dense drinks be offered in lieu of the meal provided.

WHO NEEDS A REFERRAL?

A referral is needed for a specialist opinion if there is a likely significant food allergy, coexisting chronic disease such as diabetes mellitus or cystic fibrosis, autism spectrum disorder, or if very high levels of anxiety continue in the parents despite the above advice. A clinical psychologist and paediatric dietitian may both play a key role in alleviating family stress and giving dietetic advice.

(Box 5.1)
(Box 5.2)
(Box 5.3)
(Box 5.4)

Box 5.1   **Key Points**

While breast-feeding is perfectly natural, it is still a skill that both the mother and infant need to learn.

Early skin-to-skin contact between mother and infant is optimal to establish milk supply and will increase the duration of breast-feeding.

Evidence for successful breast-feeding includes the infant being satisfied after most feeds, proper latching onto the breast, satisfactory weight gain, at least six wet nappies per day, at least three soft stools per day, and no evidence of sore nipples or breast pain.

Try to advise avoidance of 'milk roulette', or the constant switching from one formula to another, as it is very unsettling for infants.

All infants should start solids around 6 months of age.

Potentially allergenic foods (eggs, fish, nuts, soya and citrus fruits) should be introduced one by one during the first year of life to <u>reduce</u> the risk of food allergic reactions.

Gastro-oesophageal reflux or regurgitation of milk is very common (over 50 per cent of young infants) and is usually self-limiting.

Vomiting in early infancy is only significant if forceful (consider pyloric stenosis), associated with faltering growth, blood-stained (consider GORD), or bile-stained (consider small or large bowel obstruction).

Growth is an important measure of health and wellbeing in infants and children, and growth charts provide a visual representation of growth over time and are an indication of where a child's weight or length/height sits in relation to population norms for that age.

Faltering growth refers to a pattern of growth where there is slower weight gain than the expected rate for age and sex in infants and children.

If there are no signs (such as increased respiratory rate or cardiac murmur) or symptoms (such as vomiting or diarrhoea) in infants with faltering growth, then an organic cause or diagnosis is unlikely. Less than 5 per cent of cases have an organic cause.

Red flags for faltering growth include not returning to birth weight by 3 weeks, not feeding regularly from the breast or feeding frequently for long periods, not gaining appropriate weekly weight on two consecutive occasions, and any recurrent infections, recurrent vomiting or tachypnoea during feeds.

Infants and children with faltering growth should be followed up by the appropriate healthcare professionals to ensure resolution of problem.

Fussy or selective feeding is the rejection by the toddler or young child of a large proportion of familiar foods resulting in a diet with a very low variety of foods.

Distractions at mealtimes (including television), a poor routine, excessive intake of juices, a limited variety of foods, manipulative behaviour in the child, and parent anxiety can all contribute to food refusal.

In tackling food refusal, advise that the meal table should have a relaxed and positive environment free of family conflict, tensions and distractions.

Excessive intake of fluids (especially milk or juices) is probably the most common cause of food refusal.

Foods highlighted positively are more likely to be accepted by the child.

Box 5.2   **Vomiting in Early Infancy**

An 8-week-old infant presents with frequent vomits after almost all of her feeds. She is breast-fed on demand, and her mother describes her as a hungry infant. Her vomits are effortless and frequently stain her mother's clothes. Despite her frequent vomiting, she continues to gain weight, with her weight and length running along the 25th centile. Her vomit is white and never blood-stained or bile-stained. Her examination is unremarkable. Her parents are very concerned and seek professional advice.

Clinical Pearls

The most likely diagnosis is gastro-oesophageal reflux (GOR), a self-limiting condition affecting 50 per cent of infants that generally resolves by 12 months of age. A tiny minority may have gastro-oesophageal reflux disease (GORD) with symptoms of poor weight gain, unexplained crying, and symptoms of oesophagitis (excess crying, haematemesis, or melaena).

Thickening of the feeds or an alginate combination should be tried first. Detailed, repeated, and confident reassurance is required. Always look out for red flags (see above).

Placing premature infants in the left lateral position in the postprandial period can reduce GOR.

Avoid H2 antagonists and omeprazole unless food refusal, distressed behaviour or faltering growth

Interpretation of Investigations

Do **not** order a barium swallow to diagnose GOR.

Intraluminal oesophageal pH monitoring is the gold standard test to diagnose GORD but requires referral to a specialist paediatric gastroenterology service. A probe is inserted into the oesophagus to measure the frequency and duration of oesophageal acid exposure. Suspected oesophagitis is best confirmed by endoscopy with biopsy.

Pitfalls to Avoid

Red flag symptoms in terms of vomiting in early infancy include forceful or projectile vomits with associated faltering growth (consider pyloric stenosis), blood-stained vomits (consider GORD), or bile-stained vomits (consider small or large bowel obstruction).

Symptoms of pyloric stenosis include progressive non-bilious projectile vomiting, leading to dehydration and weight loss in an infant who is always hungry. The classical biochemical changes are of a hypokalemic, hypochloraemic metabolic alkalosis and occasional hypoglycaemia.

Intestinal malrotation has an incidence of about one in 500 births. Any infant or child with malrotation is at risk of midgut volvulus, which is a surgical emergency.

Up to 80 per cent of cases of malrotation present in the first month of life and in this age group the cardinal symptom is bilious vomiting.

Box 5.3   Infant With Faltering Growth

A 10-week-old female infant is bottle-fed from birth. Her birth weight was 3.0 kg, but her weight gain has been unsatisfactory, and she has gained just 600 g from birth. She is feeding well, taking six feeds of 180 mL of formula milk per day. She has no vomiting but does have over six loose bowel motions with an offensive smell per day. Her examination shows that she is not dysmorphic and that she has loose skin folds of the inner thighs. Her examination is otherwise normal, and she has been smiling for 4 weeks. Her family doctor and parents are very concerned, so she is referred for a specialist paediatric opinion.

Clinical Pearls

Faltering growth is not a disease per se, but rather a description of a relatively common growth pattern where weight gain is suboptimal.

The most likely causes of faltering growth are poor intake or undernutrition. The intake of milk is adequate for growing needs.

Organic causes of faltering growth are rare (5 per cent). If there are no symptoms or signs, then investigations are highly likely to be normal.

After establishing that intake is more than adequate, assess output (in terms of stool frequency, vomiting or polyuria), look for any dysmorphic features or developmental issues and explore family dynamics and social supports with sensitivity.

In this instance, the increased daily stool output with an offensive smell suggests malabsorption. Subsequent sweat test proved positive confirming a diagnosis of cystic fibrosis.

If faltering growth is confirmed, a dietitian will assess nutritional intake and compare to growth standards and calculated nutritional requirements. An increase in energy beyond the estimated average requirement (EAR) for age may be required. In the first instance, community-based management of faltering growth is advised.

Interpretation of Investigations:

If no symptoms (e.g. vomiting) or signs, then investigations are very likely to be normal. Therefore, embarking on a long list of investigations is futile. Let the symptom (in this instance, loose stools) steer the approach to investigation.

Pitfalls to Avoid:

Faltering growth may rarely be associated with neglect or maternal mental health issues, including addiction, and a period of time in hospital with appropriate social work input will be required to address safeguarding concerns.

Severe faltering growth in early infancy should arouse concern. Consider rare diagnoses such as Russell–Silver syndrome, severe combined immunodeficiency or diencephalic syndrome if little progress is being made despite dietetic intervention, hospitalisation and negative first line investigations.

Box 5.4   Food Refusal in a Toddler

A 20-month-old male toddler is causing great concern to his parents because they believe he is not eating enough, does not appear hungry for food and mealtimes are a constant struggle and source of conflict. It is a struggle to get him to eat even a small portion of a meal. He does like juices and milk and drinks up to 1.5 L of milk per day. His weight and height were both on the 50th centile for age but he did have intermittent constipation. His parents have unsuccessfully tried multiple strategies to get him to eat more and are now desperate for help.

Clinical Pearls

A toddler's appetite is affected by drinking too much juice or milk, grazing all day long and eating too many 'treats'. Common sense advice will clarify and hopefully resolve these issues.

Distractions at mealtimes, a poor routine, excessive intake of juices, a limited variety of foods, manipulative behaviour in the child and parent anxiety can all contribute to food refusal.

Limit milk and juice intake (if deemed excessive) to no more than 600 mL of milk or one to two small glasses of juice per day.

Advise the parents to make the meal table a relaxed and positive environment free of family conflict, tensions and distractions including television.

Avoid excessive parental pressure to eat, reduce mealtimes to 30 minutes and never punish a child for food refusal.

Role of Investigations

In general, no investigations are required if the child continues to thrive. If growth is faltering, consider coeliac disease and check coeliac serology.

Pitfalls to Avoid

Investigate if faltering growth. Eosinophilic oesophagitis is a chronic inflammatory disorder characterised by eosinophilic inflammation of the oesophagus, resulting in oesophageal dysfunction. Classical symptoms include dysphagia, food impaction, and food refusal. Diagnosis requires the presence of oesophageal eosinophilia (over 15 eosinophils per high-powered microscope field) on endoscopy. A trial of eliminating any suspected allergens from the diet is reasonable. Medical management may include swallowing puffs of corticosteroid from an asthma inhaler and the use of proton pump inhibitors.

 Video on the topic Failure to thrive is available online at Elsevier eBooks+.

Key References

Amir, L. H. (2014). Managing common breastfeeding problems in the community. *BMJ (Clinical Research Ed.)*, 348, g2954.

Bartleman, J. (2019). Infant and child nutrition. *Medicine*, 47(3), 195–198.

Drug and Therapeutics Bulletin. (2010). Managing gastro-oesophageal reflux in infants. *BMJ (Clinical Research Ed.)*, 341, c4420.

Kelly, V., Farrell, P., & Dunne, T. (2017). *Feed your child well: babies, toddlers and older children* (2nd ed.). O'Brien Press.

Feigelman, S., & Keane, V. (2018). Failure to thrive. In R. M. Kliegman, P. S. Lye, B. J. Bordini, H. Toth, & D. Basel (Eds.), *Nelson Pediatric Symptom-Based Diagnosis* (pp. 144–160). Elsevier.

Jyoti, B., & Saunders, R. (2015). *BMJ clinical review: paediatrics: study text.* BPP Learning Media.

Levene, I. R., & Williams, A. (2018). Fifteen-minute consultation: The healthy child: "my child is a fussy eater !". *Archives of Disease in Childhood, 103*(2), 71–78.

Shields, B., Wacogne, I., & Wright, C. M. (2012). Weight faltering and failure to thrive in infancy and early childhood. *BMJ, 345,* e5931.

Sicherer, S. H., Warren, C. M., Dant, C., Gupta, R. S., & Nadeau, K. C. (2020). Food allergy from infancy through adulthood. *The Journal of Allergy and Clinical Immunology in Practice, 8*(6), 1854–1864.

Online References

National Growth Charts Implementation Group. (2012, October). *Training programme for public health nurses and doctors in child health screening, surveillance and health promotion. Unit 6: Growth monitoring.* health service executive. https://www.hse.ie/eng/health/child/growthmonitoring/trainingmanual.pdf.

National Institute for Health and Care Excellence. (2017, September 27). *Faltering growth: Recognition and management of faltering growth in children.* NICE. www.nice.org.uk/guidance/ng75.

UNICEF. (2020). *The state of the world's children 2019 children, food and nutrition – growing well in a changing world.* (United Nations Publications, Ed.). UNICEF. https://www.unicef.org/reports/state-of-worlds-children-2019.

World Health Organization: Regional Office for Europe. (2016). *Growing up unequal: gender and socioeconomic differences in young people's health and well-being, Health Behaviour in School-aged Children (HBSC) study, international report from the 2013/2014 survey.* (J. Inchley, Ed.). https://www.euro.who.int/data/assets/pdf_file/0003/303438/HSBC-No.7-Growing-up-unequal-Full-Report.pdf.

6 Growth and Puberty

NIAMH MCGRATH, NUALA MURPHY and SUSAN O'CONNELL

Linear growth (height attainment) is an essential index of child wellbeing. A child's height should be measured accurately and plotted on a standardised growth chart at regular intervals. If there is a drop in the rate of growth (called the growth velocity), this needs a detailed evaluation.

Short stature is defined as a height two standard deviations below the mean for age and sex. Height follows a normal distribution curve, meaning that a small proportion of children (2 per cent) will naturally be two standard deviations both above and below the mean.

Growth failure is defined as a height velocity that is below the norm for that age. After 2 years of age, children tend to grow at a steady rate until their adolescent growth spurt.

Normal Growth

Prenatal linear growth is near zero to 50 cm in just 9 months. Infants born small for dates (under 2.5 kg) do show catch up in growth, but 10 to 20 per cent remain shorter than expected beyond infancy.

Linear growth is relatively rapid in infancy and is highly influenced by nutrition. The average growth velocity is 25 cm in the first year of life and 12 cm in the second. Thereafter, growth velocity typically proceeds along the same percentile (with a growth velocity of 5 to 6 cm/year) until the onset of the pubertal growth spurt.

Girls typically experience their pubertal growth spurt earlier than boys. However, their final adult height is typically 13 cm less than an adult male.

Measuring Children

As highlighted in Chapter 5, height is measured as supine length until 2 years of age and standing height thereafter.

Other parameters assessed include the upper to lower segment ratio (by measuring both standing and sitting heights) and the arm span.

FAMILIAL FACTORS

Parental heights and growth patterns are key influencers of growth patterns in their children. The mid-parental height (MPH) is a key measure of a child's genetic height potential and is important to calculate. The average adult male is 13 cm taller than the average adult female. To calculate the mid-parental height (MPH of a girl, add the (mother's height in cm) to the (father's height less 13 cm) and divide the result by two. Similarly, when calculating the MPH of a boy, add the (father's height) to the (mother's height plus 13 cm) and divide the result by two. The predicted adult height of the child should be plus or minus 8.5 cm around the mid-parental height.

ENDOCRINE REGULATION OF GROWTH

The anterior pituitary gland releases growth hormone (GH) in brief pulses with peak secretion in sleep. Therefore, random GH measurements are often misleading and are not useful in assessing potential GH deficiency. Insulin-like growth factor 1 (IGF-1) mediates the growth-promoting effect of GH, and IGF-1 levels are stable throughout the day. IGF can be measured as a surrogate measure of GH secretion. The gold standard for diagnosing growth hormone deficiency is growth hormone stimulation by means of an insulin tolerance test. Hypoglycaemia is induced with insulin, and serial growth hormone levels are measured. This is a hazardous test which should only be done in a specialised centre.

Growth hormone requires a normal thyroxine level to exert its full effect. Thyroxine itself also acts directly on the epiphyseal growth plate. High glucocorticoid levels are powerful inhibitors of growth. Thus, both hypothyroidism and the much rarer Cushing's syndrome are important, and treatable endocrine causes of short stature.

Sex steroids help mediate the pubertal growth spurt. Follicle stimulating hormone (FSH) is responsible for testicular or ovarian enlargement. In girls the ovarian granulosa cells produce oestradiol. Testicular Leydig cells produce testosterone in response to luteinising hormone (LH).

BONE AGE

Maturation of the wrist bones follows a very predictable pattern during growth and an X ray of the non-dominant hand is used to assess bone age. Bone age assessment is very helpful in constitutional delay in growth and puberty (CDGP) where it will be delayed and in precocious puberty, where it may be advanced.

Familial short stature and CDGP should be viewed as normal variants, and both should be easy to recognise. Neither require extensive investigations (apart from bone age X-ray) and together they account for the great majority of short children seen.

Normal Pubertal Development

Release of the gonadotrophin-releasing hormone from the hypothalamus stimulates both LH and FSH production in the anterior pituitary. Both LH and FSH are required for oestrogen production in girls, while FSH stimulates spermatogenesis and LH activates Leydig cells to produce testosterone in boys.

GIRLS

Girls begin puberty at an average of 10.5 years (range 8 to 13 years) with the first sign being breast development which may be asymmetrical. Within the next 6 months, pubic hair usually develops. The adolescent growth spurt in girls commences with the onset of breast development and lasts 2 years. By the time of first period (menarche), a girl will have reached over 95 per cent of her adult height potential.

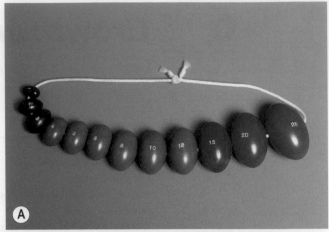

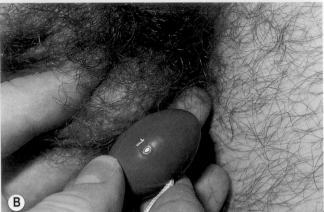

Figure 6.1 Prader orchidometer. (A) Testicular volume (in mL) may be estimated by comparison with calibrated ellipsoids. (B) Gently grip the testis in one hand and compare its volume (including the scrotal skin but excluding the epididymis) with that of the ellipsoids. The patient shown has a reduced testicular volume of 8 mL due to Klinefelter's syndrome; the normal secondary sexual hair is due to the provision of exogenous testosterone. (Reproduced with permission from Glynn, M., & Drake, W. M. (Eds.), (2017). *Hutchison's Clinical methods: An integrated approach to clinical practice* (24th ed., pp. 379–402). Elsevier.)

BOYS

Boys start puberty at an average of 11.5 years (range 9 to 14 years) with the first clinically detectable sign of puberty being testicular enlargement. Testicular volume before puberty, as measured by an orchidometer (Fig. 6.1), ranges between 1 and 2 mL. The onset of puberty in boys is signalled when at least one of the two testes has reached 4 mL in volume. It may take 5 years before the adult volume of 18 mL is reached in both testes.

Pubic hair usually develops within 6 months following testicular enlargement. Axillary hair follows the appearance of pubic hair. Penile enlargement also occurs with a prepubertal average of 3.5 cm and an adult average of 12.5 cm.

The adolescent growth spurt in boys starts later than girls when testicular volumes reach approximately 12 mL and usually occurs between 13 and 15 years of age. By the age of 15 years, a boy has attained over 95 per cent of his final adult height.

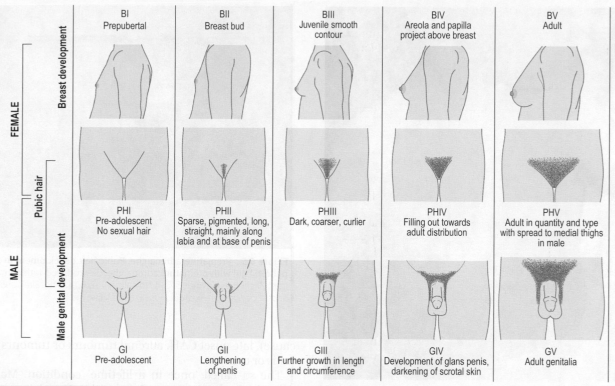

Figure 6.2 Stages of puberty in males and females. Pubertal changes according to the Tanner stages of puberty. (Reproduced with permission from Innes, J. A., Dover, R. A., & Fairhurst, K. (Eds.), (2017). *Macleod's clinical examination* (14th ed., pp. 297–318). Elsevier.)

CLINICAL STAGING OF PUBERTY

Breast development in girls, genitalia in boys and pubic hair in both are scored according to Tanner staging one to five. The chart below gives a sense of pubertal development in boys and girls and highlights the wide ranges of normal (Fig. 6.2).

Familial patterns affect the timing of puberty, including age of menarche in the mother, age at which both parents stopped growing, and age at which the father started shaving.

Early or precocious puberty is defined as occurring before 8 years of age in girls and before 9 years of age in boys (Fig. 6.3).

IDIOPATHIC PREMATURE THELARCHE

Despite generating alarm for parents, the development of breast tissue in girls at age 2 to 3 years is a common finding. Breast development is often asymmetrical (Fig. 6.4). Premature thelarche is not associated with other signs of puberty such as pubic hair, growth spurt or menarche. The bone age will not be advanced. Parents can simply be reassured, and investigations are not usually required. If performed, investigations will tend to show low FSH and LH levels and undetectable oestradiol levels. A pelvic ultrasound will show prepubertal ovaries and often multiple follicular cysts.

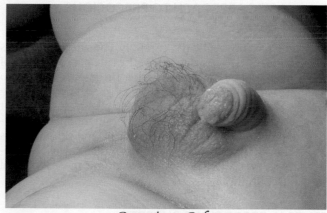

Precocious Puberty
scrotal hair in a 10 month old

Figure 6.3 Precocious puberty in a boy.

IDIOPATHIC PRECOCIOUS ADRENARCHE

In this normal variant, there is early development of pubic hair, axillary hair and body odour resulting from the premature production of adrenal androgens (Fig. 6.5). This variant is far more common in girls. Blood investigation shows elevated dehydroepiandrosterone (DHEAS) levels and a normal 17 hydroxyprogesterone level thereby excluding congenital adrenal hyperplasia (CAH).

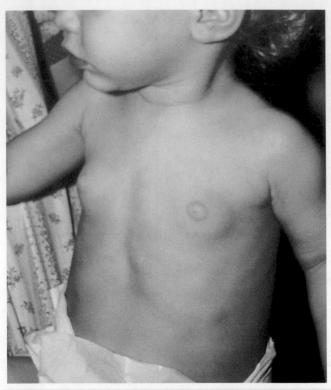

Figure 6.4 Premature thelarche. Isolated bilateral breast enlargement in a toddler with premature thelarche. (Reproduced with permission from Zitelli, B. J., McIntire, S. C., & Nowalk, A. J. (Eds.), (2018). *Zitelli and Davis' atlas of pediatric physical diagnosis* (7th ed.). Elsevier.)

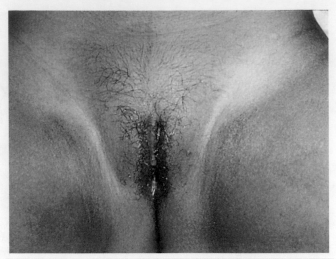

Figure 6.5 Premature adrenarche. Pubic hair development in a prepubertal girl with premature adrenarche. (Reproduced with permission from Zitelli, B. J., McIntire, S. C., & Nowalk, A. J. (Eds.), (2018). *Zitelli and Davis' atlas of pediatric physical diagnosis* (7th ed.). Elsevier.)

DIAGNOSTIC APPROACH TO PRECOCIOUS PUBERTY

First and foremost, always carefully consider precocious puberty in a boy. Try to determine the rate of progression of pubertal changes and assess whether the process is likely to originate centrally or peripherally.

Take a detailed history and family history and conduct a detailed examination looking for staging of puberty, centiles including any recent growth spurt, and skin changes of relevance (either café au lait spots indicative of Neurofibromatosis Type 1 (NF1), or 'coast of Maine' more typical of Mc Cune Albright).

CENTRAL PRECOCIOUS PUBERTY

This results from an early activation of the hypothalamic-pituitary-gonadal axis, with girls being far more likely to have central precocious puberty than boys. There are many causes of central precocious puberty including idiopathic (most common), NF 1 with optic glioma, hypothalamic hamartoma, head trauma, hydrocephalus and cranial irradiation. Investigations show a marked LH rise after LHRH stimulation in central precocious puberty.

PITUITARY GONADOTROPHIN-INDEPENDENT PRECOCIOUS PUBERTY

This is due to excessive production of androgens or oestrogens and includes precocious adrenarche (most frequent cause), late onset CAH, adrenal tumours or tumours in the testis or ovary.

The so–called 'once in a lifetime' condition, Mc Cune Albright syndrome, is associated with café au lait spots with irregular borders, precocious puberty (gonadotrophin-independent) and polyostotic fibrous dysplasia.

The main difference between central and gonadotrophin-independent precocious puberty is that there is a copious release of LH after a single dose of LHRH in central precocious puberty. On the other hand, there is no such response in gonadotrophin-independent precocious puberty – LH and FSH are suppressed, and oestradiol levels are elevated.

CONGENITAL ADRENAL HYPERPLASIA (CAH)

CAH is caused by an enzymatic defect in the biosynthesis of cortisol, most commonly 21-hydroxylase deficiency, and sometimes 11-hydroxylase deficiency. There is an overproduction of adrenal androgen precursors which causes ambiguous genitalia in affected females (Fig. 6.6).

Due to 21-hydroxylase deficiency, CAH occurs in one in 5,000 births. Affected females have ambiguous genitalia at birth. Presentation in the salt-losing form in females or males is with lethargy, vomiting and poor feeding. Clinical findings of the salt-losing form include dehydration, hypotension and hypoglycaemia. Blood investigations show hyponatraemia, hyperkalemia and an elevated plasma renin due to mineralocorticoid deficiency. An elevated 17-hydroxyprogesterone level is diagnostic.

CAH is treated with daily glucocorticoid (hydrocortisone) to replace cortisol which will reduce ACTH secretion and reverse the androgen excess. Daily mineralocorticoid (fludrocortisone) is also needed to replace aldosterone to retain salt and eradicate excess potassium. Adequate salt intake is essential, and salt supplements may be required for infants.

A referral to a paediatric endocrinology team is indicated with a multidisciplinary approach and later surgical correction of the external genitalia.

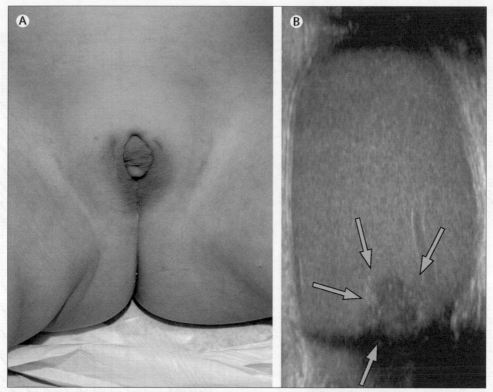

Figure 6.6 Adverse outcomes in congenital adrenal hyperplasia. (A) Atypical genitalia with clitoromegaly and posterior labial fusion of a 46,XX infant with 21-hydroxylase deficiency. (B) A right sided, lobulated echogenic focus, measuring 2.7 × 1.0× 1.1 cm, consistent with testicular adrenal rest tissue. (Reproduced with permission from El-Maouche, D., Arlt, W., & Merke, D. P. (2017). Congenital adrenal hyperplasia. *Lancet, 390*(10108), 2194–2210.)

Treatment of CAH is lifelong. At any time of stress (infections or operations, for example), increased glucocorticoids are vital and mineralocorticoids continued to prevent an adrenal crisis. Parents should be given written instructions on how to increase and then taper their dosages and, if possible, have 24-hour emergency access for telephone advice.

AMBIGUOUS GENITALIA

Children born with ambiguous genitalia may be divided into three distinct groups. These are the virilised female (no palpable gonads), the undervirilised male (who will usually have two gonads of equal size located in the scrotum, groin or labial folds), and the child with abnormal gonadal differentiation (who tend to have a single palpable gonad or asymmetrical gonads). When an infant is born with ambiguous genitalia, it is best to tell the parents that the baby's sex is uncertain and that naming of the infant should be deferred.

The most common cause of ambiguous genitalia in clinical practice is congenital adrenal hyperplasia (CAH), which causes virilisation of a chromosomal female infant (46XX) with normal reproductive organs.

Gonads are usually palpable in the undervirilised male. The major causes are inborn errors of testosterone biosynthesis, abnormal peripheral androgen activity due to 5-apha-reductase deficiency, androgen insensitivity and hypopituitariam. Complete androgen insensitivity syndrome results in female external genitalia and is the most common cause of an undervirilised male. These children are usually undiagnosed until adolescence when they fail to enter puberty or establish menses.

The two causes of abnormal gonadal differentiation are true hermaphroditism and mixed gonadal dysgenesis. True hermaphrodites have both mature testicular tissue and ovarian tissue with follicles. Mixed gonadal dysgenesis usually results from 46,XX/45XO mosaicism and often phenotypic features of Turner syndrome are seen.

Delayed Puberty

The definition of delayed puberty is the failure of development of any pubertal changes by 13 years of age in girls and 14 years of age in boys.

CONSTITUTIONAL DELAY OF GROWTH AND PUBERTY (CDGP)

CDGP is in essence a normal variant and is by far the most common cause of delayed puberty (Fig. 6.7). Always enquire about the age of menarche in the mother and any history of delayed puberty or delayed growth spurt in the father. A relevant question to ask is how tall they were compared to their classmates when entering secondary school. Height is often at or below the 3rd centile for age. The key investigation is the bone age x-ray which is moderately delayed in comparison to the child's chronological age.

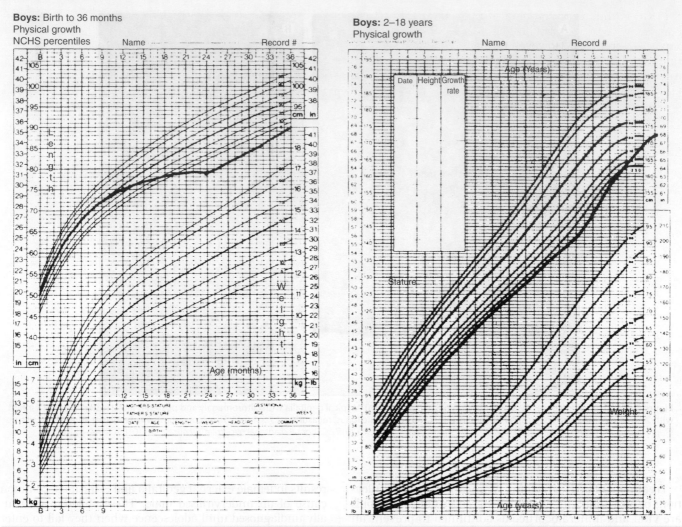

Figure 6.7 Growth charts for a patient with constitutional delay of growth. Subnormal velocity during the second year of life (left chart) followed by normal velocity through childhood and a prolonged growth period with eventual achievement of normal adult height (right chart). (Reproduced with permission from McDermott, M. T. (Ed.), (2020). *Endocrine secrets* (7th ed.). Elsevier – Health Sciences Division.)

HYPOGONADOTROPHIC HYPOGONADISM

This may relate to chronic illness, malnutrition (coeliac disease or Crohns), excessive physical activity or stress, mass lesions such as craniopharyngioma, or the ultrarare Kallmann syndrome (loss of sense of smell with gonadotrophin deficiency). LH and FSH levels will be low.

HYPERGONADOTROPIC HYPOGONADISM

Causes in boys include Klinefelter syndrome (47,XXY) with small, firm testes, pronounced gynaecomastia and frequently coordination difficulties.

The main cause in girls in Turner syndrome with elevated LH and FSH levels, short stature and ovarian insufficiency.

Evaluating a Child With Short Stature

The crucial finding of concern is a slowing in growth velocity. A bone age is a very helpful investigation, and a karyotype is a mandatory investigation in any female with significantly short stature.

True GH deficiency is rare. Characteristic features include a higher weight centile compared to height, a typical abnormal face described as being similar to a doll or cherub, delayed dentition, a high-pitched voice and decreased muscle mass.

FAMILIAL SHORT STATURE

Typically, one or both parents are 1.5 to 2 standard deviations (SD) below the mean in height, and the child has a normal growth velocity. The bone age will be as expected. This is very commonly seen.

CONSTITUTIONAL DELAY OF GROWTH AND PUBERTY (CDGP)

CDGP occurs in both sexes but is more common in boys who are noted to have both delayed puberty and a delayed bone age. These children may have a history of moderate short stature during early to middle childhood but are otherwise healthy. There is often a history of a delayed growth spurt in adolescence in either parent, but typically in the father.

CDGP is thus very common in males and, apart from bone age assessment, no investigations are required until at least 14 years of age. However, the patient must be followed until they enter puberty as hypogonadotrophic hypogonadism may present in a similar manner. Delayed puberty in girls is much less common and often has an organic cause and therefore requires investigation.

SMALL FOR GESTATIONAL AGE

Children who were born small for gestational age with subsequent poor growth in the postnatal period tend to have lower than average values of IGF-1, indicating some degree of GH resistance. Up to 10 to 20 per cent of these children fail to show catch-up growth, thus prompting the consideration of biosynthetic GH therapy for this group.

GROWTH HORMONE (GH) DEFICIENCY

Congenital GH deficiency is associated with midline craniofacial defects such as cleft palate, single central incisor, septo-optic dysplasia and holoprosencephaly. Affected newborns usually have other pituitary hormone deficiencies (hypopituitarism) and an increased incidence of hypoglycaemia. Males may have a micropenis. Associated secondary hypothyroidism (with normal or low TSH) may be missed on Guthrie card testing and can lead to hypothermia, poor growth and prolonged jaundice.

Most cases of isolated GH deficiency are idiopathic. GH deficiency may also be secondary to other conditions such head injury, cranial irradiation in oncology cases and midline tumours such as craniopharyngioma.

In idiopathic GH deficiency in childhood, poor linear growth may be evident by 3 years of age.

Bone age is classically delayed in idiopathic GH deficiency. Most will have an IGF-I level low for their age. To diagnose GH deficiency a GH stimulation test should be performed. The gold standard stimulation test is an Insulin Tolerance Test (ITT). This should only be performed in a regional endocrine centre with expertise in testing and in children over 4 years of age with no history of seizures. Glucagon, arginine, L-dopa and clonidine can also be used to stimulate GH release. A peak growth hormone of less than 7 µg/L is compatible with a diagnosis of growth hormone deficiency. All children with GH deficiency should have an MRI scan of the brain and pituitary to rule out intracranial pathology before starting GH therapy. Growth hormone treatment involves a daily subcutaneous injection and side effects are rare but include benign intracranial hypertension, slipped upper femoral epiphysis (SUFE) and insulin resistance.

GLUCOCORTICOID EXCESS

Cushing syndrome results from excessive levels of glucocorticosteroids. Physical findings include acne, virilisation, short stature, plethoric facies, hypertension, a buffalo hump and large purple striae. Diagnosis is based on a high free cortisol on a 24-hour sample (never an easy task) or an overnight dexamethasone suppression test. Give dexamethasone at 23.00 hours and measure the cortisol level the following morning. It should be normally

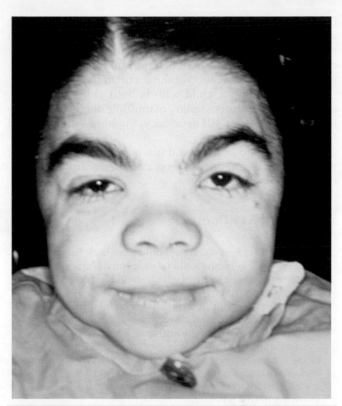

Figure 6.8 Congenital hypothyroidism (Reproduced with permission from Little, J., & Miller, C. (Eds.), (2018). *Little and Falace's dental management of the medically compromised patient* (9th ed.). Mosby.)

less than 5 ng/mL). Further investigations include measurement of adrenocorticotropic hormone (ACTH).

HYPOTHYROIDISM

Hypothyroidism is congenital (Fig. 6.8) or acquired. Newborn screening for congenital hypothyroidism (heelprick TSH levels) is performed in most countries and helps to diagnose hypothyroidism early, thus preventing neurodisability by early treatment.

Acquired hypothyroidism is usually due to autoimmune thyroiditis with an increased prevalence in children with Down syndrome, diabetes mellitus, coeliac disease, and Turner syndrome. Acquired hypothyroidism tends to present in older children and adolescents. The most common presentation is with a falloff in height gain. Other features include a goitre and relative obesity. The bone age is often significantly delayed. Blood tests in acquired hypothyroidism show an elevated thyroid stimulating hormone (TSH) and a low or normal thyroxine (T_4) level. Positive thyroperoxidase and thyroglobulin antibodies are seen in autoimmune thyroiditis. Treatment is with L-thyroxine.

EASILY MISSED

All prepubertal girls with significantly short stature should have a karyotype to rule out Turner syndrome. In Turner syndrome, the absence of one copy of the Short Stature Homeobox gene (SHOX) is believed to play a significant role. Turner syndrome is relatively common (one in 2500) and is caused by absence or abnormality of an X chromosome.

Diagnosis is frequently delayed. In addition to short stature and ovarian failure, other features include lymphoedema in newborns and a low posterior hairline, webbed neck, wide carrying angles of the arms and renal and cardiac abnormalities (especially coarctation of the aorta) in older children.

When assessing a child who is both short and obese, always consider the possibility of multiple diagnoses including hypothyroidism, GH deficiency, Cushing syndrome and Prader-Willi syndrome.

In a child who is short and has symptoms of headache, vomiting, or visual disturbance, consider craniopharyngioma as a possible diagnosis.

GH THERAPY

There are specific licensed indications for using GH therapy which include GH deficiency, Turner and Noonan syndrome, Prader-Willi syndrome, SHOX mutation, SGA children with failure to catch up by 4 years of age, and pre-transplantation chronic renal failure.

(Box 6.1)
(Box 6.2)
(Box 6.3)
(Box 6.4)
(Box 6.5)

Box 6.1   Key Points

After 2 years of age, children should have their height assessed while standing without shoes on a Harpenden stadiometer, the progress of which should be recorded on a standard growth chart.

Apart from measuring height, it is helpful to assess the upper to lower segment ratio (by measuring both standing and sitting heights) and the arm span.

Short stature is defined as height two standard deviations below the mean for age and sex. Growth velocity is a primary variable in your assessment of the short child.

Calculation of the mid-parental height is important in assessing height potential.

A bone age is a very helpful investigation, and a karyotype is mandatory in any female with significant short stature.

Girls begin puberty at an average of 10.5 years (range 8 to 13 years) with the first sign being breast development (which may be asymmetrical).

Boys begin puberty at an average of 11.5 years (range 9 to 14 years). The first clinically detectable sign of puberty is testicular enlargement.

Central precocious puberty is confirmed by a marked LH rise after LHRH stimulation.

For congenital adrenal hyperplasia, treatment is lifelong and parents must have clear instructions to increase glucocorticoids at times of stress such as acute illness or surgery.

CDGP is by far the most common cause of delayed puberty and should be considered a normal variant.

Delayed puberty in girls is much less common than boys and often has an organic cause, therefore requiring investigation.

There are several licensed indications for the use of GH therapy, including GH deficiency, Turner and Noonan syndrome, Prader-Willi syndrome, SHOX mutation, SGA children who fail to catch up by 4 years of age and pre-transplantation chronic renal failure.

Box 6.2   A Short 9-Year-Old Girl

A 9-year-old girl is brought to you by her parents, who are concerned that she is the shortest in her school class. She was born at term with a birth weight of 2.3 kg. Both parents are of above average height and there is no family history of short stature. She has a normal appetite and her physical examination is normal, apart from neck webbing. She is prepubertal (Tanner Stage 1) and her full neurological examination is normal, including visual field assessment. Her height is on the 2nd centile and her weight is on the 10th centile for age.

Clinical Pearls

Accurate height measurement using a Harpenden stadiometer is key, as is calculation of the mid-parental height, with adjustments made for a girl.

Determining height velocity requires two accurate height measurements at least 6 months apart with the normal height velocity in childhood being 5 cm/year.

Those with familial short stature all have normal growth velocity.

In this instance, the young girl is strikingly short, and you do not see any other dysmorphic features.

Calculating upper to lower body segment ratios can help spot skeletal dysplasia with disproportionate limb shortening.

Girls begin puberty at an average of 10.5 years (range 8 to 13 years) with the first sign being breast development. Pubic hair begins to develop within the next 6 months. The adolescent growth spurt in females commences with the onset of breast development and spans 2 years.

Interpretation of Investigations

X-ray of the left wrist determines her bone age. Delayed bone age and a decreased growth velocity should prompt further investigation.

Measurement of IGF-1 and IGFBP-3 can be useful screening tests for growth hormone (GH) deficiency and may help to determine whether GH provocation tests are required.

Insulin tolerance test (ITT) is the gold standard GH stimulation test in children over 4 years of age. Glucagon, arginine, L-dopa and clonidine are also used. If the peak level of GH is below 7 µg/L, then the child is considered GH deficient.

The most common presentation of acquired hypothyroidism coincides with a falloff in height gain; thyroid function tests should be performed in this case. Coeliac serology should also be performed.

Pitfalls to Avoid

Short stature may be the only manifestation in some girls with Turner syndrome, especially in those with chromosomal mosaicism. A karyotype is recommended in any girl with short stature of unknown origin and confirmed Turner syndrome in this instance.

Be aware that inflammatory bowel disease (especially Crohn disease) and coeliac disease can also lead to short stature.

Hypochondroplasia is an allelic variant of achondroplasia that may manifest as short stature with less striking dysmorphic features and quite subtle body disproportion. Features of hypochondroplasia include relatively short limbs, brachydactyly of the hands and feet, and genu varum. Again, a diagnosis that easily can be missed.

Box 6.3   A Short 15-Year-Old Boy With Pubertal Delay

A 15-year-old boy is far shorter than his peers and is very self-conscious that his voice has not broken, and he has very few signs of pubertal development. He has no history of headaches or visual symptoms. His bowel habit is normal, and he has an excellent appetite. Both his father and uncle had delayed pubertal development. He has no dysmorphic features, and his weight and height are both on the 2nd centile for age. His bone age is 3 years behind his chronological age.

Clinical Pearls

Ninety to 95 per cent of delayed puberty cases in boys are due to constitutional delay in growth and puberty (CDGP), often causing diagnosis is always the hot favourite. Characteristically, the bone age is delayed. Sexual maturity and final adult height are all achieved in CDGP, but a significant delay is quite distressing for all.

Hypogonadotrophic hypogonadism with characteristically low levels of luteinising hormone (LH) and follicle stimulating hormone (FSH) may relate to chronic illness, malnutrition (coeliac disease or Crohns), excessive physical activity or stress, mass lesions such as craniopharyngioma, or the ultrarare Kallmann syndrome (loss of sense of smell with gonadotrophin deficiency). Watchful waiting is often the best approach.

Interpretation of Investigations

In the great majority, the only investigation required is a bone age x-ray to demonstrate a delayed bone age.

Routine biochemistry should include thyroid function tests and coeliac screen, LH, FSH and testosterone. GnRH or LH-releasing hormone tests stimulate the release of FSH and LH. Elevated LH and FSH supports a diagnosis of primary gonadal failure.

Potential Pitfalls to Avoid

Screen for chronic illness such as malabsorption if suggestive symptoms occur. If visual symptoms with visual field loss or frequent headaches are present, consider craniopharyngioma and perform an MRI brain scan.

Delayed puberty in girls is much less common than in boys and often has an organic cause, therefore warranting investigation.

Look for features of Turners or Klinefelter syndromes if LH and FSH levels are high.

Turner syndrome is associated with short stature and ovarian insufficiency.

Klinefelter syndrome (47,XXY) is associated with small, firm testes, pronounced gynaecomastia and frequently coordination difficulties.

Box 6.4   A 7-Year-Old Girl With Early Pubic Hair Development

An otherwise healthy 7-year-old girl presents with early pubic hair development. She developed breast buds 6 months prior which caused minor discomfort. She was noted to be quite tall compared to her peers, and her parents noted a recent height surge. She was otherwise perfectly healthy, but her parents were very concerned and sought professional advice.

Clinical Pearls

Girls begin puberty at an average of 10.5 years (range 8 to 13 years). Breast development is the first sign and may be unilateral in the early stages. Pubic hair development usually follows breast development within 6 months but may occasionally predate it. There is an association between early sexual maturation and obesity.

Pubic hair development occurs in Tanner stage 2 in girls, and a few strands of coarse pigmented hair are visible. This should not be confused with lighter peach-coloured lanugo hair or the extension of hypertrichosis to the pubic area.

There are many causes of central precocious puberty, including idiopathic (as in this case), neurofibromatosis type 1 with optic glioma, hypothalamic hamartoma, head trauma, hydrocephalus and cranial irradiation. Secondary sexual characteristics develop in a concordant manner with the development of breast buds followed by pubic hair development and then menarche. Central precocious puberty is five to 10 times more common in girls than boys. Rates of progression of puberty may vary.

Peripheral precocious puberty is independent of activation of the hypothalamic-pituitary gonadal axis and FSH and LH levels are low. It is caused by excessive oestrogens in girls and may result in pubic and axillary hair prior to breast development.

In the initial evaluation of precocious puberty, it is necessary to establish whether it is a normal variant (e.g. breast

development in an 8-year-old), to determine the rate of progression of pubertal changes, and to establish whether it is central or peripheral in type.

Interpretation of Investigations

The first investigation is a bone age x-ray. You are most likely dealing with a normal variant if the bone age is not advanced. However, if the bone age is significantly advanced, a detailed work up is required.

If investigations are required in premature thelarche, LH and FSH levels are low and oestradiol is undetectable with an abdominal ultrasound showing prepubertal ovaries with many follicular cysts.

Premature adrenarche is characterised by the early development of pubic hair, axillary hair facial spots and adult body odour. It results from the early production of adrenal androgens and is far more common in girls. Blood investigation shows elevated dehydroepiandrosterone (DHEAS) levels and a normal 17 hydroxyprogesterone level.

Central precocious puberty is confirmed by a marked LH rise after LHRH stimulation. There is no such response in gonadotrophin-independent precocious puberty.

Potential Pitfalls to Avoid

An underlying cause of precocious puberty is far more likely in boys and investigation is mandatory. Neuroimaging may be required to exclude CNS tumours such as a hypothalamic hamartoma. A history of hydrocephalus or prior meningitis may be relevant.

Late onset CAH, adrenal tumours (or tumours in the testis or ovary) and Mc Cune Albright syndrome are all rare considerations in peripheral precocious puberty.

Box 6.5   An Acutely Ill Child With a Background History of Congenital Adrenal Hyperplasia

A 2-year-old child was referred to the emergency department with an acute viral illness with low-grade fever and vomiting. She had vomited all her routine medications that morning. She had a background diagnosis of congenital adrenal hyperplasia which had been diagnosed in the newborn period and was on maintenance therapy with regular outpatient follow up. She looked very pale on arrival with an elevated heart rate of 160 per minute and delayed capillary refill over 3 seconds. Her blood glucose was 3.0 mmol/L, and she was admitted for observation and further investigation.

Clinical Pearls:

Over 95 per cent of congenital adrenal hyperplasia (CAH) cases are due to 21 hydroxylase (OH) deficiency. This enzyme deficiency causes decreased levels of cortisol and aldosterone, and an excess of androgens.

Clinically, infants and children with 11βOH deficiency also show signs of androgen excess but have hypertension rather than salt loss.

Children with CAH should be treated with lifelong hydrocortisone given in divided doses. In salt-wasting forms of CAH, fludrocortisone is given daily to achieve a plasma renin activity in the mid-normal range. Encourage salt intake during hot weather and conditions consider seasonal adjustment of fludrocortisone dose in countries with very hot summers (for instance, the Middle East).

When oral intake is not possible (e.g. in vomiting children, such as this case), then hydrocortisone should be given by another route (intramuscular, subcutaneous or intravenous). Stress dose management with increased hydrocortisone is identical to that recommended in primary adrenal insufficiency.

One-stage surgery done in infancy for virilised females involving clitoroplasty, labioplasty and vaginoplasty is an option adopted in some countries. Surgery is more recently delayed until puberty.

Gender dysphoria is extremely rare and thus the recommended sex assignment of 46,XX infants with CAH and virilisation is female.

Children with CAH should wear an emergency bracelet, receive sick day rule education and carry an emergency hydrocortisone kit.

Bone mineral density screening should commence during early adulthood.

Interpretation of Investigations:

A 17OHP concentration above 30 nmol/L is diagnostic for 21OH deficiency. The classical biochemical features of acute adrenal crisis are hyponatraemia, hyperkalaemia and hypoglycaemia.

In X-linked adrenoleukodystrophy, an elevated level of hexacosanoic acid (a very long chain fatty acid (VLCFA)) is found.

Pitfalls to Avoid:

There is an excess mortality in infants and children with congenital adrenal hyperplasia due to adrenal crises.

Therefore, a response to acute illness in children with CAH is of paramount importance. Instruct parents and caregivers to double or triple glucocorticoid dose during intercurrent illness (acute gastroenteritis in this case), surgery or trauma, and give parenteral hydrocortisone if unable to tolerate orally.

All children with CAH who are receiving glucocorticoid therapy are at risk of growth impairment and short stature and so always aim to treat children with the lowest possible effective dose of glucocorticoids.

Over 50 per cent of girls in the UK with classic 21OH deficiency have obesity, with a third having insulin resistance; prevention of obesity is therefore vital. Long-term glucocorticoid therapy, particularly at the higher doses used to achieve tight control, is a risk factor for compromised bone health.

X-linked adrenoleukodystrophy (XLA) should be considered as a differential diagnosis for Addison's disease in young males, even if neurological symptoms are not obvious at initial examination.

XLA is characterised by intracellular accumulation of very long chain fatty acids (VLCFA). Phenotypes range from a severe progressive cerebral form in boys and Addison's disease may occur independent of a neurological presentation.

 Videos on the topic Growth & puberty and the assessment of short stature are available online at Elsevier eBooks+.

Key references

Ali, O. (2017). Short stature. In R. M. Kliegman, P. S. Lye, B. J. Bordini, H. Toth, & D. Basel (Eds.), *Nelson pediatric symptom-based diagnosis* (pp. 791–810). Elsevier – Health Sciences Division.

El-Maouche, D., Arlt, W., & Merke, D. P. (2017). Congenital adrenal hyperplasia. *Lancet, 390*(10108), 2194–2210 [published correction appears in *Lancet.* 2017;390(10108):2142].

Klein, D. A., Emerick, J. E., Sylvester, J. E., & Vogt, K. S. (2017). Disorders of puberty: An approach to diagnosis and management. *American Family Physician, 96*(9), 590–599.

Palmert, M. R., & Dunkel, L. (2012). Clinical practice. Delayed puberty. *The New England Journal of Medicine, 366*(5), 443–453.

Preedy, V. R. (Ed.), (2011). *Handbook of growth and growth monitoring in health and disease.* Springer.

Saengkaew, T., & Howard, S. R. (2020). Next-generation sequencing approach to the diagnosis of delayed puberty. *Current Opinion in Endocrine and Metabolic Research, 14*, 59–64.

Wolfgram, P. M. (2018). Disorders of puberty. In R. M. Kliegman, P. S. Lye, B. J. Bordini, H. Toth & D. Basel (Eds.), *Nelson Pediatric symptom-based diagnosis* (pp. 774–790). Elsevier.

World Health Organization. (n.d.). Child growth standards. https://www.who.int/childgrowth/standards/en/.

7 Understanding Childhood and Adolescent Obesity

SINEAD MURPHY

Historically, a well-nourished child meant a healthy child, but in the past three decades, childhood overweight and obesity have become the pressing primary paediatric health issue in most developed countries. Obesity has its origins from the outset. A longitudinal *Growing up in Ireland* study evaluated body mass index (BMI) at different ages (9 months, 3 years, and 5 years) and found that differences at birth and in infancy were strongly associated with BMI at all ages. Therefore, public health interventions should target pregnant women and families of young children to encourage healthy eating and thereby avoid excess weight gain in infancy. Factors such as ethnicity, weight status of the mother, socioeconomic status and whether breast-fed or not all had independent effects on weight status. Breast-feeding and adequate sleeping hours are beneficial in the prevention of obesity and overweight in early childhood. Recent advances in genetics have shown that genetic factors are of far greater importance than previously thought.

International Epidemic of Childhood Obesity

Childhood obesity is a global pandemic and is one of the most serious public health challenges of the twenty-first century. The problem not only affects high-income countries but is now steadily affecting many low and middle-income countries, particularly in cities. The prevalence of obesity worldwide has increased at an alarming rate – it is estimated that, by 2030, there will be 254 million people aged 5 to 19 years with obesity. Rises in obesity and overweight in children are starting to plateau in high income countries (especially in northern Europe) but they are accelerating in Asia and Africa in line with marketing of unhealthy food, reduced physical activity and increased urbanisation. In 2018, roughly three quarters of overweight children under 5 years of age lived in Asia and Africa. Almost a third of young people aged 5 to 19 years in the UK are overweight or obese, and the now retired Chief Medical Officer for England Dame Sally Davies has stated that 'children are drowning in a flood of unhealthy food and drink options'.

The WHO European Childhood Obesity Surveillance Initiative (COSI) has measured trends in in overweight and obesity in school aged children across the WHO European region for more than 10 years (Fig. 7.1). The prevalence of severe obesity is variable between included countries but is highest in Southern Europe with almost 50 per cent of Greek school children defined as overweight or obese.

Prevention of Obesity in Childhood

Prevention of childhood obesity and its comorbidities is of critical importance and will only occur if there are fundamental societal changes involving the production and availability of inexpensive healthy foods, urban planning to allow children and their families to exercise safely, education on healthy lifestyle beginning in primary schools, and a global advertising code to promote only healthy food and drink to children and adolescents. Healthcare needs to engage with policymakers worldwide to ensure we achieve this goal.

Definition of Childhood Obesity

While BMI definitions of obesity are recognised to have limitations, they are a practical way of defining paediatric overweight and obesity and BMI is now accepted as a valid indirect measure of obesity in children.

Recent clinical guidelines recommend diagnosing a child over the age of 2 years as overweight if the BMI percentile is over 85th percentile for age and sex and obese if the BMI is over 95th percentile for age and sex. The boys' and girls' BMI charts show the recommended International Obesity Task Force cut-offs for obesity and overweight in children. These correspond to the adult definitions of overweight (BMI over 25) and obesity (BMI over 30) at 18 years of age.

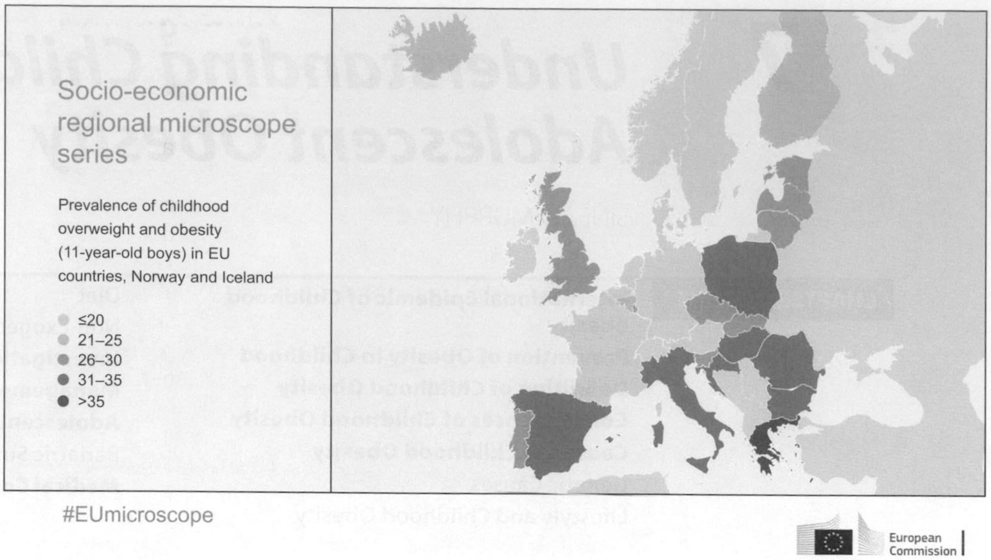

Figure 7.1 Prevalence of childhood overweight and obesity in EU countries, Norway and Iceland. (Reproduced with permission from European Commission, Joint Research Centre, Storcksdieck genannt Bonsmann, S., Carvalho, R., Safkan, S., et al., Mapping and zooming in on childhood obesity, Publications Office, 2019, https://data.europa.eu/doi/10.2760/92251.)

It is routine practice for children to have weight and height measured at every hospital visit and this provides an ideal opportunity for the child's BMI to be calculated, plotted and discussed with the family. This practice should also be incorporated into GP or clinic visits on at least an annual basis and allows early paediatric overweight to be diagnosed and addressed when lifestyle changes are most likely to be possible and impactful.

Markers of central adiposity in children, such as waist circumference, are associated with higher fasting insulin and adverse lipid profiles.

Consequences of Childhood Obesity

Childhood obesity is a multisystem disease with potentially devastating consequences. Childhood obesity is associated with significant comorbidities including hypertension, dyslipidaemia, increased blood clotting tendency, non-alcoholic fatty liver disease, sleep apnoea, polycystic ovarian syndrome and slipped upper femoral epiphysis, as well as significant and highly debilitating psychosocial morbidity. Childhood obesity is associated with premature mortality in adulthood.

Causes of Childhood Obesity

Childhood obesity is complex with a multifactorial aetiology.

GENETIC CAUSES

Childhood obesity is a condition influenced by the interactions between genetic and non-genetic mechanisms.

Common genetic variants in over 250 different sites in the genome – each with a small individual effect – have been robustly shown to influence the normal variation in adiposity across the childhood population. However, there are some genetic alterations which, alone, have a much more profound effect on body weight and the predisposition to obesity. Some of these (including mutations in specific genes or chromosome abnormalities) cause syndromes such as Prader-Willi or one of the many forms of Bardet Biedel, wherein obesity is only one of many clinical features. In recent years, a growing number of genes are being discovered. Mutations in these genes cause or strongly predispose to forms of childhood obesity in which other syndromic features are absent or less apparent. Among these are disorders of the leptin system including its downstream pathways in the brain. One of these, Melanocortin 4 receptor (MC4R) deficiency, substantially increases body weight even in the heterozygous state and has recently been established to occur at a prevalence of one in 300 people. This means that there are likely over 20 million people worldwide whose body weight is substantially increased by this single genetic cause alone. At present, if one considers children who have developed severe obesity pre-pubertally, around 10 per cent will have a currently identifiable mutation making a major contribution to their disease. Large scale genomic sequencing efforts are increasing the discovery rate for such genetic mutations and this figure is likely to rise. The clinical relevance of this growing knowledge base is becoming clear. Firstly, congenital leptin deficiency – a rare cause of severe obesity – responds dramatically to replacement therapy. Early results of trials of drugs targeting the melanocortin pathway show great promise in a range of other genetic subtypes (e.g. leptin receptor deficiency).

In the past, single gene defects have been believed to account for a small fraction of human obesity. It is now apparent that MC4R deficiency alone is more prevalent than cystic fibrosis, Duchenne muscular dystrophy and many other single gene diseases of childhood combined.

LIFESTYLE AND CHILDHOOD OBESITY

Diet and exercise (the avoidance of a sedentary lifestyle in particular) certainly play a part in the development of obesity which makes behaviour modification an essential part of any treatment programme. Education programmes about diet and exercise are important in the prevention of obesity. These should target society as well as parents and children.

DIET

The widespread consumption of nutrient poor, high calorie, high fat foods and drinks is a risk factor for the development of childhood obesity.

This is particularly relevant when it comes to the prevention of severe obesity. Children should be encouraged to increase their consumption of fruit and vegetables. Worldwide, epidemiological studies show that children eat far less than the recommended servings of fruit and vegetables.

The use of sugar-sweetened soft drinks has been shown to cause an increase in total energy intake by almost 10 per cent. It is interesting to note that children consume 40 per cent of their calories at school and therefore, the types of food and choice of drinks offered to children at school is of critical importance in addressing childhood obesity.

Increasing portion sizes are also a factor. Once again, the education of parents and families regarding appropriate portion size is essential.

NON-EXOGENOUS CAUSES

Overweight and or obesity in children rarely has a syndromic or endocrine cause. Growth hormone deficiency, Cushing's syndrome and hypothyroidism are all associated with obesity, but the distinguishing feature is the slowing of linear growth and consequent short stature. Therefore, endocrine causes for obesity should only be considered if the child is short relative to genetic potential in association with weight gain. Co-existing chronic disease also increases obesity rates.

Investigations

Children and adolescents with a BMI >85th percentile should be evaluated for potential comorbidities (Table 7.1).

Suggested laboratory screening for comorbidities includes HbA1C, fasting lipids and triglycerides, liver function tests, vitamin D levels and thyroid function tests.

The *International Task Force on Obesity* recommends against the routine measurement of fasting insulin given the lack of evidence of its usefulness in clinical practice.

Table 7.1   Evaluation of the Obese Child or Adolescent

Evaluation If BMI Over 85%

A thorough medical and family history, dietary intake and history of sedentary behaviour, history consistent with sleep apnoea

Weight, height and BMI percentile calculation

Blood pressure measurement

Check for the presence of acanthosis nigricans

Acne and/or severe hirsutism in pubertal girls (PCOS)

Consider syndromic obesity particularly if there are neurodevelopmental issues

Management

A whole-family approach is required, as parents are important role models for healthy lifestyle behaviour. Parenting programmes may help children to make healthier food choices, increase physical activity and help promote healthy behaviours. Parents play a central role in limiting sugary drinks and foods and in avoiding their use as rewards.

The earlier that intervention takes place the better, but prevention in the preschool age group is the best strategy. The goal should be to halt weight gain rather than focus on loss of excess weight.

Eating behaviours and patterns are established in the early years and these behaviours influence later food preferences, activity levels and leisure activities. Parents and families exert a great influence on young children in terms of eating behaviour and parenting plays an essential role in promoting healthy eating and in the development of healthy eating habits in young children. Therefore, prevention is key, and the early preschool years are the ideal timeframe for healthcare and education professionals to make a difference.

Adolescent Obesity

Clinicians who care for adolescents and young people will encounter a substantial number affected by obesity. Therefore, these clinicians must be able to diagnose it and its related health problems and counsel on appropriate prevention and treatment options.

Major societal changes have resulted in a greater availability of cheaper energy dense foods high in sugar and fat and a greater reliance on commercially prepared foods. At the same time, advances in technology have dramatically reduced energy expenditure both at home and in work with televisions and computers in many adolescents' bedrooms contributing to sedentary behaviour and poor sleep.

Pharmacotherapy for obesity in adolescence should only be used in conjunction with a lifestyle modification programme. There is little evidence on either safety or efficacy to support the use of pharmacotherapy in this age group.

The effects of drug therapy allied to structured lifestyle modification leads to a modest average weight loss of 5 to10 per cent, which typically plateaus at 4 to 6 months of treatment. Unfortunately, many relapse once the drug is withdrawn. Prescribing should only be by a specialist multidisciplinary team.

Some newer drugs such as liraglutide (a glucagon-like peptide 1 analogue) have shown promising results in the treatment of adult obesity, and these drugs are currently undergoing clinical trials in adolescents. They are effective because of the behaviour change they induce by reducing appetite. However, the use of pharmacotherapeutic agents in the paediatric population should be limited to large, well-controlled clinical studies.

BARIATRIC SURGERY FOR OBESITY IN ADOLESCENCE

Bariatric surgery cannot be considered in isolation but rather in collaboration with psychological assessment of the

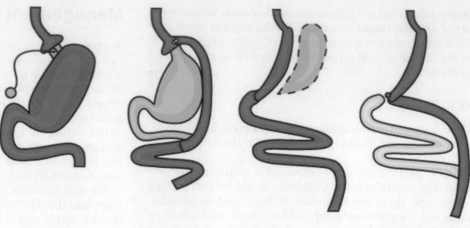

Figure 7.2 Types of bariatric surgery. (Reproduced with permission from Elsevier. (2020). *ICD-10-CM/PCS coding: Theory and practice, 2021/2022 edition.* Saunders.)

Adjustable Gastric Band (AGB)

Roux-en-Y Gastric Bypass (RYGB)

Vertical Sleeve Gastrectomy (VSG)

Biliopancreatic Diversion With a Duodenal Switch (BPD-DS)

Box 7.1   Key Points

Childhood obesity is one of the most serious global public health challenges of the twenty-first century.

Genetic causes of obesity are increasingly being identified and it is now apparent that MC4R deficiency is more prevalent than cystic fibrosis. Obesity is more likely to be a neurobehavioural disorder than a metabolic one.

Prevention is key and family interventions are necessary for success.

Generally, the aim of treatment is to help children and adolescents to maintain their weight.

In younger children, the main impact of obesity is emotional distress.

A medical cause for obesity should only be considered in children who are both short and obese for their age.

Bariatric surgery is recommended for adolescents with a BMI over 35 kg/m² with severe comorbidities (type two diabetes, pseudotumour cerebri, severe non-alcoholic steatohepatitis, severe OSA).

In Prader-Willi syndrome or leptin receptor deficiency, bariatric surgery is likely to be both ineffective and potentially dangerous.

Table 7.2   Complications of Obesity

System	Complications
Psychosocial	Low self-esteem, low mood, poor quality of life
Neurological	Benign intracranial hypertension
Cardiovascular	Dyslipidaemia, hypertension, atherosclerosis
Pulmonary	Obstructive sleep apnoea (OSA)
Gastrointestinal	Steatohepatitis, gallstones
Renal	Glomerulosclerosis, proteinuria
Endocrine	Insulin resistance, impaired glucose tolerance, polycystic ovary syndrome (PCOS)
Musculoskeletal	Slipped capital femoral epiphysis, chronic joint and back pain

Medical Complications of Obesity

Childhood obesity is associated with type two diabetes, which was previously virtually unknown in adolescence. A prediabetic state of insulin resistance is very prevalent among severely obese children regardless of ethnic background. Sleep-disordered breathing (sleep apnoea), asthma and exercise intolerance are other consequences of obesity (Table 7.2). A negative self-image can start as early as 5 years of age and worsen during adolescence with low mood and, sometimes, risk-taking behaviours.

adolescent and their family and the availability of sustainable psychological and other supports. The two bariatric surgical approaches used for adolescents are the Roux-en-Y gastric bypass and the vertical sleeve gastrectomy (Fig. 7.2). Both procedures have been shown to decrease the ghrelin hormone and increase the appetite suppressing hormones, like glucagon-like peptide 1, thereby decreasing appetite and improving insulin sensitivity. Surgery is associated with a significant improvement in comorbidities. However, lifelong monitoring for complications of surgery is essential.

In some specific conditions, such as Prader-Willi syndrome or Leptin receptor deficiency, bariatric surgery is likely to be both ineffective and potentially dangerous.

Key References

Arora, M., Barquera, S., Farpour Lambert, N. J., Hassell, T., Heymsfield, S. B., Oldfield, B., et al. (2019). Stigma and obesity: The crux of the matter. *The Lancet Public Health*, 4(11), e549–e550.

Economic and Social Research Institute and Trinity College Dublin. (n.d.). *Growing up in Ireland.* Department of Children, Equality, Disability, Integration and Youth. https://www.growingup.ie/

Fitzgerald, M. P., Hennigan, K., O'Gorman, C. S., & McCarron, L. (2019). Obesity, diet and lifestyle in 9-year-old children with parentally reported chronic diseases: Findings from the Growing Up in Ireland longitudinal child cohort study. *Irish Journal of Medical Science*, 188(1), 29–34.

Jabakhanji, S. B., Boland, F., Ward, M., & Biesma, R. (2018). Body mass index changes in early childhood. *The Journal of Pediatrics, 202,* 106–114.

Jennings, P., O'Brien, S., & O'Shea, D. (2018, May 16). *Tackling Childhood Obesity. A written submission from the Health Service Executive to the Joint Committee on Children and Youth Affairs.* Health Service Executive. https://data.oireachtas.ie/ie/oireachtas/committee/dail/32/joint_committee_on_children_and_youth_affairs/submissions/2018/2018-08-22_submission-health-service-executive_en.pdf.

Kipping, R. R., Russell, J., & Lawlor, D. A. (2008). Obesity in children. Part 2: Prevention and management. *BMJ, 337,* a1848.

The Organisation for Economic Co-operation and Development. (2019). *Heavy burden of obesity: The economics of prevention. A quick guide for policy makers.* OECD. https://www.oecd.org/health/health-systems/Heavy-burden-of-obesity-Policy-Brief-2019.pdf.

Styne, D. M., Arslanian, S. A., Connor, E. L., Farooqi, I. S., Murad, M. H., Silverstein, J. H., et al. (2017). Pediatric obesity-assessment, treatment, and prevention: An Endocrine Society clinical practice guideline. *The Journal of Clinical Endocrinology and Metabolism, 102*(3), 709–757.

Sun, J., Wang, Y., Zhang, X., & He, H. (2019). The effects of metformin on insulin resistance in overweight or obese children and adolescents: A PRISMA-compliant systematic review and meta-analysis of randomized controlled trials. *Medicine (Baltimore), 98*(4), e14249.

Willett, W., Rockström, J., Loken, B., Springmann, M., Lang, T., Vermeulen, S., et al. (2019). Food in the Anthropocene: The EAT-Lancet Commission on healthy diets from sustainable food systems. *Lancet, 393*(10170), 447–492. https://doi.org/10.1016/S0140-6736(18)31788-4.

Homepage | World Obesity Federation. (n.d.). www.worldobesity.org.

Online References

Fed to Fail: The crisis of children's diets in early life. UNICEF 2021 Child Nutrition Report. Accessed at: https://data.unicef.org/resources/fed-to-fail-2021-child-nutrition-report/#:~:text=UNICEF's%20Flagship%20Child%20Nutrition%20Report,safe%20and%20age%20appropriate%20diets.

SECTION 2

A Symptom-Based Approach

8 Common Problems in Newborns

JOHN MURPHY

Care of the newborn is an integral part of paediatrics, and this chapter will explore the common issues arising in both term and preterm infants.

Term Infants

JAUNDICE

Over 60 per cent of term infants will become jaundiced (80 per cent if preterm). Bilirubin metabolism is inefficient in the neonatal period due to immature hepatic function and excessive red cell breakdown. Physiological jaundice is usually mild, appears around day two or three of life, and disappears by the end of the first week.

Physiological jaundice may be due to an immature hepatic system and elimination pathway, increased enterohepatic circulation, a shorter RBC lifespan, a higher haematocrit or bruising during delivery.

Polycythaemia is seen in infants who are small for their gestational age and may cause symptoms of jitteriness and irritability with high colour in the first 48 hours. Polycythaemia is also associated with subsequent jaundice which may require phototherapy.

Breast milk jaundice appears within the first 2 weeks of life and may relate to poor breast milk flow. Breast milk jaundice may last several weeks and is self-limiting. Breast milk constituents may inhibit conjugation and increase enterohepatic circulation. It is a diagnosis of exclusion and no treatment is required.

Rhesus haemolytic disease occurs when a Rhesus negative mother produces antibodies to a Rhesus-positive foetus. It presents on day one of life. Sensitisation occurs via initial exposure (parturition, miscarriage, abortion and ectopic pregnancy) and re-exposure to Rh antigen during a subsequent pregnancy inducing elevation of IgG-Rh antibody. Antibodies are transported across the placenta and attach to fetal Rh + red blood cells, causing extravascular haemolysis of red cells within the foetal liver and spleen. There is a risk of erthryoblastosis fetalis with subsequent pregnancies. There has been a markedly reduced incidence since the introduction of anti-D prophylaxis.

ABO incompatibility is iso-immune haemolytic anaemia where a blood group A or B infant born to mother with blood group O with haemolysis that begins in utero. It presents with mild early-onset unconjugated hyperbilirubinaemia and is later followed by a rapidly worsening jaundice with a normal haemoglobin level. Diagnosis of ABO incompatibility is by testing the infant's blood group, the mother's blood group and the direct Coombs' test which is often only weakly positive and may even be negative.

The administration of intravenous immunoglobulin prevents haemolysis of sensitised red cells in Rhesus or ABO haemolytic disease, where bilirubin rises rapidly. It is very effective in bringing down the bilirubin and reducing the need for an exchange transfusion.

Management of ABO incompatibility is to maintain adequate hydration and evaluate for potentially aggravating factors (always consider sepsis). Phototherapy may be necessary, but thankfully exchange transfusion is now rarely needed. A follow-up haemoglobin check to exclude anaemia at the baby clinic is crucial.

Other haemolytic disorders include pyruvate kinase deficiency, hereditary spherocytosis and G6PD deficiency (with characteristic Heinz bodies on blood film) are associated with early onset jaundice. G6PD deficiency is prevalent in parts of Africa, Asia, the Mediterranean and the Middle East.

Examination

Clinical examination is essential. Undress the baby and then check the skin, sclerae and gums. The yellow colour spreads from head to toe as the bilirubin rises and is easily seen in Caucasian infants (Fig. 8.1). In infants of dark colour, the diagnosis of neonatal jaundice is even more challenging as scleral icterus may be the only clinical feature.

ESTIMATING JAUNDICE LEVEL

Although jaundice is easy to diagnose in Caucasian infants, estimating the level is more difficult, particularly in dark-skinned infants as noted above. Fortunately, the transcutaneous bilimeter is a very effective, non-invasive method of checking the baby's bilirubin, providing that the baby is greater than 35 weeks' gestation. It is used in the nursery, the baby clinic and in the community. It has greatly reduced the need for blood sampling and is reliable up to levels of 240 μmol/L. If the reading is above that, a serum bilirubin and the presence of antibodies (Rhesus or ABO incompatibility) should be checked.

The hour of life, gestational age, and the rate of rise in serum bilirubin are all relevant in assessing jaundice. If haemolysis or polycythemia are suspected, check the full blood count, a blood film (looking for spherocytosis or elliptocytosis), blood Group, and a direct Coombs test. Remember to check for G6PD in susceptible populations.

Check both total bilirubin (both conjugated and unconjugated), sometimes referred to as a 'split-bili' estimation. A high unconjugated bilirubin will most often be found. Unconjugated bilirubin is fat-soluble and thus able to cross the blood-brain barrier. If high enough, it can act as a neurotoxin (especially in the basal ganglia), causing kernicterus.

Mild symptoms of bilirubin encephalopathy include a sluggish, sleepy baby with a high-pitched cry and slightly decreased muscle tone. Severe bilirubin encephalopathy

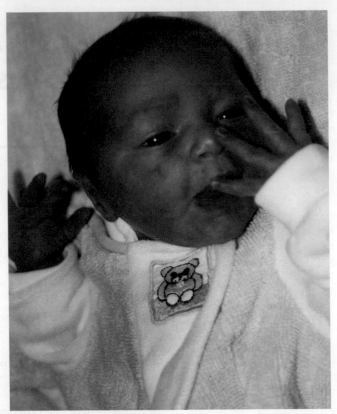

Figure 8.1 A jaundiced baby. (Reproduced with permission from Fraser, D., Cooper, M. A., & Myles, M. F. (2003). *Myles textbook for midwives.* Churchill Livingstone.)

leads to symptoms of reduced conscious level, seizures, an inconsolable infant with a weak cry, hypo- or hypertonia and, finally, opisthotonus or other posturing.

Management

Phototherapy using a 'biliblanket', or overhead phototherapy lights, enables 24-hour optimum light treatment. The light photo-isomerises the unconjugated bilirubin to a water-soluble form that is passed out in the infant's urine. Measure serial bilirubin levels over time and plot on a local or national treatment threshold graph such as the one developed by NICE. The median length of phototherapy required is about 24 hours.

Age is very important when assessing jaundice in newborns. Jaundice occurring within the first 24 hours is always of concern and is most likely related to haemolysis.

If a newborn is unwell and jaundiced, always suspect sepsis or, rarely, galactosemia.

Physiological jaundice occurs after 2 or 3 days and subsides by the end of the first week of life.

Newborns With Breathing Difficulties

Although there are several distinct neonatal respiratory disorders, the clinical assessment and investigations are common to all of them.

The key clinical observations are the infant's colour, respiratory rate with or without recession, heart rate, capillary refill time and general tone. Infants with significant respiratory distress become hypotonic.

The non-invasive respiratory support measures available include nasal prong oxygen, nasal continuous positive airway support (CPAP), humidified high flow nasal cannula therapy. Intubation and assisted ventilation are required when the infant requires an inspired oxygen level above 40 per cent to keep the FiO_2 at 91 to 95 per cent, the pH is less than 7.2, or there are episodes of apnoea.

The key investigations are pulse oximetry, blood gas and a chest x-ray.

This is a relatively common problem in both term and preterm infants. Ask about neonatal resuscitation and if breathing difficulty since delivery. Enquire whether there was meconium staining of liquor, a history of prolonged rupture of the membranes or pyrexia in labour or maternal *Group B Streptococcus* (GBS) carriage. Enquire whether the infant has just had a feed (suggests milk aspiration or possibly oesophageal atresia). In the case of oesophageal atresia, there will be a history of maternal polyhydramnios.

Observe for tachypnoea (respiratory rate over 60 breaths per minute), chest recessions, and nasal flaring and grunting. Check the heart rate and look for central cyanosis.

TRANSIENT TACHYPNOEA OF THE NEWBORN (TTN)

The most common cause of respiratory distress in a term infant, especially if born by caesarean section, is transient tachypnoea of the newborn (TTN). Another factor is being the infant of a diabetic mother. TNN is due to a delay in resorption of amniotic fluid lining the lungs with which the infant has tachypnoea rather than recession. Blood cultures should be performed and antibiotics commenced if the infant is tachypnoeic for more than 6 hours. The respiratory rate is typically over 60 breaths per minute.

If the respiratory symptoms persist, the diagnosis needs to be reviewed, and a cardiac ECHO should be performed to exclude congenital heart disease. Total anomalous venous drainage may present with a TTN picture.

Findings on a chest x-ray (CXR) include fluid in the horizontal fissure on the right side. (Fig. 8.2). TTN may initially require ambient O_2 but usually settles over the first few days of life without further treatment.

MECONIUM ASPIRATION

Meconium is passed before birth in 10 to 20 per cent of infants and increases with gestational age (25 per cent at 42 weeks). Newborn infants are at risk of inhaling and aspirating meconium when they gasp at birth, and meconium causes both mechanical obstruction and chemical pneumonitis and predisposes to infection. This condition is now less common due to the avoidance of post maturity (over 42 weeks) and improved detection of fetal distress in labour.

Suctioning after birth is not helpful and therefore is no longer recommended. Many cases settle with nasal oxygen or continuous positive airways pressure, intravenous fluids, and intravenous antibiotics, but more severe cases require assisted ventilation and nitric oxide. Pressors may be needed to maintain an adequate system blood pressure.

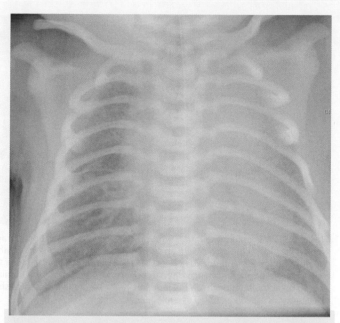

Figure 8.2 Typical chest x-ray of an infant with transient tachypnoea of the newborn (TTN) taken at 4 hours after delivery. This shows perihilar streaky appearances, fluid in the horizontal fissure and well-expanded lung fields to positive end expiratory pressure (PEEP) applied exogenously. (Reproduced with permission from Reynolds, P. (2010). Foetal to neonatal transition – what can go wrong? *Surgery, 28*(1), 5–8.)

Clinical signs in support of the diagnosis including meconium staining of the nails and the umbilicus.

The CXR in meconium aspiration shows overinflated lungs with more than six anterior ribs with patches of collapse and consolidation (Fig. 8.3). There is a high incidence of air leak (pneumothorax and pneumomediastinum), and some develop persistent pulmonary hypertension of the newborn (PPHN) with consequent difficulty in oxygenation despite high ventilatory pressures. Severe cases are associated with increased morbidity and mortality. ECMO (extracorporeal membrane oxygenation) is required for severe cases. The oxygenation index (OI) is a critical assessment tool calculated by measuring the mean airway pressure, inspired oxygen concentration and arterial PaO2. ECMO is indicated if the OI is over 40.

CONGENITAL PNEUMONIA

Risk factors include prolonged rupture of membranes (PROM) or chorioamnionitis (inflammation of the fetal membranes secondary to infection, usually bacterial), maternal pyrexia in labour or history of maternal GBS, and being of low birth weight or preterm. Presentation is often non-specific but can present with signs of respiratory distress. The infant with congenital pneumonia typically has tachypnoea with recession and a heart rate over 160 per minute. If there is associated sepsis, the capillary refill time will be over 2 seconds, and hypotension is common.

The investigations include a blood culture, peripheral swabs, a full blood count, C-reactive protein, CXR, placental swabs and placental histology. The white cell count is frequently low, and the C-reactive protein is raised. The CXR may show opacities (Fig. 8.4). Treatment is carried out with broad-spectrum antibiotics.

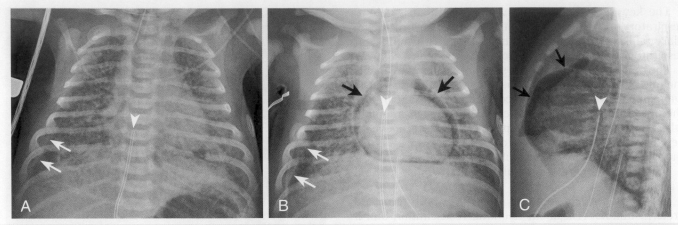

Figure 8.3 Meconium aspiration syndrome. (A) Newborn chest radiograph shows normal to large lung volumes and bilateral, coarse, ropy markings. Note right pleural effusion (white arrow). Also note umbilical venous catheter with tip (arrowhead) into right atrium. Tip should be at the junction of the right atrium and inferior vena cava. (B) Frontal and (C) lateral views of the chest obtained a few days later due to clinical deterioration show interval development of pneumopericardium (black arrows). Note that the umbilical venous catheter tip terminates deep in the right atrium (arrowhead). Tip should be at the inferior cavoatrial junction. Right pleural effusion persists (white arrows). (Reproduced with permission from Donnelly, L. F. (Ed.). (2021). *Fundamentals of pediatric imaging* (3rd ed.). Academic Press.)

Management depends on whether there is respiratory compromise or not. If simple with no respiratory compromise, give supplemental oxygen. Ventilatory support with either CPAP or assisted ventilation is required in more severe cases.

PNEUMOTHORAX

Pneumothorax occurs spontaneously in up to one in 50 deliveries and is usually asymptomatic. It may also be secondary to meconium aspiration, respiratory distress syndrome and mechanical ventilation. Diagnosis is by transillumination and CXR (Fig. 8.5). Transillumination works well for preterm infants because of their thin chest wall.

Significant clinical findings include cyanosis, prolonged capillary refill time (due to reduced cardiac output), tachycardia (over 160 per minute), hypotension (Blood pressure (BP) under 40 mm Hg) and chest asymmetry with greater prominence of the affected side.

Management depends on whether there is respiratory compromise or not. If it is a small pneumothorax with no respiratory compromise, give supplemental oxygen. If it is a tension pneumothorax, a needle thoracentesis (20 mL syringe attached to butterfly needle, 2ICS MCL and aspiration) may be required. Needle aspiration reduces the need for a chest drain by 50 per cent. If tension or a large pneumothorax, one should intubate, ventilate and insert a chest drain in the fourth or fifth intercostal space midaxillary line. A pig-tail catheter is preferred.

TIME OUT is very important before doing a needle aspiration or inserting a pig-tail drain. You must be certain that the **correct side** of the chest is being aspirated.

PERSISTENT PULMONARY HYPERTENSION OF THE NEWBORN (PPHN)

After birth, there is normally a progressive fall in pulmonary vascular resistance (PVR) and an immediate rise in systemic vascular resistance.

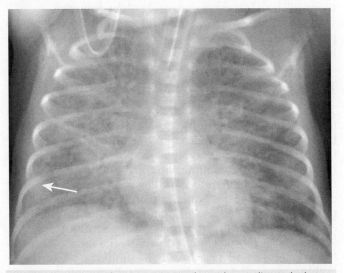

Figure 8.4 Neonatal pneumonia. Newborn chest radiograph shows large lung volumes and coarse, bilateral perihilar markings. Notice the small associated pleural effusion (arrow). (Reproduced with permission from Donnelly, L. F. (Ed.). (2017). *Fundamentals of pediatric imaging* (2nd ed.). Academic Press.)

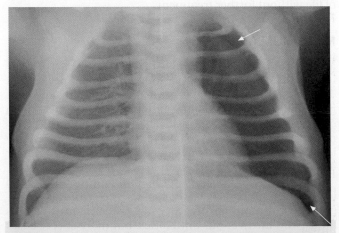

Figure 8.5 Pneumothorax left side (arrows) in intubated premature baby on day two of life. (Courtesy Prof. Stephanie Ryan.)

Measure the oxygen saturations on the right hand and either foot. They should be similar, but the foot can be 0.8 per cent lower. The difference is significant if greater than 3.0 per cent and can be indicative of PPHN.

A cardiac echocardiogram is very helpful. It will show mitral regurgitation and right-to-left or bidirectional shunting and rule out a cardiac cause.

Conditions that interfere with the normal postnatal decline in the PVR can lead to PPHN include birth asphyxia, meconium aspiration, septicaemia and respiratory distress syndrome.

High pulmonary vascular resistance causes right to left shunting of deoxygenated blood within the lungs, at the level of the atria through a patent foramen ovale, and through the persistent ductus arteriosus (PDA).

A key aim in managing PPHN to achieve adequate oxygenation is by maintaining systolic blood pressure while reducing pulmonary arterial pressure. Inhaled NO causes selective pulmonary vessel vasodilation, thereby reducing the pulmonary pressures to levels below systemic pressures to allow reversal of the right to left shunting of blood. High-frequency oscillatory ventilation (HFOV) is recommended in some cases. Extracorporeal membrane oxygenation (ECMO) may be required in severe cases (when the OI exceeds 40).

MILK ASPIRATION

Milk aspiration occurs more frequently in infants who are preterm and those with neonatal encephalopathy, respiratory distress of any cause, bronchopulmonary dysplasia, gastroesophageal reflux, or cleft palate. If it occurs soon after birth, exclude oesophageal atresia by passing an orogastric tube into the stomach. The usual scenario is that the infant will become cyanosed after a feed with choking-type respirations. Management of milk aspiration is immediate oropharyngeal suctioning and administration of oxygen if required. Manage the underlying aetiology to prevent recurrence. Preterm infants start oral feeding at 32 to 33 weeks' corrected age gestation. It takes them 2 to 3 weeks to become competent. Speech and language therapists play a primary role in the management of infants with persisting feeding problems.

RESPIRATORY DISTRESS SYNDROME (RDS)

RDS usually presents in preterm infants due to a deficiency in surfactant production by type II pneumocytes. Clinical signs include tachypnoea, intercostal and subcostal recessions, expiratory grunting, and cyanosis out of oxygen. In moderate and severe RDS cases, these features become more marked over a few hours. The occurrence of apnoea is an indication for ventilation.

The incidence of RDS is inversely related to gestational age. The more preterm the infant, the greater the risk of RDS. Antenatal steroids play a key role in the prevention of RDS in preterm infants with the result that many preterm infants may only require continuous positive airway pressure (CPAP). Caffeine is administered from the outset.

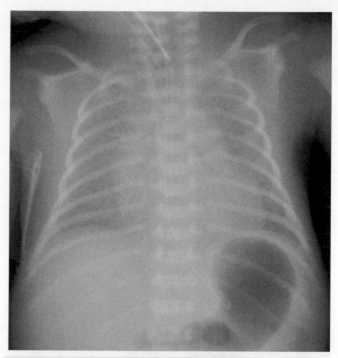

Figure 8.6 Respiratory distress syndrome (RDS). Chest radiograph day zero of baby born at 27 weeks' gestation. (Courtesy Prof. Stephanie Ryan.)

The initial treatment is nasal CPAP. Assisted ventilation will be required if the infant develops increasing respiratory difficulties with an FiO_2 above 40 per cent, capillary pH < 7.2, or apnoea. Volume cycle ventilation is now the preferred form of ventilation because it reduces pulmonary barotrauma.

Following intubation, the infant should be administered surfactant, which improves pulmonary compliance and rapidly reduces ventilation requirements. Its other advantage is that it significantly reduces the risk of a pneumothorax. The infant's respiratory condition tends to improve quickly, and overventilation is a risk. It is important to monitor the pCO2 carefully in order avoid hypocarbia (pCO2 under 4.0 kPa).

RDS is a clinical diagnosis with signs of respiratory distress and risk factors for RDS. CXR shows a homogenous ground glass appearance bilaterally with an air bronchogram [Fig.8.6].

Neurological Problems

A typical newborn infant will sleep for around 20 hours/day but wakes for feeds. A healthy newborn should latch onto a teat and suck, cry but be consolable, and have symmetrical facial movements. Infants fix their eyes on faces by 6 weeks but may have horizontal strabismus. They startle to a loud noise. They have a semi-flexed posture and a little head lag. They move all limbs spontaneously and by roughly the same amount and occasionally may have some movements that appear unusual. Finally, they demonstrate primitive reflexes that resolve as cortical control develops (usually 8 to 12 weeks after birth).

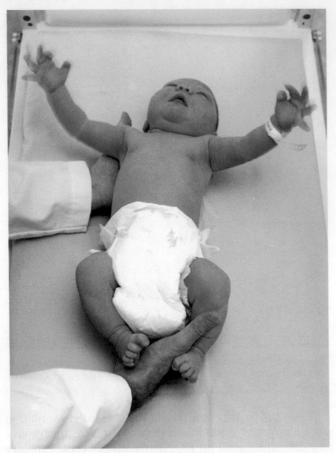

Figure 8.7   First phase of the Moro reflex: arms and fingers are opened and stretched. (Reproduced with permission from Förg, T. (Ed.). (2019). *Basics pädiatrie* (4th ed.). Elsevier.)

INFANT REFLEXES

Some primitive reflexes should **_always_** be present (the sucking and Moro reflex) (Fig. 8.7), and their absence is very significant.

Some primitive reflexes are not consistently demonstrable in the first few days after birth and their significance lies in their abnormal persistence, an example being the asymmetric tonic neck reflex (ATNR).

Most primitive reflexes disappear around 4 months of age, making persistence past 6 months is of significant concern. Deep tendon reflexes are normally brisk in newborns, making absent or reduced deep tendon reflexes a concern. The plantar reflex is upgoing in newborns.

MEASUREMENT OF HEAD CIRCUMFERENCE

The head circumference in a normal term newborn should be between 32 and 38 cm (Fig. 8.8). A sloping forehead is evident in microcephaly. Microcephaly has a myriad of causes including congenital infections (most commonly CMV), trisomy 13 and 18, Seckel syndrome, Smith-Lemli-Opitz, Cornelia de Lange, Wolf-Hirschhorn, and cri-du-chat syndromes, lissencephaly, schizencephaly, polymicrogyria and pachygyria, untreated maternal phenylketonuria, and fetal alcohol syndrome.

Perinatal insults (hypoglycaemia, hypoxic ischaemic encephalopathy and neonatal meningitis) may cause a failure of head growth after birth (secondary microcephaly).

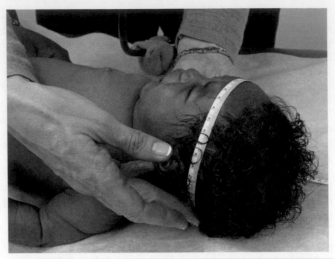

Figure 8.8   Accurate measurement of head circumference. (Reproduced with permission from Duderstadt, K. G. (Ed.). (2019). *physical examination: an illustrated handbook* (3rd ed.). Elsevier.)

The best initial tests are a cranial ultrasound and a brain MRI. These will identify any brain malformation. Other investigations include an eye examination (looking for optic atrophy), a hearing test (to exclude deafness), a brain MRI, TORCH titres, and blood microarray and urine for cytomegalovirus (CMV).

MACROCEPHALY

Macrocephaly is a head circumference 2 standard deviations (SD) above the mean.

Macrocephaly (head size above 38 cm at birth) may be familial or relate to hydrocephalus where a ventriculoperitoneal shunt may be required for drainage. In hydrocephalus, the skull sutures are separated, and the fontanelle is full. Always sit the infant up when assessing the anterior fontanelle. The so-called 'sun set sign' occurs when a rim of sclera is clearly visible between the cornea and the upper eyelid [Fig. 8.9].

The clinical definition of hydrocephalus is an occipitofrontal circumference (OFC) increase greater than two cm/week and a cranial ultrasound showing ventricular dilatation. A brain MRI is required for detailed analysis.

Common causes of hydrocephalus in newborns include post-haemorrhagic (especially preterm), associated with the Arnold-Chiari malformation in myelomeningocoele, post-meningitis, and, rarely, due to aqueduct stenosis or a Dandy-Walker cyst of the fourth ventricle. Hydrocephalus is very rarely due to excessive CSF production due to a choroid plexus papilloma.

NEONATAL ENCEPHALOPATHY (NE)

Neonatal encephalopathy is a condition seen in term infants with an altered level of consciousness and is often accompanied by seizures and a failure of spontaneous breathing. The incidence is 1.1 cases per 1000 births. At birth, the infant is typically pale, limp, has poor respiratory effort, a slow heart rate, and no suction response. The Apgar score and cord pH are low.

The causes are diverse, but many cases are due to decreased delivery of blood or oxygen to the foetal brain during labour (hypoxic-ischemic encephalopathy).

Recognised sentinel events include uterine rupture, shoulder dystocia, prolapsed cord, placental abruption and maternal eclamptic seizures.

MANAGEMENT OF NE

An early neurological examination is imperative. If the infant demonstrates the features of neonatal encephalopathy, therapeutic hypothermia (TH) is the standard of care.

TH involves the reduction of the infant's rectal temperature to 33.5°C using a servo-controlled cooling jacket (Fig. 8.10). After 72 hours, the infant is slowly rewarmed over a 12-hour period.

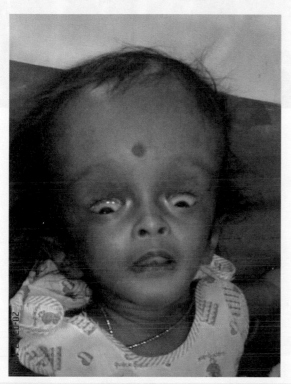

Figure 8.9 Positive 'sun set' sign. (Reproduced with permission from Thirunavukkarasu, A. B. (2018). *Pediatrics for medical graduates.* Elsevier.)

The infant is monitored for seizures with an aEEG. Phenobarbitone is the preferred anticonvulsant.

The infant's neurological status is assessed with the Sarnat score.

Other important measurements include blood pressure control and blood glucose monitoring.

There is very good evidence that TH prevents adverse motor outcomes at 18 months in moderate to severe NE.

MRI SCANNING IN NE

MRI scanning is based on the principle that following a hypoxic brain insults the normal diffusion or flow of water and the brain tissue is disturbed. This abnormal diffusion shows up as bright areas on the MRI (Fig. 8.11). They are most clearly seen in the first week of life. Two patterns are seen – a deep basal ganglia pattern is more severe and is associated with dyskinetic cerebral palsy (CP). The other is the parasagittal pattern associated with a milder, nondyskinetic form of CP.

These early MRI diffusion changes resolve in a matter of a few weeks. There is a period of 'pseudo-normalisation' before the permanent abnormal brain MRI changes appear.

Long-Term Outcomes of NE

Possible adverse outcomes of NE include death, cerebral palsy (CP), epilepsy, sensory deficits, cognitive impairment and behavioural problems.

In the precooling period for those with severe NE, the majority died and almost all survivors had CP. Few with moderate NE died but roughly 20 per cent had CP and most had obvious cognitive deficits. There were no obvious abnormalities in mild NE.

The brain MRI undertaken in the first week of life is quite predictive. If the brain MRI is normal, the incidence of subsequent deficits is low with 8 per cent having motor deficits, 8 per cent having cognition issues, and 25 per cent having speech and language issues.

If the brain MRI is abnormal, the incidence of subsequent deficits is 30 per cent motor deficits, 39 per cent cognition issues and 48 per cent speech and language issues.

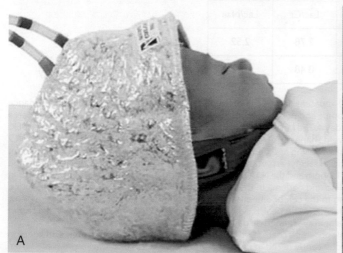
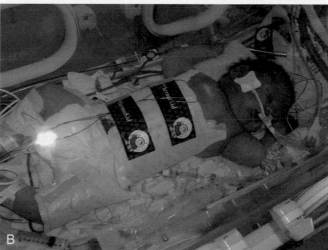

Figure 8.10 Therapeutic hypothermia – two approaches to hypothermia. (A) Selective head cooling with head wrap and chin straps. (B) Infant receiving whole body therapeutic hypothermia via body wrap. (Reproduced with permission from Volpe, J. J., Terrie, E. I., et al. (2018). *Volpe's neurology of the newborn* (pp. 510–563.e15). Elsevier.)

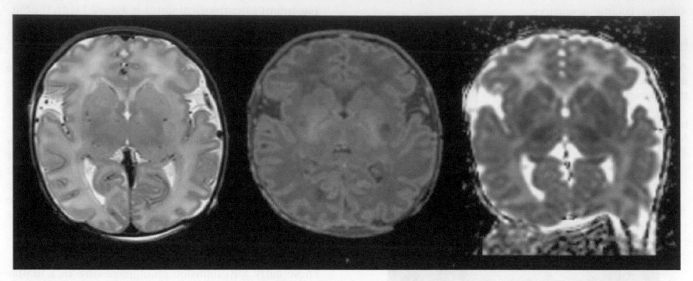

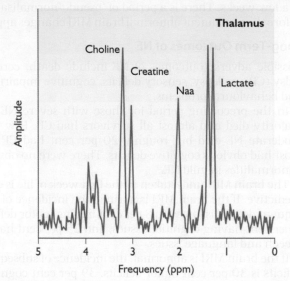

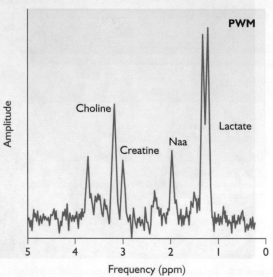

	Naa/Cho	Naa/Cr	Cho/Cr	Lac/Cho	Lac/Cr	Lac/Naa
Thalamus	0.68	1.10	1.63	1.71	2.78	2.52
PWM	0.65	2.07	3.20	2.65	8.48	4.10

Figure 8.11 T1-weighted image (top left), T2-weighted image (top centre) apparent diffusion coefficient map (top right). Proton magnetic resonance spectroscopy (MRS) (PRESS, TE 288ms) spectra from basal ganglia and thalamus and posterior white matter (PWM). The 1H MRS metabolite peak area ratios are shown in the table. (a) Normal full-term infant scanned at 1.5 T on day 4. The MRI and MRS findings are within the normal range. A normal PLIC is seen as high signal on T1-weighted images and low signal but a more ovoid shape on T2-weighted images. (b) Full-term infant with Sarnat Stage 2 neonatal encephalopathy scanned on day 4. Bilateral moderate basal ganglia swelling and oedema with restricted diffusion are seen on the apparent diffusion coefficient map. 1H MRS peak area ratios demonstrate a raised lac/ N -acetyl aspartate (NAA) peak area ratio in both the basal ganglia and thalamus (BGT) and PWM; the upright lactate doublet can be seen clearly at 1.3 ppm and the NAA peak height is reduced. (c) Full-term infant with Sarnat Stage 3 neonatal encephalopathy scanned on day 6. There is marked swelling and oedema in the BGT, midbrain and pons, in keeping with profound hypoxic -ischaemic brain injury. There are also diffuse oedema and swelling in the cerebral hemisphere white matter. 1H MRS peak area ratios show markedly raised lactate/NAA ratios due to a markedly raised lactate and reduced NAA. A peak is seen also at 1.1 ppm due to propan-1,2 diol, the carrier for phenobarbital. (d) Full-term infant with Sarnat Stage 3 neonatal encephalopathy scanned on day 1. There are bilateral BGT infarction (including lentiform and caudate nuclei), infarction of the perirolandic cortex and both hippocampi. There is involvement of both cerebral hemispheres, in keeping with very severe global hypoxic -ischaemic injury. The lactate doublet is significantly raised in both BGT and PWM. (Reproduced with permission from Rennie JM (Ed) (2012) *Rennie & Roberton's Textbook of Neonatology*, Fifth Edition. Elsevier Ltd)

NEONATAL SEIZURES

Neonatal seizures can be difficult to recognise, and the most common types are clonic, subclinical and subtle.

Diagnosis of newborn seizures is therefore frequently problematic and may require continuous EEG. Seizures may be missed or over-diagnosed with clinical judgement alone. If the EEG is normal, the seizures are presumed to be non-epileptic.

An important cause of neonatal seizures is a perinatal stroke. The incidence is one in 3500 births. The affected baby is typically normal at birth with seizures developing during the first day of life. The area of infarction on the MRI is most commonly in the distribution of the left middle cerebral artery.

Overall, the prognosis is good, but some develop a hemiplegia or seizures in childhood. If the baby develops a hemiplegia, motor deficits such as reaching and grasping at 4 to 6 months will become noticeable. Speech and language and cognitive development will need to be assessed.

Neonatal brain malformations are another group of disorders causing seizures.

Inborn errors of metabolism associated with seizures in newborns include maple syrup urine disease, organic acidurias (such as glutaric aciduria, propionic aciduria and methylmalonic aciduria), urea cycle disorders, nonketotic hyperglycinemia and pyridoxine dependent seizures.

JITTERINESS

It is important to be able to distinguish between a jittery infant and an infant who is having a seizure. Jitteriness is common while seizures are rare.

Jitteriness is characterised by fast, fine movements that stop with gentle pressure. These movements are peripheral, and the infant remains alert with a normal colour, heart rate and respiratory rate.

On the other hand, seizures will continue despite gentle pressure. An infant having a seizure will be unresponsive, may become cyanosed, will have an increased heart rate, and may develop apnoea.

Jitteriness is therefore defined as a tremor that can be brought on with stimuli and stopped with restraint of the affected limb. It is very common in the first 3 days of life and occurs in normal, healthy babies. Further investigation is unwarranted if the infant is otherwise normal, the tremor is not severe, and glucose is normal (over 2.6 mmol/L).

BENIGN NEONATAL SLEEP MYOCLONUS

This is very common and onset occurs within the first few weeks of life. It is characterised by a flurry of myoclonic movements of the arms and legs *exclusively during sleep*. These movements do not distress or wake the baby and disappear spontaneously by 4 months of age. They only occur during sleep, so a helpful test is to wake the infant up and they then disappear. No investigations are required.

ERB'S PALSY

Erb's palsy is where C5, C6, C7 and C8 nerve roots are affected, and the risk is increased if there is shoulder dystocia prior to delivery. C5 and C6 are the most affected roots, and C7 is involved in 50 per cent of cases.

Presentation is with decreased movement, a 'waiter's tip' posture, and an asymmetrical Moro reflex. When placed in ventral suspension, the affected arm 'hangs down' while the other arm flexes.

Early physiotherapy passive exercises are important in the prevention of contractures while waiting for function to return.

Most recover spontaneously, with only 10 per cent having any deficit by 3 months of age. The Toronto score is a clinical scoring system used to predict the outcome.

Erb's may be associated with clavicle fracture, Horner's syndrome or phrenic nerve palsy. Request a chest x-ray to out rule fractures or phrenic nerve palsy, physiotherapy to aid recovery and early referral to neurosurgery (using Toronto criteria) if injury fails to resolve.

KLUMPKE'S PALSY

Klumpke's is rare and involves the C8 and T1 nerve roots and may relate to a breech delivery or traction on an outstretched arm. It results in a 'claw hand'.

FACIAL NERVE PALSY

Facial nerve palsy in newborns may follow a forceps delivery. It is typically a temporary injury. Eye drops are needed to avoid a corneal abrasion if the eyelid on the affected side does not close properly.

It is important not to confuse facial palsy with the relatively common, benign condition of hypoplasia of the depressor anguli oris. In this condition, there is asymmetry of the mouth when the baby is crying, but the eye closes normally, and the nasolabial fold is intact. No treatment is needed, and it resolves spontaneously over time.

Vitamin K Deficiency Bleeding (VKDB) of the Newborn

Vitamin K deficiency is a particular problem in newborns previously called haemorrhagic disease of the newborn.

All babies should receive vitamin K intramuscularly after birth. It is important to carefully document that it has been administered.

Vitamin K ensures that the clotting factors 2, 7, 9 and 10 can bind to a surface and thereby enable a normal clotting cascade. The most sensitive indicator of vitamin K deficiency is a prolonged prothrombin time (PT).

The breast-fed newborn is at high risk for vitamin K deficiency, as breast milk is relatively vitamin K-deficient, the newborn liver is relatively immature, and the gut of a newborn requires several days to develop normal bacterial flora. Severe vitamin K deficiency in newborns (haemorrhagic disease of the newborn) can occur in breast-fed infants who have not received vitamin K prophylaxis. It can lead to diffuse bleeding and even CNS haemorrhage, thus making use of vitamin K prophylaxis universally recommended. If prophylaxis is refused, parents should be given very clear advice about the potential for catastrophic bleeding. In the absence of prophylactic vitamin K, the incidence of vitamin K deficiency bleeding (VKDB) ranges from 0.25 to 1.7 per cent.

Vitamin K administration restores the prothrombin time rapidly. Fresh, frozen plasma may be required in cases of severe bleeding.

Congenital Cytomegalovirus (CMV) Infection

Congenital CMV is by far the most common congenital infection (affects one in 200 newborns) with the true incidence far higher, as 90 per cent of infants with congenital CMV are asymptomatic at birth.

Either universal or targeted screening of asymptomatic newborns with congenital CMV might enable early antiviral treatment and the earlier identification of hearing loss. If started within 4 weeks of birth, antiviral therapy reduces deterioration in hearing in infants with symptomatic congenital CMV infection.

In most countries without newborn CMV screening, the diagnosis of congenital CMV infection is based on clinical suspicion. Symptoms of concern include a failed newborn hearing screening test, being small for gestational age, primary microcephaly, seizures, and the finding of jaundice, chorioretinitis, petechiae or hepatosplenomegaly on newborn examination. Congenital CMV is the most frequent non-genetic cause of sensorineural hearing loss and may be progressive in up to 50 per cent of cases wherein the initial newborn hearing screen may have been passed.

There is evidence that 6 weeks of therapy with ganciclovir improves or maintains hearing outcomes and 6 months of therapy with valganciclovir has even greater effects in improving \ hearing and neurocognitive outcomes.

There is no evidence to suggest antiviral treatment is needed in a newborn with asymptomatic CMV who has passed their newborn hearing screen.

There is no current data to support treatment with antivirals in CMV-related hearing loss developing after 1 month of age.

In conclusion, screening for congenital CMV using urine PCR testing would enable earlier detection of CMV-related sensorineural hearing loss. However, antiviral therapy treatment in affected infants remains controversial.

Care of the Preterm Infant

Preterm birth is defined as delivery before 37 weeks' gestation, and occurs in 5 to 6 per cent of all pregnancies. Preterm births have increased by 20 per cent in the United States over the past 20 years, mainly because of the increase in twin births.

Extremely preterm births (23 to 26 weeks' gestation) account for less than 1 per cent of all births, but advances in neonatal care mean that more of these infants are surviving. However, they are at greater risk of long-term complications and frequent hospital admissions, especially in the first 2 to 3 years of life.

Obstetrical complications that cause spontaneous preterm delivery include rupture of membranes, chorioamnionitis, placental abruption, polyhydramnios and multiple pregnancy. Planned early delivery may occur due to maternal illness (such as renal disease or decompensation of congenital heart disease), severe pre-eclampsia or foetal distress.

IMPROVED INTACT SURVIVAL

The first few hours are vital for survival and long-term outcome of the premature newborn. The attendance of a specialist neonatal team at delivery ensures skilled resuscitation and avoids hypoxia, hyperoxia and hypothermia. High oxygen saturation is avoided to reduce lung inflammation from oxygen toxicity. Glucose levels and acid-base balance must be kept within normal ranges. Ventilation strategies have changed as use of continuous positive airway pressure has increased and and use of mechanical ventilation has decreased.

The long-term outcome for preterm infants has therefore improved greatly. CP has become particularly less common. Antenatal steroids have significantly reduced the incidence of intraventricular haemorrhage. The optimal management and prevention of hypotension has reduced the rate of periventricular leukomalacia (PVL). Volume-targeted ventilation has been an important advance and has reduced both PVL and IVH, with a number of 11 needed for treatment.

SURVIVAL STATISTICS FOR MARKEDLY PRETERM INFANTS

The British Association of Perinatal Medicine (BAPM) statistics show that, at 23 weeks, four in 10 survive and one in four have disability; at 24 weeks, six in 10 survive and one in seven have disability; at 25 weeks, seven in 10 survive and one in seven have disability; and, at 26 weeks, eight in 10 survive and one in 10 have disability.

The most important variable affecting mortality in extremely preterm infants is gender (yet again, girls do better!). Therefore, for infants born at under 26 weeks of gestation, postnatal survival increases steeply in the first few postnatal days and varies by gestational age in days, even within a category of completed gestational age in weeks, meaning each day in utero counts.

CARE OF THE PRETERM INFANT IN THE DELIVERY ROOM

In delivery room management of a preterm infant under 28 weeks' gestation, delayed cord clamping for 1 minute and placement in a polyurethane bag to maintain temperature are the first steps.

Gentle resuscitation with a Neopuff and blended oxygen are given, as is early nasal CPAP, with later administration of surfactant if the infant has increasing respiratory difficulties.

MANAGEMENT IN NEONATAL INTENSIVE CARE UNIT (NICU)

Check the blood glucose and blood gases on arrival into the NICU. Start monitoring to facilitate minimal handling. Establish intravenous access and then vascular access via umbilical venous and arterial line with or without a peripherally inserted central catheter (PICC) line. Fluid management is very important. Consider both immaturity of the kidneys and insensible losses.

Respiratory Distress Syndrome (RDS)

RDS may lead to early respiratory failure and is prevented by means of antenatal steroids and the delivery room administration of artificial surfactant. The risk of RDS is 60 per cent in infants born before 28 weeks and under 5 per cent in infants born at 35 weeks' gestation. RDS with respiratory failure requires either CPAP or mechanical ventilation with additional temperature control and maintenance of normal blood pressure.

Continuous positive airways pressure (CPAP) is commenced at birth. Once admitted to the NICU, caffeine citrate is recommended in all infants at risk of RDS (under 30 weeks of gestation) until their clinical status can be assessed. In infants that require mechanical ventilation, aim to ventilate for as short a time as possible to avoid hyperoxia, hypocarbia and barotrauma. Continue caffeine in infants with apnoea or to facilitate weaning from mechanical ventilation.

Avoid hypocarbia (pCO_2 under 4.0 Kp) when providing assisted ventilation. Hypocarbia is a risk factor for periventricular leukomalacia (PVL).

Apnoea of Prematurity

Apnoea is defined as a cessation of breathing for more than 20 seconds and may be associated with a drop in O_2 saturation and heart rate. It is very common in preterm infants and affects almost all those born under 28 weeks' gestation. Incidence drops to less than 10 per cent in infants born at 34 weeks or more of gestation. Thus, apnoea monitoring is recommended for infants under 34 weeks' gestation.

Apnoea is graded based on three categories. Grade 1 shows no change in heart rate or colour, grade 2 shows a change in colour but a normal heart rate, and grade 3 shows changes in both colour and bradycardia.

Apnoea is primarily managed and prevented with caffeine citrate. The next step is CPAP if the infant is unresponsive. Less commonly, the infant may require intubation and assisted ventilation.

Patent Ductus Arteriosus

The ductus arteriosus normally closes by day 2 but remains open in preterm infants. The clinical signs appear on day four when the pulmonary vascular resistance falls, resulting in a left-to right shunt. The infant develops a murmur and full pulses. There is tachycardia and a widening of the pulse pressure. Pulse pressure is the difference between the systolic BP and the diastolic BP, the normal range being 15 to 20 mmHg.

Medical treatment is considered for symptomatic infants. Ibuprofen, a prostaglandin inhibitor, is commonly administered. Ibuprofen may cause renal impairment, reduced urinary output and hyponatraemia. A strict fluid balance must be maintained. If hyponatraemia occurs, reduce the infant's fluid intake.

Paracetamol is being increasingly administered because of fewer side effects.

A ductal ligation may be required if the infant remains dependent on oxygen or ventilator despite medical treatment.

No treatment is required if the PDA is small and there are no symptoms.

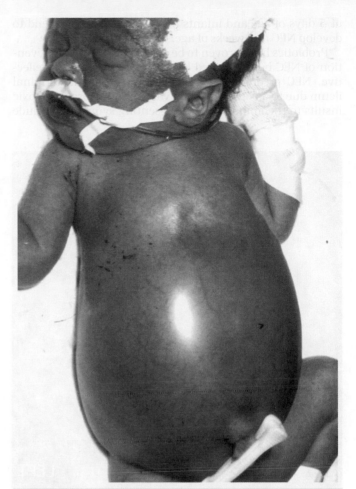

Figure 8.12 A distended abdomen in necrotising enterocolitis. (Reproduced with permission from Fraser, D., Cooper, M. A., & Myles, M. F. (2003). *Myles textbook for midwives*. Churchill Livingstone.)

Nutrition

Preterm infants have an immature suck and swallow until at least 32 weeks' gestation. Early nasogastric feeding is advised and is protective of the gut. Expressed breast milk is preferred. Total parenteral nutrition may be required but may also be associated with cholestasis.

Metabolic Bone Disease of Prematurity

Metabolic bone disease of prematurity (or rickets of prematurity) was frequently seen in the past, particularly in infants with extremely low birth weight (under 1000 g) whose primary problem was phosphate deficiency. It is no longer seen as modern total parenteral nutrition and oral feeds have sufficient phosphate to prevent it.

Necrotising Enterocolitis (NEC)

NEC is characterised by patchy necrosis of the small and large bowel often accompanied by sepsis. The infant may show systemic signs of sepsis with a distended abdomen and rectal bleeding (Fig. 8.12). The abdominal films in NEC typically show dilated bowel loops with pneumatosis (Fig. 8.13). Perforation may occur (Fig. 8.14). The incidence of NEC is inversely related to birth weight and gestation. Term infants tend to develop NEC in the first 1 to 2 days of life. Over 34-week gestation, infants tend to develop NEC at 5 days of age and infants born before 30 weeks tend to develop NEC at 3 weeks of age.

Probiotics have proven to be disappointing in the prevention of NEC but expressed breast milk appears to be effective. NEC predominantly affects the colon and terminal ileum due to a combination of vascular, mucosal and toxic insults to the immature gut. Presenting symptoms include abdominal distension, apnoea, intolerance of feeds, bile-stained aspirates and blood in the stools.

NEC may be associated with a later development of strictures. Infants with NEC may also have complications relating to TPN including thrombophlebitis, hyperglycaemia, hepatic cholestasis, osteopenia, acidosis, or electrolyte imbalance.

INTRAVENTRICULAR HAEMORRHAGE (IVH)

Intraventricular haemorrhage (IVH) is a condition in preterm infants characterised by bleeding into the lateral ventricles of the brain.

The haemorrhage arises from the germinal matrix lining the lateral ventricle. The matrix is a highly vascularised structure containing future neuronal and glial cells. In the extremely preterm infant, it surrounds the whole ventricular system. It is predisposed to haemorrhage as the blood vessels are thin-walled and fragile. The germinal matrix structure is vulnerable to hypoperfusion-reperfusion injury. By 36 weeks' gestation, the germinal matrix has involuted and IVH is uncommon after that time. Ninety per cent of IVH occurs within the first 72 hours after birth with small bleeds of little consequence. Large bleeds may result in death or handicap. Portable cranial ultrasound through the anterior fontanelle is used to diagnose IVH and assess its severity.

A grading system based on the ultrasound findings is used to describe the extent of the IVH. In Grade 1, there is a small bleed in the subependymal plate only. In Grade 2, there is blood in the lateral ventricles, but they are not distended. In Grade 3, there is a large amount of blood in the lateral ventricles, and they are distended. In Grade 4, there is a large amount of blood in the lateral ventricles, the ventricles are distended, and the bleed has extended into the surrounding brain tissue.

The incidence of IVH is gestational age-dependent; the more preterm the infant, the higher the risk of IVH. The incidence of IVH – particularly severe grades – has decreased over the past 2 decades. IVH grading provides guidance on the prognosis for the infant. For grade 1 or 2 IVH, particularly those markedly preterm, have a 5 per cent increased risk of disability compared to those of the same gestation without IVH. In contrast, infants with Grade 3 IVH have a

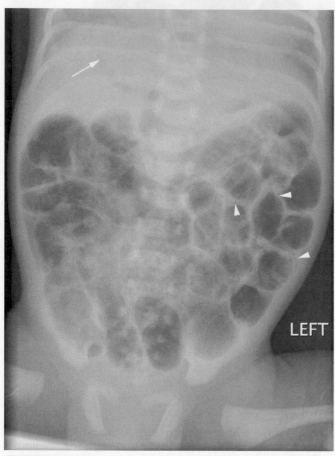

Figure 8.13 Abdominal x-ray showing extensive intramural gas in a neonate with necrotising enterocolitis (arrowheads). Note also portal venous gas (arrow). (Reproduced with permission from Rennie, J. M. (2012). *Rennie & Roberton's textbook of neonatology* (5th ed.). Elsevier.)

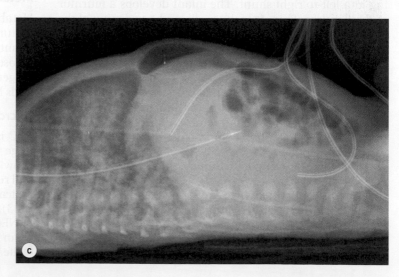

Figure 8.14 Abdominal x-ray of infant with necrotising enterocolitis showing perforation with free intra-abdominal air on lateral film. (Reproduced with permission from Paterson-Brown, S. (2013). *Core topics in general and emergency surgery: a companion to specialist surgical practice* (5th ed.). Elsevier.

50 per cent risk of neurodevelopmental issues. Infants with grade 4, particularly if bilateral, have a poor outcome with a 30 per cent incidence of post-haemorrhagic hydrocephalus. In those with hydrocephalus, the head circumference starts to expand excessively within 7 to 21 days after the bleed. The clinical features depend on the size of the bleed. If grade 1 or 2 IVH, the infant is often asymptomatic. If grade 3 or 4, the infant may present with pallor due to anaemia, apnoea, or hypotension, and may require increased respiratory support. They may have reduced body movements, reduced responsiveness, seizures and a full fontanelle.

Between 30 and 50 per cent of infants under 30 weeks' gestation with IVH will develop ventricular dilatation with a number developing post-haemorrhagic hydrocephalus (Fig. 8.15). Clinical features of raised intracranial pressure with progressive ventriculomegaly are indicators for ventriculoperitoneal shunt insertion, but earlier treatment may have potential benefits and is being further studied in a multi-centre trial. Antenatal steroids play an important role in preventing IVH and are recommended if preterm delivery is anticipated between 23 and 34 weeks' gestation. For optimal benefit, they should be administered more than 24 hours but less than 7 days before birth. Magnesium sulphate, administered to mothers in preterm labour, has additional benefits in reducing the risk of both CP and IVH in the infant.

Periventricular Leukomalacia (PVL)

PVL is a major predictor of CP, in particular spastic diplegia, in preterm infants. PVL is diagnosed by ultrasound or MRI (Fig. 8.16). PVL is caused by white matter injury due to impairment of the immature oligodendrocyte. It may be asymptomatic. It is usually identified as a white matter flare on ultrasound at 2 to 3 weeks of age.

The periventricular white matter is the watershed area in preterm infants between 23 and 32 weeks' gestation.

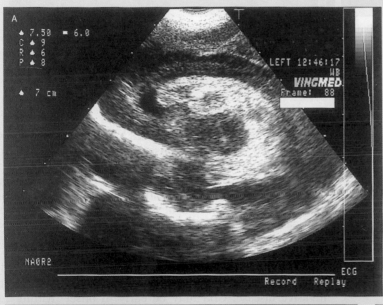

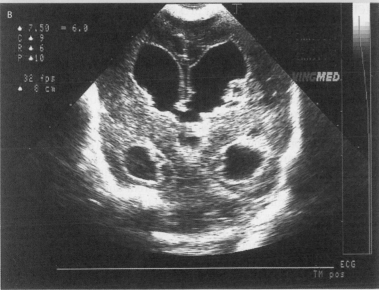

Figure 8.15 (A) A parasagittal neonatal cranial ultrasound scan showing extensive intraventricular haemorrhage. (B) Coronal ultrasound scan of a neonatal brain with hydrocephalus. (Reproduced with permission from Kapoor, R., & Barnes, K. (2016). *Crash course: paediatrics* (4th ed.). Elsevier.)

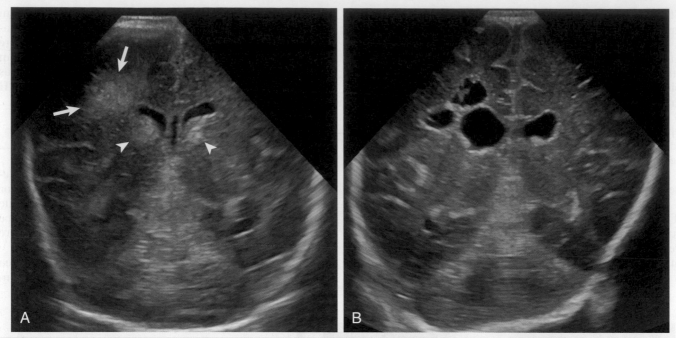

Figure 8.16 Evolution of periventricular leukomalacia in a preterm infant. (A) At 1 day of age, there is increased echogenicity in the right periventricular white matter (arrows), along with bilateral grade I IVH (arrowheads). Note the narrow cavum septum pellucidum between the frontal horns. (B) Six weeks later, cystic leukomalacia has developed in the right periventricular white matter, and volume loss on the right has caused the right lateral ventricle to enlarge more than the left. (Reproduced with permission from McGahan, J. P., Schick, M. A., & Mills, L. (2020). *Fundamentals of emergency ultrasound.* Elsevier – Health Sciences Division.)

PVL may be either cystic or non-cystic, with the cystic form being more severe. The cystic form has become less common with better perinatal care including antenatal steroids and optimal neonatal blood pressure control.

Risk factors for PVL include chorioamnionitis, sentinel events prior to delivery (such as abruptio placentae), recurrent apnoea, and either hypocarbia (low pCO2) or hyponatraemia.

Infants with PVL need careful neurodevelopmental follow-up for early diagnosis and management of cerebral palsy.

EARLY AND LATE ONSET SEPSIS

Sepsis is always a possibility for preterm infants in the NICU. Intravenous antibiotics are often commenced after birth for the first 48 hours until cultures return.

The *Neonatal Early Onset Sepsis (NEOS) Calculator* is a helpful clinical decision support tool in determining which infants need blood cultures and antibiotics. It uses a composite of risk factors: gestation age, maternal temperature, GBS status, duration of ROM and the infant's clinical examination. It is available on a mobile application.

Preterm infants have a greater susceptibility to infection due to low birth weight, an immature immune system, invasive procedures in the NICU, and overcrowding in the NICU with consequent understaffing.

Suspect sepsis if an infant has a poor colour, prolonged capillary refill time, tachycardia (over 160 per minute), a drop in BP (under 30 mmHg if preterm), abdominal distension due to ileus or a periumbilical flare, apnoea or tachypnoea (over 60 breaths per minute).

Low or high blood sugar may be evident.

EARLY ONSET SEPSIS

Early onset sepsis occurs within 48 hours of birth and may be associated with a rapid onset of fulminant multisystem disease. Pneumonia is a prominent feature and over 75 per cent of cases are associated with maternal risk factors for infection. These include a prolonged rupture of the membranes, maternal pyrexia in labour, foul-smelling liquor, GBS carriage or bacteriuria, or a history of GBS in prior delivery.

Twenty to 30 per cent of pregnant women are GBS carriers. Fifty per cent of infants born to untreated carriers will be colonised and just 1 to 2 per cent of these will develop invasive disease. GBS may be early in onset (within 24 hours) or have a later presentation (typically 3 to 4 weeks of age). There is universal GBS screening in pregnant women in USA but not in Ireland or the United Kingdom due to a lower incidence of GBS carriage. Indications for intrapartum antibiotics include a previous infant born with GBS disease, preterm delivery under 37 weeks, premature rupture of the membranes, pyrexia during labour, multiple births and rupture of the membranes for over 18 hours.

Listeria monocytogenes is a less common but nonetheless important cause of early onset sepsis. Transmission occurs via transplacental spread from the mother, who may acquire the infection from eating soft cheeses during pregnancy. The amniotic fluid may be discoloured, and the infant presents with similar features to GBS early onset sepsis, but respiratory distress is more prominent, and a rash may be noted.

Penicillin and gentamycin are the antibiotics of choice for early onset sepsis. Add cefotaxime is meningitis is suspected. Antibiotics are continued for 7 to 10 days and, if uncomplicated meningitis, for 14 to 21 days in total.

LATE ONSET SEPSIS

This is where the onset occurs after 48 hours of age and is usually associated with in-dwelling devices (such as a PICC line). Pneumonia is uncommon. Late onset sepsis may be due to GBS, *Escherichia coli* and *Listeria monocytogenes*, but is more likely due to *Staphylococcus epidermidis* with methicillin-resistant staphylococcus aureus (MRSA) now seen less frequently.

The antibiotic regimen for late onset sepsis is guided by local antibiotic sensitivities and may include flucloxacillin and gentamicin with the addition of cefotaxime if meningitis is suspected or likely.

Bronchopulmonary Dysplasia

Bronchopulmonary dysplasia (BPD) is a chronic lung disorder affecting preterm infants. Typically, the infant has breathing difficulties, is oxygen-dependent, has poor growth, feeding problems and an abnormal CXR with hyperinflation, streaky infiltrates, and cystic changes (Fig. 8.17). The most useful of the many definitions for the condition is a preterm infant still requiring supplemental oxygen at 36 weeks of postmenstrual age.

BPD mostly affects preterm infants less than 28 weeks' gestation; the more preterm the infant, the higher the rate of BPD. The incidence ranges from 94 per cent at 23 weeks, 71 per cent at 24 to 25 weeks, 44 per cent at 26 to 27 weeks, and 21 per cent at 28 to 29 weeks of gestation.

Prematurity is the main reason for the development of BPD. If the infant suffered from intrauterine growth retardation (IUGR), this is an independent risk factor. IUGR infants have rates two to three times greater than infants of normal weight.

Chorioamnionitis is another factor associated with BPD. Foetuses exposed to chorioamnionitis are at increased risk of developing a systemic inflammatory response. This inflammation causes adverse remodelling in the fetal lung, leading to subsequent BPD.

The severity of the BPD can be assessed by the concentration of inspired oxygen that the infant requires and whether the infant needs high flow oxygen or CPAP. When the concentration of oxygen required is under 30 per cent, the BPD can be considered mild. When over 30 per cent, it is considered moderate or severe. Poor weight gain is another feature.

Several strategies are employed to reduce the incidence and severity of BPD in preterm infants. Blended oxygen, rather than 100 per cent oxygen, is used at birth. It is recommended to start with FiO_2 30 per cent and increase as required to reach the target oxygen saturation.

Ventilation causes barotrauma to the infant's lungs. It is no longer advised to routinely intubate and ventilate preterm infants at birth. A more selective approach is now employed and non-invasive ventilation is used whenever possible. Many preterm infants have a good respiratory drive and can cope with CPAP and caffeine citrate. If they do require assisted ventilation, the duration on the ventilator should be kept to the shortest time possible.

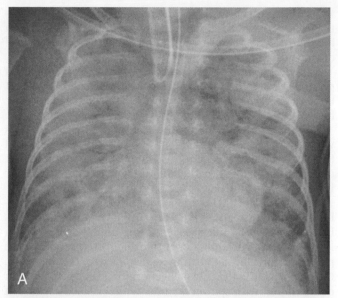
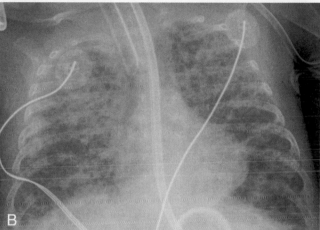
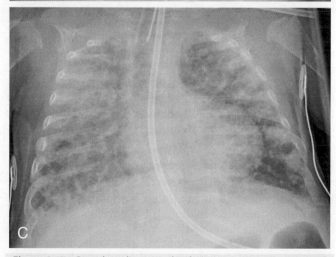

Figure 8.17 Bronchopulmonary dysplasia in a premature neonatal girl. (A) Chest radiograph at 20 days of life shows persistent bilateral lung opacities. (B) Chest radiograph at 35 days of life shows coarsening of the lung markings. (C) Chest radiograph at 60 days of life shows increased coarse lung markings and development of diffuse bubble-like lucencies. (Reproduced with permission from Donnelly, L. F. (Ed.). (2017). *Fundamentals of pediatric imaging* (2nd ed.). Academic Press.)

Another recommended measure is to use volume-targeted ventilation rather than pressure-cycle ventilation in infants who require ventilation as this reduces risk of developing BPD.

Caffeine citrate which is primarily used to treat apnoea of prematurity but is also beneficial in the treatment of BPD. It is more effective if commenced within the first 3 days after birth.

It is important to enhance the postnatal growth in infants with BPD as weight gain tends to be suboptimal because of their excess energy expenditure due to the increased effort of breathing. Therefore, they require fortified breast milk or high energy formulae.

Infants with BPD experience interstitial and alveolar oedema due to pulmonary inflammation. Diuretics improve the pulmonary oedema; the choice is between a loop diuretic (frusemide) or a thiazide. Frusemide is more potent than thiazide but may cause a metabolic alkalosis. Chlorothiazide is the thiazide generally prescribed, often in combination with spironolactone, which is used because of its potassium-sparing effects.

Steroids have been an important tool in the treatment of infants with significant, persistent BPD, as steroids reduce bronchial and pulmonary oedema, inflammation and bronchospasm. Dexamethasone is the most commonly used steroid with current lower dosage regimens than previously because of concerns about PVL. When an infant is on steroids, monitor for hyperglycaemia, hypertension, electrolyte imbalance, neutrophilia, lymphopenia and faltered growth.

Twenty per cent of infants with BPD develop pulmonary arterial hypertension. Pulmonary hypertension (PH) should be suspected when the BPD is complicated by increased oxygen requirements and episodes of cyanosis. It is diagnosed by cardiac echocardiography with typical features of tricuspid regurgitation and a mean pulmonary systemic pressure above 0.5.

When managing infants with BPD complicated by PH, it is important to keep oxygen saturations in the 92 to 95 per cent range to help prevent reactive pulmonary vasoconstriction.

Sildenafil is commonly used as a selective phosphodiesterase inhibitor, which causes pulmonary vasodilatation. If the infant with BPD is still being ventilated, inhaled nitric oxide (NO) is commonly administered.

Retinopathy of Prematurity

Retinopathy of prematurity (ROP) is an important cause of visual impairment in children. It is a developmental vascular proliferation disorder (Fig. 8.18). If not identified and treated promptly, its more severe form can lead to macular dragging, retinal detachment and blindness. Fortunately, blindness has become rare with the advent of screening, early detection and effective therapies.

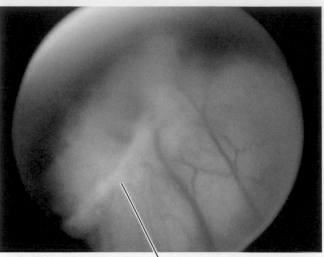

Extraretinal fibrovascular proliferation

Figure 8.18 Retinopathy of prematurity (ROP) demonstrating extraretinal fibrovascular proliferation along the ridge (stage 3 ROP). (Reproduced with permission from Friedman, N. J., Kaiser, P. K., Pineda, R., & Massachusetts Eye and Ear Infirmary. (2021). *The Massachusetts eye and ear infirmary illustrated manual of ophthalmology*. Elsevier.)

ROP affects infants under 32 weeks' gestation. Infants at 28 to 31 weeks' gestation usually have mild ROP. More severe types of ROP are encountered in preterm infants under 28 weeks' gestation.

In addition to prematurity, predisposing factors include hyperoxia, hypoxia, hypotension and free radical formation. New blood vessels grow abnormally out of the retina into the vitreous of the eye.

There is a complex interplay between insulin growth factor 1 (IGF1) and vascular endothelial growth factor (VEGF) in the regulation of retinal vessel growth. IGF1 promotes normal vessel growth. IGF1 levels are low in preterm infants, possibly leading to reduced vascularization and hypoxia in areas of the retina. VEGF, produced in response to the retinal ischaemia, subsequently causes abnormal vessel growth.

The screening for ROP is performed at 31 weeks corrected gestation age. It is a complex procedure undertaken by a skilled ophthalmologist with a special interest in ROP. When ROP is present, the decision to treat is based on the zone involved, the stage of the process, and the presence of plus disease.

The two available options are laser treatment or bevacizumab. Bevacizumab is less invasive, easier to administer, and causes less myopia. It requires more prolonged monitoring due to the risk of ROP recurrence, cataract formation, and endophthalmitis.

(Box 8.1)
(Box 8.2)
(Box 8.3)
(Box 8.4)

Box 8.1   Key Points

Physiological jaundice is usually mild, appears around day two or three of life, and disappears by the end of the first week. Haemolytic disease usually presents on day one of life.

The transcutaneous bilimeter is a very effective, non-invasive method of checking the baby's bilirubin, providing that the baby is born past than 35 weeks' gestation. It is especially helpful in babies of colour in whom jaundice can be difficult to clinically detect.

In Rhesus or ABO haemolytic disease, the administration of intravenous immunoglobulin is very effective in bringing down the bilirubin and reducing the need for an exchange transfusion.

If a newborn is unwell and jaundiced, always suspect sepsis or, rarely, galactosemia.

The most common cause of respiratory distress in a term infant – especially those born by caesarean section – is transient tachypnoea of the newborn (TTN).

Suctioning after birth is <u>not</u> helpful to prevent meconium aspiration and therefore is no longer recommended.

The infant with congenital pneumonia typically has tachypnoea (over 60 breaths per minute) with recession and a heart rate over 160 per minute.

Pneumothorax can occur spontaneously in up to 2 per cent of deliveries and is usually asymptomatic. It may also be secondary to meconium aspiration, respiratory distress syndrome and mechanical ventilation. Diagnosis is by transillumination and CXR.

Extracorporeal membrane oxygenation (ECMO) may be required in severe cases of persistent pulmonary hypertension of the newborn.

Antenatal steroids play a key role in the prevention of RDS in preterm infants and now many preterm infants only require continuous positive airway pressure.

Most primitive reflexes disappear from around 4 months of age, making persistence past 6 months of age highly concerning.

The clinical definition of hydrocephalus is an OFC increase greater than 2 cm/week and a cranial ultrasound showing ventricular dilatation. A brain MRI is required for detailed analysis.

The treatment of neonatal encephalopathy (NE) is supportive management and, for babies with moderate or severe hypoxic-ischaemic encephalopathy, therapeutic hypothermia. There is very good evidence that 'cooling' prevents adverse motor outcomes at 18 months in moderate to severe NE (Number Needed to Treat (NNT) is seven). The brain MRI undertaken in the first week of life is very predictive.

With jitteriness, there are fast, fine movements that will stop with gentle pressure. These movements are peripheral, and the infant remains alert with a normal colour, heart rate and respiratory rate. Seizures, on the other hand, will continue despite gentle pressure.

Organised neonatal networks and categorisation of neonatal units in utero and postnatal transport lead to improved survival of preterm infants.

In the delivery room management of a preterm infant under 28 weeks' gestation, the first steps are delayed cord clamping for 1 minute and placement in a polyurethane bag to maintain temperature.

CPAP with early rescue surfactant should be considered the optimal management of infants with RDS. Apnoea monitoring is recommended for infants under 34 weeks' gestation.

No treatment is required if the persistent ductus arteriosus is small and there are no symptoms. If persistent, treat with ibuprofen or paracetamol and perform surgical ligation if ventilator-dependent.

Probiotics have proven to be disappointing in the prevention of necrotising enterocolitis (NEC) but expressed breast milk appears to be effective.

In the management of NEC, stop feeds and starting intravenous fluids, start intravenous antibiotics including metronidazole, nasogastric aspiration and inotropic support if needed for hypotension. Surgery is required if obstruction occurs, and insertion of a Penrose drain is recommended if perforation occurs secondary to NEC.

Group B *Streptococcus* (GBS) is the most common cause of neonatal sepsis in the developed world.

Suspect sepsis if an infant has a poor colour, prolonged capillary refill time, tachycardia (over 160 per minute), a drop in BP (under 30 mmHg if preterm), apnoea or tachypnoea (over 60 breaths per minute).

Use volume-targeted ventilation rather than pressure-cycle ventilation in infants who require ventilation, as this reduces risk of developing bronchopulmonary dysplasia (BPD). When infants with BPD are oxygen-dependent, it is important to maintain the oxygen saturation at 92 per cent to 95 per cent. This prevents rebound pulmonary vasoconstriction.

Retinopathy of prematurity (ROP) affects infants under 32 weeks' gestation. Infants born at 28 to 31 weeks' gestation usually have mild ROP. The more severe types of ROP are encountered in preterm infants under 28 weeks' gestation.

Infants under 32 weeks (31 weeks and 6 days) gestation or under 1500 g should be screened for ROP.

When ROP is present, the decision to treat is based on the zone involved, the stage of the process, and the presence of plus disease. The treatment modalities are laser photocoagulation or the anti-vascular endothelial growth factor (VEGF) agent Bevacizumab administered by intravitreal injection.

Box 8.2   Respiratory Distress in a Term Infant

A male infant is born at 41 weeks' gestation by spontaneous vertex delivery weighing 3 kg. His mother is a 30-year-old primigravid but was found to be colonised with Group B *Streptococcus* (GBS) on high vaginal swab at 36 weeks' gestation. She went into spontaneous labour at 40 weeks and had a spontaneous rupture of the membranes with clear liquor. His Apgar score was 8[1] and 9[5]. At 4 hours of age, just after a feed, he is noted to be pale and to have a raised respiratory rate of 70 breaths per minute and moderate recession. His heart rate is 170 per minute, his temperature 35.8°C, his oxygen saturation is 89 per cent and his capillary refill time is 3 seconds. He is admitted to the special care baby unit, commenced on oxygen and observed in an incubator where his temperature returns to normal, but he remains tachypnoeic. He is commenced on intravenous fluids, intravenous antibiotics (post-blood cultures), and a chest x-ray is ordered.

Clinical Pearls

Symptoms of early onset sepsis in newborns are often non-specific and may be insidious. They may present with a high or low temperature, poor feeding, irritability or lethargy, and occasionally with circulatory collapse.

Risk factors for congenital pneumonia include prolonged rupture of membranes (PROM), strong-smelling liquor due to chorioamnionitis, maternal pyrexia in labour or history of maternal GBS.

Continued

Box 8.2   Respiratory Distress in a Term Infant—cont'd

The low temperature, tachypnoea and tachycardia in this instance all point to sepsis with congenital pneumonia. Therefore, the right course of action is to promptly start intravenous penicillin and gentamicin.

Severe respiratory distress with cyanosis soon after birth points to a congenital diaphragmatic hernia or pneumothorax. Marked tachypnoea post-Lower Segment Caesarean Section (LSCS) points to transient tachypnoea of the newborn. Marked respiratory distress at the first feed may relate to oesophageal atresia or milk aspiration. If preterm (under 37 weeks), consider respiratory distress syndrome and, if postmature, meconium aspiration syndrome.

Persistent pulmonary hypertension of the newborn (PPHN) may develop as a complication of meconium aspiration syndrome or congenital pneumonia.

Interpretation of Investigations

Chest x-ray is the key investigation but initial changes in congenital pneumonia may be non-specific, so empirical treatment is warranted if risk factors are present.

Blood gases are helpful to demonstrate impending respiratory failure (high pCO2), but look out for metabolic acidosis with a high anion gap. Measure the serum lactate as values above 4 mmol/L are significant.

C-reactive protein (CRP) is helpful if elevated and may point to sepsis at the cause.

Failure to oxygenate the infant despite increased support including artificial ventilation may indicate PPHN. For PPHN, the key test is to measure the preductal (right hand) and postductal oxygen (foot) saturation concentrations. A difference of more than 10 per cent between the two readings is indicative of right-to-left shunting. Cardiac echocardiography is very helpful in assessing the severity of the PPHN. Tricuspid regurgitation is one of the common findings.

Pitfalls to Avoid

For the administration of antibiotics, **Prescribe** them, **Get** them, and **Give** them with the goal that the infant should receive the antibiotics within **1 hour** of first contact or admission.

Once the infant stabilises, a lumbar puncture should be performed if meningitis is suspected.

Peripartum infection with herpes simplex or varicella zoster can cause devastating infections in newborns. If varicella exposure occurs between 5 days before delivery and 2 days postdelivery, give VZIG (varicella zoster immunoglobulin) to the infant and commence acyclovir. If evidence of herpes fix type 2 infection is present in the mother, deliver by caesarean section and give acyclovir to the newborn infant. Remember, however, that acyclovir can cause transient renal impairment.

Consider an inborn error of metabolism in the presence of a history of consanguinity, a well period before deterioration, metabolic acidosis with a raised anion gap, ketosis, hypoglycaemia and unusual odours (which classically include the smell of maple syrup in maple syrup urine disease, or the smell of sweaty feet reported in isovaleric acidemia).

The ultrarare total anomalous pulmonary venous connection (TAPVC) with obstruction should be suspected if the presentation is later (after 12 hours of age), or if there is evidence of cyanosis and tachypnoea, reduced pulses and significant hepatomegaly. Diagnosis is by echocardiography.

Box 8.3   A Term Infant With Neonatal Encephalopathy

A female infant was born in a small maternity unit by emergency LSCS at term due to significant foetal distress due to abruptio placentae. Her mother is a 25-year-old primigravid with no relevant history. She is born flat with no spontaneous breaths and a heart rate of 70 per minute. Her Apgar scores are 1[1] and 3[5]. She is intubated by a consultant paediatrician, the neonatal transport team is contacted, and advice is sought. She is passively cooled, placed on intravenous fluids, and subsequently transferred to a tertiary neonatal centre for therapeutic hypothermia. Soon after arrival in the tertiary centre, she has repetitive jerking of all four limbs and is commenced on phenobarbitone. Over the next 3 days she has further seizures, and her parents are very concerned about her neurodevelopmental outcome.

Clinical Pearls

Clinical examination, the Sarnat score, and the amplitude-integrated electroencephalogram (aEEG) are used to assess neonatal encephalopathy (NE) as mild (hyperalert), moderate (lethargic) or severe (comatose).

Following the original insult, apnoea, seizures, and multiorgan dysfunction may result in further brain injury.

The treatment of NE is supportive management and therapeutic hypothermia for babies with moderate or severe hypoxic-ischaemic encephalopathy.

In NE, the initial injury sets off processes which, after a few hours, result in neuronal apoptosis and therapeutic hypothermia (TH) works by decreasing apoptosis. Maintain the infant at a temperature of 33°C to 34°C for 72 hours.

During the cooling period, TH has been found to decrease mortality and rates of cerebral palsy (CP). Some data suggests that cooling improves cognitive outcomes.

The timing of the seizures is important in determining the cause, as seizures due to neonatal encephalopathy develop shortly after birth and are associated with perinatal asphyxia and abnormal neurological behaviour.

Treatment of neonatal seizures is supportive treatment first and then treatment of underlying causes (**do not forget glucose**), and empirical intravenous antibiotics are given until the infant is proven not to have sepsis or meningitis.

Anticonvulsants for neonatal seizures include phenobarbitone (as first line) and then levetiracetam.

Interpretation of Investigations

Full EEG monitoring is desirable to detect subclinical seizures.

Brain MRI is used to help predict the likelihood of possible adverse outcomes which include death, CP, epilepsy, sensory defects, cognitive impairment and behavioural problems.

Brain MRI may also point to another pathology besides HIE. A diffusion-weighted MRI is the imaging of choice.

Pitfalls to Avoid

Transfer to a level three neonatal intensive care unit is required for TH.

Adverse effects of TH include an exacerbation of PPHN, coagulopathy with a low fibrinogen, and subcutaneous fat necrosis with hypercalcaemia. Parents may find the procedure both physically and psychologically upsetting.

Neonatal meningitis (most often due to Group B *Streptococcus*) should always be considered in the differential diagnosis of neonatal seizures.

Seizures may relate to HIE, neonatal stroke or brain haemorrhage, but can also occur due to hypoglycaemia, hyponatraemia, hypocalcaemia or hypomagnesemia.

Box 8.4   A Markedly Preterm Infant

A male infant is born by LSCS at 25 weeks' gestation weighing 650 g. He cries at birth and is placed in a polyurethane bag to keep him warm. He is transferred from the delivery suite on CPAP, where he remains intermittently on CPAP for 4 weeks. He has umbilical lines inserted and receives both total parenteral nutrition and a small amount of early breast milk via nasogastric tube. On day four of life, he is noted to have full pulses and a hyperdynamic praecordium and echocardiography confirms a patent ductus arteriosus. He receives ibuprofen with good effect and his ductus closes. He has several cerebral ultrasound scans which are all reassuring.

At 5 weeks of age, he is still oxygen-dependent and his chest x-ray is consistent with chronic lung disease. He has regular top-up transfusions and two episodes of suspected sepsis requiring cessation of feeds and intravenous antibiotics. He is shown to have mild ROP on ophthalmology screening.

The team has been very supportive of his parents throughout and, 6 months postdelivery, he is to be discharged home.

Clinical Pearls

The administration of maternal antenatal corticosteroids is associated with increased survival of both moderately preterm and extremely preterm infants.

Organised neonatal networks and categorisation of neonatal units in utero and postnatal transport all lead to improved survival.

Improved neonatal nutrition practices, the use of caffeine and the curtailment of the use of postnatal corticosteroids have all helped to reduce morbidity.

CPAP with early rescue surfactant should be considered optimal management of infants with RDS.

If a PDA is persistent, treat with ibuprofen or paracetamol and consider surgical ligation if ventilator dependent.

In the management of NEC, stop feeds and start intravenous fluids and intravenous antibiotics including metronidazole, nasogastric aspiration and inotropic support if needed for hypotension.

The treatment modalities for retinopathy of prematurity (ROP) are laser photocoagulation or the anti-VEGF agent bevacizumab administered by intravitreal injection.

A focus on the developmental environment of the preterm infant in intensive care has resulted in minimal handling and a reduction in noise levels.

Interpretation of Investigations

The renal blood supply in markedly preterm infants may be compromised by even relatively brief systemic hypotension resulting in acute renal failure. Check the urea and electrolytes regularly and monitor urinary output (should be at least 2 mL/kg/h) and watch out for hyperkalaemia.

Ibuprofen can cause renal impairment with water retention and hyponatraemia. It is imperative when prescribing ibuprofen that the infant is weighed daily, that the urine output is measured, and that the serum sodium is monitored. Hyponatraemia is also a risk factor for periventricular leukomalacia (PVL).

Plain abdominal x-ray in NEC shows typically dilated bowel loops with pneumatosis.

Coagulase negative *Staphylococcus* (CONS) is the predominant pathogen in late onset sepsis and hand hygiene is a key factor in prevention.

The screening assessment for ROP looks at the zone, the stage, the extent and the presence of plus disease.

Pitfalls to Avoid

Preparation is key in the delivery of a markedly preterm infant. Ensure all equipment needed is at hand and that experienced staff arrive prior to delivery. Thermoregulation is critical to prevent hypothermia. Delayed cord clamping for 1 minute is now widely practiced.

Use blended oxygen (start at 30 per cent) and avoid high oxygen saturation to reduce the chance of lung inflammation from oxygen toxicity.

If the gut perforates in NEC, the mortality is 20 to 40 per cent. Surgery is required if obstruction occurs and insertion of a Penrose drain is recommended if perforation occurs secondary to NEC.

To reduce the risk of bronchopulmonary dysplasia, use blended oxygen at birth, optimise caloric intake, use CPAP and caffeine citrate with minimal time on ventilation, maintain saturations between 92 and 95 per cent, and use preferentially volume-targeted ventilation if needed.

Infants under 32 weeks' (31 weeks and 6 days) gestation or under 1500 g should be screened for ROP.

Key References

Bordini, B., Toth, H., & Basel, D. (Eds.). *Nelson pediatric symptom-based diagnosis* (pp. 682–700). Elsevier.

British Association of Perinatal Medicine. (n.d.). British Association of Perinatal Medicine: leading excellence in perinatal Care. https://www.bapm.org/

British Association of Perinatal Medicine. (2019). *Perinatal management of extreme preterm birth before 27 weeks of gestation: A framework for practice.* https://www.bapm.org/resources/80-perinatalmanagement-of-extremepreterm-birth-before-27-weeksof-gestation-2019.

Buonocore, G., Bracci, R., & Weindling, A. M. (Eds.). (2020). *Neonatology: A practical approach to neonatal diseases.* Springer Nature.

Flood, V. H., & Scott, J. P. (2018). Bleeding and thrombosis. In R. M. Kliegman & P. S. Lye (Eds.). *Nelson pediatric symptom-based diagnosis.* Elsevier.

Fox, G. F. (2020). Controversies and discussion of the BAPM Framework for the perinatal management of extreme preterm birth before 27 weeks of gestation. *Archives of Disease in Childhood – Education and Practice, 106*(3), 160–161.

Hilditch, C., Liersch, B., Spurrier, N., et al. (2018). Does screening for congenital cytomegalovirus at birth improve longer term hearing outcomes? *Archives of Disease in Childhood, 103*(10), 988–992.

Jones, I. H., & Hall, N. J. (2020). Contemporary outcomes for infants with necrotising enterocolitis – a systematic review. *The Journal of Pediatrics, 220,* 86–92.

Loughlin, L., Knowles, S., Twomey, A., & Murphy, J. F. A. (2020). The neonatal early onset sepsis calculator; in clinical practice. *Irish Medical Journal, 113*(4), 57.

National Collaborating Centre for Women's and Children's Health. (2010). *Neonatal jaundice.* https://www.nice.org.uk/guidance/cg98/evidence/full-guideline-245411821.

Prasad, M., & Babiker, M. O. (2016). Fifteen-minute consultation: when is a seizure not a seizure? part 1, the younger child. *Archives of Disease in Childhood – Education and Practice, 101*(1), 15–20.

Sachdeva, M., Murki, S., Oleti, T. P., & Kandraju, H. (2015). Intermittent versus continuous phototherapy for the treatment of neonatal non-hemolytic moderate hyperbilirubinemia in infants more than 34 weeks of gestational age: a randomized controlled trial. *European Journal of Pediatrics, 174*(2), 177–181.

Shah, P. S., Rau, S., Yoon, E. W., et al. (2020). Actuarial survival based on gestational age in days at birth for infants born at <26 weeks of gestation. *The Journal of Pediatrics, 225,* 97–102.

Yeaney, N. K., Murdoch, E. M., & Lees, C. C. (2009). The extremely premature neonate: Anticipating and managing care. *BMJ, 338,* b2325.

9 Evaluating the Dysmorphic Child

ALF NICHOLSON and JAMES O'BYRNE

One child in 40 (2.5 per cent) is born with a significant major congenital anomaly. This may be a malformation, deformation, disruption or dysplasia, and such anomalies account for a significant percentage of perinatal and childhood mortality and may indicate an underlying syndrome. Evaluating for dysmorphic features is a challenging area heavily reliant on training, experience and a great sense of old-fashioned 'gestalt', which is essentially the recognition of patterns of dysmorphic features. It takes time to acquire and sharpen the skills needed to recognise patterns of malformations and dysmorphism. These dysmorphic features may be subtle and, although they can be supported by dysmorphology databases, it may seem overwhelming for students encountering paediatrics for the first time. However, most clinicians and examiners will only expect an undergraduate to recognise the most common dysmorphic syndromes, particularly Down syndrome (discussed in detail later in this chapter).

A *syndrome* is a description of a group of signs and symptoms and a pattern of anomalies wherein there is often a *known cause* or *an assumption about causation*. The term can include chromosomal disorders such as Down syndrome, single gene disorders such as Noonan syndrome, or non-genetic causes such as foetal alcohol spectrum disorder. An *association* can be defined as a clustering of anomalies occurring more frequently than by chance but with no prior assumption about causation. An example is the association of Vertebral anomalies, Anal anomalies, TracheooEsophageal fistula, Renal anomalies, and Limb anomalies (VATERL association). A *sequence* can be defined as a primary malformation resulting in secondary deformations. For instance, Pierre Robin sequence is a grouping of cleft palate, micrognathia or retrognathia, and glossoptosis, which can have at least 20 different causes.

Many of the syndromes, described before the genomic era, are eponymous or named after those who described them (singly or as a group) – Klippel–Trenaunay–Weber syndrome is one example. More recently, the trend has been to name the syndrome to reflect the molecular defect, such as PIK3CA-related overgrowth spectrum. Features of a syndrome can evolve over time, and some conditions that may be difficult to recognise in the neonatal period or early infancy may become more apparent as the child gets older.

Karyotype analysis is traditionally used to confirm the diagnosis of a trisomy such as Down, Edwards or Patau syndrome, or sex chromosome disorders such as Turner syndrome (45 X0). However, this technique is used less and less as newer technologies such as microarray or whole exome or genome sequencing have far higher diagnostic yields for genetic disorders. Despite the advent of multi-omics technologies, genetic testing will not always provide a molecular diagnosis. It is also important to bear in mind that new technology has limitations, and karyotype analysis is more likely to detect apparently balanced translocations rather than whole exome sequencing. If a malformation syndrome diagnosis is made, it is important to remember that syndromes can be caused by chromosomal, single gene (monogenic), multiple gene (polygenic) disorders or by environmental agents. A clinical genetic opinion should also be sought, as a clinical geneticist can often help greatly in achieving a diagnosis and in counselling parents about the likelihood of similar problems occurring in other family members.

Inheritance Patterns

Recognised patterns of inheritance include autosomal dominant, autosomal recessive, X-linked, and mitochondrial. Some autosomal dominant conditions, for instance neurofibromatosis type 1 (NF1), can either be due to a significant variant (mutation) on the *NF1* gene or be due to a de novo or new mutation that has occurred in the patient. Patients may display variability in *penetrance* (whether features of the condition develop) and *expression* (how the features of the condition manifest). Penetrance is very high in someone with a significant variant on the *NF1* gene; however, different people with NF1 can express the condition in different ways, with some showing mild expression with a few skin lesions and others with severe intracerebral complications. Thus, the *expression* of NF1 is highly variable.

In autosomal recessive inheritance (e.g. sickle cell anaemia) both parents are usually unaffected carriers and there is a one in four risk of a child being affected, whether male or female.

In X-linked recessive disorders (e.g. Duchenne muscular dystrophy), there is often a relatively high de novo mutation rate and affected boys may not have any family history of the condition. If a female carries the gene variant, she is usually either unaffected or mildly affected due to the presence of a second 'healthy' X chromosome but can also sometimes be severely affected.

Components of a Dysmorphic Evaluation

HISTORY

Take a family history and construct a three-generation family tree. Enquire about obstetrical history, including assisted reproduction, prior miscarriages, stillbirths or neonatal deaths, viral illnesses (such as cytomegalovirus) during pregnancy, exposure to potential teratogens (noting the timing in pregnancy), and gestational diabetes. Ask about birth history and behaviour in the neonatal period. Chart developmental progress to date and take a detailed developmental history. Ask about consanguinity in a sensitive manner.

EXAMINATION

Start with a general observation. An experienced eye may be able to diagnose a syndromic child on initial observation alone; however, a systematic approach can help the less experienced examiner to reach the correct diagnosis. Note whether features are unilateral or bilateral. Examination of the parents should also be considered, and it should be noted whether the features are familial or not.

GROWTH PARAMETERS

Always measure the head circumference, weight and length, chart on the age-appropriate centile chart and look for prior measurements to assess growth trends if available. Check if stature is proportionate or disproportionate. If disproportionate, this should prompt further measurements (e.g. upper vs lower segment and height and/or arm span). Note the build of the child and describe any abnormalities such as central obesity.

FACE

Allowing for ethnic features, note if the overall facial features are normal or familial. Note if face is symmetrical or not during rest or when crying. Poor muscle tone of the facial muscles may indicate primary muscle disease.

CRANIUM

Prominence of the metopic ridge is seen in 10 per cent of infants, but it may also indicate exposure to valproate use in pregnancy.

Macrocephaly, frontal bossing and a large chin are characteristic of Sotos syndrome.

At birth, the anterior fontanelle size varies from 1 to 5 cm in diameter. A very large anterior fontanelle may indicate Zellweger syndrome or cleidocranial dysostosis. Zellweger syndrome may present with features of profound neonatal hypotonia, epicanthic folds, Brushfield spots and early onset seizures. Cleidocranial dysostosis may present with features of frontal and parietal bossing and a groove along the metopic suture along with hypoplastic or absent clavicles.

Severe craniosynostosis with syndactyly of hands and feet may indicate Apert syndrome.

EARS

The finding of low set ears is a common observation often made inaccurately. To assess the position of the ears, draw an imaginary horizontal line through the outer canthi of both eyes – the ears are judged to be low set if the root of the helix of the pinna falls below this line. Low set ears are a very non-specific feature and can indicate one of many syndromes; examples include Noonan syndrome (Fig. 9.1), Smith–Lemli–Opitz syndrome and 22q11 deletion.

Microtia (a small, underformed ear) can be a feature of Treacher Collins syndrome and CHARGE (C-coloboma of eye, H-heart defects, A-atresia choanae, R-retarded growth,

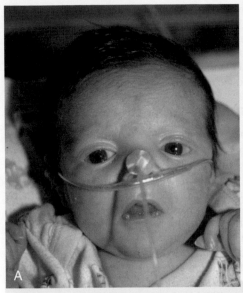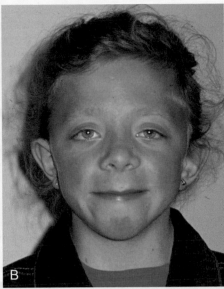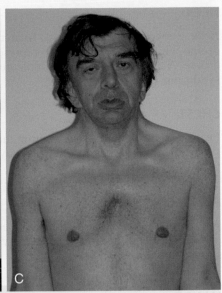

Figure 9.1 Noonan syndrome: (A) in a baby presenting with cardiomyopathy at birth (which later resolved); (B) in a child; and (C) in a 57-year-old man. (Reproduced with permission from Ellard S, Cleaver R et al (Eds) Emery's Elements of Medical Genetics and Genomics, Sixteenth Edition. Elsevier Ltd, 2022.)

G-genital abnormalities, and E-ear abnormalities) syndrome. Many other syndromes are associated with unusual ear shapes. Ear lobe creases and preauricular pits are a feature of Beckwith–Wiedemann syndrome. While a single preauricular skin tag can be normal, multiple preauricular skin tags may indicate Goldenhar or Townes–Brocks syndrome.

EYES

Although newborns may have periorbital oedema over the first few days of life due to delivery, it is important to examine each eye to ensure it is present and normally formed.

Prominent epicanthic folds are characteristic of Down syndrome, and in Stickler syndrome may present in late childhood. Prominent epicanthic folds may also be a normal variant.

Almond shaped eyes are classically associated with Prader–Willi syndrome with other presentations including hypotonia and severe feeding issues in early infancy.

Proptosis is a feature of Crouzon, Apert and Pfeiffer syndromes, where an abnormal head shape will also be seen due to craniosynostosis. Bilateral ptosis is a feature of Moebius syndrome (sixth and seventh cranial nerve palsies), myotonic dystrophy and Noonan syndrome. Carefully measure the interpupillary distance to assess for hypertelorism where the distance may be increased (e.g. in Robinow syndrome, often occurring with anteverted nares) or hypotelorism where the distance is reduced (e.g. in Smith–Lemli–Opitz syndrome, often occurring with second/third toe syndactyly).

Blue sclerae are a feature of osteogenesis imperfecta, Ehlers–Danlos syndrome, Russell Silver syndrome (small size with hemihypertrophy) and Kabuki syndrome.

EYEBROWS

Synophrys (eyebrows meeting in the middle) is a feature of mucopolysaccharidoses, Cornelia de Lange syndrome and Sanfilippo syndrome (which can be associated with sleep and behavioural issues). An interrupted or arched eyebrow may indicate Kabuki syndrome.

NOSE

A widened nasal bridge or increased intercanthal distance may indicate Waardenburg syndrome and is associated with a white forelock, deafness and heterochromia irides. A high nasal bridge in infancy may suggest Wolf–Hirschhorn syndrome, while a depressed nasal bridge may suggest Stickler syndrome. Extension of the nasal columella below the level of the alae nasi is characteristic of Rubinstein–Taybi syndrome (with associated broad thumbs). Anteverted nares are characteristic of Williams Beuren syndrome, where supravalvular aortic stenosis, hypercalcaemia and a stellate iris are often observed, and Robinow syndrome.

MOUTH

A smooth philtrum is characteristic of foetal alcohol syndrome while a long philtrum with infraorbital skin creases may indicate foetal valproate syndrome. Spotty pigmentation on the lips may indicate Peutz-Jeghers syndrome while lip pits may indicate Van der Woude syndrome.

TONGUE

Macroglossia may indicate Beckwith–Wiedemann or Simpson–Golabi–Behmel syndrome.

CHIN

Micrognathia or retrognathia (a small or displaced backwards lower jaw) may indicate Pierre Robin sequence (usually with midline cleft palate due to the failure of the fusion of the palatal shelves and backward displacement of the tongue) and Stickler syndrome (high myopia, retinal detachment, and early onset arthropathy).

NECK

Neck webbing is a feature of Turner and Noonan syndrome while a short neck may represent Klippel-Feil syndrome. A branchial sinus may indicate branchio-oto-renal syndrome.

CHEST

Pectus excavatum and carinatum may indicate Marfan syndrome while accessory nipples may indicate foetal valproate syndrome.

ABDOMEN

An omphalocoele may indicate Beckwith-Wiedemann syndrome while inguinal hernias may be seen in William syndrome.

HANDS

Post-axial polydactyly (extra digit on the ulnar side) may run in families or be associated with Trisomy 13, Ellis-van-Crefeld syndrome (heart murmur and multiple oral frenula), or Jeune asphyxiating thoracic dystrophy (very narrow thorax and immediate respiratory distress after birth). Pre-axial polydactyly (extra digit on the radial side) is a feature of Robinow syndrome with other features being anteverted nares, cleft palate and hypertelorism.

Overlapping fingers with syndactyly and small nails are characteristic of Trisomy 18 (Edwards syndrome). Clinodactyly may indicate Russell Silver syndrome. Hypoplastic thumbs may indicate VACTERL association, thrombocytopaenia-aplastic radii (TAR), Holt–Oram syndrome or Fanconi anaemia. Deep palmar creases with redundant skin may indicate Costello syndrome.

FEET

Toe syndactyly (second and third digit) may be a familial trait but in the context of other medical issues might indicate Smith–Lemli–Opitz or Pallister–Hall syndromes. Foot oedema in the newborn period may indicate Turner or Noonan syndromes.

SKIN

Multiple café-au-lait patches may signify NF1 or Russell-Silver syndrome.

Down Syndrome

Down syndrome (DS) is the most common human chromosomal disorder with a birth prevalence of one in 1000 overall, but its incidence increases markedly with maternal age, increasing from one in 1500 at 17 years of age to one in 100 at 40 years of age. Ninety-five per cent of trisomy 21 cases are due to non-disjunction during meiosis. Three per cent are due to translocation (usually long arm of chromosome 21 attached to chromosome 14). In translocation there is no maternal age

effect. Seventy-five per cent of translocations arise de novo, but in the remaining 25 per cent it may be maternal or paternal in origin. Two per cent of cases of trisomy 21 are due to mosaicism, where a non-disjunction event takes place during early cell division and does not affect all cells. The fraction of cells affected varies widely, as does phenotypic expression.

CLINICAL FEATURES

Many cases of Down syndrome are identified antenatally, but for others the diagnosis is usually made rapidly after birth, as features are readily recognisable by experienced midwifery staff. As Down syndrome has lifelong implications, communication of the diagnosis should be by an experienced doctor (specialist registrar or consultant paediatrician) who can address parental concerns. Where possible, this sensitive consultation should take place with both parents and the newborn present in a private setting. It is preferable if another person can hold the pager and mobile phone so that there are no disruptions.

The discussion should always start with congratulations on the birth of their baby. Parents will remember how the diagnosis was disclosed. It is not appropriate to withhold the diagnosis until the chromosomal analysis is available, and so parents are counselled that there is a clinical suspicion of DS, but that the final definitive diagnosis may take 2 weeks or more. Discussion should focus on the features seen, the immediate health concerns (if present), and likely developmental and other long-term progress. It is essential to communicate the diagnosis to all healthcare practitioners who will be caring for the infant and to refer to early intervention services who can provide community based multidisciplinary developmental support to the family. Parents are often anxious for an early confirmation of the diagnosis. FISH (fluorescent in situ hybridisation) analysis can give results in 24 to 48 hours but will only detect an extra copy of chromosome 21 (non-disjunction), and not a translocation. It is prudent to counsel parents on the importance of waiting for the complete chromosomal analysis report, which may take up to 2 weeks to produce.

Classical features of Down syndrome include epicanthic folds, Brushfield spots of the iris, a depressed nasal bridge, a protruding tongue, and brachycephaly (Fig. 9.2).

The most important clinical feature during the newborn period is marked hypotonia, although this varies between infants.

Other observable features include a single palmar crease, fifth finger clinodactyly and a wide sandal gap between the hallux and second toe.

Down syndrome is rarely associated with other abnormalities such as gastrointestinal problems, duodenal atresia or stenosis, Hirschsprung disease (less than 1 per cent), tracheo-oesophageal fistula and imperforate anus may occur. Infant feeding may be poor even without a structural gastrointestinal problem.

HEALTH SURVEILLANCE FOR CHILDREN WITH DS

Growth

Short stature is a recognised characteristic of most people with Down syndrome. Across nearly all ages, the average

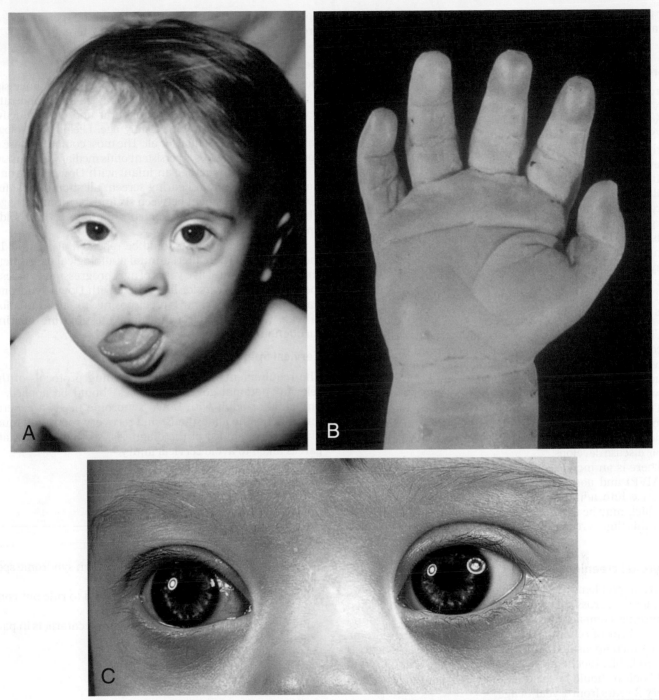

Figure 9.2 Down syndrome. (A–C) Young infant. Flat facies, straight hair, protrusion of tongue, single crease on inturned fifth finger. (Reproduced with permission from del Campo, M., Lyons Jones, K., et al. (Eds.), (2022). *Smith's recognizable patterns of human malformation* (8th ed.). Elsevier Inc.)

height of children with Down syndrome is equivalent to the second centile for the general population. National Down syndrome specific growth charts are essential for assessing linear growth. Regular surveillance of growth, general health, and nutritional and thyroid status allow early identification of pathological causes of growth retardation.

Clinical observation and the body mass index (BMI) data included on charts aid in the assessment of those who are overweight, and for the prevention of obesity. Although there is a high prevalence of overweight and obesity among people with Down syndrome, it is not inevitable. As with

the general population, weight is influenced by environment as well as biological factors.

Measurements should be recorded at least annually throughout childhood and at regular intervals in adult life. Regular measurements detect early indicators of many of the medical problems over-represented in people with Down syndrome.

Those with DS do have an adolescent growth spurt, but it is usually less marked than in the general population. Puberty may occur at an earlier age and requires anticipation together with education and support for parents and for the child. Early onset of puberty has a limiting effect on final height.

Cardiac Screening

Between 40 and 50 per cent of babies with Down syndrome have congenital heart defects and of these, 30 to 40 per cent have complete atrioventricular septal defects (AVSD). Most AVSDs can be successfully treated if the diagnosis is made early and the baby is referred for full corrective surgery before irreversible pulmonary vascular disease (PVD) is established.

It is highly desirable to establish the cardiac status of every child with Down syndrome by 6 weeks of age. Early cardiac surgery is desirable for children with Down syndrome with surgically correctable cardiac lesions to optimise outcomes. It is important to note that some cardiac defects such as ventricular septal defect (VSD) or atrial septal defect (ASD) may not present with a murmur on examination in the first few weeks of life.

The following course of action is advised to detect all serious cardiac abnormalities:

- Clinical examination, electrocardiogram (ECG) and echocardiogram (ECHO) should be performed by someone with appropriate paediatric cardiological training for all newborns with Down syndrome, ideally by the age of 6 weeks (particularly those with a superior QRS axis on ECG).
- Those with suspected problems should be referred for immediate paediatric cardiology review so that intervention, if necessary, can take place before pulmonary vascular disease develops.
- There is an increased incidence of mitral valve prolapse (MVP) and aortic regurgitation (AR) from late adolescence into adulthood in people with Down syndrome, which may be asymptomatic. Repeat cardiac evaluation at this time is recommended.

Thyroid Screening

Thyroid problems (usually hypothyroidism) occur more frequently across all age groups of children with Down syndrome compared to the general population. Around 10 per cent of school age children with Down Syndrome have uncompensated hypothyroidism. Clinical diagnosis is unreliable. Biochemical screening (T4, TSH and thyroid antibodies) should be lifelong and carried out at least once every 2 years from 1 year of age.

Ophthalmology

Refractive errors and strabismus (squint) may occur at an early age and persist into childhood. Over 50 per cent of children with Down syndrome will require glasses in primary school; however, screening begins much earlier.

All newborns with Down syndrome should have an eye examination carried out at 4 to 6 weeks to exclude urgent problems such as congenital glaucoma, cataract and other eye abnormalities.

Between 18 months and 2 years of age, all children with Down syndrome should have a formal ophthalmological examination. This should include orthoptic assessment, refraction and fundus examination. A further formal ophthalmological examination should be performed at around 4 years of age and every 2 years thereafter.

Hearing Impairment

Over 50 per cent of people with Down syndrome have significant hearing impairment, which may be mild, moderate, severe, or profound, and sensorineural and/or conductive hearing loss may be present at any age. Lifelong audiological surveillance is essential for all. The most common cause of conductive hearing loss is persistent otitis media with effusion.

Irrespective of whether an infant with Down syndrome has passed a neonatal hearing screen, all should have full audiological assessment between six and 10 months of age. This should include measurement of auditory thresholds, impedance testing and otoscopy.

All three assessments should be repeated at around 18 months of age. Thereafter, annual audiological assessment should be done until five years of age, progressing to assessment every two years for life. People with Down syndrome have narrow ear canals predisposing to accumulation of wax, which can affect impedance testing and hearing throughout life.

Cervical Spine Disorders

The requirements and clinical screening protocols of the relevant national governing bodies should be applied. If any child or adult with Down syndrome needs a general anaesthetic, the anaesthetist and recovery room staff must always be reminded of the diagnosis, so that appropriate care is taken to avoid cervical injury.

Summary of Management Guidelines

AT 6 WEEKS

- Assess feeding and chart growth on Down syndrome specific charts
- Ensure cardiac assessment has occurred to rule out congenital heart disease
- Recheck eye examination for congenital cataracts in particular
- Monitor head growth

FOR THE FIRST 2 YEARS

- regular routine clinical reviews
- formal audiology review
- growth and developmental assessment at each visit
- check for early onset squint
- check thyroid function tests (T4, TSH) annually

PRESCHOOL AGE GROUP (UNDER 5 YEARS OF AGE)

- growth assessment and chart on specific centile charts
- use BMI conversion charts over 2 years of age if concerns about being overweight
- dental examination
- eye examination (look for refractive errors, formal fundoscopy and orthoptic screening)

- annual thyroid function tests (TFT) and coeliac screening tests
- full audiological review

SCHOOL-AGE GROUP (5 TO 18 YEARS OF AGE)

- annual review
- echocardiography in early adult life to rule out mitral valve prolapse
- two yearly audiological review and ophthalmological examination including refraction and fundal examination and focusing ability
- two yearly T4 and TSH (venous) or TSH (finger prick) annually

Dysmorphic Features and Recognition of Selected Other Syndromes

ANGELMAN SYNDROME

Typical facial appearance is with a wide, smiling mouth, prominent chin and deep-set eyes, profound speech impairment, ataxia, wide based and stiff legged gait, excitable personality, inappropriately happy affect and microcephaly (Fig. 9.3). Angelman syndrome is usually due to a deletion on the maternal copy of chromosome 15q11–13.

DIGEORGE SYNDROME (22Q11 DELETION)

Typical facial appearance includes short palpebral fissures, wide and prominent nasal bridge and squashed nasal tip, delayed speech milestones, congenital heart disease (classically conotruncal defects such as the tetralogy of Fallot), cleft palate, submucosal cleft palate or bifid uvula, short stature, polymicrogyria, neonatal hypocalcaemia and poor problem-solving skills in school-aged children with later risk of psychiatric symptoms (Fig. 9.4).

EDWARDS SYNDROME (TRISOMY 18)

Edwards syndrome is a condition that is usually lethal in the newborn period. It occurs in about one in 3000 births.

Affected children are usually extremely small and have congenital heart disease, exomphalos, renal anomalies, clenched hands with overlapping fingers (Fig. 9.5), and rocker bottom feet. Over 95 per cent are new genetic events in the affected infant.

FOETAL ALCOHOL SYNDROME (FAS)

Classical features include a history of maternal alcohol misuse with both pre- and postnatal growth restriction. The combination of three facial features (short palpebral fissures, smooth philtrum and thin upper lip) is characteristic of FAS (Fig. 9.6), with impairment in at least three of the following domains: motor function, cognition, language, academic achievement, memory and attention, executive function (including impulse control and hyperactivity) and social skills or communication.

FRAGILE X SYNDROME

Fragile X syndrome, previously thought to be the most common inherited cause of intellectual disability, is now estimated to affect between one in 4000 to 7000 males and one in 6000 to 11,000 females. Fragile X syndrome occurs because of unstable DNA in the *FMR1* gene of the X chromosome (hence the name!). Males with more than 200 triplet repeats will be symptomatic and have intellectual disability. Common presentations are with delayed speech and language, autism spectrum disorder, anxiety and issues with attention. Characteristic physical features are difficult to identify in infants and young children. Characteristic features in older children include large and protruding ears, a prominent jaw, a high forehead, and personality features such as shyness, lack of eye contact followed by friendliness, verbosity and echolalia, stereotypical hand movements, and macroorchidism (Fig. 9.7).

KLINEFELTER SYNDROME (47, XXY)

Boys with Klinefelter syndrome rarely present in childhood. However, a significant number can have delayed puberty, teenage gynaecomastia or fertility issues in later life.

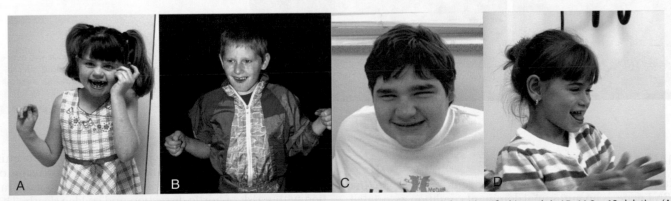

Figure 9.3 Pictured are individuals with genetic test-proven Angelman syndrome. The UBE3A defect identified in each is 15q11.2–q13 deletion (A and B), UBE3A mutation (C), and paternal uniparental disomy (D) (Reproduced with permission from Pascual, J. M., & Rosenberg, R. N. (2020). *Rosenberg's molecular and genetic basis of neurological and psychiatric disease* (6th ed.). Elsevier.)

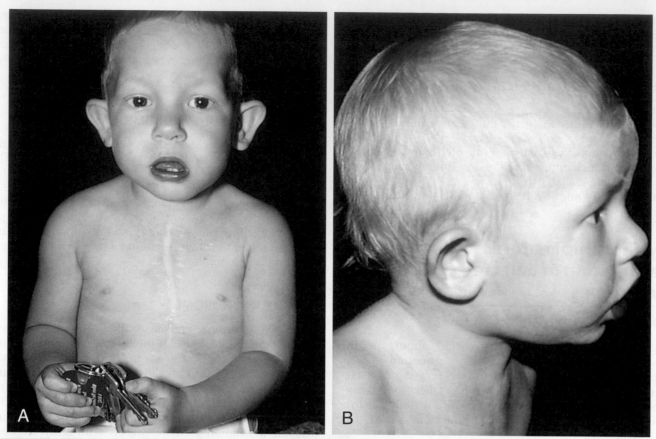

Figures 9.4   22q11 syndrome. Characteristic facial features: frontal (A) and lateral (B) views. Note the micrognathia; hypertelorism; low-set, malformed ears; and smooth philtrum. Also note the midline scar from repair of a cardiac defect. (Reproduced with permission from Chong, H., Green, T., et al. (2018). Allergy and immunology. In *Zitelli and Davis' atlas of pediatric physical diagnosis* (pp. 101–135). © 2018.)

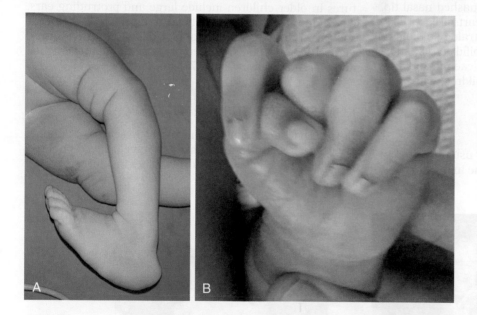

Figure 9.5   (A, B) Rocker bottom foot and overlapping fingers in Edward's syndrome. (Reproduced with permission from Pediatrics for Medical Graduates. Thirunavukkarasu AB (Ed) Elsevier, a division of RELX India, Pvt. Ltd, 2017)

MARFAN SYNDROME

Marfan syndrome, due to a pathogenic variant on the *FBN1* gene, is an autosomal dominant condition associated with an increased arm span (exceeding the child's height), joint laxity, arachnodactyly, ectopia lentis and aortic root dilatation (Fig. 9.8). Other features seen include pectus carinatum, scoliosis, pes planus and medial protrusion of the hip acetabulum. It is associated with aortic root dilatation with a risk of aortic dissection and sudden death. The revised Ghent criteria (2010) are the current diagnostic criteria for Marfan.

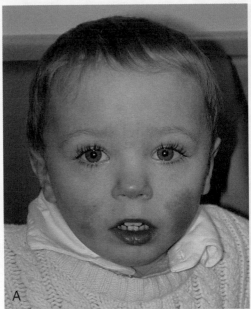

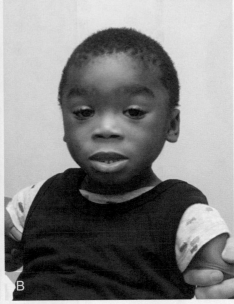

Figure 9.6 (A) A 2-year-old child with foetal alcohol syndrome (FAS). Note the depressed nasal root, short palpebral fissures, smooth philtrum and thin upper lip vermilion. (B) FAS in an African American child. Note short palpebral fissures, smooth philtrum and relatively thin upper lip vermilion compared to the lower. (Reproduced with permission from Jorde, L. B., Carey, J. C., & Bamshad, M. J. (2020). *Medical genetics* (6th ed.). Elsevier – Health Sciences.)

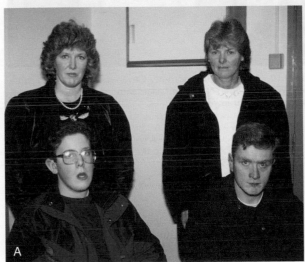

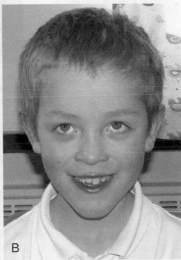

Figure 9.7 (A) A family affected by fragile X syndrome. Two sisters, both carriers of a small *FRAXA* mutation inherited from their father, have had affected sons with different degrees of learning difficulty. (B) A young boy with typical facial features of fragile X syndrome, showing a long face, long ears and slightly large head. (Reproduced with permission from Turnpenny, P. D., Ellard, S., & Cleaver, R. (2021). *Emery's elements of medical genetics and genomics* (16th ed.). Elsevier – Health Sciences.)

PATAU SYNDROME (TRISOMY 13)

Patau syndrome is a condition that is usually lethal in the newborn period. Affected children have congenital heart disease, polydactyly, cleft lip and palate, microcephaly, and often a single frontal lobe in their brain (holoprosencephaly) (Fig. 9.9). Like Down syndrome, 95 per cent are new genetic events, but there are rare translocation forms which can run in families.

PRADER–WILLI SYNDROME

Features of Prader–Willi syndrome (PWS) include truncal hypotonia with early feeding difficulties, typical facial appearance (almond shaped eyes, narrow forehead, triangular shaped upper lip), rapid weight gain from 1 to 6 years of age, moderate learning disabilities, small hands and feet

with short stature, typical behavioural phenotype with ritualistic behaviours, temper outbursts and stubbornness (Fig. 9.10). PWS is usually due to a deletion on the paternal copy of chromosome 15q11–13.

RETT SYNDROME (MECP2 PATHOGENIC VARIANTS)

Girls with Rett syndrome have relatively normal early development with later loss of skills (especially in communication and speech), deceleration in head growth, dyspraxia, small, cold feet, stereotyped motor mannerisms (hand flapping or complex whole-body movements), social withdrawal with little or no speech, spontaneous outbursts of laughing or crying and reduced responses to pain (Fig. 9.11).

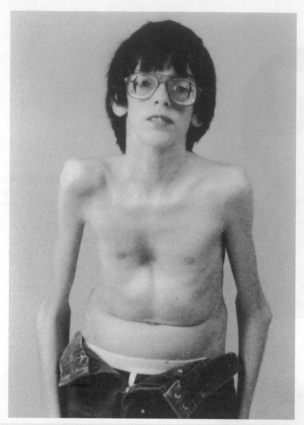

Figure 9.8 Clinical appearance of a patient with Marfan syndrome. Note the extreme myopia (represented by thick corrective lenses), severe pectus excavatum, long limbs and arachnodactyly. The patient also has scoliosis and severe planovalgus feet. This appearance is typical of patients with florid manifestations of the syndrome. (Reproduced with permission from Herring, J. A. (2021). *Tachdjian's pediatric orthopaedics: From the Texas Scottish Rite Hospital for Children* (6th ed., 2 vols). Elsevier – Health Sciences.)

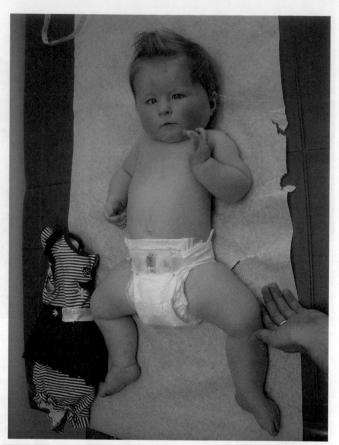

Figure 9.10 Prader–Willi syndrome. Eleven-month-old child with Prader–Willi syndrome. Note the facial features and the hypotonic posture of hips and lower extremities. (Reproduced with permission from Hickey, S. E., Thrush, D. L., Walters-Sen, L., Reshmi, S. C., Astbury, C., Gastier-Foster, J. M., & Atkin, J. (2013). A case of an atypically large proximal 15q deletion as cause for Prader–Willi syndrome arising from a de novo unbalanced translocation. *European Journal of Medical Genetics*, *56*(9), 510–514.)

TURNER SYNDROME (45,X)

Girls with Turner syndrome are more prone to congenital heart disease, classically coarctation of the aorta, and may also have renal anomalies. They may present in the newborn period with these anomalies in the presence or absence of 'puffy hands and feet' caused by lymphoedema. Short stature is a feature and spontaneous puberty is unlikely, due to ovarian dysgenesis (Fig. 9.12).

WILLIAMS–BEUREN SYNDROME

Characteristic facial features of Williams–Beuren syndrome include periorbital fullness, long philtrum, flattened nasal bridge, wide mouth, full lips, full cheeks, widely spaced teeth and stellate irises of the eyes (Fig. 9.13).

Other features include variable learning disabilities, congenital heart disease (75 per cent supravalvular aortic stenosis), hyperacusis, phonophobia, hypercalcaemia in early infancy, renal artery stenosis, and a very friendly personality with a short attention span and high distractibility. Williams–Beuren syndrome is usually due to a deletion of chromosome 7q11 encompassing the *ELN* gene.

(Box 9.1)
(Box 9.2)

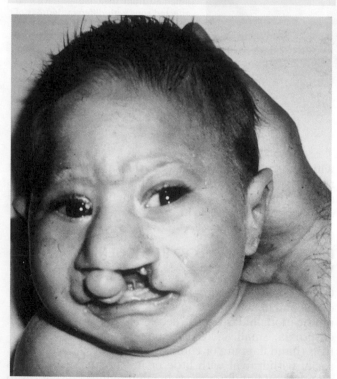

Figure 9.9 Facial features of trisomy 13 (Patau syndrome). (Reproduced with permission from McIntosh, N., Helms, P. J., Smyth, R. L., & Logan, S. (2008). *Forfar and Arneil's textbook of pediatrics* (7th ed.). Churchill Livingstone.)

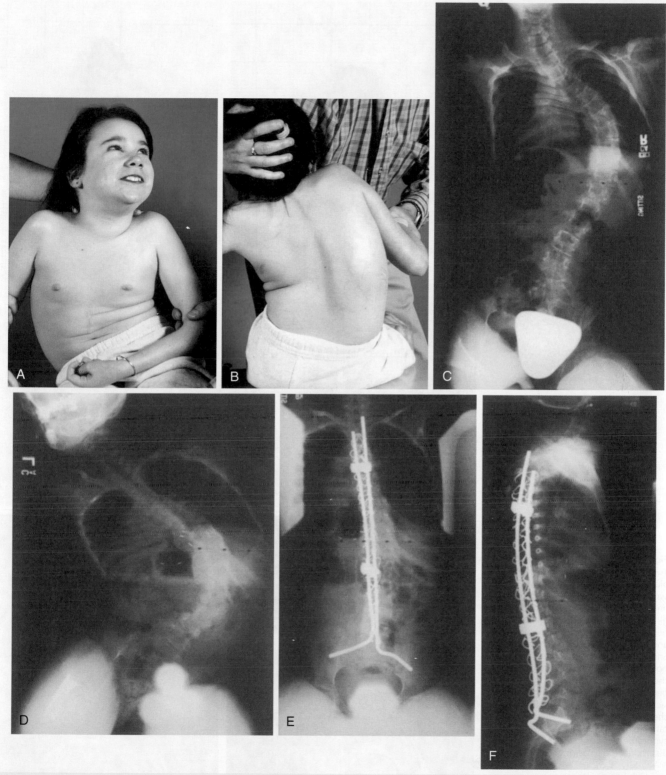

Figure 9.11 (A and B) Clinical appearance of a 10-year, 7-month-old girl with scoliosis secondary to Rett syndrome. (C) Radiograph obtained at 7 years, 9 months of age. (D) The curve had worsened by 10 years, 6 months of age. (E and F) Posterior spinal fusion with Luque-Galveston instrumentation was performed. (Reproduced with permission from Herring, J. A. (2021). *Tachdjian's pediatric orthopaedics: From the Texas Scottish Rite Hospital for Children* (6th ed., 2 vols). Elsevier – Health Sciences.)

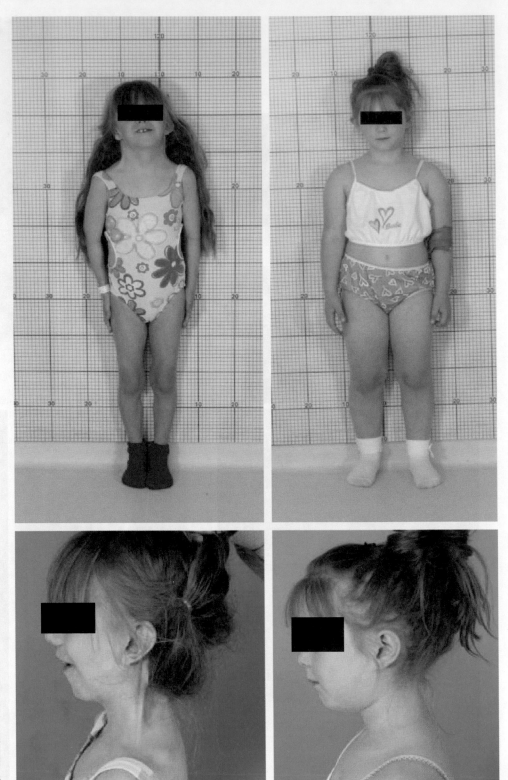

Figure 9.12 Phenotypic variability in Turner syndrome. Both of these 7-year-old girls with short stature have Turner syndrome with a 45, X karyotype confirmed in analysis of 50 lymphocytes. The girl on the left was diagnosed at birth because of prominent neck webbing and low-set and posteriorly rotated ears. She also has micrognathia and a low posterior hairline. In contrast, the girl on the right was diagnosed at age 7 years because of short stature without "classical" stigmata of Turner syndrome, and she is more typical of the clinical presentation of the majority of girls with Turner syndrome diagnosed in the 21st century. (Reproduced with permission from Sperling MA (2021) *Sperling Pediatric Endocrinology*, Fifth Edition Elsevier Inc.)

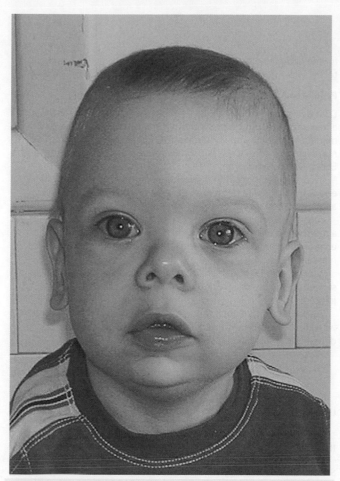

Figure 9.13 Presenting phenotype and clinical evaluation in a cohort of 22 patients with Williams–Beuren syndrome. Broad forehead with bitemporal narrowing, low nasal root, bulbous nasal tip, periorbital fullness, stellate iris pattern, malar flattening, full lips. (Reproduced with permission from Giovanni, B., Biamino, E., et al. (2007). *European Journal of Medical Genetics, 50*(5), 327–337. © 2007.)

Box 9.1   Key Points

It takes time to learn to recognise patterns of malformations and dysmorphism, and it may seem overwhelming for students encountering paediatrics for the first time. Hence a systematic approach is required.

Karyotype analysis will confirm trisomies such as Down, Edwards or Patau syndrome, or sex chromosome disorders such as Turner syndrome (45 X0). More sophisticated technologies, such as next generation sequencing, are increasingly being used to establish the diagnosis at a molecular level.

Take a family history and construct a three-generation family tree. Enquire about obstetric history, including prior miscarriages, viral illnesses (such as cytomegalovirus (CMV)) during pregnancy, exposure to potential teratogens and gestational diabetes.

An undergraduate student would be expected to recognise the features of Down syndrome (DS). For the postgraduate student, focus on elements of good practice relating to the initial review and meeting with the family, which will involve counselling (see case scenario above).

Ninety-five per cent of DS cases are due to non-disjunction during meiosis, and 3 per cent are due to translocation (usually long arm of chromosome 21 attached to chromosome 14). In translocation, there is no maternal age effect. The most important clinical feature during the newborn period is marked hypotonia, although this varies between infants.

Other observable features in DS include a single palmar crease, fifth finger clinodactyly and a wide sandal gap between the hallux and second toe.

It is highly desirable to establish the cardiac status of every child with Down syndrome by 6 weeks of age. Cardiac defects occur in 40 per cent of cases, the most common of which are endocardial cushion defects, followed by VSD, secundum ASD, and Fallot's tetralogy.

Around 10 per cent of school-age children with Down syndrome have uncompensated hypothyroidism.

Classical features of foetal alcohol syndrome (FAS) include a history of maternal alcohol misuse with both pre- and postnatal growth restriction. The combination of three facial features (short palpebral fissures, smooth philtrum and thin upper lip) is characteristic of FAS.

BOX 9.2   A Newborn With Down Syndrome

A live female infant was delivered weighing 3 kg at birth to a 32-year-old para [2+0] mother with an uneventful antenatal history. Her two older children are perfectly healthy and no first trimester screening took place. In the delivery suite, the midwives were concerned about some facial features suggestive of Down syndrome (DS) and called the on-call paediatric team. The most obvious feature evident was profound hypotonia and the on-call team contacted the paediatrician on-call seeking advice. Both parents were very anxious to know if anything was amiss, and the consultant came immediately to the hospital to assess the infant and speak to both parents.

Clinical Pearls

The initial meeting with the parents is one they will remember forever, and key good practice points (following feedback from parents and adapted from Smith et al) include the following:

Speak to parents about the diagnosis of DS as soon as appropriate to do so, after the birth. Introduce yourself properly to both parents and explain your concerns clearly.

Ensure that both parents are present or, if a single parent, that a friend or family member is invited to the conversation.

Ensure the environment provides privacy and confidentiality. Firstly, congratulate parents on the birth of their child and give the baby to the parents to hold if possible.

Refer to the baby by name. If the baby has not been named yet, parents recommended to address the baby as 'your daughter' or 'your son'. Emphasise that first and foremost their newborn infant will require the very same care as any other baby: feeding, bathing, burping, cuddles and so on.

Tell parents that their child will meet their milestones (walking, talking, attending school) but will just need extra help to do so.

Continued

BOX 9.2   A Newborn With Down Syndrome—cont'd

Acknowledge that this is a shock and a change in their expectations and that they will of course require time to adjust to this unexpected news and that they will feel confused, upset or frightened.

Emphasise that help is available and that they will be linked with support services. Offer to provide written information and reliable internet resources and a list of parents with children with DS to contact.

Designate a point-of-contact person to be available in the first few weeks to offer support, direct to relevant services and provide advice.

Speak slowly and simply. Do not be rushed; and give time for the parents to ask questions and return to check in on the family predischarge home to answer questions and offer support.

Interpretation of Investigations

95 per cent of trisomy 21 cases are due to non-disjunction during meiosis. Three per cent are due to translocation (usually long arm of chromosome 21 attached to chromosome 14).

FISH (fluorescent in situ hybridisation) analysis can give results in 24 to 48 hours but will only detect an extra copy of chromosome 21 (non-disjunction) and not a translocation. It is preferable to wait for the complete chromosomal analysis report which may take up to 2 weeks.

Pitfalls to Avoid

DS is usually clinically obvious from birth with marked hypotonia a major feature, but other syndromes may also be associated with marked hypotonia and should be distinguishable. Epicanthic folds may also be a normal variant, for example in Stickler syndrome and Ehlers-Danlos syndrome.

Cardiac defects occur in 40 per cent of cases, most commonly endocardial cushion defects and thereafter VSD, secundum ASD and Fallot's tetralogy.

Cardiac defects such as VSD or ASD may not present with a murmur on examination in the first few weeks of life and so echocardiogram is required even If the newborn cardiac exam is reassuring.

Cervical spine x-rays in children have **no** predictive validity for subsequent acute dislocation or subluxation at the atlantoaxial joint.

Cardiac evaluation including echocardiography for all people with Down syndrome should be repeated early in adult life to detect mitral valve prolapse

 Video on the topic Assessment of dysmorphic features is available online at Elsevier eBooks+.

Key References

Down's Syndrome Association. (n.d.). www.downs-syndrome.org.uk

Fisher, P. G. (2020). Who should care for children with Down syndrome? *The Journal of Pediatrics, 218,* 1–4.

Green, A. J., & O'Byrne, J. J. (2020). *Pediatric clinical genetics.* In P. Puri (Ed.), *General principles and newborn surgery.* Springer-Verlag.

Horridge, K. A. (2011). Assessment and investigation of the child with disordered development. *Archives of Disease in Childhood – Education and Practice, 96*(1), 9–20.

Ivan, D. L., & Cromwell, P. (2014a). Clinical practice guidelines for management of children with Down syndrome: Part I. *Journal of Pediatric Health Care, 28*(1), 105–110.

Ivan, D. L., & Cromwell, P. (2014b). Clinical practice guidelines for management of children with Down syndrome: Part II. *Journal of Pediatric Health Care, 28*(3), 280–284.

O'Byrne, J. J., Sweeney, M., Donnelly, D. E., Lambert, D. M., Beattie, E. D., Gervin, C. M., et al. (2017). Incidence of fragile X syndrome in Ireland. *American Journal of Medical Genetics. Part A, 173*(3), 678–683.

Reardon, W. (2015). *The bedside dysmorphologist* (2nd ed.). Oxford University Press.

Smith, A. M., O'Rahelly, M., & Flanagan, O. (2019). Disclosing the diagnosis of Down syndrome: The experience of 50 Irish parents. *Archives of Disease in Childhood, 104*(8), 820–821.

Online References

Management guidelines for children and adolescents with Down syndrome in Ireland. https://downsyndrome.ie/wp-content/uploads/2018/05/Medical-Management-Guidelines-for-Children-and-Adolescents-with-Down-Syndrome-with-updates-2009-and-2015.pdf

SIGN guidelines for foetal alcohol syndrome (2019). https://www.sign.ac.uk/media/1092/sign156.pdf

10 Anaemia – The Pale Child

AENGUS O'MARCAIGH

Newborn infants have relatively high circulating haemoglobin, which reaches its lowest point (usually 10 g/dL) at 2 to 3 months of age. The mean haemoglobin level rises gradually during childhood (equally for boys and girls) until puberty, when the level in boys is 20 per cent higher than in girls.

The main reasons for a child to become anaemic divide into three main categories:

- acute blood loss usually obvious from the history
- impaired bone marrow production of red blood cells
- increased peripheral destruction by haemolysis of red blood cells with a key feature is an increase in reticulocytes

History

A full dietary history is very important. At-risk groups include preterm infants or those exclusively breast-fed. Children who consume high levels of cow's milk and too little meat or green vegetables are also at risk.

A congenital haemolytic anaemia is suggested by a neonatal history of significant hyperbilirubinaemia. A positive family history of anaemia, splenectomy or cholecystectomy is relevant. Certain drugs (such as antimalarials and sulphonamides) may lead to acute haemolysis in children if they are deficient in glucose-6-phosphate dehydrogenase (G6PD).

HISTORICAL CLUES IN ASSESSING ANAEMIA

- Age – Iron deficiency presents in toddlers while sickle cell anaemia and beta thalassaemia tend to present as foetal haemoglobin disappears at 4 to 8 months of age.
- Family history – Hereditary spherocytosis (HS) is autosomal dominant, G6PD is X-linked recessive and sickle cell anaemia and beta thalassaemia are autosomal recessive with ethnicity playing an important role. Hereditary spherocytosis is seen in North America and northern and western Europe. Beta thalassaemia is seen especially in the Mediterranean, the Middle East and the Far East, while sickle cell anaemia is seen in Africa, African Americans and those from the Caribbean.
- Nutrition – Strict vegetarian diets or excess cow's milk in the diet, especially in toddlers, can predispose to iron deficiency.
- Drugs – especially acute haemolysis precipitated by drugs in G6PD
- Poor weight gain and diarrhoea – Consider malabsorption in both coeliac disease and Crohn's disease.
- Overt GI blood loss – Consider a Meckel's diverticulum or ulcerative colitis.

EXAMINATION

General assessment includes assessing weight and height and charting on appropriate centile charts. Look for conjunctival pallor (Fig. 10.1), pale palmar creases, leukonychia and koilonychia and scleral icterus. General examination also includes assessment for bruising and ecchymoses, lymphadenopathy and hepatosplenomegaly.

In thalassaemia major, features of extramedullary haematopoiesis may present as 'chipmunk facies' with prominent cheekbones, frontal bossing and dental malocclusion (Fig. 10.2). Signs of haemolysis in hereditary spherocytosis may include pallor, scleral icterus and splenomegaly. The infiltrative process in the bone marrow such as leukaemia may present with lymphadenopathy and/or hepatosplenomegaly. Children with Fanconi anaemia are usually of short stature and can have hyperpigmentation, hypoplastic thumbs and radial aplasia.

LABORATORY EVALUATION

The reticulocyte count is essential to categorise anaemia (Fig. 10.3). An elevated reticulocyte count is suggestive of a bone marrow response to either acute blood loss (usually clinically obvious) or increased red cell destruction or haemolysis. In the setting of a normal haemoglobin, the absolute reticulocyte count is approximately 40 to 160 $\times$ 10^9/L.

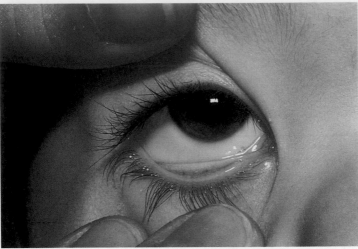

Figure 10.1 Child with severe anaemia. Pale conjunctiva may be seen in the patient with severe anaemia. (Reproduced with permission from Zitelli, B. J., McIntire, S. C., & Nowalk, A. J. (2012). *Zitelli and Davis' atlas of pediatric physical diagnosis: Expert consult – online and print* (6th ed.). Saunders. Fig. 11.4A.)

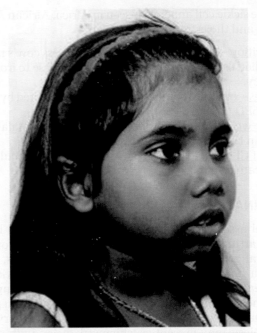

Figure 10.2 A young girl with beta-thalassaemia demonstrating mild frontal bossing of the right forehead with prominent cheekbones, and dental malocclusion. (Reproduced with permission from Hockenberry, M. J., & Wilson, D. (2006). In C. Jackson (Ed.), *Wong's nursing care of infants and children* (8th ed.). Mosby.)

The mean corpuscular volume (MCV) can be used to classify anaemia, with a high MCV indicating macrocytosis while a low MCV suggests microcytosis. Normal ranges of MCV are age-related.

Microcytosis in childhood is associated with iron deficiency, thalassaemia and rare conditions such as sideroblastic anaemia and lead poisoning (Fig. 10.4).

Macrocytosis is rare in childhood and may relate to vitamin B12 or folate deficiency, Fanconi and Blackfan-Diamond anaemias, and, rarely, severe hypothyroidism. Vitamin B12 and folate deficiencies are rarely seen in childhood. Check RBC folate to measure folate levels. B12 deficiency can be seen in children on strict vegan diets,

congenital pernicious anaemia and terminal ileitis in Crohn disease.

Evaluation of the white cell count (WBC), WBC differential and platelet count are imperative in the setting of anaemia. Consider bone marrow aspiration or biopsy if either neutropenia or thrombocytopenia in addition to anaemia.

An elevated indirect (unconjugated) bilirubin and elevated LDH can be seen in acute or chronic haemolysis. The direct Coombs test will be positive in autoimmune haemolytic anaemia.

Haemoglobin electrophoresis will identify haemoglobinopathies such as sickle cell disease or thalassaemia.

If there is acute haemolysis, check red blood cell enzyme levels (e.g. G6PD).

Iron Deficiency Anaemia

By far the most common type of anaemia is iron deficiency, in which nutritional intake of iron lags behind the increased demands linked to growth or there is excessive blood loss. Toddlers and adolescent females are at highest risk of iron deficiency. Delayed weaning onto solids, prolonged breast-feeding and excessive cow's milk intake are major causative factors in toddlers. Excessive bleeding with menses may predispose to anaemia in adolescent females. Severe iron deficiency can have other effects apart from clinical features of anaemia, including pica, impaired cognitive development, koilonychia (spoon-shaped nails), angular stomatitis, glossitis and marked irritability. Supplemental iron for 3 months is the treatment of choice.

Transient erythroblastopaenia of childhood is rare, occurs mainly in infants and toddlers, and is in essence a transient arrest in erythropoiesis with a striking fall in haemoglobin. The full blood count shows a normocytic anaemia and a very low reticulocyte response. Recovery is spontaneous and very few require blood transfusion.

Blackfan-Diamond anaemia is a red cell aplasia typically presenting with severe anaemia in infancy and a low reticulocyte count. Treatment is with corticosteroids and some may require repeated blood transfusions.

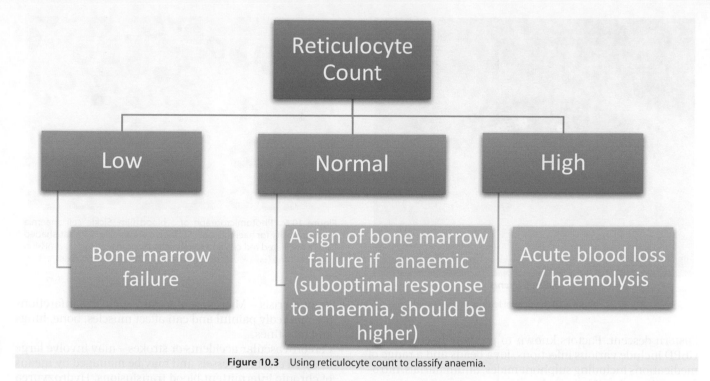

Figure 10.3 Using reticulocyte count to classify anaemia.

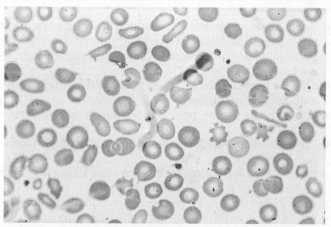

Figure 10.4 The blood in iron deficiency: microcytic, hypochromic anaemia. There is central pallor of the erythrocytes and poikilocytosis with elongated (pencil or cigar cells). (Reproduced with permission from Cross, S. (2018). *Underwood's pathology: A clinical approach* (7th ed.). Elsevier – Health Sciences.)

In Fanconi anaemia, overt haematological manifestations may not present until 4 to 5 years of age although thumb abnormalities and radial changes may be picked up much sooner. Increased chromosomal breakages are seen, and bone marrow transplantation is the treatment of choice.

Beta Thalassaemia

In beta thalassaemia, a deficiency of beta globin chain production leads to the precipitation of alpha globin chains with consequent ineffective erythropoiesis.

Children with beta thalassaemia typically present with severe anaemia at six to 12 months of age, when haemoglobin

production transitions from the foetal (HbF) to the adult form (HbA). Typical presentation is with fatigue, irritability, pallor, jaundice and marked hepatosplenomegaly. Expansion of the marrow space leads to both frontal bossing and prominent cheekbones with most patients being of Mediterranean or Asian descent.

Laboratory tests show a severe anaemia, a low MCV and target cells on peripheral blood smear. Long term blood transfusions (to maintain haemoglobin over 10 g/dL) and chelation to prevent iron overload are the mainstays of treatment. Ultimately, bone marrow transplantation is curative.

Hereditary spherocytosis

HS is typically seen in children and adults of northern European descent and is inherited largely as an autosomal dominant condition. There is often a family history of anaemia and splenectomy or cholecystectomy.

Classical features include anaemia, mild icterus and splenomegaly. Spherocytes are evident on blood smear. There is an elevated reticulocyte count. Diagnosis is made via the eosin-5-maleimide (EMA) binding test, which is far less onerous than the traditional osmotic fragility test.

Newborns may present with jaundice on day 1 of life, requiring either phototherapy or occasionally exchange transfusion. There is a broad spectrum of severity of HS with viral illnesses sometimes worsening haemolysis and thereby precipitating anaemia.

G6PD

G6PD should always be considered if a presentation with acute haemolytic anaemia and scleral icterus (Fig. 10.5) in a boy, especially if of African, Mediterranean or Middle

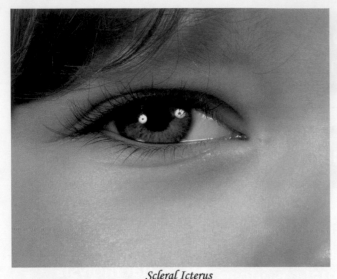

Scleral Icterus

Figure 10.5   Scleral Icterus.

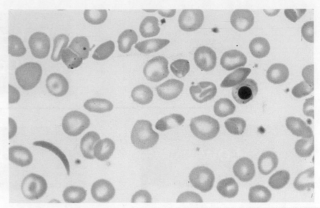

Figure 10.6   Photomicrograph of a blood film. Sickle cell anaemia (homozygosity for haemoglobin S). Shown are a sickle cell boat-shaped cells, a nucleated red cell and target cells. (Reproduced with permission from *Dacie and Lewis Practical Haematology* (12th ed.). (2016). Elsevier.)

Eastern descent. Factors known to promote haemolysis in G6PD include various infections, fava beans and a range of medications including sulphonamides, antimalarials, nitrofurantoin and nalidixic acid.

Sickle Cell Anaemia (SS Disease)

A single amino acid substitution in the beta globin chain, namely valine for glutamic acid in the number six position, is the change seen in sickle haemoglobin. Sickle cell anaemia is inherited as an autosomal recessive condition. Carriers have what is termed sickle cell trait. Carriers have a normal blood film and are not anaemic but may occasionally experience haematuria.

In sickle cell anaemia, children are invariably anaemic, have a high reticulocyte count, and sickle cells can be seen on blood film (Fig. 10.6). The haemoglobin solubility test (Sickledex) should not be used to make the diagnosis but rather haemoglobin electrophoresis.

The three key manifestations of sickle cell anaemia are chronic haemolytic anaemia, vaso-occlusion with consequent ischaemic injury to tissues and an increased susceptibility to infection. Infants under 4 to 6 months of age often show no clinical manifestations due to high foetal haemoglobin. Thus, selective neonatal screening is important in at-risk populations.

CLINICAL MANIFESTATION OF SS DISEASE

- Anaemia – a chronic anaemia from 4 to 6 months of age. In older children, folate supplements are required due to excess haemolysis.
- Aplastic crisis – tends to be acute and may be precipitated by parvovirus infection. A key marker is a drop in reticulocyte count.
- Sequestration crisis – is life-threatening and rapid in onset with shock, pallor, and massive splenomegaly.
- Haemolytic crisis – may be associated with coincident G6PD deficiency.
- Dactylitis – is a presentation seen in infancy and may be a presenting feature of SS disease (Fig. 10.7).

- Painful crisis – Microvascular vaso-occlusive infarctions are markedly painful and can affect muscles, bone, lungs and intestines.
- Cerebrovascular accidents or strokes – may involve large or small cerebral vessels and may be managed by means of chronic intermittent blood transfusions. Hydroxyurea and a blood transfusion programme reduces the risk of stroke in SS disease.
- Acute chest syndrome – Presents with cough and need for oxygen due to hypoxia which may progress to hypoventilation, with severe hypoxia and marked pulmonary infiltrates (Fig. 10.8).
- Chronic lung disease – relates to restrictive lung disease with pulmonary fibrosis.
- Cholelithiasis – may present with biliary colic or acute cholecystitis.
- Priapism – very painful and may be associated with eventual impotence.
- Renal – may have a renal concentrating defect and may present with a microscopic haematuria.
- Growth failure – may be helped by nutritional supplements and may have associated pubertal delay.
- Propensity to infections – Autoinfarction of the spleen due to microvascular occlusion leads to a functional asplenia by 3 to 4 years of age. This predisposes the child to infections such as *Streptococcus pneumoniae*, *Haemophilus influenzae*, *Salmonella*, severe *Mycoplasma pneumoniae* and *Escherichia coli*.
- Psychological problems – relate to the chronic nature of the condition and frequent episodes of severe pain.

The newborn screening programme in selected populations helps to identify homozygous sickle cell anaemia and complex heterozygotes such as haemoglobin SC. The key risks of SS disease include invasive pneumococcal disease, acute splenic sequestration, acute chest syndrome and stroke.

SS disease has a 600-fold increased risk of pneumococcal infection. For the prevention of infection, lifelong penicillin prophylaxis (no easy task), pneumococcal vaccination and annual influenza vaccination are recommended.

Transcranial doppler detects cerebral vascular changes and annual transcranial doppler screening is an accepted international standard from the age of 2 to 3 years. If a child with SS disease experiences a stroke, there is an increased risk of a recurrence of stroke. Regular blood transfusions can reduce this risk and should continue throughout childhood.

Hydroxyurea should be considered in children and adults who have frequent painful episodes or who have had acute chest syndrome.

Acute Leukaemia

Acute leukaemia is the most common form of childhood cancer. The risk of leukaemia is increased in Down syndrome, Fanconi anaemia, ataxia telangiectasia, neurofibromatosis type 1, Wiskott-Aldrich syndrome and Noonan syndrome.

Infants and children with Down syndrome are at increased risk of transient abnormal myelopoiesis (TAM). Common findings in TAM include an elevated number of circulating immature myeloid cells, nucleated red cells, megakaryocyte fragments and either a high or low platelet count. TAM tends to present in the neonatal period and, in most cases, tends to resolve spontaneously without intervention. If there are severe symptoms due to TAM, low

dose cytarabine chemotherapy is recommended – however, be aware that about 20 per cent will develop acute megakaryocytic leukaemia by 4 years of age.

There are **two** key presenting features in acute leukaemia:

■ Bone marrow failure – leading to anaemia, neutropenia and thrombocytopenia
■ Tissue infiltration – leading to bone pain, lymphadenopathy and hepatosplenomegaly

About 80 per cent of childhood leukaemia is acute lymphoblastic (ALL) with the remainder being acute myeloid (AML).

Common presenting features include pallor, petechiae and unexplained bruising, tiredness, lethargy, bone pain or a limp, lymphadenopathy, hepatosplenomegaly or enlarged testes.

DIAGNOSIS

Definitive diagnosis is via the detection of leukaemic blast cells on either blood film or bone marrow aspirate. Bone marrow aspirate or biopsy is the definitive test in which one looks for morphology (presence of blast cells), immunophenotyping and cytogenetic analysis.

There are a few differential diagnoses to be considered including infections (in particular, EBV or parvovirus), aplastic anaemia, idiopathic thrombocytopenic purpura and juvenile idiopathic arthritis.

TREATMENT OF LEUKAEMIA

Standardised treatment protocols, which are internationally agreed upon, have led to an overall excellent prognosis. Age over 10 years or a WBC over 50 are adverse prognostic factors. Chemotherapy is the mainstay of treatment. Rarely, bone marrow transplantation is required for children who do not enter remission or who later relapse. The overall treatment plan for ALL lasts up to 3 years. Treatment for AML is shorter in duration (under 6 months) but more intensive and highly myelosuppressive. A poor response to treatment in AML requires bone marrow transplantation for cure.

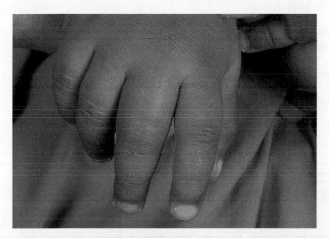

Figure 10.7 Sickle cell dactylitis. (With permission from Hoffbrand. (2010). *Color atlas of clinical hematology.* Elsevier.)

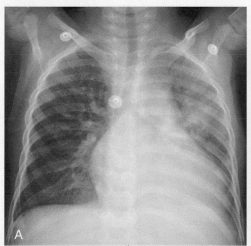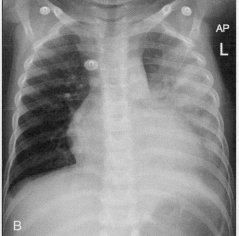

Figure 10.8 Acute chest syndrome in a 4-year-old boy with sickle cell anaemia. (A) Chest radiograph obtained at admission shows focal retrocardiac and faint left upper lobe airspace opacity. There is moderate cardiomegaly. (B) Chest radiograph obtained 1 day later shows consolidation near the entire left lung. (Reproduced with permission from Donnelly, L. (Ed.). (2021). *Fundamentals of pediatric imaging* (3rd ed.). Academic Press.)

COMPLICATIONS OF LEUKAEMIA

- Febrile neutropenia is defined as a neutrophil count under 0.5 and fever above 38 degrees. Treatment is with urgent broad-spectrum intravenous antibiotics after taking blood and line cultures.
- Opportunistic infections include *Pneumocystis carinii*, fungal infections and both gram-positive and gram-negative organisms.
- Anaemia and thrombocytopaenia require transfusions.

- Tumour lysis syndrome is characterised by hyperkalaemia, hyperphosphataemia, hyperuricaemia and hypocalcaemia, and may occur spontaneously or soon after starting treatment. This may lead to urate nephropathy.

Currently, well over 90 per cent of ALL children achieve complete remission and the vast majority will be cured.

(Box 10.1)

(Box 10.2)

(Box 10.3)

Box 10.1   Key Points

When assessing for anaemia, look for conjunctival pallor, pale palmar creases, leukonychia and koilonychia and scleral icterus. General examination includes assessment for bruising and ecchymoses, lymphadenopathy and hepatosplenomegaly.

A neonatal history of significant hyperbilirubinaemia may point to a possible diagnosis of a congenital haemolytic anaemia which may be further supported by a positive family history of anaemia.

A raised reticulocyte count suggests a bone marrow response to either increased haemolysis or acute blood loss.

Haemoglobin electrophoresis identifies haemoglobinopathies such as sickle cell disease or thalassaemia.

Assessment of red blood cell enzyme levels (e.g. G6PD) may be necessary if acute haemolysis is evident.

Severe iron deficiency can have other effects apart from clinical features of anaemia not least pica, impaired cognitive development, koilonychia (spoon-shaped nails), angular stomatitis, glossitis and marked irritability.

Typical presentation of beta thalassaemia is with fatigue, irritability, pallor, jaundice and marked hepatosplenomegaly. Frontal bossing and prominent cheekbones are typically seen. Most patients are of Mediterranean or Asian descent.

Classical features of hereditary spherocytosis include anaemia, mild icterus and splenomegaly.

In sickle cell anaemia (SS disease), children are invariably anaemic, have a high reticulocyte count and sickle cells can be seen on blood film. Diagnosis is made by haemoglobin electrophoresis.

Complications of SS disease include invasive pneumococcal disease, acute splenic sequestration, acute chest syndrome and stroke.

Common presenting features of acute leukaemia include pallor, petechiae and unexplained bruising, tiredness, lethargy and bone pain or a limp, lymphadenopathy, hepatosplenomegaly or enlarged testes.

Currently well over 90 per cent of acute lymphoblastic leukaemia (ALL) children achieve complete remission.

Box 10.2   A Pale Toddler

A 3-year-old presents with a history of a pallor and repeated viral infections. He is well grown and consumes over 1 L of milk per day. He is noted to have mild speech delay. He has significant pallor, but his height and weight are both on the 75th centile. His family doctor requested a full blood count, the results of which showed a haemoglobin of 7.0 g/dL with a microcytic picture on blood film.

Clinical Pearls

This young toddler has dietary iron deficiency anaemia (IDA).

There is a higher risk of IDA in infants (especially preterm), toddlers and adolescent females.

Ingesting cow's milk in large quantities leads to IDA because cow's milk is low in iron, it promotes occult blood loss in the gut, and non-haem iron absorption is inhibited by the casein in cow's milk.

Parental advice should be to avoid cow's milk in large quantities and in tea.

IDA is treated with a daily iron supplement and continued for 2 to 3 months post a normal Hb level to replenish iron stores. Compliance with treatment is a significant issue.

Interpretation of the Blood Film

The presence of hypochromic, microcytic red cells most often suggests iron deficiency anaemia, but this picture may also be seen in beta thalassaemia.

Decreased ferritin levels are helpful in diagnosing iron deficiency.

In iron deficiency, the mean corpuscular haemoglobin concentration (MCHC) is low and the MCHC is often normal in beta thalassaemia, where target cells are often seen.

In hereditary spherocytosis, spherocytes are evident on blood smear and there is an elevated reticulocyte count. In sickle cell anaemia, a high reticulocyte count and sickle cells seen on the blood film are typical features.

Potential Pitfalls

Be aware that serum ferritin is an acute phase reactant and can be falsely normal in an intercurrent viral illness.

Transient erythroblastopaenia of childhood is rare and represents a transient arrest in erythropoiesis with a striking fall in haemoglobin. The full blood count shows a normocytic anaemia and a very low reticulocyte response.

Iron deficiency anaemia may be one of the presenting features of coeliac disease with coincident presentation with severe failure to thrive.

In sickle cell anaemia, infants younger than 4 to 6 months usually show no clinical manifestations due to high foetal haemoglobin. Thus, selective neonatal screening is important in at-risk populations.

In leukaemia, the peripheral blood film will usually show blast cells, but may be normal if blast cells are confined to the bone marrow. If leukaemia is clinically suspected, a bone marrow aspiration and biopsy should be performed.

Box 10.3   12-Month-Old With Sickle Cell Anaemia

A 12-month-old male had a positive sickle screen at birth and was being followed up at the specialist haematology clinic. He had been fully immunised and had normal developmental milestones. He presented with an episode of collapse with marked pallor and looked markedly unwell. His examination revealed circulatory shock with marked tachycardia and delayed capillary refill time of 5 seconds. He had a 6 cm spleen palpable on abdominal examination. A diagnosis of acute splenic sequestration was made, and urgent transfusion was required.

Clinical Pearls

Sickle cell disease is a common and life-threatening haematological disorder that affects millions of people worldwide.

Outcomes for children with sickle cell disease have improved considerably due to newborn screening, penicillin prophylaxis, pneumococcal immunisation, and education about disease complications.

An acute drop in haemoglobin levels can occur in acute splenic sequestration (as above) and transient red cell aplasia from parvovirus B19 infection.

In infancy, vaso-occlusion leads to dactylitis, whereas older children and adults develop pain affecting bones in the extremities, chest, and back. Non-steroidal anti-inflammatory drugs and opioids are used for pain relief.

Functional asplenia increases the risk of life-threatening infections.

Stroke predominantly affects children. For acute stroke, the treatment is prompt exchange transfusion followed by regular transfusions to prevent stroke recurrence.

Hydroxycarbamide given orally once daily is effective in reducing the number of painful crises per year in children and in adults. Stem cell transplantation is currently the only cure in sickle cell disease, with an HLA-matched sibling transplantation enabling an overall survival approaching 90 per cent.

Interpretation of Investigations

Diagnosis of sickle cell anaemia is by haemoglobin electrophoresis.

Transcranial Doppler allows measurement of the mean velocity of blood flow in the intracranial arteries and identifies children with abnormal velocities who are at the highest risk of developing stroke.

In children with sickle cell anaemia, presentation with a rapid onset of neurological symptoms warrants investigation with both brain MRI and magnetic resonance angiography (MRA).

Microalbuminuria is an early sign of sickle nephropathy and may progress to nephrotic syndrome.

Pitfalls to Avoid

Both stroke and acute chest syndrome are potentially life-threatening and require prompt specialist care.

Primary stroke prevention identifies children at highest risk using transcranial Doppler screening followed by a transfusion programme.

Quantification of liver iron content using MRI helps in picking up iron overload relating to repeated transfusions.

Both diastolic cardiac dysfunction and pulmonary hypertension are associated with increased mortality in adults.

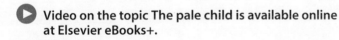 **Video on the topic The pale child is available online at Elsevier eBooks+.**

Key References

Brandow, M. (2018). Pallor and anemia. In R. M. Kliegman, P. S. Lye, B. Bordini, H. Toth, & D. Basel (Eds.), *Nelson pediatric symptom-based diagnosis* (pp. 661–681). Elsevier.

Dick, M. C. (2008). Standards for the management of sickle cell disease in children. *Archives of Disease in Childhood. Education and Practice Edition, 93*(6), 169–176.

Hanna, M., Fogarty, M., Loughrey, C., Thompson, A., Macartney, C., Thompson, A., et al. (2019). How to use… iron studies. *Archives of Disease in Childhood. Education and Practice Edition, 104*(6), 321–327.

McNaughten, B., Thompson, A., Macartney, C., & Thompson, A. (2018). How to use… a blood film. *Archives of Disease in Childhood. Education and Practice Edition, 103*(5), 263–266.

National Heart, Lung, and Blood Institute. (2020, September 1). *Sickle cell disease: Overview*. Department of Health and Human Services, National Institutes of Health. https://www.nhlbi.nih.gov/health-topics/sickle-cell-disease.

Needs, T., Gonzalez-Mosquera, L. F., & Lynch, D. T. (2020, May 23). Beta Thalassemia. In *StatPearls*. Treasure Island: StatPearls Publishing.

Olusanya, B. O., Kaplan, M., & Hansen, T. W. R. (2018). Neonatal hyperbilirubinaemia: a global perspective. *The Lancet. Child & Adolescent Health, 2*(8), 610–620.

Ware, R. E., de Montalembert, M., Tshilolo, L., & Abboud, M. R. (2017). Sickle cell disease. *The Lancet, 390*(10091), 311–323.

11 Congenital Heart Disease

TERENCE PRENDIVILLE

The birth prevalence of congenital heart disease (CHD) is seven to eight per 1000 liveborn infants, accounting for nearly one-third of all major congenital malformations. Approximately 30 per cent of CHD is thought to be related to genetic syndromes and is frequently accompanied by additional extracardiac manifestations. It is an important cause of morbidity and mortality during infancy and childhood, and early detection makes a significant impact on the outcome. Pulse oximetry screening of newborn infants has been proven to assist in the diagnosis of CHD along with a careful newborn clinical examination prior to discharge. In the current era, once diagnosed, the prognosis for most children with CHD is excellent with a longer-term focus on optimising neurodevelopmental outcome. A diagnosis of CHD frequently causes significant psychological distress for parents that a multidisciplinary approach to care delivery can help ameliorate.

Antenatal Screening for Congenital Heart Disease

It is now recommended that all foetuses be screened for congenital heart disease at 20 weeks' gestation. Those with a concern for CHD raised on ultrasound will be seen promptly by a paediatric cardiologist. Parents who have congenital heart disease or a previous child with congenital heart disease have an increased risk (2 to 3 per cent) of an affected child. Over 50 per cent of serious congenital heart lesions are now detected antenatally, allowing planned delivery and elective transfer to a specialist cardiology service soon after birth. In a large population-based longitudinal study of severe congenital heart disease in Norway published in 2020, over 80 per cent of preoperative deaths occurred in a palliative care setting, and significant comorbidities and univentricular congenital heart defects were commonly seen.

Newborn Examination for Congenital Heart Disease

The identification of congenital heart disease is one of the essential aspects of the newborn examination. Ideally, the heart should be examined between 6 and 48 hours after birth to allow time for the ductus arteriosus to close and for the pulmonary vascular resistance to start to fall. The current reality is, however, that most newborn examination is performed prior to discharge on day one of life.

Parents should be aware that symptoms of poor feeding, lethargy, or tachypnoea after discharge from the postnatal ward should prompt urgent medical review, as haemodynamically significant CHD can present at any time over the first few weeks of life.

Infants with clinically significant congenital heart disease (most notably, duct-dependent lesions) may present

113

with tachypnoea, persistent recession, excessive sweating, poor feeding and central cyanosis. These infants should be referred for urgent paediatric cardiology opinion.

Murmurs can be heard in 2 per cent of newborns but only 30 to 40 per cent of these will have congenital heart disease. Pulse oximetry performed on all infants pre-discharge improves the pickup rate for congenital heart disease and thus pulse oximetry is a simple, safe and acceptable test that adds value to existing screening and helps identify critical congenital heart disease that would otherwise go undetected.

SPECIFIC CONDITIONS ASSOCIATED WITH CONGENITAL HEART DISEASE

It is known that 40 per cent of children with Down syndrome have associated congenital heart disease, typically atrioventricular septal defects, and clear protocols for identifying congenital heart disease are now in place.

Children with Marfan's syndrome can develop aortic root dilatation (60 to 80 per cent) or mitral valve prolapse (40 to 80 per cent), requiring medical therapy or surgical repair throughout their lifetime. Noonan syndrome is classically associated with pulmonary valve stenosis, atrial septal defects or hypertrophic cardiomyopathy. Turner syndrome is associated with coarctation of the aorta (12 per cent) along with a bicuspid aortic valve (30 per cent). Williams syndrome (a microdeletion syndrome including the Elastin gene, ELN) is associated with supravalvar aortic stenosis (45 to 75 per cent) or pulmonary artery stenosis (40 per cent). 22q11.2 microdeletion syndrome, also known as DiGeorge syndrome, is associated with CHD in up to 75 per cent of cases, classically tetralogy of Fallot, truncus arteriosus or an interrupted aortic arch.

Heart Murmurs

A murmur is due to turbulent blood flow within the heart or great vessels. It is important in diagnosis to note the timing and the site of all murmurs (Figs 11.1 and 11.2). Just under 1 per cent of children born have a structural heart defect, and most have a murmur. It is, however, important to note that an infant can have significant CHD with a relatively normal cardiac auscultatory exam. Frequently, those same infants will have other clinical indicators of CHD, including cyanosis (saturation less than 95 per cent), tachypnoea, relative tachycardia, an active praecordium, a gallop rhythm or a 3-cm palpable liver edge.

INNOCENT MURMURS

Many children (up to 50 per cent) will have innocent murmurs (no underlying cardiac anomaly), most often noted at the time of an intercurrent fever or anaemia. These murmurs, when noted, can be a source of significant anxiety and concern to parents.

PULMONARY FLOW MURMUR

This low intensity murmur is ejection systolic and is heard over the left sternal border with radiation to the pulmonary area. This murmur is best heard in the supine position and is louder on expiration and the murmur is diminished by sitting up or holding breath in inspiration. This murmur is

similar in quality to the murmur associated with an atrial septal defect but without the accompanying fixed splitting of S_2 from right ventricular volume overload.

PERIPHERAL PULMONARY ARTERIAL STENOSIS MURMUR

Physiological turbulence at the proximal origins of the left and right pulmonary arteries may lead to this murmur. The murmur is typically grade 1 or 2 in intensity and often radiates to the posterior lung fields and axillae. It is an ejection systolic murmur beginning in early to mid-systole.

VIBRATORY STILL MURMUR

This is the most frequently seen innocent murmur of childhood, is confined to early systole, and is best heard at the lower left sternal border. The key feature of a Still murmur is its vibratory, musical and harmonious character.

VENOUS HUM

A venous hum is the most frequently encountered continuous murmur, thus heard into both systole and diastole in an otherwise healthy child. It is best heard in the neck and in the infraclavicular area of the anterior chest. The murmur is best discerned when the child is sitting and looking away from the examiner and is reduced by gentle compression of the jugular vein or turning the child's head towards the side of the murmur. The murmur tends to resolve on lying down. The murmur is described as low-pitched, rumbling, whirring and roaring in character.

Acyanotic Congenital Heart Disease

Ventricular Septal Defect

A ventricular septal defect (VSD) is a hole in the septum that separates the ventricles, the lower chambers of the heart (Figs 11.3 and 11.4). As the peripheral vascular resistance (PVR) naturally falls over the first weeks of life, a ventricular septal defect results in oxygen-rich (red) blood being ejected from the left ventricle, through the septal defect, into the right ventricle and augmenting the volume of blood flow to the lungs.

VSDs in the muscular septum represent most defects with a high spontaneous closure rate. Perimembranous or outlet VSDs are located underneath the aortic valve and have a 50 per cent rate of requiring interventional closure by surgery or catheter-delivered occlusion device.

Symptoms of ventricular septal defect

The size of the ventricular septal opening dictates both the type and severity of symptoms as well as the age they first occur. A VSD results in additional blood volume shunting from the left ventricle through to the right ventricle. A small defect in the ventricular septum allows only a relatively small amount of blood to pass from the left ventricle to the right ventricle but leads to a loud and harsh murmur from the accelerated jet of flow.

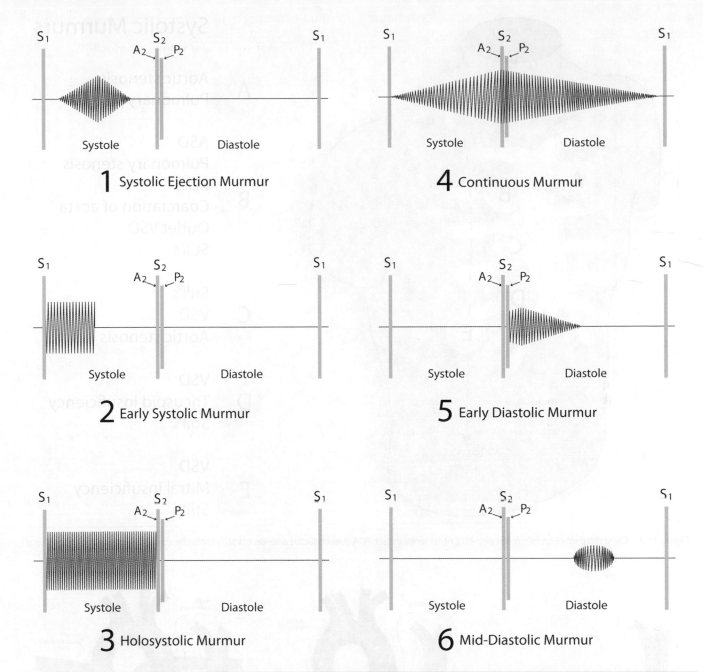

Figure 11.1   Timings of heart murmurs. (Courtesy Dr W Evans.)

The larger the defect, the greater the degree of shunting and the earlier presentation and severity of the symptoms of CHF. Symptoms of heart failure include fatigue, sweating, rapid breathing and tiredness during feeds with consequent reduced oral intake.

Chronic pulmonary over-circulation results in both thickened and muscularised pulmonary vasculature, which are the hallmarks of longstanding pulmonary arterial hypertension.

How loud the murmur is related to both flow and pressure gradient across the ventricular septal defect. Small VSDs may be very loud, moderate VSDs may have a harsh murmur along with a palpable thrill. Large VSDs may have a deceptively soft murmur but additional features including tachycardia, an active praecordium, a gallop (S3) rhythm and a palpable liver edge.

Treatment for ventricular septal defect

Periodic cardiology review aims to pick up congestive heart failure (CHF) and to monitor the VSD over time. Medical treatment may include pre-load reduction (diuretics), inotropes (digoxin). or afterload reduction (angiotensin-converting enzyme (ACE) inhibitors).

Infants with a haemodynamically significant VSD with CHF may tire during feeds and thereby have faltering growth. In these instances, high-calorie formula, fortified breast milk or supplemental nasogatric (NG) tube feeds may be required.

An infant or child's VSD may be repaired by a cardiac catheterisation procedure using a septal occluder if they are deemed a favourable candidate from an anatomical perspective, or by surgical closure if not.

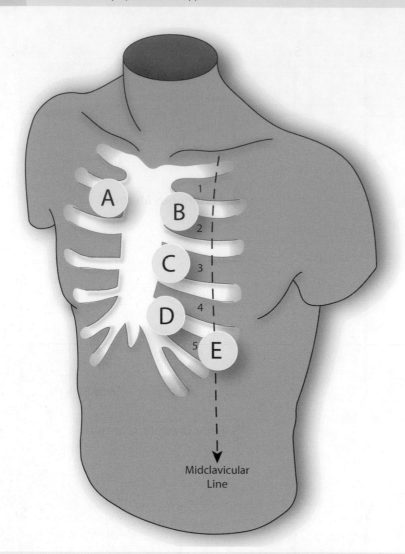

Systolic Murmurs

A Aortic stenosis
Pulmonary stenosis

B ASD
Pulmonary stenosis
PDA
Coarctation of aorta
Outlet VSD
Still's

C Still's
VSD
Aortic stenosis

D VSD
Tricuspid insuficiency
Still's

E VSD
Mitral insuficiency
Still's

Figure 11.2   Chest diagram of systolic murmurs. *ASD,* Atrial septal defect; *PDA,* patent ductus arteriosus; *VSD,* ventricular septal defect. (Courtesy Dr W Evans.)

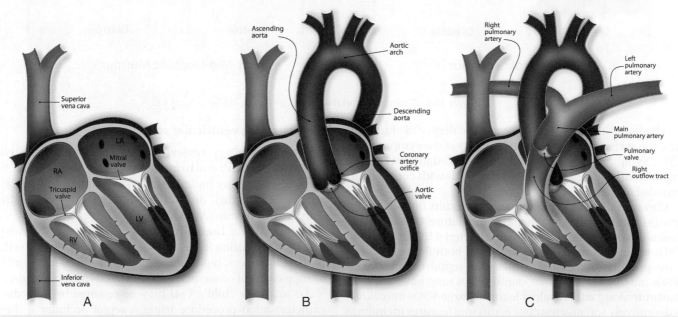

Figure 11.3   Normal heart. (Courtesy Dr W Evans.)

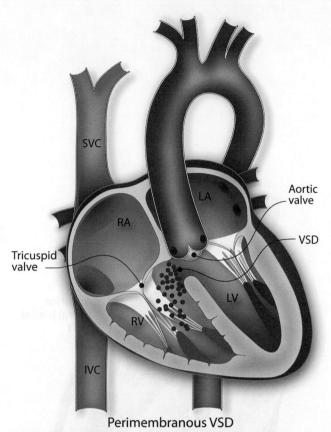

Figure 11.4 Perimembranous ventriculo-septal defect. (Courtesy Dr W Evans.)

Atrial Septal Defect (ASD)

An ostium secundum defect is the commonest form of ASD (Fig. 11.5). The auscultatory findings relate to the increased shunting from left to right at atrial level during diastole with consequent right heart volume overload and a resultant pulmonary flow murmur during systole. This additional blood shunted from the left atrium through the ASD leads to a higher volume of blood that fills the right heart in diastole. Thus, the P_2 component of the second heart sound (HS_2) is delayed with the result that the HS_2 becomes widely split and fixed. A low intensity ejection systolic murmur is heard. Surgical or device closure of ASD in the catheterisation laboratory is the treatment of choice.

Patent Ductus Arteriosus (PDA)

In this condition, the ductus arteriosus that normally spontaneously closes within the first few weeks of birth remains patent with a burden of left (aorta) to right (pulmonary artery) shunting resulting in left heart volume overload (Fig. 11.6).

A loud machinery murmur is heard in the pulmonary or left infra-scapular region. This murmur is harsh sounding and continues into diastole. The peripheral pulses tend to be bounding to palpation secondary to a wide pulse pressure from a lower diastolic value with the PDA runoff into the pulmonary artery.

PDA is frequently seen in preterm infants and may be associated with congestive heart failure with a hyperdynamic praecordium from left heart volume overload, and the infant may have difficulty weaning off ventilation. Treatment in preterm infants includes ibuprofen and fluid restriction. If this treatment is unsuccessful, surgical ligation may be indicated.

Beyond the neonatal period, treatment of PDA is by surgical ligation or device closure during cardiac catheterisation.

Pulmonary Valve Stenosis (PS)

Key auscultatory findings in PS include an ejection systolic murmur which is best heard in the pulmonary area. With higher levels of valvular obstruction, the murmur becomes louder and higher pitched and tends to peak later in systole (Fig. 11.7). An ejection click is frequently heard. As pulmonary valve stenosis becomes more severe, the ejection click tends to be softer and tends to be earlier in systole.

A thrill in the pulmonary area and a prominent right ventricular impulse may be evident. Balloon valve dilatation in the catheterisation laboratory is the treatment of choice.

Aortic Valve Stenosis (AS)

AS leads to increased afterload on the left ventricle due to outflow tract obstruction that can result in left ventricular hypertrophy and, on occasion, acute cardiovascular collapse as the PDA closes after birth (Fig. 11.8). Clinical features of AS include a thrusting apex beat relating to left ventricular hypertrophy, a suprasternal thrill and a harsh ejection systolic murmur in the aortic area with possible extension both into the neck and throughout the praecordium. On auscultation, an ejection click may also be evident at the apex.

An ejection systolic click is not present in supravalvular aortic stenosis.

Treatment of severe AS is by either open heart surgery or balloon valvotomy with some children requiring valve replacement.

Coarctation of the Aorta

The pathophysiology in coarctation of the aorta is secondary to a markedly elevated afterload on the heart due to discrete narrowing within the arch of the aorta (Fig. 11.9). The femoral pulses are typically absent, diminished or delayed in older children. The four-limb blood pressure may show a difference between the arms and legs.

The patient often presents on day 3 to 5 of life with acute cardiogenic shock as the left ventricle struggles to cope with the sudden development of downstream obstruction. Coupled with this, distal perfusion past the arch obstruction is severely impaired, resulting in lactic acidosis.

The murmur of coarctation is best heard in the interscapular area posteriorly.

Surgical management of coarctation of the aorta in the neonatal period is through a left thoracotomy approach. Aortic coarctation angioplasty is a safe alternative to surgery in children.

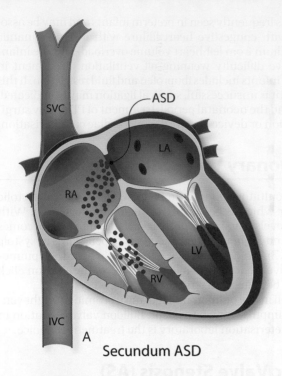

A
Secundum ASD

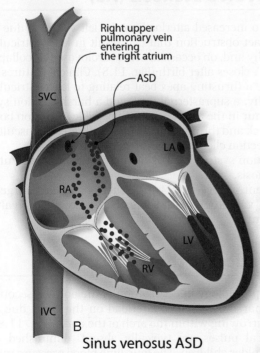

B
Sinus venosus ASD

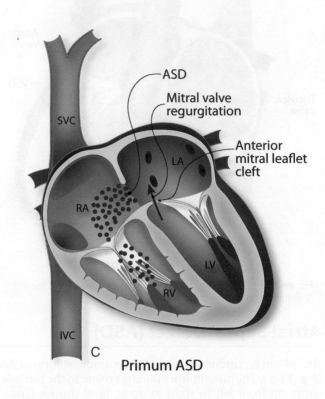

C
Primum ASD

Figure 11.5   Types of atrial septal defect. (Courtesy Dr W Evans.)

Cyanotic Congenital Heart Disease

These are best remembered by the mnemonic 'five Ts and an H'.

T: Tetralogy of Fallot (the most common accounting for 5 per cent of all congenital heart disease)

T: Transposition of the great arteries (TGA) (2 per cent of all congenital heart disease)

T: Total anomalous pulmonary venous drainage (TAPVD)

T: Truncus arteriosus

T: Tricuspid atresia

H: Hypoplastic right heart syndrome

The hyperoxia test helps to differentiate between cardiac and respiratory causes of cyanosis in the newborn period. The infant is placed in 100 per cent oxygen for 10 minutes, and the saturations will rise if the pathology is primarily respiratory. If saturations do not rise and an arterial blood gas shows an arterial PaO_2 of less than 20 kPa, this indicates a high likelihood of cyanotic heart disease.

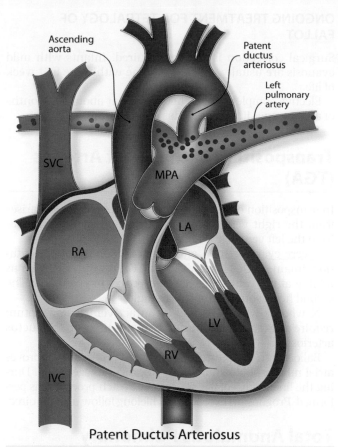

Patent Ductus Arteriosus

Figure 11.6   Patent ductus arteriosus. (Courtesy Dr W Evans.)

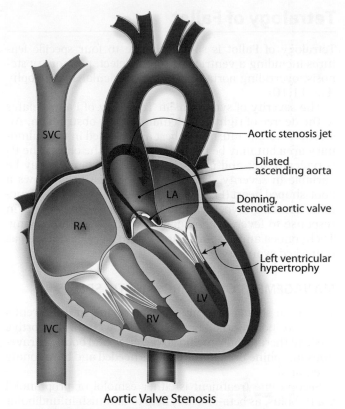

Aortic Valve Stenosis

Figure 11.8   Aortic valve stenosis. (Courtesy Dr W Evans.)

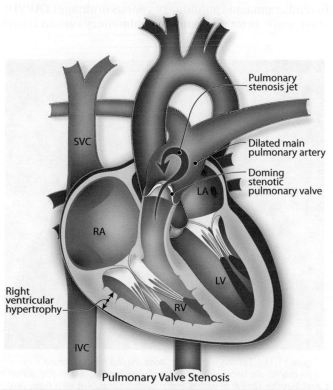

Pulmonary Valve Stenosis

Figure 11.7   Pulmonary valve stenosis. (Courtesy Dr W Evans.)

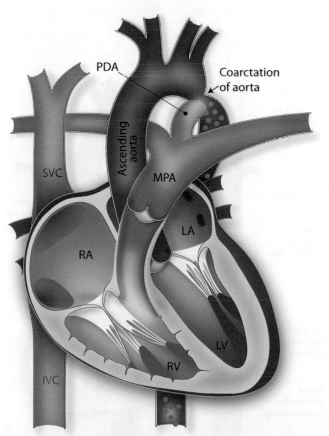

Coarctation of Aorta and Patent Ductus Arteriosus

Figure 11.9   Coarctation of the aorta. (Courtesy Dr W Evans.)

Tetralogy of Fallot

Tetralogy of Fallot is so-named due to four specific features including a ventricular septal defect, pulmonary stenosis, overriding aorta and right ventricular hypertrophy (Fig. 11.10).

The severity of symptoms in Tetralogy of Fallot relates to the degree of right ventricular outflow obstruction. An ejection systolic murmur is best appreciated in the pulmonary area but may be heard throughout the chest. The P_2 is typically soft and may not be heard. Cyanosis may be variable in severity. The chest x-ray classically shows a boot-shaped heart (Fig. 11.11). A sudden reactive obstruction, termed a 'hypercyanotic' or 'tet spell', may occur in response to fever, illness, dehydration or intense crying. Tachypnoea and dyspnoea are seen in a typical tet spell as is marked cyanosis.

MANAGEMENT OF HYPERCYANOTIC SPELLS

The infant should be kept calm and secure in the parent's arms, positioning the knees close to the chest. Supportive medical therapy may include oxygen, a fluid bolus, intravenous morphine to calm the child as needed and bicarbonate if required.

Second line treatment is either esmolol or propranolol via IV bolus, as beta-blockers help to diminish infundibular obstruction by both decreasing the heart rate and prolonging diastolic filling.

ONGOING TREATMENT FOR TETRALOGY OF FALLOT

Surgical correction is always required. Infants with mild cyanosis are usually able to go home within the first week of life.

Elective complete repair takes place at about six months of age – sooner if the infant has severe cyanosis.

Transposition of the Great Arteries (TGA)

In transposition of the great arteries (TGA), the aorta arises from the right ventricle and the pulmonary artery arises from the left ventricle (Fig. 11.12).

Severe cyanosis soon after birth is the typical presentation. Infants with a large VSD and TGA may present later as mixing at the ventricular level improves oxygenation. The second heart sound is typically single.

Newborns with TGA and an intact ventricular septum require prostaglandin infusion to maintain open the ductus arteriosus.

Balloon atrial septostomy (Rashkind procedure) improves atrial mixing of blood and thus improves oxygenation. During the first 7 days of life, an arterial switch procedure is performed. Prognosis is excellent but lifelong follow up is required.

Total Anomalous Pulmonary Venous Drainage (TAPVD)

In total anomalous pulmonary venous drainage (TAPVD), also known as total anomalous pulmonary venous return

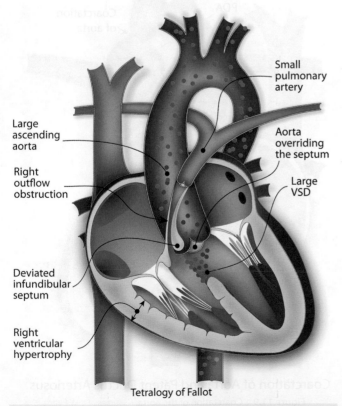

Large ascending aorta

Right outflow obstruction

Deviated infundibular septum

Right ventricular hypertrophy

Small pulmonary artery

Aorta overriding the septum

Large VSD

Tetralogy of Fallot

Figure 11.10   Tetralogy of Fallot. (Courtesy Dr W Evans.)

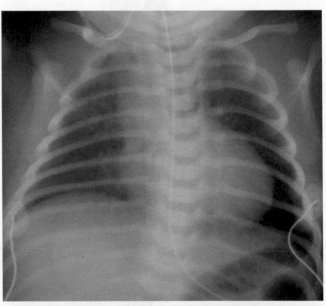

Figure 11.11   Tetralogy of Fallot. Boot shaped heart on chest x-ray in a six-month-old baby with cyanosis during feeding. Heart size is normal, but the apex is elevated and rounded consistent with right ventricular hypertrophy (toe of boot). There is a right sided aortic arch (heel of boot to right of trachea). Absence of left arch and small pulmonary arteries account for the instep appearance of the 'boot' left of the trachea. Pulmonary vascularity is reduced. (Courtesy Prof. Stephanie Ryan.)

(TAPVR), the pulmonary veins drain into the right atrium instead of the left atrium (Fig. 11.13). There are four types: in the supracardiac type, the pulmonary veins drain into the superior vena cava; in the cardiac type, the pulmonary veins drain into the right atrium or the coronary sinus; in both cardiac and supracardiac types, cyanosis is mild and the infant presents with congestive heart failure.

In the infracardiac type, the pulmonary veins drain into the inferior vena cava or the portal vein. Presentation is in the neonatal period with marked cyanosis and collapse due to obstruction. A murmur is invariably absent.

Finally, there is a mixed type of the above three. Surgical correction is required for all four types of TAPVD.

Truncus Arteriosus

In truncus arteriosus, one artery arises from the heart (Fig. 11.14) If there is associated pulmonary valve atresia, cyanosis follows ductal closure and examination also reveals a systolic murmur and a single second heart sound. Truncus arteriosus is associated with 22q11 deletion.

Tricuspid Atresia

Tricuspid atresia is due to abnormal formation of the tricuspid valve and presents with severe cyanosis and tachypnoea after birth (Fig. 11.15). Examination reveals a systolic murmur at the left sternal border, a single second heart sound and a dynamic left ventricular impulse. The electrocardiogram

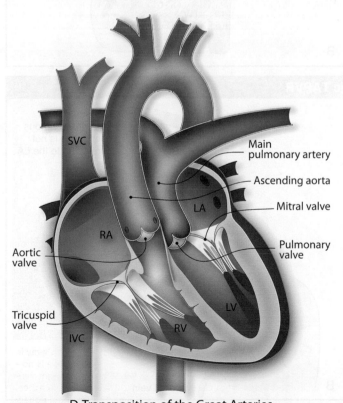

D-Transposition of the Great Arteries

Figure 11.12 Transposition of the great arteries. (Courtesy Dr W Evans.)

(ECG) shows left axis deviation. Initial treatment is with a prostaglandin E_1 infusion with later a Fontan procedure.

Hypoplastic Left Heart Syndrome

Hypoplastic left heart syndrome consists of left heart hypoplasia or atresia whereby the left ventricle is unable to support the systemic circulation (Fig. 11.16). Hypoplastic left heart syndrome is often picked up on antenatal scanning or presents on day 2 of life with cyanosis, tachypnoea, and very poor peripheral perfusion with life-saving improvement following intravenous prostaglandin E_1. Advice about a staged Norwood repair is given following a multidisciplinary team discussion (MDT) and consultation with the family.

Chest Pains in Childhood

Chest pain is relatively common in childhood and adolescence and is a source of great concern. Only a tiny minority of all cases of chest pain in children (without known congenital heart disease) are found to have a cardiac cause despite these heightened concerns within the family.

The great majority of chest pain in childhood and adolescence is idiopathic, psychogenic or musculoskeletal. A detailed history and examination are required.

Chest pain or syncope brought on by exercise should be taken seriously, especially if there is a family history of sudden cardiac death, cardiomyopathy or inherited arrhythmia.

Key points in the history are the duration of pain, aggravating or relieving factors and associated symptoms.

RED FLAG symptoms increasing the likelihood of a cardiac cause for chest pain:

- chest pain on exercise
- exertional syncope
- pain awakening the child or adolescent from sleep
- association with concomitant palpitations
- family history of sudden death, inherited arrhythmias or long QT syndrome
- prior history of congenital heart disease
- prior history of Kawasaki disease

Cardiac Causes of Chest Pain

SEVERE PULMONARY OR AORTIC VALVE STENOSIS

Severe aortic or pulmonary valve stenosis, if undiagnosed, may present with chest pain with typical auscultatory findings and echocardiography being vital to the diagnosis. The treatment is either surgical or ballooning of the valve in the catheterisation laboratory.

ANOMALOUS CORONARY ARTERIES

This includes a coronary artery fistula, coronary aneurysms related to Kawasaki disease or an anomalous origin of the left or right coronary arteries.

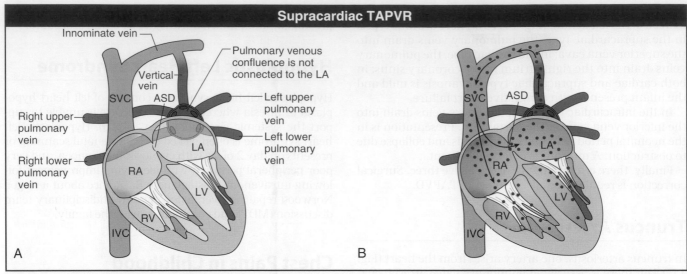

Supracardiac TAPVR

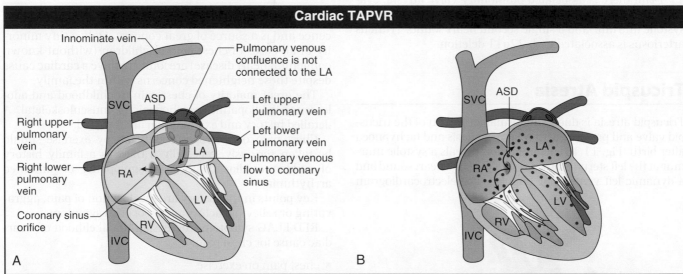

Cardiac TAPVR

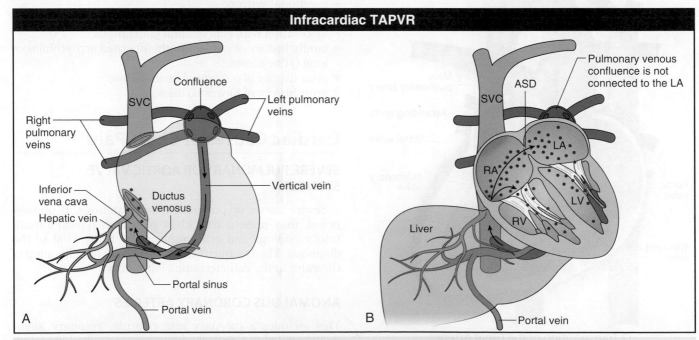

Infracardiac TAPVR

Figure 11.13 Total anomalous pulmonary venous drainage (TAPVD). (Courtesy Dr W Evans.)

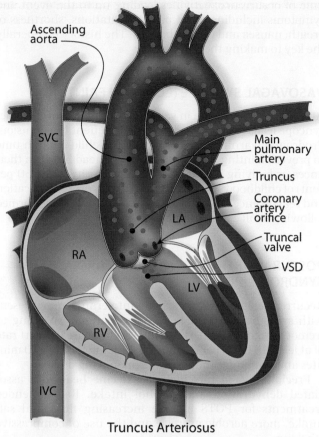

Truncus Arteriosus

Figure 11.14   Truncus arteriosus. (Courtesy Dr W Evans.)

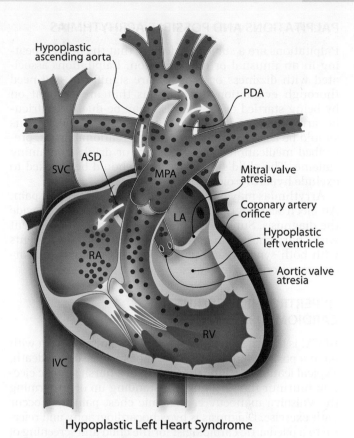

Hypoplastic Left Heart Syndrome

Figure 11.16   Hypoplastic left heart syndrome. (Courtesy Dr W Evans.)

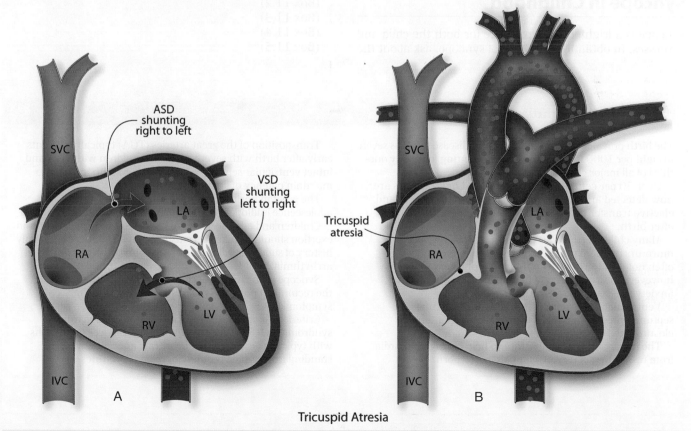

Tricuspid Atresia

Figure 11.15   Tricuspid atresia. (Courtesy Dr W Evans.)

PALPITATIONS AND POSSIBLE ARRHYTHMIAS

Palpitations are a subjective feeling that the heart is beating in an unusual or quick fashion. Palpitations associated with dizziness or syncope are significant and need thorough evaluation. Palpitations that are brought on by being startled or by exercise may be due to ventricular arrythmias. Adolescents who experience palpitations should be asked about the use of recreational drugs, prescribed medications, energy drinks or drinks containing caffeine. The child's thyroid status should be checked to exclude hyperthyroidism.

Arrythmias may be interpreted by a child as chest pain. An electrocardiogram (ECG) or a Holter monitor provide the diagnosis. Supraventricular tachycardia may present with sharp chest pain and palpitations. If a child presents with both syncope and palpitations, 24-hour home cardiac monitoring is indicated.

HYPERTROPHIC OBSTRUCTIVE CARDIOMYOPATHY (HOCM)

HOCM is inherited in an autosomal dominant pattern with often a positive family history or a history of sudden death. Typical features include the finding of a harsh systolic ejection murmur that is louder on standing up or performing the Valsalva manoeuvre. Ischemic chest pain may occur with exercise. Diagnosis is by echocardiography and referral to a paediatric cardiologist for the child and screening of the family should take place.

Syncope in Childhood

Syncope is a frightening experience for both the child and witnesses. In obtaining a history of syncope, ask about the time of occurrence, activities leading up to the event and symptoms including chest pain, palpitations, shortness of breath, nausea and visual changes. The history is generally the key to making the diagnosis.

VASOVAGAL SYNCOPE (COMMON FAINTING)

Autonomic dysfunction in vasovagal (or neurocardiogenic) syncope leads to bradycardia and subsequent hypotension. Prodromal warning signs may give the child enough time to prevent fainting by sitting with their head between their knees or by lying supine. The great majority (over 60 per cent) of childhood syncope is vasovagal in origin. Education and reassurance are required. An ECG should be performed following a full examination.

POSTURAL ORTHOSTATIC TACHYCARDIA SYNDROME (POTS)

Recurrent episodes of orthostatic intolerance may present with symptoms of light headedness, fatigue, sweating or tremor. Diagnostic criteria include an increase in heart rate of at least 40 beats per minute on standing for over 10 minutes and symptoms that improve upon lying down.

Precipitating factors include extreme heat with associated dehydration and alcohol intake. Recommended treatments for POTS include increasing fluid and salt intake, more aerobic exercise and the use of compressive stockings.

(Box 11.1)
(Box 11.2)
(Box 11.3)
(Box 11.4)
(Box 11.5)

Box 11.1 **Key Points**

The birth prevalence of congenital heart disease (CHD) is seven to eight per 1000 liveborn infants, accounting for nearly one-third of all major congenital malformations.

Over 50 per cent of serious congenital heart lesions are now detected antenatally, allowing planned delivery and elective transfer to a specialist cardiology service soon after birth.

Many children (up to 50 per cent) will have innocent murmurs (with no underlying cardiac anomaly) most often noted at the time of an intercurrent fever or anaemia–however, these murmurs, when noted, can be a cause of anxiety and concern to parents.

Ventricular septal defects (VSDs) in the muscular septum represent most defects with a high spontaneous closure rate.

The hyperoxia test is important to help distinguish cardiac from respiratory causes of cyanosis in newborn.

Transposition of the great arteries (TGA) typically presents early after birth with severe cyanosis. Children with TGA and intact ventricular septum require prostaglandin infusion to maintain patency of ductus arteriosus.

The great majority of chest pain in childhood and adolescence is idiopathic, psychogenic or musculoskeletal.

Children and adolescents who have chest pain or syncope on exertion should be taken seriously, especially if there is a family history of sudden cardiac death, cardiomyopathy or inherited arrhythmia.

Syncope occurs in the upright or sitting position and the recumbent position often results in resolution of symptoms.

Criteria to diagnose postural orthostatic tachycardia syndrome (POTS) include symptoms lasting over six months with typically an increase in heart rate after assuming a standing from supine position for over 10 minutes.

Box 11.2   A Murmur Picked up Incidentally in a Well Child

An active six-year-old boy has an intercurrent viral illness and is seen by his family doctor. He is pyrexial, and his doctor picks up a soft systolic murmur at the upper left sternal border. Despite being reassured, the child's parents have become worried and are seeking an opinion from a paediatric cardiologist. The family live in a rural community over 100 miles from the nearest tertiary cardiac centre.

Clinical Pearls

The vast majority of murmurs in childhood are benign and <u>not</u> indicative of CHD.

Innocent murmurs are soft, systolic, have no associated symptoms, may vary with posture and respiration and are localised.

Innocent murmurs are typically of low intensity (less than grade 2/6), short duration, present in systole only, located along the left sternal edge without radiation, associated with normal splitting of S_2 and with no additional cardiac findings such as an active praecordium, gallop rhythm or palpable liver edge.

The likelihood of finding significant cardiac pathology from a murmur found on examination decreases after the first year of life with up to <u>40 to 50 per cent</u> of healthy, school-aged children having innocent murmurs on careful cardiac auscultation.

A vibratory Still murmur (the diagnosis in this case) is the most common innocent murmur of childhood and is typically audible between the ages of 2 and 6 years old. The murmur is loudest when the child is in the supine position, and the most characteristic feature of the murmur is its vibratory, musical and harmonious quality, often described as a twanging sound with the intensity of the murmur decreasing with upright positioning.

If a murmur is deemed innocent, then no endocarditis prophylaxis is required.

Interpretation of Investigations

A chest x-ray and electrocardiogram (ECG) rarely assist in the diagnosis of heart murmurs in children and should clinical judgement indicate concern, a referral to paediatric cardiology for echocardiography is indicated.

Pitfalls to Avoid

The key pitfall is over-investigation of innocent cardiac murmurs with consequent overwhelming of paediatric cardiology services.

Structural heart disease is more likely when murmurs have certain characteristics such as a holosystolic, grade 3 or higher in intensity with a harsh-sounding quality, associated with a systolic click or present in diastole.

Box 11.3   VSD With Heart Failure

A male infant is born by spontaneous vertex delivery and weighs 3.5 kg at birth. He had a normal cardiovascular examination in the newborn period and was discharged home at 48 hours of age. At 8 weeks of age, he attends his family doctor with concerns about diminished feeding over the prior 2 weeks. He is irritable, upset and constantly sweating. His mother also states that he is breathing quickly and looks pale. An active praecordium, loud pansystolic murmur and a 4-cm liver are noted on examination.

Clinical Pearls

VSDs are either muscular or perimembranous and account for 30 per cent of all congenital heart disease (CHD).

The experienced clinician will recognise that these are worrisome symptoms that suggest congestive heart failure (CHF), and that the most likely diagnosis is a ventricular septal defect.

As the peripheral vascular resistance (PVR) naturally falls during the first 6 weeks of life to approximately 20 per cent of the SVR, a significant increase in left to right shunting through the ventricular septal defect will develop. This results in clinically significant pulmonary over-circulation presenting with signs and symptoms of congestive heart failure (CHF).

Examination findings in CHF include tachypnoea, tachycardia, an S3 gallop rhythm, a left parasternal heave and hepatomegaly.

In an infant with a large <u>VSD</u>, heart failure may develop at <u>4 to 6 weeks</u> of age.

On the other hand, CHF that develops in the <u>first week of life</u> (especially the first 3 days) is usually due to an obstructive lesion–typically critical aortic stenosis, hypoplastic left heart syndrome or coarctation of the aorta.

The optimal time of repair of VSD is around 4 to 6 months of age.

Interpretation of Investigations

Chest x-ray may show cardiomegaly and pulmonary plethora (Fig. 11.17).

Electrocardiogram (ECG) may show evidence of right ventricular hypertrophy (RVH) or p pulmonale if pulmonary hypertension.

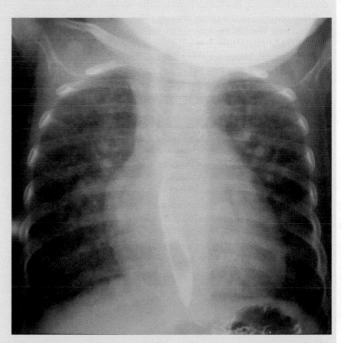

Figure 11.17 Pulmonary plethora. Chest x-ray in a six-month-old boy with Trisomy 21. There is increased pulmonary vascularity due to left to right shunt. Enlargement of the right heart border indicates right atrial enlargement due to an atrial septal defect. A little contrast in the oesophagus shows oesophageal deviation by an enlarged left atrium indicating a ventricular septal defect. Echocardiography confirmed an endocardial cushion defect–an atrioventricular septal defect. (Courtesy Prof Stephanie Ryan).

Continued

BOX 11.3   VSD With Heart Failure—cont'd

Echocardiogram shows the position of the defect within the ventricular septum and determines its size and relation to surrounding cardiac structures.

Pitfalls to Avoid

Ventricular septal defects usually become symptomatic at 4 to 6 weeks of age, and a murmur is often **not** evident on the newborn discharge examination.

If left untreated, a VSD can cause progressively irreversible pulmonary hypertension. This can manifest as a prominent S_2 (P_2) on cardiac auscultation (Fig. 11.18). Longstanding pulmonary hypertension may eventually lead to reversal of shunt flow with consequent cyanosis and secondary polycythaemia.

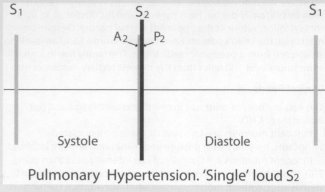

Figure 11.18   Single P_2 in pulmonary hypertension. (Courtesy Dr W Evans.)

Box 11.4   Cyanosis in the Newborn Period

A 2-day-old infant is not feeding well and is noted to be off colour. Pulse oximetry detects desaturation down to 82 per cent and the oxygen saturation does not improve with oxygen administration via nasal prongs.

Clinical Pearls

There are many types of cyanotic congenital heart disease (CHD), and the following key features help differentiate them.

Transposition of the great arteries (TGA) with an intact ventricular septum manifests as <u>profound cyanosis on day 1</u>. Saturations do not significantly improve with oxygen administration (the hyperoxia test). There may be a faint ejection murmur, but often no murmur is heard. The P_2 is often not heard.

Tetralogy of Fallot is the most seen cyanotic congenital heart disease and may present with hypercyanotic spells in later infancy.

In tricuspid valve atresia, the tricuspid valve does not develop, the right ventricle is very small and a diffuse left ventricular cardiac impulse may be palpated.

In truncus arteriosus, one sees cyanosis with a rapid onset of congestive heart failure (CHF) usually in the first 2 days of life.

In hypoplastic left heart syndrome, deterioration occurs when the ductus arteriosus closes and as the pulmonary vascular resistance falls within a day or two of birth (favouring pulmonary blood flow at the expense of systemic perfusion). The affected newborn becomes tachypnoeic, blue and poorly perfused. Prostaglandin E_1 is lifesaving in this instance.

Interpretation of Investigations

The hyperoxia test helps to differentiate between cardiac and respiratory causes of cyanosis in the newborn period.

In longstanding, unrepaired tetralogy of Fallot, a characteristic 'boot-shaped' heart with pulmonary oligemia is seen on chest x-ray and right axis deviation and right ventricular hypertrophy are seen on ECG.

In transposition, the chest x-ray may show an 'egg on its side' appearance with pulmonary oligaemia.

In tricuspid valve atresia, the ECG reveals characteristic superior left axis deviation.

In total, anomalous pulmonary venous drainage (TAPVD) investigations show a normal ECG with the chest x-ray showing a cardiac outline termed 'snowman in a snowstorm' appearance.

Echocardiography provides the definitive diagnosis with increasingly diagnoses being made antenatally following routine 20-week foetal anomaly scans.

Pitfalls to Avoid

Cyanosis may be difficult to pick up clinically on the newborn examination and thus both antenatal scans and newborn pulse oximetry have helped to pick up cases prior to further clinical deterioration.

If cyanotic congenital heart disease is suspected post-hyperoxia test, start a prostaglandin E_1 infusion to keep the ductus open, maintain oxygen saturations in the mid 80s and seek prompt transfer to a paediatric cardiology tertiary centre.

Box 11.5   A Fainting Episode in a 10-Year-Old

A 10-year-old girl presents to her family doctor with two episodes of apparent fainting. Each episode occurred in a crowded environment and on each occasion she became very pale, started to sweat and fell to the ground without sustaining any injury. She made a quick recovery within 5 minutes. Her past and perinatal history were unremarkable. There is no family history of epilepsy or cardiac disease. Her neurological and cardiac examinations were normal. She went on to have a normal ECG.

Clinical Pearls

Vasovagal syncope or simple fainting is seen frequently and is typically short-lived; there is typically a loss of postural tone with the child slumping to the floor. The child tends to recover quickly without intervention.

Prior to the episode, the child may have obvious pallor and sweating and a sense of nausea. Vasovagal syncope has a few well known triggers (for instance, prolonged standing) and is usually short-lived. The pulse rate during the episode tends to be slow. In contrast, postural orthostatic tachycardia syndrome (POTS) is associated with tachycardia when the child stands up, and there is also a drop in blood pressure which may lead to a feeling of faintness or actual collapse.

Trigger avoidance and increasing both salt and water intake are essential strategies in managing vasovagal syncope; however, if very frequent, beta blockers or fludrocortisone may be required.

Interpretation of Investigations

Cardiac causes of syncope can be excluded by appropriate history taking, clinical examination and an ECG.

ECG will rule out prolonged QT syndrome.

Brugada syndrome has typical ECG finding of ST elevation in the right precordial leads as well as right bundle branch block type picture.

Echocardiography will pick up hypertrophic cardiomyopathy or aortic stenosis.

Tilt table testing is not particularly useful in children and adolescents with syncope. If there is a family history of sudden cardiac death or arrhythmias, referral to a paediatric cardiologist and echocardiography is warranted.

Pitfalls to Avoid

Patients with prolonged QT syndrome are prone to ventricular arrhythmias that may present as syncope or sudden death. It is a familial condition inherited in an autosomal dominant fashion. Triggers that induce arrhythmias include medications that prolong the QT interval (including commonly prescribed antibiotics such as erythromycin and clarithromycin), swimming or exercise (QT1), auditory stimuli and emotional stress (QT2) and rest or sleep (QT3).

Brugada syndrome is typically seen in adults but may present in a child with syncope and preceding fever.

Hypertrophic cardiomyopathy or severe aortic stenosis may also present with syncope.

Exercise may precipitate syncope in children with an abnormal origin of coronary arteries.

 Videos on the topic Congenital heart disease and Heart murmur are available online at Elsevier eBooks+.

Key References

Abdulla, R. (Ed.). (2011). *Heart diseases in children: A pediatrician's guide.* Springer.

Baumgartner, H., De Backer, J., Babu-Narayan, S. V., Budts, W., Chessa, M., et al. 2021). 2020 ESC Guidelines for the management of adult congenital heart disease. *European Heart Journal, 42*(6), 563–645.

Cohen, G. (2018). Syncope and dizziness. In R. M. Kliegman, P. S. Lye, B. Bordini, H. Toth, & D. Basel (Eds.), *Nelson pediatric symptom-based diagnosis* (pp. 83–103). Elsevier.

da Cruz, E., Dunbar, I., Hraska, V., & Jaggers, J. (Eds.). (2013). *Pediatric and congenital cardiology, cardiac surgery and intensive care* (2014th ed.). Springer.

Kang, O., & Schmid, J. (2020). Five Ts of cyanotic congenital heart disease (mnemonic). Radiopaedia.org https://radiopaedia.org/articles/five-ts-of-cyanotic-congenital-heart-disease-mnemonic.

Kolinski, J. M. (2018). Chest pain. In R. M. Kliegman, P. S. Lye, B. Bordini, H. Toth, & D. Basel (Eds.), *Nelson pediatric symptom-based diagnosis* (pp. 104–115). Elsevier.

Pelech, A. N. (2018). Murmurs. In R. M. Kliegman, P. S. Lye, B. Bordini, H. Toth, & D. Basel (Eds.), *Nelson pediatric symptom-based diagnosis* (pp. 116–143). Elsevier.

Plana, M. N., Zamora, J., Suresh, G., Fernandez-Pineda, L., Thangaratinam, S., & Ewer, A. K. (2018). Pulse oximetry screening for critical congenital heart defects. *Cochrane Database of Systematic Reviews, 3*(3), CD011912.

The Down Syndrome Medical Interest Group. (n.d.). Guidelines for picking up congenital heart disease. www.dsmig.org.uk.

Wik, G., Jortveit, J., Sitras, V., Døhlen, G., Rønnestad, A. E., & Holmstrøm, H. (2020). Severe congenital heart defects: Incidence, causes and time trends of preoperative mortality in Norway. *Archives of Disease in Childhood, 105*(8), 738–743.

12 *The Child With a Cough*

MICHAEL WILLIAMSON

Coughing is a primary defence mechanism that allows the clearance of secretions and particles from the airways and protects against aspiration of foreign materials. Most coughing in childhood is due to an acute respiratory infection and will improve or disappear within 3 weeks. Preschool children may experience between 6 and 10 respiratory tract infections per year and coughing may affect up to 30 per cent of children at any one time.

Clues From the History

The history should focus on the age of onset, duration of the cough, and whether it is dry or wet, barking or honking in nature. Ask if there are any triggering or alleviating factors, and if there has been any response to prior therapy (such as the use of a bronchodilator). Ask whether the cough is constant or paroxysmal, and whether sleep-related or not. Coughing due to asthma is generally worse at night, whereas a habit cough disappears during sleep. Seek information about exposure to cigarette smoke or other aeroallergens and any other associated symptoms. Seek a family history (perhaps asthma or cystic fibrosis) and a full immunisation history.

Clues from the Examination

The examination should focus on a comprehensive respiratory examination. Note height and weight on an age-appropriate centile chart. Observe whether the child is in respiratory distress and look for use of the accessory muscles of respiration (subcostal or intercostal recession or flaring of the nostrils, grunting, or an audible wheeze). Check the vital signs. Check carefully for clubbing in the fingers. Observe the chest for features of hyperinflation and auscultate the lungs. Carefully examine the nose, looking for features of allergic rhinitis or nasal polyposis. Perform a 'sniff test' to assess if any nasal obstruction is present.

Specific Clinical Pointers to a Diagnosis

Sudden onset of a cough with a possible choking episode should prompt consideration of an inhaled foreign body. Bronchoscopy is the investigation of choice.

A classical paroxysmal cough or coughing spasms with associated cyanosis or apnoea in a young infant may be related to *Bordetella pertussis* infection and a pernasal swab should be requested.

A history of nocturnal or exercise-induced coughing with associated wheezing should prompt consideration of an asthma diagnosis. Assess bronchodilator responsiveness and perform spirometry, if the child is over six years of age.

A harsh, honking cough that disappears during sleep may indicate a habit cough.

A wet cough with purulent sputum, poor growth, nasal polyposis, and features of malabsorption should prompt consideration of cystic fibrosis. Sweat tests and genotyping are the appropriate investigations.

A history of recurrent infections or hospitalisations for pneumonia should prompt consideration of a primary immunodeficiency such as common variable immunodeficiency, and serum immunoglobulins should be requested.

A progressive cough, weight loss, night sweats and haemoptysis should prompt consideration of tuberculosis.

A wet cough, symptoms from early infancy, purulent sputum, nasal obstruction, and hearing loss should prompt consideration of primary ciliary dyskinesia. Nasal brushing for ciliary motion and electron microscopy are the investigations of choice.

Children with choking episodes relating to feeds or post-feed chestiness with or without developmental delay may have recurrent aspiration. The investigations of choice are chest x-ray, feeding studies and videofluoroscopy.

If exertional dyspnoea or an abnormal cardiac examina the then congenital or acquired heart disease should be suspected, and an echocardiography and cardiology referral be coordinated.

The most common scenario is that of a child with a chronic cough, a normal chest x-ray and spirometry, and no clinical pointers of underlying disease. In this scenario, the most important diagnostic clue is whether the cough is dry or wet.

If the cough is dry and the child remains well, then an expectant approach and parental reassurance are appropriate. Coughing relating to acute respiratory infection may persist for 4 to 6 weeks. Exposure to aero irritants should be explored and, if similar to prior episodes, asthma should be considered. A trial of bronchodilators may be indicated. Persistent bacterial bronchitis should be considered if a persistent wet cough lasts for over 4 weeks,

Red flags prompting specialist referral include:

- neonatal or early infancy onset of cough (consider primary ciliary dyskinesia (PCD))
- chronic moist, wet, or productive cough (consider cystic fibrosis or PCD)
- recurrent confirmed cases of pneumonia (consider primary immunodeficiencies)
- coughing during or after feeding (consider aspiration or H-type tracheoesophageal fistula)
- significant comorbidity or neurodevelopmental delay (consider aspiration pneumonia)
- presence of finger clubbing (consider chronic lung suppurative disease)

Habit or psychogenic cough is disruptive, bizarre, honking in type and puzzling as it is not responsive to bronchodilators or oral corticosteroids. It decreases at night or on distraction and tends to be more prominent at school. The secondary gain of time off school may increase the cough. Behaviour modification regimens are helpful, and investigation should be kept to a minimum. Tourette's syndrome should be considered if features other than an isolated cough are present.

Asthma

Asthma is a condition characterised by variable airflow obstruction and symptoms of recurrent episodes of wheeze, cough, and breathlessness. Risk factors include a positive family history of asthma and atopy, maternal smoking in pregnancy, and sensitisation to aeroallergens. Prevalence of asthma does vary in different countries but is at least 15 per cent of the child population in Europe.

PRESENTATION OF ASTHMA

Main symptoms are dry cough, wheeze and breathlessness. Symptoms tend to be worse at night. Associated triggers include viral upper respiratory infections, exercise, exposure to cigarette smoke, or aeroallergens. Rarely, children may have cough-variant asthma.

Confirming the Diagnosis

Asthma in children younger than 6 years is largely a clinical diagnosis considering possible differential diagnosis and noting a typical dry cough. Nocturnal predominance with response to bronchodilators is critical.

Lung function testing in children with asthma is often normal as the obstruction is reversible. If spirometry shows obstruction in children over 6 years of age, a useful test to confirm variable airflow obstruction is the improvement in the Forced expiratory volume (FEV1) by at least 12 per cent, 15 minutes after administration of salbutamol via large-volume spacer.

Peak flow variability of at least 15 per cent over two to four weeks is strongly suggestive of asthma. A routine chest x-ray is not required to make the diagnosis.

Referral for specialist paediatric opinion is justified if the diagnosis is in doubt or if treatment is not working despite apparently good compliance.

MEASUREMENT OF THE PEAK EXPIRATORY FLOW RATE

The peak expiratory flow rate (PEFR) is the maximum rate of flow in forced expiration, starting from full inspiration and is measured in litres per minute. PEFR reflects the calibre of the large proximal airways with a diameter of over 2 mm. PEFR monitoring is helpful in the assessment of acute asthma and the long-term monitoring of asthma. Most children over 6 years of age can have their peak flow measured with appropriate training.

To perform measurement of the PEFR, ensure that the mouthpiece used is correctly fitted. The indicator should be set at zero and the child should be standing or sitting up straight. Ask the child to take a deep breath in and to hold it. Place the mouthpiece in the child's mouth and ask the child to close their lips around it to make a seal. Then ask the child to blow out as hard and fast as possible, and note the number that appears on the meter.

Children with a poor perception of asthma symptoms may benefit from home PEFR monitoring. Peak flow diaries may help to identify trends and to assess the response to therapy. Peak flow recordings persistently under 80 per cent of that predicted suggest that adequate asthma control has not been achieved. Children should be encouraged to measure pre- and postbronchodilator PEFR when possible. A change of more than 15 per cent after the administration of bronchodilator suggests that asthma control is suboptimal. Early morning dips in PEFR indicate suboptimal control.

MANAGEMENT OF CHRONIC ASTHMA

Preventive treatment in the first instance should be with inhaled corticosteroids, as there is no evidence to support the use of combination inhalers as the first line treatment in treating children with asthma. Children must be shown how to use inhalers and their technique should be checked regularly.

Aerochambers are recommended under 3 years of age, and large volume spacer devices are appropriate from 3 to 6 years or during exacerbations.

Any tobacco smoking in the household has an adverse effect on asthma outcomes. Consider a skin-prick test to identify allergies to household pets. Reduction of house dust mite measures is very popular but unproven.

Comorbidities such as obesity, rhinosinusitis, food allergies, vocal cord dysfunction and psychosocial issues may all worsen asthma symptoms.

Vocal cord dysfunction may be difficult to diagnose and may be associated with stridor, hoarseness and a sore throat, and confirmation may be by video recording of the attack and subsequent laryngoscopy.

DRUG THERAPY IN ASTHMA

Treatment goals in childhood asthma include the control of interval symptoms, the maintenance of lung function and the prevention of acute exacerbations, with minimal or no adverse effects. There are several national and international guidelines that should be followed.

Medications are delivered by aerosol inhalation, and spacers are recommended for children of all ages when using a metered inhaler or when having an acute exacerbation. A spacer device helps reduce the need to coordinate inhalation, and with the actuation of the metered-dose inhaler, increases medication delivery to the airways and decreases deposition in the mouth.

Inhaled corticosteroids are the cornerstone of treatment for asthma. They include beclomethasone dipropionate, budesonide, and fluticasone propionate, with fluticasone having twice the potency of budesonide and beclomethasone. Low to medium doses of inhaled corticosteroids (up to 400 µg/day) have a minimal effect on growth velocity, but the final adult height is unaffected.

Salbutamol and terbutaline are used for day-to-day reliever treatment in asthma. Long-acting drugs such as salmeterol or formoterol are useful as add-on treatments for improved control.

Montelukast is a leukotriene receptor antagonist which confers an add-on benefit when given with inhaled corticosteroids. There is considerable individual variation in the effectiveness of montelukast, but it is generally well tolerated. It can occasionally cause sleep disturbance and headaches.

The recombinant monoclonal antibody omalizumab acts by inhibiting the binding of IgE to the mast cell and basophil surface receptors, thereby preventing the release of inflammatory mediators. The use of omalizumab is restricted to a very small group of asthmatics who are compliant, attending a specialist respiratory service but have failed other therapies.

ASTHMA TREATMENT PLAN

All children with asthma should have a **personal treatment plan.**

An asthma treatment plan guides both parents and children in terms of maintenance treatment, the avoidance of triggers, and what actions to take if symptoms worsen, indicating acute asthma.

Regular follow-up is essential to the assessment of ongoing symptoms and asthma control. Always check the child's inhaler technique, as the most common reason for treatment failure is either an incorrect diagnosis or poor compliance with treatment. After an acute attack, determine if there are ongoing reversible problems that may have contributed to the episode (such as passive smoking) and review the acute management of the episode. To improve background control, use optimal doses of inhaled corticosteroids and attempt to reduce exposure to environmental allergens.

ACUTE EXACERBATION OF ASTHMA

A personal action plan for an acute episode may advise giving up to 10 puffs of salbutamol (depending on age) via a large-volume spacer, and seeing a nurse or the family doctor on the same day if the symptoms are improved. Medical attention should be sought if relief lasts for under 4 hours. If severe symptoms persist despite salbutamol puffs, the parents should call an ambulance and continue to give further salbutamol puffs every 15 minutes prior to the ambulance's arrival.

As part of the medical assessment of an acute exacerbation, it is reasonable for a chest x-ray to be performed after a first episode to out rule other causes. Atelectasis is frequently evident on chest x-rays in acute asthma, and pneumothorax is a potential complication in acute severe asthma.

A small number will present with severe symptoms (inability to speak or count, a silent chest, or cyanosis), and these patients require intensive care admission.

The acute management plan for severe asthma includes high flow oxygen via mask or nasal cannula to achieve normal saturations and nebulised salbutamol. Repeat every 20 minutes if the child has a poor response, and add nebulised ipratropium bromide. Give oral prednisolone or intravenous hydrocortisone if the child is unable to tolerate oral medication. If pulsus paradoxus is present, there is a higher relative risk of the child requiring magnesium sulphate or aminophylline or being admitted to intensive care (see chapter 26 on Severe illness).

AIMS OF TREATMENT IN CHILDHOOD ASTHMA

The critical aims should be no daytime symptoms, no asthma-related nighttime awakening, no need for rescue medication, no exacerbations, and no limitation in activity including exercise and normal lung function (Peak expiratory flow (PEF) > 80 per cent predicted).

Acute Respiratory Infections

Many infants and children develop upper respiratory tract symptoms of coughing, coryza and fever. When faced with these symptoms, the key issue is to decide whether this is an upper or a lower respiratory infection. To make this distinction, always seek signs of respiratory distress such as tachypnoea, grunting, the use of accessory muscles of respiration, leading to either intercostal or subcostal recession or nasal flaring. A lower respiratory tract infection should be suspected if any of these signs are present.

If a child is under 12 months of age, acute bronchiolitis is the most likely cause of a lower respiratory infection.

The most important lower respiratory infection symptom in an older child is tachypnoea with grunting, and the most important sign is the presence of a raised respiratory rate with evidence of respiratory distress. Dullness to percussion may or may not be evident. Signs of consolidation (reduced air entry with increased vocal fremitus and possibly bronchial breathing) or effusion (marked dullness, reduced air entry and reduced vocal fremitus) may be challenging to elicit.

It is perfectly reasonable to treat with antibiotics when community-acquired pneumonia is suspected but equally important to review after 48 hours to ensure that progress is being made and the child is improving.

The dominant cause in children with bacterial pneumonia is *Streptococcus Pnemoniae*, for which amoxycillin or co-amoxiclov can be used. Staphylococcal pneumonia may occur in infants and young children with the risk of pneumatocoeles. They require an appropriate course of intravenous antibiotics. In the school age child, Mycoplasma must also be considered, and a macrolide prescribed.

BRONCHIOLITIS

In infants, bronchiolitis is by far the most frequent cause of cough and acute respiratory distress. Bronchiolitis is a lower respiratory tract infection seen in winter and is most often due to respiratory syncytial virus. Indications for hospital admission include SpO2 measurement (significant if under 92 per cent), tachypnoea over 60 breaths per minute, apnoea and severe respiratory distress with inadequate fluid intake.

Evidence-based treatments include supplemental oxygen via nasal prongs and nasogastric feeds, if oral intake is inadequate. High flow oxygen is preferred to continuous positive airway pressure. Following inpatient care, consider discharge if the infant is tolerating feeds and has had SpO2 over 92 per cent for at least 4 hours, including a period of sleep. Chest x-rays are <u>not</u> routinely performed. Nasal suctioning is recommended in infants with coincident nasal blockage causing respiratory distress. Infants with chronic lung disease, congenital heart disease, neuromuscular disease and immunodeficiency are more likely to have severe disease, as are preterm infants born before 32 weeks' gestation. There is no evidence that hypertonic saline provides an added benefit.

Chronic Respiratory Conditions

PULMONARY TUBERCULOSIS

Tuberculosis (TB) is seen in the great majority of cases in developing countries. Consider this diagnosis in a child with unexplained respiratory symptoms, in a child who has come from an endemic area, or in a child known to have been exposed to an adult with active tuberculosis. Request a Mantoux test, a QuantiFERON test, a culture of sputum, an early morning gastric aspirate, or bronchoalveolar lavage to make the diagnosis. The usual pattern of illness is firstly primary pulmonary tuberculosis with subsequent inactivation and later reactivation in adolescence. Primary tuberculosis often presents as a lower or middle lobe infiltrate. With impaired immune function, these changes may either progress to miliary tuberculosis (Fig. 12.1) or reactivate at distal sites causing tuberculous, meningitis, or osteomyelitis. Upper lobe reactivation may cause cavitation with consequent 'open tuberculosis' similar to the disease among adults.

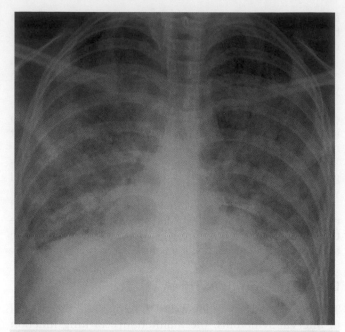

Figure 12.1   Miliary Tuberculosis. A 5-year-old girl has a fever, headache, weight loss and hepatosplenomegaly. There is a diffuse nodular pattern in both lungs. Miliary TB is the most likely diagnosis in this clinical setting. This child was found to have nodules in the brain, liver and spleen. (Courtesy Prof. Stephanie Ryan.)

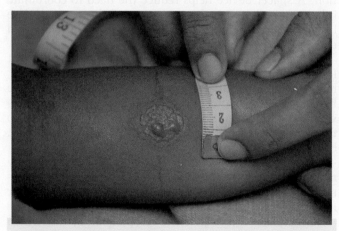

Figure 12.2   Mantoux test. (Reproduced with permission from Lakshmanaswamy, A. (Ed.). (2022). *Textbook of pediatrics* (1st ed.). Elsevier Inc.)

The Mantoux Test

Five (5) tuberculin units (TU) per test dose of 0.1 mL is the standard strength used for intradermal (Mantoux) testing. A tense pale wheal should appear over the needle after injection.

The skin test should be read within 48 to 72 hours after administration. Inspect the site, palpate, and measure the induration in millimetres (Fig. 12.2). If induration is greater than 10 mm, then the Mantoux is considered positive if the child is under 5 years of age, is a recent immigrant from an endemic country or has been exposed to an adult at high risk of active tuberculosis.

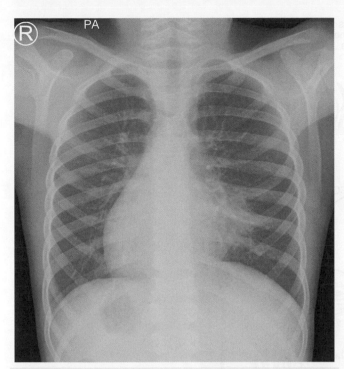

Figure 12.3 Primary ciliary dyskinesia. A 7-year-old boy with recurrent respiratory tract infection. He has situs inversus (note the heart and the stomach bubble are on the right). Density in the left middle lobe blurring the left heart border is due to bronchiectasis. (Courtesy Prof. Stephanie Ryan.)

PERSISTENT BACTERIAL BRONCHITIS

A wet cough in the absence of other concerning features may be due to persistent bacterial bronchitis (PBB).

PBB is a clinical diagnosis with a typical history of a chronic wet cough present for at least 4 weeks that responds well to antibiotics in the absence of any other underlying pathology. A 3-week course of a broad-spectrum antibiotic such as co-amoxiclav is the appropriate treatment. The child should be reviewed after 3 weeks, as recurrence of symptoms is common and may require a second course of antibiotics. The likelihood of underlying bronchiectasis or airway abnormality is increased if the wet cough is persistent despite antibiotic treatment. If still symptomatic after two courses of antibiotics, referral to a paediatric respiratory team is recommended.

PRIMARY CILIARY DYSKINESIA

Primary ciliary dyskinesia (PCD) is a rare autosomal recessive condition where abnormal ciliary function interferes with normal mucociliary clearance. A recent review in England showed that children with PCD have worse lung function than those with cystic fibrosis. Hearing loss is common in PCD but appears to improve with age. In this review, the median age at diagnosis of PCD was 2.6 years (IQR: 0.5 to 7.2 years). *Haemophilus influenzae* is the most frequent respiratory pathogen cultured in children with PCD.

Children with PCD who have a lower BMI tend to have impaired lung function, making nutritional support crucial in managing the condition.

Management of PCD is largely based on expert opinion and consensus guidelines and is extrapolated from the evidence base available for patients with CF.

In primary ciliary dyskinesia (PCD), cilia found mostly in the airways, nasal lining and reproductive tract have impaired movement. This leads to poor airway clearance, recurrent infections, a chronic wet cough from an early age and subsequent bronchiectasis. Presentation in the neonatal period with unexplained neonatal respiratory distress may occur. Nasal obstruction and rhinorrhoea are common, and up to 80 per cent of cases have persistent otitis media with middle ear effusion and associated conductive hearing loss. Approximately 50 per cent of children with PCD have situs inversus; therefore any child with dextrocardia should be investigated for PCD (Fig. 12.3). Sperm immobility leads to male infertility. Females with PCD also have reduced fertility.

The diagnosis of PCD is based on ciliary sampling from nasal or lower airway brushing. High-speed video can show abnormal or static ciliary motion while electron microscopy can elicit abnormal internal ciliary structure. Genetic testing has become increasingly useful as the genetic mutations causing PCD are described. Treatment is by means of physiotherapy, airway clearance techniques, nasal lavage and a low threshold for treatment with antibiotics. Hearing loss is generally treated with hearing aids rather than grommet insertion, which can lead to chronic discharge. Early diagnosis is essential to prevent a poor prognosis.

CYSTIC FIBROSIS

Cystic fibrosis (CF) occurs due to mutations in the cystic fibrosis transmembrane conductance regulator (CFTR) gene on chromosome 7. Gene mutations lead to an imbalance in chloride ion transport across cell surfaces with consequent alterations in sodium chloride and water absorption and secretion across multiple systems (see Fig. 12.4). The lungs are most obviously affected with thick, viscous secretions, and consequently reduced mucociliary clearance. This in turn leads to later bronchiectasis and colonisation with opportunistic pathogens (Fig. 12.5). Blocked pancreatic ducts cause pancreatic exocrine function with consequent steatorrhoea, failure to thrive and malabsorption of fat-soluble vitamins.

Over 100,000 people worldwide have a diagnosis of CF, with a high prevalence in Caucasian populations. Prior to neonatal screening, CF often presented with recurrent respiratory tract infections and failure to thrive. Life expectancy has improved remarkably with current life expectancy in the mid-30s to early 40s in Europe.

Since the discovery of the CFTR gene in 1989, there have been over 2100 causal mutations (and rising) identified, with the *F508del* being the most common mutation. Gating or conductance mutations diminish the functioning of the CFTR channels, with the most common gating mutation being *G551D*.

Presentation and Diagnosis of CF

Cystic fibrosis CF has a wide spectrum of clinical manifestations, not least of which is a chronic, moist cough with purulent sputum production, nasal polyposis, meconium

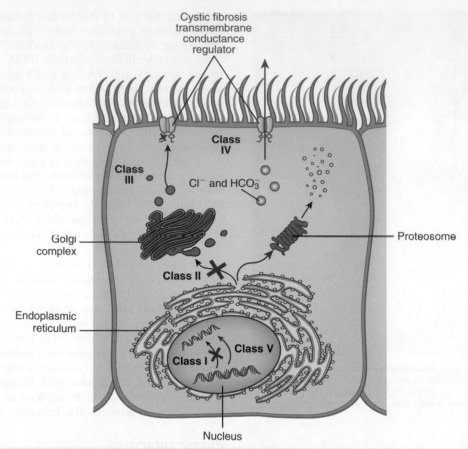

Figure 12.4 Cystic fibrosis transmembrane conductance regulator (CFTR) gene mutations and molecular consequences. Classes of defects in the CFTR gene product include the absence of synthesis (class I); defective protein maturation and premature degradation (class II); disordered regulation, such as diminished adenosine triphosphate binding and hydrolysis (class III); defective chloride conductance or channel gating (class IV); and a reduced number of CFTR transcripts due to a promoter or splicing abnormality (class V). Another class of defect has reduced protein stability at the cell surface (class VI, not shown). (Reproduced with permission from Lazarus SC, Ernst JD et al (Eds) (2022) *Murray & Nadel's Textbook of Respiratory Medicine, Seventh Edition.* Elsevier Inc.)

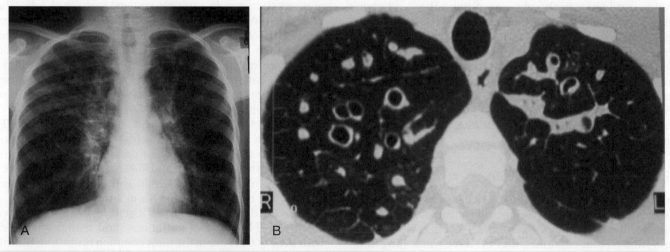

Figure 12.5 Bronchiectasis. A 16-year-old girl with cystic fibrosis. (A) CXR showing increased perihilar density and bilateral bronchiectasis most severe in the right upper lobe. (B) On CT, several of the right upper lobe bronchi are seen to be dilated significantly more than their adjacent vessels, a signet ring sign. (Courtesy Prof. Stephanie Ryan.)

ileus, prolonged neonatal jaundice, pseudo-Bartter syndrome, and failure to thrive with pale, bulky, offensive stools, rectal prolapse, unexplained clubbing, heat exhaustion, short stature, and male infertility.

Almost all cases are now picked up on newborn screening (blood immunoreactive trypsin followed by a sweat test and DNA genotyping analysis if raised). The gold standard diagnostic investigation is the sweat test with a sweat chloride of over 60 nmol/L being diagnostic. Other conditions with an elevated sweat chloride include untreated adrenal insufficiency, type one glycogen storage disease, hereditary nephrogenic diabetes insipidus, and ectodermal dysplasia.

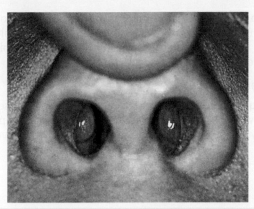

Figure 12.6 Cystic fibrosis. Nasal polyps in a patient with cystic fibrosis. (Reproduced with permission from Szentpetery, S., Weiner, D.J., et al. (2018, January 1). *Zitelli and Davis' atlas of pediatric physical diagnosis* (pp. 593–615). Elsevier.)

Respiratory infections in early life are with *Staphylococcus aureus*, *H.influenzae*, *Escherichia coli* and *Klebsiella* species. Subsequently, mucoid *Pseudomonas aeruginosa*, *Burkholderia cepacia* (may cause rapid deterioration in lung function) *Aspergillus fumigatus* (associated with bronchopulmonary aspergillosis), and atypical mycobacteria are the other respiratory pathogens.

Other Manifestations of CF

CF may present at birth with meconium ileus (10 to 15 per cent) or later in infancy and childhood with faltering growth and steatorrhoea, despite a voracious appetite. CF may also present early in life with prolonged neonatal jaundice. The most common presenting symptom after the neonatal period is cough, which may be dry, productive or paroxysmal.

Hepatomegaly may be a presenting sign secondary to fatty infiltration of the liver. Gallstones are more common in CF. The peak presentations of CF-related liver disease and CF-related diabetes occur in adolescence.

Examination features seen on physical examination include a low weight for height (seen in over 50 per cent), finger clubbing (80 per cent), nasal polyps (20 per cent) (Fig. 12.6), chest hyperinflation, hepatomegaly (10 per cent), recurrent rectal prolapse (10 per cent), and right lower quadrant faecal masses due to distal intestinal obstruction syndrome (DIOS) (5 to 10 per cent). Almost all males (95 per cent) have bilateral atresia or absence of the vas deferens with consequent infertility.

Management of Cystic Fibrosis

The two essential elements of therapy for CF are respiratory and nutritional management.

Respiratory management attempts to clear thick, viscous secretions from the airways. This is initially achieved using basic chest tapping in infants, and oscillation devices such as acapella in older children and adolescents. Inhaled rhDNAse helps to reduce the viscosity of airway secretions. Inhaled hypertonic saline has a similar effect.

Respiratory pathogens are targeted through prophylaxis (most commonly for S Areus) Global standards of care include eradication of early P aeruginosa. Inhaled antipseudomonal antibiotics such as tobramycin help lessen the impact of chronic infection with *Pseudomonas* species. Acute exacerbations are heralded by worsening respiratory symptoms or a falloff in weight, and some patients require portacath placement to enable the frequent courses of IV antibiotics.

Pancreatic enzyme replacement therapy and fat-soluble vitamins (ADEK) both play a key role in management. High-calorie diets to promote adequate growth are recommended for children and adolescents with CF.

Pancreatic endocrine dysfunction in adolescence may lead to diabetes mellitus requiring insulin treatment. This is termed CF-related diabetes, and low doses of insulin may be sufficient to achieve excellent glycaemic control.

Respiratory failure is the leading cause of mortality in end-stage CF, with an option of lung transplantation to improve quality of life.

Newer therapies that target the underlying pathophysiological mechanisms of CF have the potential to further improve prognosis in CF. The restoration of CFTR function via new small molecules modulator drugs has transformed the disease for many CF patients.

Targeting CFTR Channels

CFTR protein modulators have been developed to improve CFTR function by several mechanisms. Ivacaftor potentiates the abnormal protein channel at the cell surface, whereas lumacaftor and tezacaftor both correct protein transfer to the cell surface. CFTR modulators have been approved by the European Medicines Agency and the US Food and Drug Administration for use in patients with CF and certain genotypes.

Triple combinations of tezacaftor, elaxacaftor and ivacaftor could have the potential to transform health outcomes for CF patients with at least one *F508del* mutation

The introduction of CFTR modulators at an early age may improve both life expectancy and quality of life.

Minimal Standards of Care

Newborn Screening. A two-tier newborn screening programme based on the heel prick test is now the norm in most European countries, and diagnosed infants are referred to a specialist CF centre. Parents are also referred for genetic counselling. Thus, the majority of newly diagnosed children with CF are referred directly to a specialist CF centre at a very early age.

Specialist CF Teams. CF children and adolescents should be regularly followed up in a designated specialist CF centre, often in partnership with a designated locally shared CF care centre. A team of CF specialist health professionals provide this service with staffing levels determined by the size of the CF population at a given centre.

Role of the CF MDT. A multidisciplinary team (MDT) approach is key in managing CF. Respiratory physiotherapy with airway clearance and physical exercise are key elements of care. Likewise, nutritional support is crucial for all, regardless of age. Psychosocial support improves outcomes and should be routinely available to all CF patients and their families.

Clinical pharmacists play a significant role, especially following the advent of CFTR modulators and the potential for complex drug interactions. Pulmonary function studies should be regularly performed as they help to monitor lung function.

The CF team also monitors for developing complications such as liver disease and CF-related diabetes. Vascular access and issues of antibiotic resistance also require skilled management.

Annual Reviews

All patients with CF should have an annual review with all members of their CF multidisciplinary team (MDT) for a full review of progress over the previous year. Annual review testing is age-appropriate and includes blood tests and imaging such as an annual chest x-ray or biennial CT thorax, liver ultrasound scan and DEXA scan. Microbiology samples are a fundamental aspect of CF care and require considerable expertise.

Changes in values obtained in pulmonary function testing require taking many measurements – preferably over time in the same centre – using highly trained respiratory physiology scientists.

Inpatient Facilities

Key requirements for inpatient facilities include isolation rooms with en-suite facilities, access to paediatric physiotherapy and access to same-day therapeutic drug levels.

(Box 12.1)
(Box 12.2)
(Box 12.3)
(Box 12.4)

Box 12.1   **Key Points**

An acute cough usually resolves within 3 to 4 weeks and chronic cough persists for more than 8 weeks.

Most cases of acute cough in healthy children are due to a self-limiting viral upper respiratory infection. In a quarter of cases, children continue to have symptoms for at least 4 to 6 weeks after the onset of symptoms.

An isolated cough without wheeze or breathlessness is rarely due to asthma.

A wet cough is a significant symptom and prompts further investigation.

The absence of tachypnoea is the best single finding to rule out pneumonia in a child with a cough.

There is no evidence for the use of over-the-counter drugs (such as an antihistamine or decongestant preparations) in acute cough.

When assessing a child with cough, the history should focus on the age of onset, duration of the cough, and whether the cough is dry or wet, barking or honking in nature.

A sudden onset of cough with a possible choking episode should prompt consideration of an inhaled foreign body; bronchoscopy is the investigation of choice.

A history of nocturnal or exercise-induced coughing with associated wheezing should prompt consideration of an asthma diagnosis. Assess bronchodilator responsiveness and perform spirometry if the affected child is over 6 years of age.

A wet cough, symptoms from early infancy, purulent sputum, nasal obstruction, and hearing loss should prompt consideration of primary ciliary dyskinesia.

The diagnosis of tuberculosis is made by skin testing (purified protein derivative), a positive QuantiFERON test, a history of contact with a person who has tuberculosis and

recovery of the organism from sputum, bronchoalveolar lavage, pleural fluid, or early morning gastric aspirates.

Persistent bacterial bronchitis (PBB) is a clinical diagnosis with a typical history of a chronic wet cough present for at least 4 weeks that responds well to antibiotics in the absence of any other underlying pathology.

Asthma is suggested by symptoms of dry cough, wheeze, and breathlessness.

The goals of treatment in childhood asthma are the control of interval symptoms, maintenance of lung function and prevention of acute exacerbations with minimal or no adverse effects.

Low to medium doses of inhaled corticosteroids (up to 400 μg/day) have a small effect on growth velocity, but the final adult height is unaffected.

Primary ciliary dyskinesia (PCD) is a rare autosomal recessive condition where abnormal ciliary function leads to impaired mucociliary clearance.

Most CF cases are now diagnosed in the neonatal period, allowing for earlier treatment and prevention of complications.

CFTR protein modulators have been developed to improve CFTR function via several mechanisms. Ivacaftor potentiates the abnormal protein channel at the cell surface, whereas lumacaftor and tezacaftor both correct protein transfer to the cell surface.

With the routine implementation of CFTR modulators at an early age for patients with CF, there is the potential to enhance the quality of life for longer periods of time and to reduce the need for lung transplantation at an early age.

All patients with CF should have an annual review with all members of their CF multidisciplinary team (MDT) for a full review of progress over the previous 12 months.

Box 12.2   **Pneumonia**

A 4-year-old boy presents with a high fever, tachypnoea and pleuritic chest pain. His respiratory rate is 50 per minute with moderate intercostal recession. He has an audible grunt and his respiratory examination reveals dullness to percussion and reduced air entry on the right side.

Clinical Pearls

Pneumonia is very common in childhood and presents with fever, tachypnoea, respiratory distress (grunting, subcostal and intercostal recession with nasal flaring), and – rarely – hypoxia.

In young children, pneumonia is often viral (respiratory syncytial virus (RSV), rhinovirus, parainfluenza, adenovirus, and influenza)

but may also be due to *Streptococcus pneumoniae*, *Haemophilus influenzae* and *Staphylococcus aureus*. *Mycoplasma pneumoniae* is a common cause in school-aged children.

The absence of tachypnoea is the best single finding to rule out pneumonia in a child with a cough.

Key Investigations

Patchy infiltrates and atelectasis are more suggestive of atypical or viral pneumonia. Lobar consolidation (Fig. 12.7) or large pleural effusions (Fig. 12.8) are likely bacterial in origin. A repeat chest x-ray should be performed 6 weeks post-discharge to ensure resolution of consolidation (especially if lobar) (Fig. 12.9).

Continued

Box 12.2   **Pneumonia – cont'd**

The indications to perform a chest x-ray include lower respiratory symptoms with tachypnoea, grunting, high fever and use of accessory muscles of respiration.

Pitfalls to Avoid

Children with lower lobe pneumonia may also present with abdominal pain mimicking acute appendicitis.

If there have been recurrent cases of pneumonia requiring intravenous antibiotics, consider common variable immunodeficiency (CVID). Children with CVID are susceptible to frequent respiratory tract infections due to *S. pneumoniae, H. influenzae* type b, and *Mycoplasma*. Bronchiectasis is a frequent complication in CVID.

Complicated pneumonia should be suspected if a child with pneumonia is not responding to appropriate antibiotic treatment within 48 to 72 hours.

Children with complicated pneumonia should be referred to a tertiary care centre. Initial imaging should include a chest x-ray and an ultrasound with a chest CT reserved for selected patients.

Complicated pneumonia is characterised by a parapneumonic effusion or empyema, necrotising pneumonia, or a lung abscess, with the child also being highly pyrexial and quite unwell.

Most require chest drain insertion with a minority requiring intrapleural fibrinolytic therapy. Complicated pneumonia is thus characterised by severe illness and prolonged hospitalisation. Most children make a full recovery, and pneumococcal conjugate vaccine (PCV) 13 immunisation has considerably reduced the burden of complicated pneumonia in children.

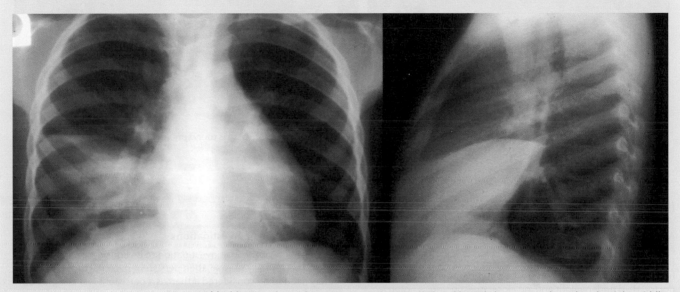

Figure 12.7   Lobar pneumonia. A 3-year-old with a cough and fever. (A) posteroanterior (PA) and lateral chest x-rays show that the right middle lobe is dense with little or no volume loss consistent with consolidation. (Courtesy Prof. Stephanie Ryan.)

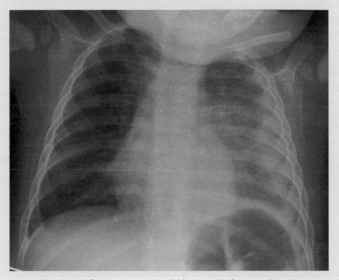

Figure 12.8   Pneumococcal pneumonia with pleural fluid. A 7-month-old baby with fever and tachypnoea. Dense left lower lobe and large left pleural effusion at presentation. (Courtesy Prof. Stephanie Ryan.)

Continued

Box 12.2   Pneumonia – cont'd

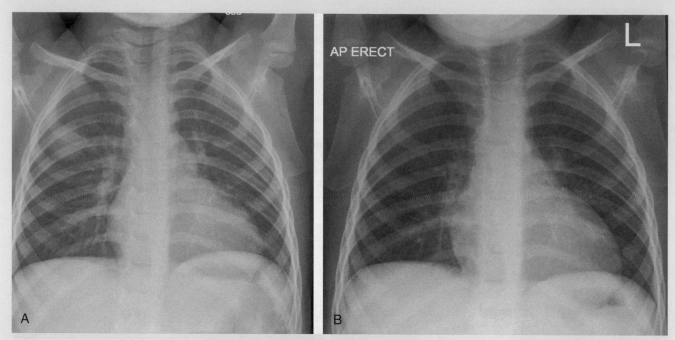

Figure 12.9   Round pneumonia. A 6-year-old with a fever and acute respiratory infection. (A) There is round pneumonia in the right mid lung. (B) A radiograph 2 weeks later shows complete resolution of pneumonia. (Courtesy Prof. Stephanie Ryan.)

Box 12.3   All That Wheezes Is Not Asthma

A 4-year-old child presents with a history of intermittent nocturnal and exercise-induced coughing. Each coughing episode is preceded by a viral infection and the cough remains for 3 to 4 weeks. He also has a frequent wet cough and has had numerous visits to his family doctor. He is underweight and, on closer questioning, is noted to have had symptoms from infancy. Intravenous antibiotic therapy was required in all three admissions with pneumonia. His family history is negative for atopy or asthma. He has repeated episodes of otitis media and significant conductive hearing loss with prior grommet insertion and now hearing aids in situ.

Clinical Pearls

Beware of the second diagnosis, as red flags in this instance include symptoms from infancy and three prior hospitalisations for pneumonia requiring intravenous antibiotics.

The presence of a <u>chronic wet cough is abnormal</u> and should prompt investigation into causes of bronchiectasis. Newborn cystic fibrosis (CF) screening is in place in most EU countries, but consideration of CF as a diagnosis may depend on the child's age, as some of those presenting were born prior to national screening.

Interpretation of Investigations

A chest x-ray is the first investigation to be considered. If the chest x-ray is essentially normal, then persistent bacterial bronchitis (PBB) may need to be considered if there is a persistent wet cough. PBB requires at least 3 weeks of an antibiotic such as co-amoxiclav.

In this instance, both primary ciliary dyskinesia (PCD) and common variable immunodeficiency (CVID) need to be considered. Immunoglobulins were normal and vaccine responses appropriate. Nasal brushings were sent to a supra-regional laboratory-confirmed PCD.

Pitfalls to Avoid

Beware of the <u>second diagnosis,</u> as this boy had both asthma <u>and</u> PCD.

In PCD, cilia are found mostly in the airways, nasal lining, and reproductive tract and have impaired movement. This leads to poor airway clearance, recurrent infections, a chronic wet cough from an early age and subsequent bronchiectasis.

Look out for red flags. As a result of neonatal CF screening, PCD and CVID are the two diagnoses to consider if the presentation is atypical.

Box 12.4 Foreign Body Inhalation

A 3-year-old presents to his family doctor with a 4-week history of a dry and persistent cough. His mother recalled an acute, violent episode of coughing while eating popcorn 4 weeks earlier. His family doctor commences him on inhalers and oral antibiotics, but he is largely unresponsive. He is referred to hospital for a chest x-ray and specialist opinion.

Clinical Pearls

An inhaled foreign body in a child can easily be missed, particularly if a history of choking or coughing is not forthcoming.

Consider foreign body inhalation in any child with a witnessed choking episode.

Foreign bodies tend to lodge in the main or lobar bronchi.

Foreign body inhalation is mostly seen in children aged 1 to 4 years. The most common objects inhaled include popcorn, peanuts, seeds, carrots, beans, small toy parts, and baby teeth. Inhalation of peanuts, raisins, or popcorn kernels can cause an intense local inflammatory response.

Wheezing is typically unilateral as the foreign body lodges into the main or lobar bronchi.

Interpretation of Investigations

When considering foreign body inhalation, inspiratory and expiratory chest x-ray films should be requested. Obstructive air trapping and hyperinflation of the affected side are the most important signs to identify (Fig. 12.10).

CXR will only detect radio-opaque foreign bodies.

Collapse/consolidation beyond the obstruction may not always be present.

Pitfalls to Avoid

A normal chest x-ray does <u>not</u> rule out foreign body aspiration.

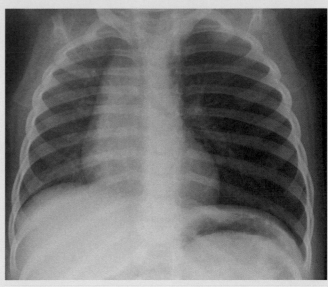

Figure 12.10 Inhaled foreign body. An 18-month-old toddler had dyspnoea after eating peanuts. Chest x-rays show expansion and hyperlucency of the left lung with a mediastinal shift to the right. A bit of peanut was found in the left main bronchus on bronchoscopy. (Courtesy Prof. Stephanie Ryan.)

Rigid bronchoscopy is the investigation of choice, and the foreign body can be removed.

Chest x-ray post-removal should demonstrate resolution of changes.

Key References

Alviani, C., Ruiz, G., & Gupta, A. (2018). Fifteen-minute consultation: A structured approach to the management of chronic cough in a child. *Archives of Disease in Childhood. Education and Practice Edition, 103*(2), 65–70.

Amos, L. B. (2018). Cough. In R. M. Kleigman, P. S. Lye, B. Bordini, H. Toth, & D. Basel (Eds.), *Nelson pediatric symptom-based diagnosis* (pp. 15–38). Elsevier Health Sciences Division.

Anderson, M., & Thomas, D. A. (2010). Drug therapy for chronic asthma in children. '*Archives of Disease in Childhood*'. *Education and Practice Edition, 95*(5), 145–150.

Attieh, S. (2017). Targeting cystic fibrosis pathophysiology is changing the future for children worldwide. Royal College of Surgeons in Ireland Student Medical Journal, 1, 99–104.

Brodlie, M., Graham, C., & McKean, M. C. (2012). Childhood cough. *BMJ (Clinical Research Ed.), 344*, e1177.

Bush, A., & Fleming, L. (2015). Diagnosis and management of asthma in children. *BMJ (Clinical Research Ed.), 350*, h996.

Dobra, R., & Equi, A. (2018). How to use peak expiratory flow rate. *Archives of Disease in Childhood. Education and Practice Edition, 103*(3), 158–162.

Heijerman, H., McKone, E. F., Downey, D. G., Van Braeckel, E., Rowe, S. M., Tullis, E., et al. (2019). Efficacy and safety of the elexacaftor plus tezacaftor plus ivacaftor combination regimen in people with cystic fibrosis homozygous for the F508del mutation: a double-blind, randomised, phase 3 trial [published correction appears in Lancet. 2020 May 30;395(10238):1694]. *Lancet* (London, England), *394*(10212), 1940–1948.

Krishnan, S. G., Wong, H. C., Ganapathy, S., & Ong, G. Y. (2020). Oximetry-detected pulsus paradoxus predicts for severity in paediatric asthma. *Archives of Disease in Childhood, 105*(6), 533–538.

Rey, M. M., Bonk, M. P., & Hadjiliadis D. (2019). Cystic fibrosis: Emerging understanding and therapies. *Annual Review of Medicine, 70*, 197–210.

Rubbo, B., Best, S., Hirst, R. A., Shoemark, A., Goggin, P., Carr, S. B., et al. (2020). Clinical features and management of children with primary ciliary dyskinesia in England. *Archives of Disease in Childhood, 105*(8), 724–772.

Shteinberg, M., Haq, I. J., Polineni, D., & Davies, J. C. (2021). Cystic fibrosis. *Lancet* (London, England), *397*(10290), 2195–2211.

Werner, C., Lablans, M., Ataian, M., Raidt, J., Wallmeier, J., Große-Onnebrink, J., et al. (2016). An international registry for primary ciliary dyskinesia. *The European Respiratory Journal, 47*(3), 849–859.

Zemanick, E. T., & Accurso, F. J. (2019). Entering the era of highly effective CFTR modulator therapy. *Lancet* (London, England), *394*(10212), 1886–1888.

Online References

British Thoracic Society Guidelines https://www.brit-thoracic.org.uk/quality-improvement/guidelines/asthma/works for british thoracic society

Cystic Fibrosis Mutation Database (CFTR1) maintained by the Cystic Fibrosis Centre at the Hospital for Sick Children in Toronto. http://www.genet.sickkids.on.ca/Home.html.

HS Clement Clarke International. (2004, October 7). Paediatric normal values – Peak expiratory flow rate. www.peakflow.com/paediatric_normal_values.pdf.

National Institute for Health and Care Excellence. (2021, August 9). Bronchiolitis in children: diagnosis and management. NICE guideline [NG9]. www.nice.org.uk/guidance/ng9.

National Clinical Programme for Cystic Fibrosis. (2019). *Cystic fibrosis – A model of care for Ireland*. https://www.hse.ie/eng/about/who/cspd/ncps/cystic-fibrosis/resources/ncpcf-model-of-care-final-september-2019.pdf.

13 The Child With Diarrhoea

MICHAEL COSGROVE

Gastrointestinal (GI) disease remains a very important health issue in childhood with acute gastroenteritis being a leading cause of mortality and morbidity in low-income countries where oral rehydration therapy is truly lifesaving.

Inflammatory bowel disease (IBD) is an ever-increasing problem in high-income countries. Other important issues in paediatric gastroenterology are recurrent abdominal pain (covered in Illness without disease chapter 34) and constipation (covered in Frequent flyers in the toddler years chapter 29).

Acute Gastroenteritis

Acute gastroenteritis is a very common presentation in infancy and childhood and the landscape in high-income countries has been changed by the successful introduction of rotavirus vaccination. Rotavirus was previously the leading cause of gastroenteritis, accounting for over 40 per cent of presentations. Other common causes of gastroenteritis in young children are adenoviruses and noroviruses. Bacterial gastroenteritis is much less common and more likely to cause bloody diarrhoea, high fever and systemic illness. Causative bacterial pathogens include Salmonella species, Shigella species, *Campylobacter jejuni* and enteropathogenic *E. coli*.

Gastroenteritis usually begins with an acute onset of fever and vomiting followed by frequent watery stools. Vomiting usually lasts for 1 to 2 days and diarrhoea may persist for up to 14 days.

TREATMENT OF GASTROENTERITIS

The management of acute gastroenteritis focuses on the prevention and treatment of dehydration. Several scoring systems have been devised to assess dehydration, but most are problematic and tend to overdiagnose the degree of dehydration. The key measurement is weight on admission to hospital and weight post-rehydration to retrospectively calculate the degree of dehydration. However, dehydration greater than 3 per cent is quite rare in developed countries in the post-rotavirus vaccination era.

ORAL REHYDRATION THERAPY

Rehydration with oral rehydration solution (ORS) is the preferred method of rehydration in both hospital and community settings. Along with vaccination, it is arguably one of the great global developments to improve child survival of gastroenteritis. For every 25 children treated with oral rehydration therapy, one will not respond and will require intravenous therapy. The World Health Organisation recommends the use of an ORS (with an osmolality of 224 mmol/L containing sodium, potassium and sugar content of 2 g/100 mL) in treating gastroenteritis with dehydration or for maintaining hydration in children. Additional ORS should be given after each loose stool to try to correct dehydration over 4 hours. Breast-feeding should continue throughout the rehydration and maintenance phases of the treatment of gastroenteritis. Non-breast milk feeding should also be restarted as soon as possible and usually by 24 hours as this reduces both the duration and severity of diarrhoea. Avoid carbonated drinks as the sugar content of some is far too high at 11 g/100 mL and the low-calorie versions are even more unsuitable as they do not contain sugar at all. Also avoid anti-diarrhoeal or anti-emetics drugs, except ondansetron in the emergency department setting, which may increase tolerance of ORS and avoid hospitalisation. Lactose-free diets are not routinely recommended post-gastroenteritis as secondary lactose intolerance is very rare. Rotavirus vaccination is extremely effective in preventing rotavirus infection in both low- and high-income countries.

Chronic Non-Specific Diarrhoea (or Toddler Diarrhoea)

Toddler diarrhoea typically affects 1- to 3-year-olds and presents with frequent watery and unformed stools. Stools tend to become loose as the day progresses. Undigested vegetables (especially peas and carrots) may be seen. Blood, mucus and excessive fat are not typically found, and the child continues to gain weight normally.

The pathophysiology involves abnormal intestinal motility with a rapid gut transit time. Consumption of fruit juices is often implicated and may overwhelm the carbohydrate absorptive capacity of the gut. In general terms, the toddler is healthy with plenty of energy, is gaining weight and shows no other symptoms apart from frequent watery stools.

Strategies to improve symptoms and reduce stool frequency are achieved by adopting the 'three Fs' approach (fat, fruit juice and fluid).

The fat content of the diet should be increased by providing full-fat milk (200 mL three times daily), cheese and full-fat yoghurt, but not by resorting to junk foods. Fruit juices (much loved by toddlers) may contain fructose or sorbitol and may significantly contribute to diarrhoea if taken in large amounts daily. Thus fruit juice intake should be restricted. Drinking large volumes of fluid is another contributor to toddler diarrhoea. A child 1 to 5 years old should drink at most between 1200 and 1500 mL/day. Parental reassurance is important, and they should be encouraged to avoid dietary restrictions (for example, gluten exclusion). Symptoms usually improve with increasing age.

Lactose Intolerance

Toddler diarrhoea must be distinguished from temporary lactose intolerance, which may follow acute gastroenteritis. Enzymes required for digestion of carbohydrates are located in the brush border epithelium of the small bowel. In lactose intolerance, frequent watery acidic stools are passed. Primary lactose intolerance is rare in northern Europeans but very common in other ethnic groups. Presentation is with osmotic diarrhoea, pain, abdominal distension and faltering growth from birth.

A similar inherited disorder of carbohydrate digestion is sucrase-isomaltase deficiency, which classically presents at 9 to 18 months of age with severe watery diarrhoea, irritability and poor weight gain following exposure to sucrose and starch. Diagnosis requires an upper GI endoscopy and biopsy which shows normal small bowel morphology and a marked reduction in sucrase and maltase activity.

Coeliac Disease

Coeliac disease is a very common immune-mediated disorder (population screening studies suggest as many as 1 per cent in some countries) brought on by exposure to gluten and tends to run in families. The concordance in monozygotic twins is 100 per cent, indicating a strong genetic factor. First-degree relatives, children with type 1 diabetes mellitus or auto-immune thyroid disease, children with Down syndrome, Turner syndrome and William syndrome all have a higher risk of coeliac disease.

To develop coeliac disease first requires exposure to gliadin found in wheat, rye and barley. Typical endoscopic small intestinal biopsy findings include villous atrophy, elongation of crypts and intraepithelial lymphocytosis (Fig. 13.1). Targeted screening of asymptomatic children with a strong family history or other risk factors is by serology testing. Elevated anti-tissue transglutaminase (TTG) IgA

antibodies and typical biopsy changes are diagnostic. A rise greater than 10-fold in TTG IgA antibodies with positive anti-endomysial IgA antibodies can confirm the diagnosis without need for small intestinal biopsy.

The classical presentation in the first 2 years with severe failure to thrive and chronic diarrhoea is now rarely seen (Fig. 13.2). Many other symptoms are associated with coeliac disease, including recurrent abdominal pain, steatorrhea, constipation, fatigue, mouth ulcers, rash and short stature. Children experience a resolution of symptoms when placed on a strict gluten-free diet. T-cell lymphoma and adenocarcinoma of the jejunum may rarely occur in untreated coeliac disease later in life.

Inflammatory Bowel Disease

Inflammatory bowel disease (IBD) comprises both ulcerative colitis (UC) and Crohn's disease (CD) with classical symptoms of abdominal pain, diarrhoea with blood in the stools and weight loss. The prevalence of IBD is increasing in the paediatric population, although the reason for this is unknown.

Mucosal inflammation restricted to the colon is seen in UC. UC may involve the whole colon, often starting in the rectum with proximal extension. In children with UC, pancolitis is the most frequent presentation.

A characteristic feature of CD is transmural inflammation affecting all layers of the intestinal wall and may involve any portion of the gastrointestinal tract. Skip lesions in which areas of normal mucosa are interspersed with inflammatory lesions are seen in CD. Clinical features suggestive of CD include perianal disease and evidence of bowel fistulae.

On physical examination, establish the nutritional status of the child or adolescent and their pubertal status (often delayed in Crohn's disease), and review recent growth on the centiles. Check for features of anaemia, finger clubbing and aphthous ulcers (Fig. 13.3) in the oral cavity (seen in 10 per cent of CD patients). Check the eyes for episcleritis and request a formal ophthalmological assessment for anterior uveitis. Look for features of erythema nodosum, which is a painful red rash typically seen over the anterior tibial surfaces (Fig. 13.4). Pyoderma gangrenosum is a severe ulcerating rash typically seen in UC (Fig. 13.5). Carefully examine the abdomen for masses and tenderness and check the perianal area which is typically involved in CD (Fig. 13.6).

SUGGESTED INVESTIGATIONS IN IBD

- FBC – look for iron deficiency anaemia and for a high platelet count suggestive of inflammation.
- Erythrocyte sedimentation rate (ESR) and C-reactive protein (CRP) may be elevated.
- Serum albumin and liver function tests. Hypoalbuminemia is typically seen in small intestinal CD.
- Stool microbiology for enteric pathogens, including *Clostridium difficile*, *Yersinia* and for ova, cysts and parasites.
- Faecal calprotectin level should precede endoscopy and is a good screening test for bowel inflammation.
- Magnetic resonance (MR) enterography.
- Upper and lower gastrointestinal endoscopy and biopsies.

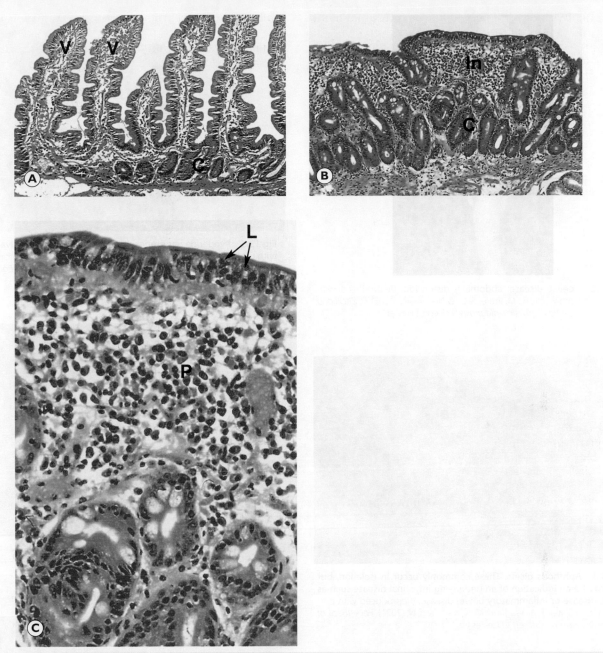

Fig 13.1 Coeliac disease (gluten-sensitive enteropathy). (A) Normal jejunal mucosa (medium power MP); (B) atrophic jejunal mucosa (MP); (C) atrophic jejunal mucosa (high power). (Reproduced with permission from O'Dowd, G., Bell, S., & Wright, S. (2019). *Wheater's pathology: A text, atlas and review of histopathology* (6th ed.). Elsevier.)

CROHN'S DISEASE (CD)

CD has a peak incidence in the mid-teenage years and most often presents with diarrhoea. Stool passed may contain microscopic blood, and nocturnal diarrhoea with urgency is a characteristic feature. Other features include anorexia, weight loss, abdominal pain and fatigue. Symptoms in CD evolve in a relapsing and remitting manner. CD may involve all segments of the gastrointestinal tract with the terminal ileum and colon most commonly affected. Complications frequently occur and include strictures, fistulae and abscess formation, all of which may require surgery.

The prevalence of CD is highest in Europe, Canada and the United States. The prevalence of CD is also rising in urbanised parts of Asia.

Diagnosis is confirmed by MR enterography and endoscopy with typical histology showing transmural inflammation and skip lesions (Fig. 13.7).

Due to the side effects of corticosteroids, exclusive enteral nutrition is generally the recommended first-line treatment to help induce remission in CD. However, there may be circumstances in which steroids are preferred, particularly in severe colonic disease.

Immune-modulating drugs, such as azathioprine or methotrexate, are increasingly used earlier after diagnosis in an attempt to reduce the risk of some of the longer-term complications related to ongoing inflammation such as strictures, perforation and fistulae. If these drugs are ineffective in controlling inflammation, or cause unacceptable

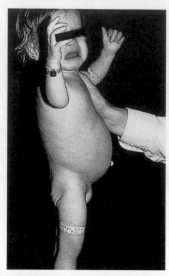

Fig 13.2   Coeliac disease: abdominal distension. (Reproduced with permission from Zitelli, B., McIntire, S. C., & Nowalk, A. J. (2017). *Zitelli and Davis' atlas of pediatric physical diagnosis* (7th ed.). Elsevier.)

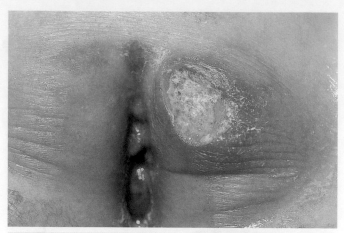

Fig 13.5   Pyoderma gangrenosum. Painful ulcer on the vulva of a girl with Crohn's disease. (Reproduced with permission from Mancini, A. J., & Paller, A. S. (2021). *Hurwitz clinical pediatric dermatology: A textbook of skin disorders of childhood and adolescence* (6th ed.). Elsevier Inc.)

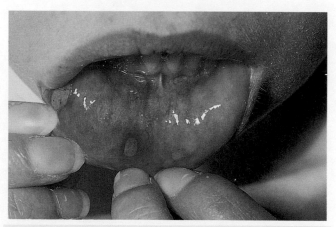

Fig 13.3   Aphthous ulcers. These commonly occur in isolation, but they may be an indication of an underlying intestinal disease such as coeliac disease or inflammatory bowel disease. (Reproduced with permission from Slater, T. A., Waduud, M. A., & Ahmed, N. (2021). *Pocketbook of differential diagnosis* (5th ed.). Elsevier.)

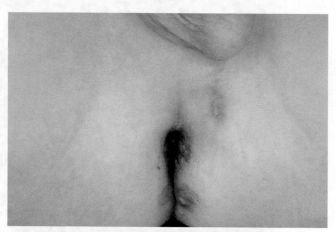

Perianal disease in Crohns
perianal abscess formation

Fig 13.6   Perianal involvement in Crohn's disease.

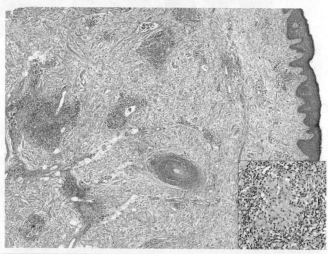

Fig 13.7   Crohn's disease. There is superficial and deep chronic granulomatous inflammation. The granulomas (inset) are typically noncaseating. (Reproduced with permission from, Nucci, M. R. (2020). In C. Parra-Herran (Ed.), *Gynecologic pathology: A volume in foundations in diagnostic pathology series* 2nd ed.). Elsevier Inc.)

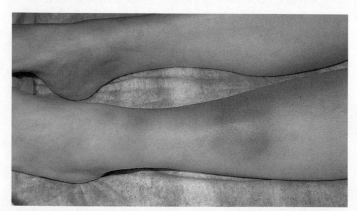

Fig 13.4   Erythema nodosum. (Reproduced with permission from Swartz, M. H. (2020). *Textbook of physical diagnosis: History and examination* (8th ed.). Elsevier Inc.)

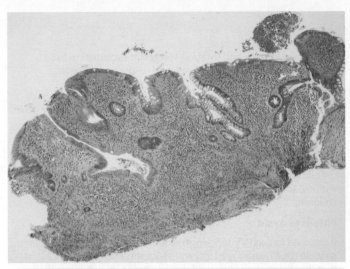

Fig 13.8 Ulcerative colitis. A 14-year-old girl with pancolitis. Photomicrograph of colonic biopsy demonstrating polypoid surface and diffuse inflammatory cell infiltration of the lamina propria mucosae. The crypts are short and very distorted. (Reproduced with permission from Sebire, S., Malone, M., Ashworth, M., & Jacques, T. S. (2010). *Diagnostic pediatric surgical pathology* (1st ed.). Elsevier.)

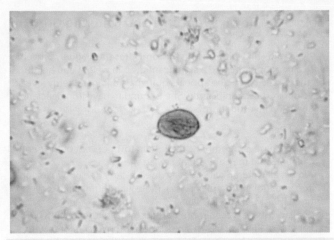

Fig 13.9 Cyst of Giardia species. A small ovoid-shaped cyst with distinct periphery is shown. (Reproduced with permission from Bassert, J. M. (2021). *McCurnin's clinical textbook for veterinary technicians and nurses* (10th ed.). Saunders.)

side effects, biologic agents such as infliximab and adalimumab are now widely used. Infliximab is effective in the treatment of perianal disease. Antibiotics may also be used for perianal disease in CD. For severe CD, especially with strictures, parenteral nutrition may be required. Surgical intervention may be required for strictures, fistulae or uncontrolled inflammation despite escalation of treatment.

ULCERATIVE COLITIS (UC)

Bloody diarrhoea is almost always seen in UC. Rectal bleeding, tenesmus and faecal urgency are the major symptoms. UC in children most commonly affects the whole colon, and 'backwash' ileitis affecting the terminal ileum is possible. The histology of UC is of inflammation affecting only the mucosa and submucosa. Typical histology shows crypt architecture distortion, crypt abscesses and ulceration (Fig. 13.8).

Children and adolescents with UC require prompt treatment with steroids or aminosalicylates. The child diagnosed with acute severe colitis should be urgently admitted to hospital for intravenous fluids, high-dose intravenous methylprednisolone and close monitoring by surgeons, as an urgent colectomy may be required. If the child is not responding to steroids, infliximab may be given to try salvaging the colon.

Maintenance treatment in UC is with aminosalicylates, escalating to thiopurines and biologic agents such as infliximab if required.

Giardiasis

Giardia intestinalis is a flagellated protozoan that can cause symptoms of diarrhoea, abdominal cramps or malabsorption, but infected children may also have no symptoms. Symptoms occur generally 1 to 3 weeks after exposure and may appear similar to those seen in acute gastroenteritis. A chronic illness subsequently develops with intermittent diarrhoea, abdominal bloating and weight loss. Many develop secondary lactose intolerance. Diagnosis is by examination of fresh stool samples for cysts (Fig. 13.9), or by PCR of stool. Treatment is with metronidazole.

(Box 13.1)
(Box 13.2)
(Box 13.3)

Box 13.1 Key Points

Acute gastroenteritis is a very common presentation in infancy and childhood, and the landscape in high-income countries has been changed by the successful introduction of rotavirus vaccination.

Oral rehydration solution (ORS) is the preferred method of rehydration in both hospital and community settings.

For every 25 children treated with oral rehydration therapy, one will not respond and will require intravenous therapy.

Clinical assessment of dehydration tends to overestimate it (degree mainly under 3 per cent).

Diarrhoea can last for up to 2 weeks in gastroenteritis and is lessened by early reintroduction of solids.

There is <u>no</u> role for carbonated drinks or antiemetics except ondansetron in an ED setting to avoid admission.

Toddler diarrhoea typically affects 1- to 3-year-olds with several watery and unformed stools per day. The stools often contain undigested vegetables but lack blood, mucus or excessive fat.

Coeliac disease is a very common immune-mediated disorder (population screening studies suggest as many as 1 per cent in some countries) brought on by exposure to gluten and tends to run in families.

A greater than 10-fold rise in TTG IgA antibodies with positive anti-endomysial IgA antibodies can confirm the diagnosis without need for duodenal biopsy.

The prevalence of both UC and CD has risen significantly over the past 30 years in all high-income countries.

Investigations suggestive of IBD include a negative stool microscopy and culture, high inflammatory markers (CRP+ESR), a low serum albumin, elevated transaminases, a high platelet count and low haemoglobin (especially in ulcerative colitis).

The likelihood of an IBD diagnosis increases as the level of faecal calprotectin gets higher.

Giardia intestinalis is a flagellated protozoan that can cause weight loss, diarrhoea, abdominal pain and malabsorption, but infection can also be asymptomatic.

Box 13.2   Down Syndrome and Faltering Growth

A 9-year-old child with Down syndrome presents vaguely unwell with a poor appetite and a significant drop in weight and height on the centile chart. She appears quite pale and her energy levels have diminished significantly. She is found to have iron deficiency anaemia on investigation.

Clinical Pearls

Coeliac disease is common, affecting up to 1 per cent of the general population, and may present at any age.

Almost all children with coeliac disease carry one of two major histocompatibility complex class II molecules (human leukocyte antigen [HLA]-DQ2 or -DQ8).

Coeliac disease is seen more frequently in children with type 1 diabetes mellitus or Down syndrome (as above). Children with Down syndrome have a _six-fold_ increased risk of coeliac disease.

Classic coeliac disease presents with symptoms and signs of malabsorption, including diarrhoea, steatorrhoea, weight loss or growth failure, abdominal pain and discomfort and associated fatigue.

After diagnosis, the child should be referred to a dietician with specific training in coeliac disease to start a gluten-free diet.

Interpretation of Investigations

Young children with a first-degree relative with coeliac disease have a 7 per cent risk of coeliac disease and, for this reason, serological testing should be considered before the onset of symptoms in children with a positive family history. Immunoglobulin A-tissue transglutaminase (IgA-tTG) titre is the serological test of choice.

Anti-endomysial antibody (EMA) has greater specificity but lower sensitivity than IgA-tTG and is more expensive.

A normal IgA-tTG and total IgA test result excludes coeliac disease if there is a low clinical index of suspicion for coeliac disease.

Children with symptoms consistent with coeliac disease, a high IgA-tTG titre (above 10 times the normal range), and a positive EMA may be diagnosed _without_ a small intestinal biopsy.

The presence of typical coeliac changes on duodenal histology with clinical improvement on a gluten-free diet confirms the diagnosis.

Following a gluten-free diet, IgA-tTG titres should normalise within 6 to 9 months, but it may take up to 3 years in some children.

Pitfalls to Avoid

If the child has an IgA deficiency, request IgG-deamidated gliadin peptide (DGP) serology or IgG anti-tTG antibodies but be aware that the diagnostic accuracy of these tests is somewhat less than that of IgA-tTG.

Giardiasis may present with very similar symptoms. Multiple stool specimens may be required to diagnose giardiasis.

Common variable immunodeficiency (CVID) can present with similar symptoms to coeliac disease.

Dermatitis herpetiformis is the skin manifestation of active coeliac disease but can occur even if on a strict gluten-free diet.

Intestinal and extraintestinal lymphoma and carcinomas of the digestive tract are more common in patients with coeliac disease.

Hyposplenism has been associated with coeliac disease, thereby increasing the risk of infections from encapsulated bacteria such as _Streptococcus pneumoniae_.

Box 13.3   A Teenager With Delayed Puberty and Nocturnal Diarrhoea

A 14-year-old boy presents with short stature and delayed pubertal development. He has vague abdominal pains and has had significant weight loss over the past 3 months. He has had loose stools for 3 weeks with nocturnal diarrhoea for the last five nights. He is noted to have aphthous ulcers in the mouth. His faecal calprotectin is elevated at 1000 µg/mg.

Clinical Pearls

Early and effective treatment in Crohn's disease (CD) aims to control symptoms, minimise impact on nutrition and growth and enable the child to function well.

Symptoms typical of inflammatory bowel disease (IBD) include diarrhoea for over 2 weeks without another cause (particularly no recent travel), bloody diarrhoea, weight loss (Crohn's disease only) and persistent abdominal pain for more than 2 weeks. A positive family history of IBD should heighten concern.

Important signs include perianal disease such as fistulae, fissures and skin tags, frequent severe mouth ulcers (Crohn's disease only), and extraintestinal manifestations such as uveitis, erythema nodosum and large joint arthritis.

Interpretation of Investigations

Investigations suggestive of IBD include a negative stool microscopy and culture, high inflammatory markers, a drop in serum albumin, elevated transaminases, an elevated platelet count and anaemia.

Faecal calprotectin is a sensitive marker for inflammatory bowel disease (IBD). The likelihood of a diagnosis of IBD increases as the level of faecal calprotectin gets higher with values above 800 indicate that over 90 per cent will have a diagnosis of IBD.

Diagnosis is confirmed by MR enterography and endoscopy with histology of biopsies showing transmural inflammation and skip lesions in Crohn's disease.

Pitfalls to Avoid

Bearing in mind the frequency of functional abdominal pain, confusion may exist with the diagnosis of Crohn's disease being thereby delayed. Oral or perianal manifestations and recent weight loss should always raise concern about the possibility of IBD, particularly Crohn's disease.

One of the main acute complications of UC is acute severe colitis, which may progress to toxic megacolon (dilatation of the colon above six cm in diameter detected on plain abdominal x-ray) and risk of bowel perforation.

Key References

Al-Toma, A., Volta, U., Auricchio, R., Castillejo, G., Sanders, D. S., Cellier, C., et al. (2019). European Society for the Study of Coeliac Disease (ESsCD) guideline for coeliac disease and other gluten-related disorders. *United European Gastroenterol Journal, 7*(5), 583–613.

Ashton, J. J., Ennis, S., & Beattie, R. M. (2017). Early-onset paediatric inflammatory bowel disease. *The Lancet Child & Adolescent Health, 1*(2), 147–158.

Ashton, J. J., Harden, A., & Beattie, R. M. (2018). Paediatric inflammatory bowel disease: Improving early diagnosis [published correction appears in *Archives of Disease in Childhood, 104(9):925*]. *Archives of Disease in Childhood, 103*(4), 307–308.

Ashton, J. J., Gavin, J., & Beattie, R. M. (2019). Exclusive enteral nutrition in Crohn's disease: Evidence and practicalities. *Clinical Nutrition, 38*(1), 80–89.

BMJ Best Practice. (n.d.). Coeliac disease. https://bestpractice.bmj.com/topics/en-gb/636/aetiology#referencePop1

European Society for Paediatric Gastroenterology, Hepatology and Nutrition. (n.d.). Knowledge Center. http://www.espghan.org/guidelines/gastroenterology/

Gurram, B. (2018). Diarrhea. In R. M. Kliegman, P. S. Lye, B. Bordini, H. Toth, & D. Basel (Eds.), *Nelson pediatric symptom-based diagnosis* (pp. 182–203). Elsevier.

Ruemmele, F. M., Veres, G., Kolho, K. L., Griffiths, A., Levine, A., Escher, J. C., et al. (2014). Consensus guidelines of ECCO/ESPGHAN on the medical management of pediatric Crohn's disease. *Journal of Crohn's & Colitis, 8*(10), 1179–1207.

The Royal Children's Hospital Melbourne. (2020, December). *Clinical practice guidelines: Diarrhoea and vomiting.* https://www.rch.org.au/clinicalguide/guideline_index/Diarrhoea_and_vomiting/.

Torres, J., Mehandru, S., Colombel, J. F., & Peyrin-Biroulet, L. (2017). Crohn's disease. *Lancet, 389*(10080), 1741–1755.

van Rheenen, P. F., Aloi, M., Assa, A., Bronsky, J., Escher, J. C., Fagerberg, U. L., et al. (2020). The medical management of paediatric Crohn's disease: An ECCO-ESPGHAN guideline update. *Journal of Crohn's & Colitis, 15*(2), 171–194. https://doi.org/10.1093/ecco-jcc/jjaa161.

Ye, Y., Manne, S., Treem, W. R., & Bennett, D. (2020). Prevalence of Inflammatory bowel disease in pediatric and adult populations: Recent estimates from large national databases in the United States, 2007–2016. *Inflammatory Bowel Diseases, 26*(4), 619–625.

14 Diabetes Mellitus in Childhood and Adolescence

NUALA MURPHY, NIAMH McGRATH and SUSAN O'CONNELL

The vast majority of diabetes mellitus in childhood is type 1 characterised by autoimmune T-cell-mediated damage to the islet cells of the pancreas leading to insulin deficiency. Insulin deficiency leads to elevated blood glucose concentrations. Genetic factors are particularly relevant with a concordance between identical twins of 30 to 50 per cent. The HLA-DR3 and HLA-DR4 regions of the genome are associated with an increased risk of diabetes. Studies have indicated that exposure to certain viruses (enteroviruses such as coxsackie B) may be environmental triggers. Diabetes autoimmunity is present in 85 to 98 per cent.

Clinical Features

Most patients with new-onset diabetes have a short history of classical symptoms (polyuria, polydipsia, weight loss and fatigue), but if the osmotic symptoms are unrecognised, the first presentation may be with diabetic ketoacidosis (DKA). Drinking a lot and passing a lot of urine may not be noticed by parents, especially in younger children who are unable to articulate their symptoms and in whom the symptoms may be non-specific. Another concerning symptom is when the child starts wetting the bed, having previously been dry at night for some time. Symptoms of DKA include abdominal pain, vomiting, and drowsiness with unexplained tachypnoea. Infants under 2 years of age may be very challenging to diagnose, and this age group often present with diabetic ketoacidosis.

Management

Children and adolescents with type 1 diabetes mellitus require insulin, which is started on the day of referral. The child will be managed by the diabetes multidisciplinary team consisting of a paediatric endocrinologist (or paediatrician with a special interest in diabetes), a dietician, a diabetes clinical nurse specialist, a psychologist and a social worker. An insulin regimen is started and consists of multiple daily injections, with other treatment options such as insulin pump therapy in the future. Blood glucose is monitored at regular intervals with intermittent or continuous blood glucose monitors, aiming for target blood glucose readings of 4 to 8 mmol/L. Long-term control is monitored by measuring HbA1c levels, and levels <7.0 per cent (53 mmol) are associated with a lower risk of diabetes-related complications.

Education in Newly Diagnosed Diabetics (Table 14.1)

EDUCATION

Essential competencies include home glucose and ketone monitoring, administering injections, and how to address low blood glucose readings. Significant support with a multidisciplinary approach is required for the child and family as this is a life-changing diagnosis requiring initial daily contact with staff and other resources. It is important to stress from the outset that excellent blood glucose control significantly reduces long-term complications.

Table 14.1 Key areas to be discussed with children and families of newly diagnosed diabetics

- administering insulin injections while focusing on correct dose, correct technique, and rotating injection sites to avoid insulin lipohypertrophy (Fig. 14.1)
- dietetic advice and carbohydrate counting
- measuring blood glucose and blood glucose targets
- recognising symptoms of hypoglycaemia (which can be quite variable) and treatment of hypoglycaemia
- sick day rules and perioperative adjustments
- prevention of long-term complications

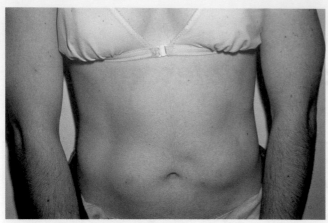

Figure 14.1   Insulin-induced lipohypertrophy. (Reproduced with permission from James, W. D., Elston, D., Treat, J., Rosenbach, M., & Micheletti, R. G. (2019). *Andrews' diseases of the skin: Clinical dermatology* (13th ed., pp. 485-495). Elsevier.)

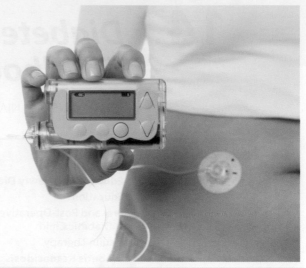

Figure 14.2   Insulin pumps push insulin from a refillable cartridge in the pump through tubing into a diabetic patient's body. (Reproduced with permission from Privitera, M.B. (Ed.). (2019). *Applied human factors in medical device design* (1st ed.). Academic Press..)

The **Five Sick Day Rules** in diabetes management (as per ISPAD) are:

1. Sick day guidelines, including insulin adjustments, should be taught soon after diagnosis and reviewed at least annually with patients and family members to reduce the risk of DKA and severe hypoglycaemia.
2. More frequent blood glucose and blood ketone monitoring.
3. DO NOT STOP INSULIN. However, the dose will likely need to be adjusted.
4. Monitor and maintain hydration with adequate salt and water balance.
5. Treat any underlying, precipitating illness.

PRE- AND POST-OPERATIVE CARE OF THE DIABETIC CHILD

Surgery involving children and adolescents with diabetes should be performed in hospitals with appropriate staff and facilities to care for children with diabetes.

Collaboration is required between surgical, anaesthetic and children's diabetes care teams before hospital admission for elective surgery and as soon as possible after admission for emergency surgery.

Elective surgery should preferably be scheduled in the morning, with the child ideally being first on the list. Careful blood glucose monitoring is required with hourly blood glucose checks in the pre-, intra-, and post-operative periods to ideally maintain blood glucose in the range of 5 to 10 mmol/L during surgical procedures in children.

Dextrose 5 per cent with 0.9 per cent saline is often sufficient, but dextrose 10 per cent may be necessary if there is an increased risk of hypoglycaemia.

Additional insulin is required if blood ketone and blood glucose concentrations are elevated.

INSULIN THERAPY

Type 1 diabetes requires the lifelong administration of exogenous insulin. The goals of treatment are to maintain near-normoglycaemia through intensive insulin therapy, avoid

acute complications and prevent long-term complications while attempting to facilitate as close to a normal life as possible. The choice of insulin regime will depend on the child's age, family, patient and physician preferences. There are many different options, all with advantages and disadvantages, as none are truly physiological. Options include pre-meal fast-acting subcutaneous injections combined with a once-daily long-acting subcutaneous injection in a multiple injection daily regime or continuous subcutaneous insulin pump therapy (Fig. 14.2).

It is noteworthy that there is often a 'honeymoon period' after initial diagnosis where insulin requirements reduce for a period, and some children may even come off insulin completely, but insulin requirements will later rise again.

Post-diagnosis regular review at the diabetes clinic occurs every 3 months with a formal annual review and a series of blood tests. Each visit assesses HbA1c and home monitoring record, recognition, treatment and occurrence of hypoglycaemia, injection sites and technique, diet (carbohydrate counting), insulin dose adjustment with exercise, school issues and psychosocial adjustment.

Annual review incorporates a growth check and comorbidity screening to include blood pressure measurement, blood lipid screening, thyroid function tests, coeliac screening, foot neuropathy screening, retinopathy and nephropathy screening.

Diabetic Ketoacidosis

Diabetic ketoacidosis (DKA) is a triad of hyperglycaemia (blood glucose is usually over 11 mmol/L), acidosis (pH less than 7.3), and ketosis in the blood (greater than 2.5 mmol/L), with the high blood glucose leading to osmotic diuresis, causing fluid and electrolyte imbalance. Most deaths in DKA occur because of cerebral oedema. We should aim to prevent DKA with earlier diagnosis at the onset of diabetes, immediate hospital referral once diabetes is suspected and by providing additional support for those challenged by diabetes self-care.

GENERAL RESUSCITATION

As always, ensure that the airway is patent, and secure the airway if the child has a diminished level of consciousness. If coma or persistent vomiting are present, a nasogastric tube should be passed.

An initial bolus of 0.9 per cent saline is recommended if a child is volume-depleted but not shocked. If the child is shocked, seek senior advice before repeat boluses. Quickly measure the child's weight to calculate accurately fluid and insulin requirements.

Admit to paediatric intensive care (PICU) if severe DKA (pH below 7.1), shock, depressed level of consciousness, persistent vomiting or a DKA episode in a child under 2 years old.

FLUID MANAGEMENT

Calculate the fluid deficit and then add maintenance fluids to this calculated deficit, subtracting any initial emergency rehydration and giving the total volume evenly over 48 hours.

Normal saline (0.9 per cent) is the recommended initial fluid type. Add dextrose to the normal saline as required when the glucose falls as in guidelines.

POTASSIUM

Total body potassium is always depleted in DKA, although initial serum potassium levels may be low, normal or elevated. Potassium levels will tend to fall once insulin is commenced.

After initial resuscitation, start potassium supplements as soon as possible unless anuria is suspected or peaked T-waves on ECG. Serum electrolytes should be monitored; 2 hourly initially and then 2 to 4 hourly until DKA has corrected and adjust the potassium replacement accordingly. Continue ECG monitoring during resuscitation.

INSULIN THERAPY

Continuous low-dose insulin infusion is recommended following current local or national guidelines.

Consider reduction of the insulin infusion rate if the blood glucose drops when the child is maintained on 0.9 per cent saline and 10 per cent dextrose.

Excessive ongoing losses may need to be replaced if dehydration is not improving after review. Delay insulin therapy until shock (if present) has been reversed by resuscitation and wait until intravenous fluids have been running for 1 hour.

ORAL FLUIDS

Keep children nil by mouth initially. Once there is significant clinical improvement and acidosis has been corrected, gradually reintroduce oral fluids and subtract oral intake from the total fluid required.

Complications of DKA: Cerebral Oedema

Cerebral oedema is **A LIFE-THREATENING EMERGENCY.** The cause of cerebral oedema during treatment of DKA remains unclear. Cerebral oedema occurs most often within the first 24 hours of treatment – usually 4 to 12 hours after initial treatment but may occur 24 to 48 hours afterwards.

Cerebral oedema is more likely in younger children, during the first presentation, if severe dehydration or acidosis is present and with a longer duration of symptoms.

When managing children at high risk of cerebral oedema, the appropriate dose of mannitol or 3 per cent saline should be calculated, drawn up, and left at the bedside.

IDIOPATHIC CEREBRAL OEDEMA (TABLE 14.2)

Give mannitol or hypertonic saline if there are signs of cerebral oedema. A repeat dose may be required if no response. Nurse with the head up at a 30-degree angle and in the midline. Transfer to a tertiary PICU as intubation and invasive ventilation may be required. Intubation should be performed by the most experienced operator available with the aim of maintaining low $PaCO_2$ and high PaO_2 throughout to prevent a further rise in intracranial pressure.

Neuroimaging (CT/MRI) is indicated as other intracerebral pathology (e.g. cerebral venous thrombosis) may occur and present similarly.

Long-Term Management of Type 1 DM

The long-term goals are to maintain a healthy lifestyle, optimise metabolic control and prevent microvascular complications. The relative risk of long-term complications increases with elevated HbA1c levels.

Future directions include prevention trials (enterovirus vaccination), regeneration of beta cells (using stem cell technology) and technological approaches (closed-loop pumps with continuous blood glucose monitoring to mimic normal pancreatic function).

Type 2 Diabetes

The vast majority of diabetes mellitus (DM) in childhood is type 1; however, type 2 diabetes is emerging and should be considered particularly in obese adolescents who may show signs of insulin resistance (acanthosis nigricans) and negative diabetes autoantibodies. Initial strategies relate

Table 14.2 Warning signs of Idiopathic cerebral oedoma

- slowing of the heart rate
- headache
- change in neurological status (irritability, restlessness, or increasing drowsiness)
- rise in BP

to modification of risk factors, especially obesity (no easy task!), and the addition of first-line medication with met-formin. There is a trend towards considering bariatric sur-gery in markedly obese adolescents with type 2 DM. There is a worldwide epidemic related to increasing obesity (30 per cent of new cases of diabetes in the second decade in the US) with a higher risk in non-Caucasian populations.

Maturity-Onset Diabetes in the Young (MODY)

This is a rare type of diabetes that usually presents under 25 years of age. It has an autosomal dominant mode of inheritance (thus a positive family history in three genera-tions may be found) due to a variety of genetic mutations affecting insulin production. It is important to recognise, as affected individuals may have improved diabetes con-trol with oral agents and understanding the genetic cause can predict future course. Consider MODY in children with positive family history of diabetes, negative diabetes

autoantibodies, low insulin requirements and an elevated c-peptide outside the honeymoon period.

Cystic Fibrosis Related Diabetes (CFRD)

CFRD occurs in approximately 20 per cent of adolescents with cystic fibrosis (CF) and is caused by pancreatic dam-age causing insulin deficiency. In addition, CF can lead to insulin resistance. Annual screening for diabetes in CF starts from 10 years of age. The goal of treatment is to main-tain normal blood glucose readings to maintain weight and improve muscle mass, lung function and wellbeing.

Neonatal Diabetes

Neonatal diabetes is very rare and usually presents under 6 months of age. It can be transient or permanent. It is caused by a single gene disorder. All children diagnosed with

---

Box 14.1 **Key Points**

Twenty-five per cent of newly diagnosed children/adolescents with diabetes present in diabetic ketoacidosis (DKA) with a higher incidence in toddlers and younger children in severe DKA or at first presentation.

Most have a short history of classical symptoms (fatigue, weight loss, polydipsia and polyuria), but if the osmotic symptoms are unrecognised, the first presentation may be with diabetic ketoacidosis (DKA).

Incidence of DKA episodes complicated by cerebral oedema is 0.3 to 1.0 per cent and the mortality from cerebral oedema is 20 to 25 per cent.

Delay in diagnosis is the lead cause of DKA in young children while omission of insulin is the leading cause in adolescents.

Education immediately following diagnosis is key. Signifi-cant support is required for the child and family as this is a

life-changing diagnosis, involves recent technology and is very resource- and staff-intensive with initial daily contact required.

At each visit, assess HbA1c and home monitoring record, recognition, occurrences and management of hypoglycaemia, injection sites and technique, diet (carbohydrate counting), dose adjustment with exercise, and school issues.

Annual review incorporates a growth check and comor-bidity screening, including blood pressure measurement, a blood lipid screen, thyroid function tests and coeliac screen, foot neuropathy, retinopathy and nephropathy screening.

Type 2 diabetes should be considered, particularly in obese adolescents who may have signs of insulin resistance (acan-thosis nigricans) and negative diabetes autoantibodies.

Box 14.2 **A 6-Year-Old With Tiredness and Secondary Enuresis.**

A 6-year-old girl presents with vague tiredness and malaise over the previous 3 weeks. She is constantly tired and over the past week has started wetting the bed, despite keeping dry at night for a number of years. She is constantly thirsty and is losing weight despite increased appetite. Her parents are very concerned about her. Her family history is negative for diabetes mellitus, but there is a positive family history of coeliac disease. Her astute GP checks a finger prick glucometer reading and finds a glucose level of 18.5 mm/L and promptly sends her to hospital for assessment and management.

Clinical Pearls

The incidence of type I diabetes mellitus is increasing, especially in younger children in whom diagnosis can be more challenging. Consider and rule out diabetes in all unwell toddlers and young children.

Secondary nocturnal enuresis, as in this case, is a very common presenting symptom. Twenty-five per cent of children still present with diabetic ketoacidosis (DKA) at diagnosis with many having had earlier contact with a healthcare professional.

Differential diagnoses include urinary tract infection (UTI), appendicitis (as may present with abdominal pain) and pneumonia (where DKA with tachypnoea or Kussmaul's respiration is evident).

Interpretation of Investigations

Diabetes mellitus is defined as either a random blood glucose over 11.1 mmol/L or a fasting blood glucose over 7.0 mmol/L.

Urinalysis or point-of-care blood glucose allows the diagnosis to be made in most instances without delay. Refer all children with elevated blood glucose on the same day they present to primary care.

HbA1c levels are used to evaluate glycaemic control over the preceding 2 to 3 months, the aim of which is to keep HbA1c levels below 7.0 (53 mmol).

Pitfalls to Avoid

Firstly, consider the diagnosis in an unwell child and perform point-of-care urinalysis and blood glucose testing.

Cerebral oedema is **A LIFE-THREATENING EMERGENCY.** Its occurrence is more likely in younger children, during the first presentation, if severe dehydration or acidosis is present and with a longer duration of symptoms. Warning signs of idiopathic cerebral oedema include slowing of the heart rate, a headache, change in neurological status (irritability, restlessness or increasing drowsiness), and rising blood pressure in the child.

diabetes under 6 months of age should undergo genetic screening as optimal therapy requires a specific diagnosis.

(Box14.1)

(Box14.2)

 Video on the topic Diabetes mellitus is available online at Elsevier eBooks+.

Key references

Health Service Executive & Royal College of Physicians of Ireland. (2021, April). *National Clinical Guideline: Care of the child newly diagnosed with type 1 diabetes without DKA (Guideline reference: CDI005/2-21.* https://www.hse.ie/eng/about/who/cspd/ncps/paediatrics-neonatology/resources/care-of-the-child-newly-diagnosed-with-type-1-diabetes-without-dka.pdf.

Health Service Executive & Royal College of Physicians of Ireland. (2018, December). *National Clinical Guideline: Management of Paediatric Diabetic Ketoacidosis.* https://olchc.ie/Healthcare-Professionals/Clinical-Guidelines/Diabetes-National-Clinical-Guidelines-for-the-Management-of-Diabetic-Ketoacidosis.pdf.

International Society for Pediatric and Adolescent Diabetes. (2018). *ISPAD Clinical Practice Consensus Guidelines 2018*. https://www.ispad.org/page/ISPADGuidelines2018.

Laffel, L. M., Limbert, C., Phelan, H., Virmani, A., Wood, J., & Hofer, S. E. (2018). ISPAD Clinical Practice Consensus Guidelines 2018: Sick day management in children and adolescents with diabetes. *Pediatric Diabetes, 19*(Suppl 27), 193–204.

Leach, D., Barton, J., & British Society for Paediatric Endocrinology and Diabetes (2020, March). *Integrated care pathway for the management of children and young people with diabetic ketoacidosis.* https://www.bsped.org.uk/media/1742/dka-icp-2020-v1_1.pdf.

NICE Pathways. (n.d.). Diabetes in children and young people overview. National Institute for Health and Care Excellence. https://pathways.nice.org.uk/pathways/diabetes-in-children-and-young-people

Our Lady's Children's Hospital. (n.d.). Newly Diagnosed Education Competency Checklist. http://www.olchc.ie/Healthcare-Professionals/Nursing-Practice-Guidelines/Diabetes-New-Patient-Competency-Checklist.pdf

Rodriguez-Saldana, J. (Ed.). (2019). *The diabetes textbook: clinical principles, patient management and public health issues* (1st ed.) Springer International Publishing.

Tasker, R. C. (2020). Fluid management during diabetic ketoacidosis in children: Guidelines, consensus, recommendations and clinical judgement. *Archives of Disease in Childhood, 105*(10), 917–918.

15 | *The Child With a Fever*

KARINA BUTLER

As over 30 per cent of consultations in general practice relate to children, the presentation of infants and children with fever is an everyday occurrence. The most frequent illnesses associated with fever are outlined below.

Fever in Children Under 2 Years Old

Fever is very common in young children and is certainly one of the most common reasons for consultation with a healthcare professional. The great majority of feverish illnesses in young children are due to self-limiting viral illnesses; however, amongst this large group is a small number with serious bacterial illness.

The Traffic Light system developed by the National Institute of Clinical Excellence is very helpful for recognizing acutely ill febrile infants and children in the community and ascertaining who needs urgent referral and who can be safely managed at home.

MEASUREMENT OF TEMPERATURE IN INFANTS AND CHILDREN

In infants under 4 weeks of age, temperature should be measured with an electronic thermometer in the axilla. From 4 weeks to 5 years of age, the temperature should be measured by an electronic thermometer in the axilla, a chemical dot thermometer in the axilla or an infrared tympanic thermometer (favoured in hospitals).

INFANTS UNDER 3 MONTHS OF AGE

In general, these young infants are at higher risk of invasive bacterial infection, and thus merit at least 6 hours of observation in an observation ward or admission to hospital. Regular assessment of the vital signs (heart rate (HR), respiratory rate (RR) and temperature) should take place. There should be a low threshold for investigation and admission. First line investigations include urinalysis and urine culture, stool culture (if diarrhoea), blood cultures, CRP and full blood count. Lumbar puncture should be considered if the infant is unwell or if under 2 months of age. Intravenous broad-spectrum antibiotics are empirically started while awaiting cultures. Rates of serious bacterial infection in febrile infants under 2 months are as high as 12 to 14 per cent with clinical examination alone being a poor determinant of risk. Several clinical guidelines (including the Rochester, Philadelphia, Boston and Pittsburgh criteria) have been used to stratify infants into risk categories. Higher rates of serious bacterial infection were seen in those infants who had fever documented in the emergency department (ED) compared to those with fever at home who were afebrile in the ED.

INFANTS OVER 3 MONTHS OF AGE

First, look for any life-threatening features such as a decreased level of consciousness, shock with delayed capillary refill time, tachycardia and cold peripheries or airway compromise. If fever and shock is evident, give an intravenous bolus of 0.9 per cent saline and start immediate parenteral antibiotics.

Use the Traffic Light system to assess the risk of serious illness with infants and children without any of the amber or red features, which may remain at home with appropriate advice to parents as to when to seek further attention.

Recognition of Sepsis

Among those with fever, who have self-limiting illnesses is a small but very important group of infants and children who have sepsis. It is important to be able to recognise and speedily treat this group. The recognition and prompt management of sepsis has been helped by the introduction of Paediatric Early Warning Scores (PEWS), greater situational awareness, more robust handover and the Sepsis 6 algorithm.

Both in primary care and in hospital, prompt recognition of sepsis is essential to improve outcomes. In this regard, attention to the level of parental concern is a key factor as are regular observation of vital signs, identifying and responding to concerns of the nursing staff and excellent communication between the whole team.

High immunisation uptake has happily led to a striking fall in the rates of invasive meningococcal and pneumococcal disease. However, cases still occur and need early recognition and prompt treatment for better outcomes. There has been an increase in invasive group A streptococcus (GAS) infections. This condition also requires prompt recognition and treatment.

Latest evidence advises against the routine use of paracetamol and ibuprofen together, the use of antipyretics simply to lower temperature or being reassured that a temperature drop with antipyretics excludes sepsis. One should check a urine sample for culture if an infant under 6 months of age is pyrexial. Reassess any infant or child with amber or red features after a minimum of 1 to 2 hours. Carefully monitor the heart rate as tachycardia is a critical – and often overlooked – sign of sepsis (Table 15.1).

PAEDIATRIC EARLY WARNING SYSTEM (PEWS) SCORES

Paediatric early warning system scores have been in existence for over 10 years. In essence, PEWS scores convert clinical observations into a score and combine them with the concerns of nurses or family at the bedside. This information helps clinicians recognise and intervene to rescue a sick child before they deteriorate. The total PEWS score should never undermine or replace clinical judgement.

Standard observation charts help prompt good decisions, as does situational awareness in frontline healthcare staff. There should be a clear escalation pathway available to all treating staff. Finally, in the detection of the deteriorating child, clinical acumen is imperative. Always consider the family, who are best placed to recognise when children are 'not right' or 'not themselves'.

Core parameters are parental or professional concern, respiratory rate and effort, oxygen therapy, heart rate and level of consciousness.

SEPSIS 6 ALGORITHM

Paediatric Sepsis 6 involves two elements: firstly, the recognition of the child at risk (a child with suspected or proven infection,

Table 15.1 Ranges of Tachycardia Causing Concern

Under 12 Months Over 160 Beats per Minute (bpm)

12 to 24 months over 150 bpm
2 to 5 years over 140 bpm

and at least two of the following: a core temperature of under 36°C or above 38.5°C [38.0°C if immunocompromised], tachycardia or altered mental state [sleepiness, irritability, lethargy, floppiness]); and prolonged capillary refill (over 2 seconds).

And/Or

Red flag signs with any one of hypotension, a lactate over 2.0 mmol/L, extreme tachycardia or tachypnoea, SpO_2 under 90 per cent/grunting/cyanosis/apnoea, being just responsive to pain or unconscious, if immunocompromised, or a non-blanching, rash/mottled skin.

If the criteria are met, the sepsis 6 guideline should be activated and investigation and treatment for sepsis should start immediately. Cold peripheries marked tachycardia and prolonged capillary refill time are all key observations in assessing the sick infant or child for sepsis.

Common Causes of Fever in Infants and Children

ACUTE OTITIS MEDIA

Acute otitis media is the most common cause of otalgia or ear pain in children. Over 80 per cent of children will experience at least one episode of otitis media in the first 3 years of life. Younger children tend to present with fever, irritability and ear pulling.

Risk factors for acute otitis media (AOM) include prior episodes or a family history of AOM, Down syndrome, household cigarette smoke, male gender, social disadvantage, presence of a cleft palate, presence of other siblings in the household and attendance at day care.

Otoscopy enables the examiner to view the tympanic membrane. Proper positioning of the child is essential for this. Findings show the middle ear, filled with fluid, with a tympanic membrane that is opaque and bulging (Fig. 15.1). Rarely, perforation with otorrhoea is noted.

The leading causes of AOM are often viral. Common bacterial causes include *Streptococcus pneumoniae*, non-typable *Haemophilus influenzae* and *Moraxella catarrhalis*.

The goals of treatment are to relieve discomfort and to prevent infectious complications such as acute mastoiditis. As there is a very high rate of spontaneous resolution, a period of observation (up to 48 hours) with adequate analgesia is preferable to the immediate commencement of antibiotics. Amoxicillin is the antibiotic of choice, used at an appropriate dose for AOM. Oral cephalosporins may be an alternative if there is a history of non-urticarial penicillin rash. Cephalosporins should be avoided if there is a history of serious penicillin allergy (anaphylaxis, angioedema, acute urticaria, wheezing or breathing difficulty), unless allergy testing has indicated tolerance of specific cephalosporins.

Acute mastoiditis is a potentially serious complication of AOM. Features include otalgia, fever and otorrhoea with displacement of the pinna anteriorly (such that it sticks out rather than lying back against the skull), posterior auricular tenderness and erythema. Mastoiditis accompanied by periosteitis means the infection has spread to the periosteum of the mastoid process and intravenous antibiotics are required. Indications for mastoidectomy include severe osteitis, mastoid abscess formation and intracranial suppurative complications.

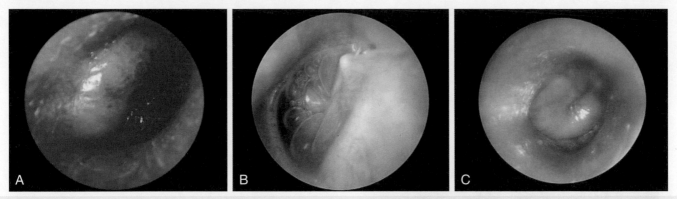

Figure 15.1   Acute otitis media. (a) This is the textbook picture: an erythematous, opaque, bulging tympanic membrane. The light reflex is reduced, and the landmarks are partially obscured. Mobility is markedly reduced. (b) In this acutely febrile child who complained of otalgia, the presence of both air and fluid formed bubbles separated by greyish-yellow menisci. Even though the drum was not injected, this finding, combined with fever and otalgia, is consistent with acute infection. (c) In this child the tympanic membrane was injected at the periphery, and a yellow purulent effusion caused the inferior portion to bulge outwards. Mobility was markedly reduced. (Reproduced with permission from (a) Hawke M, Yellon RF (Eds) (2012) *Zitelli and Davis' atlas of pediatric physical diagnosis, 6th edn*. Philadelphia: Saunders) (b) and (c) Talley NJ, O'Connor S (Eds) (2018) *Clinical examination: A systematic guide to physical diagnosis*, *Eighth Edition*. Elsevier Australia (a division of Reed International Books Australia Pty Ltd.)

OTITIS EXTERNA

Otitis externa (sometimes referred to as Swimmer's ear) is an infection of the external ear canal. Risk factors include warm, humid weather, moisture in the canal, and swimming. Main symptoms are intense pain and otorrhoea. The peak age of occurrence is 7 to 12 years of age. Otitis externa can present with ear pain with discharge, and manipulating the tragus and pinna will lead to discomfort and pain. In otitis externa, the external ear canal is red, and there is typically an ear discharge, making it readily distinguishable from AOM. Treatment is topical (e.g. a topical suspension of ofloxacin and hydrocortisone) with most children responding in a few days.

ACUTE FOLLICULAR TONSILLITIS

Acute pharyngitis or tonsillitis in children is most often viral in origin but may be due to group A streptococcus (*Streptococcus pyogenes*). The tonsils are enlarged, symmetrical and red, with patchy exudates on their surfaces (Fig. 15.2). Treatment is with oral penicillin.

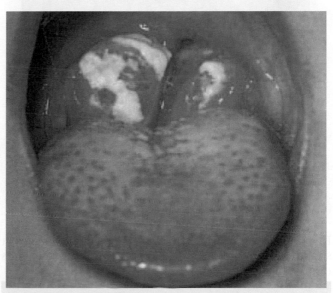

Figure 15.2   Acute tonsillitis. (Reproduced with permission from Atkinson, P., Kendall, R., & van Rensburg, L. (Fds.). (2010). *Emergency medicine: An illustrated colour text*. Churchill Livingstone.)

Fever with a Rash

CHICKENPOX (VARICELLA)

Varicella has an incubation period of 10 to 21 days and is spread by close contact and respiratory droplets. Initial red macules evolve through papular, vesicular and pustular changes over a period of 24 to 48 hours. During the early vesicular stage, the skin lesions are described as 'dew drops on a pink rose petal'. Crops of lesions (up to 100 or more) in various stages of development are typical of varicella. The skin lesions (Fig. 15.3) are accompanied by fever and general malaise. Varicella can be more extensive in those with pre-existing atopic dermatitis. Most often, the diagnosis is clear-cut based on clinical appearance alone. However, if required, confirmatory tests include PCR, immunofluorescent staining and viral culture. Varicella is highly contagious and secondary cases in the same family tend to be more severe. Aciclovir is not required for otherwise healthy children who have varicella. Immunocompromised children who have been exposed to varicella should receive zoster immune gammaglobulin (ZIG) as soon as possible and no later than 72 hours following exposure. For those who miss this window period, prophylactic aciclovir can be used.

While the great majority of children with varicella have a relatively mild illness, complications such as secondary bacterial infection (cellulitis, lymphadenitis), varicella pneumonia, hepatitis, encephalitis and hemorrhagic chickenpox can occur. One may rarely see stroke as a late complication of varicella.

A feared complication is the development of invasive group A streptococcal (GAS) illness during varicella. Fever due to uncomplicated varicella rarely persists for more than 2 to 3 days. Persistence of fever, new onset or higher fever – particularly if associated with a new rash or redness extending around the lesions – should always raise concerns and prompt evaluation for the presence of secondary bacterial infection.

Many countries have introduced the varicella vaccine into their recommended primary immunisation schedules.

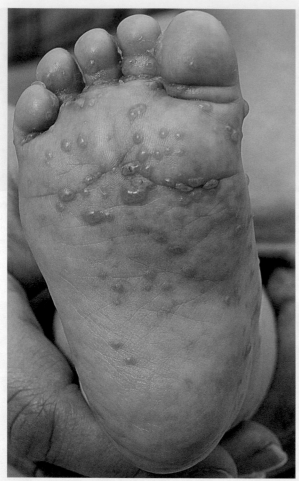

Figure 15.3   Varicella of the foot.

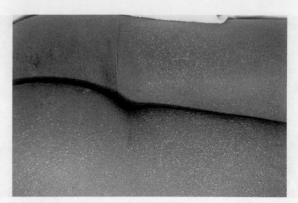

Figure 15.4   Scarlet fever caused by *Streptococcus* pyogenes. The skin has a sandpaper appearance and feel in this black patient. In a white patient, the rash presents as a fine, erythematous, macular and papular eruption. (Reproduced with permission from Paller, A. S., & Mancini, A. J. (2015). *Hurwitz clinical pediatric dermatology: A textbook of skin disorders of childhood and adolescence* (5th ed.). Elsevier – Health Sciences Division.)

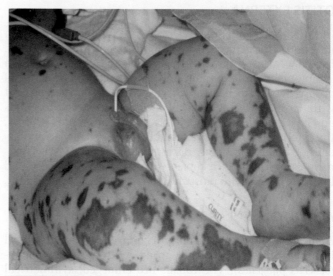

Figure 15.5   Purpura fulminans in meningococcal septicaemia.

In our view, countries who have not yet introduced it should do so mainly because of the risk of complications (especially invasive GAS).

SCARLET FEVER

The rash of scarlet fever is caused by a strain of group A streptococcus that contains a bacteriophage that produces exotoxin A. The scarlet fever rash has a texture like sandpaper and blanches on pressure (Fig. 15.4). The rash usually begins on the face, and then becomes generalized after 24 hours. The cheeks are red, but there is a rim of circumoral pallor that is quite characteristic. Erythema is more marked at flexor skin creases, especially the anterior cubital fossae with linear, petechial appearance, so-called Pastia's lines. There is often a strawberry tongue. The erythema fades within a few days. Fine desquamation begins within a week of onset on the face and progresses all over the body, resembling a mild sunburn.

The main differential diagnoses are Kawasaki disease (KD), staphylococcal toxic shock syndrome and measles. Treatment is with oral penicillin.

ACUTE MENINGOCOCCAL SEPSIS

Now thankfully rare in Europe, acute meningococcal sepsis requires prompt recognition and treatment. As trainees are less likely to see this condition because of immunisation, there is a risk that they will struggle to recognise it when seen for the first time. The adage 'how do you recognise Auntie May – because you have seen her before!' rings true in this instance. If meningococcal infection is suspected, urgent transfer to hospital is required with pre-hospital parenteral penicillin administered where feasible. The administration of intramuscular or intravenous penicillin should never delay transfer. Key presenting features are of a sick child with fever and a spreading petechial or purpuric rash (Fig. 15.5). In the earliest phases of infection, the rash may be absent or a very non-specific erythematous macular rash. The initial symptoms are remarkably similar to those of a viral illness. A child who is thought to have a viral syndrome with a nonspecific rash but who also has leg pains, cold hands and feet or abnormal skin colour, warrants close observation, monitoring and consideration of the possibility of meningococcal infection. If sending a child with febrile illness to continue their care at home, always emphasise to their caretakers that they should not hesitate to seek further medical attention if their concern increases or if the child's condition deteriorates.

Confirmation of the diagnosis is by detection of meningococci either by culture of blood and/or cerebrospinal fluid (CSF) or by polymerase chain reaction (PCR) testing. Gram staining of skin scrapings taken from a purpuric lesion may reveal the characteristic Gram-negative diplococci but is rarely used now for diagnostic purposes. Fluid boluses and inotropes are often required and children with meningococcal sepsis often require paediatric intensive care. Mortality is 3 to 5 per cent and can be much higher if diagnosis is delayed.

INVASIVE GROUP A STREPTOCOCCAL INFECTION (GAS)

There has been an increase in invasive group A streptococcal infection in the past number of years, especially in young children under 2 years of age.

There are three overlapping clinical presentations, including focal disease (cellulitis, lymphadenitis, osteoarticular infection), bacteraemia, and necrotising fasciitis (Fig. 15.6). Definitive diagnosis requires isolation of GAS from a normally sterile body site. Some group A streptococcal strains, in addition to capacity for direct bacterial invasion, are associated with virulent toxin production and cause toxic shock syndrome. This is associated with sudden rapid deterioration, hypotension, multiorgan failure and high mortality if not promptly treated.

Treatment of invasive GAS is with intravenous antibiotics such as penicillin or a cephalosporin. Clindamycin is generally added if there is serious infection or concern about toxin production. The combination of high dose penicillin with clindamycin is recommended for treatment of necrotising fasciitis with the addition of IVIG in severe cases. IVIG is postulated to reduce circulating toxin, and its use has been associated with a lower overall mortality.

STAPHYLOCOCCAL SCALDED SKIN SYNDROME

Staphylococcal scalded skin is caused by staphylococcal exfoliative toxins and is generally seen under 5 years of age.

Fever, skin tenderness and marked irritability often precede the rash. Crusting and fissuring are seen around the mouth, eyes and nose. Flaccid bullae and a positive Nikolsky sign (sloughing of the skin with light pressure) are characteristic features (Fig. 15.7). Healing occurs within 2 weeks with no scarring. Characteristically, the mucosal surfaces are spared.

Treatment is with an anti-staphylococcal antibiotic according to local sensitivities. When methicillin-resistant *Staphylococcus aureus* (MRSA) infection is suspected, an antibiotic with MRSA activity must be selected.

Systemic corticosteroids are contraindicated. Ensure appropriate management of heat and fluid losses and adequate pain management.

ERYTHEMA MULTIFORME

Erythema multiforme is a hypersensitivity eruption which may follow herpes simplex or other viral infection, mycoplasma or medications.

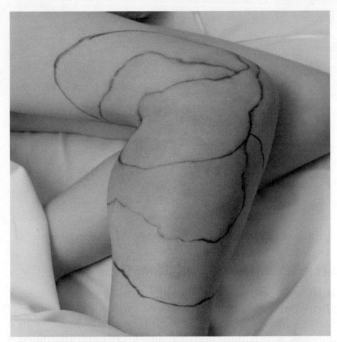

Figure 15.6   Invasive group A *Streptococcus* infection on treatment.

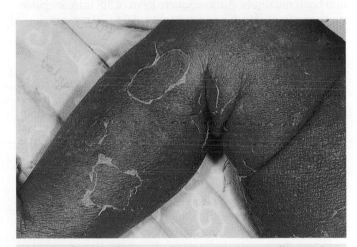

Figure 15.7   Staphylococcal scalded skin syndrome. Diffuse peeling and erythema in a 4-week-old African American infant girl who also had *Staphylococcus aureus* isolated from her blood. (Reproduced with permission from Paller, A. S., & Mancini, A. J. (2015). *Hurwitz clinical pediatric dermatology: A textbook of skin disorders of childhood and adolescence* (5th ed.). Elsevier – Health Sciences Division.)

It is generally a relatively mild, self-limiting condition associated with a low-grade fever. Skin lesions start as red macules or urticaria and some later develop into characteristic target lesions (Fig. 15.8). Mucosal involvement is not uncommon.

The skin rash starts abruptly and symmetrically, and parents are often concerned regarding a new striking rash on a background of apparent mild illness and fever. The skin lesions are usually round or oval, and all are present within the first few days.

Management involves removal or treatment of the offending trigger if identified coupled with symptomatic support.

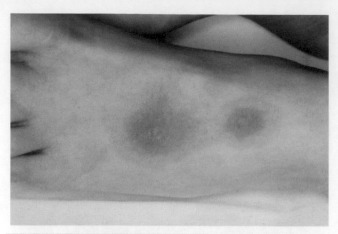

Figure 15.8 Erythema multiforme with classical target lesions.

STEVENS JOHNSON SYNDROME (SJS)

Medications (including sulphonamides, carbamazepine, phenytoin and lamotrigine) are the most common causes of Stevens Johnson Syndrome in childhood. SJS begins with a non-specific prodrome and thereafter to crusting of the mucous membranes of the mouth, nose, eyes and genitalia (Fig. 15.9). Complications include dehydration, electrolyte disturbance and bacterial sepsis. A more severe form of SJS is toxic epidermal necrolysis, which has a mortality of 5 to 20 per cent.

DENGUE FEVER

Dengue fever is a globally important airborne infection transmitted by the *Aedes* genus of mosquito (Fig. 15.10). It is a notifiable disease endemic in over 120 countries, especially in Southeast Asia, the Caribbean and Latin America. The last 50 years have seen the emergence of epidemic arboviral diseases transmitted by the urban mosquito *Aedes aegypti*. High population growth and density in urban tropical and subtropical centres provides the ideal ecology for arboviral diseases. Recommendations by a recent *Lancet* commission include improved house screening, the prevention of construction of structures that hold water accessible to mosquitoes thereby reducing the aquatic habitats of *A. aegypti*, the provision of sewage waste management and reliable piped water.

Approximately one in four people who contract dengue are symptomatic. These symptoms may be mild or severe and can last 2 to 7 days. Severe infection is more likely if there is a history of prior infection with dengue virus, if the patient is under 1 year of age, or if the patient is pregnant. Dengue shock syndrome is the most severe form of dengue haemorrhagic fever. Severe disease is also associated with a marked thrombocytopenia, severe haemorrhage, organ impairment with shock and respiratory distress due to pulmonary oedema

Diagnosis is confirmed by finding viral antigen or nucleic acid detection or via serology. The main differentials are Zika and Chikungunya infections.

There is currently no specific antiviral agent for dengue, and treatment involves careful fluid management and the prompt identification of those with severe disease and associated shock. Paracetamol (acetaminophen) can be used for fever management. Aspirin and non-steroidal anti-inflammatory drugs should not be used because of their antiplatelet effect and associated bleeding risk. Several candidate vaccines are in development.

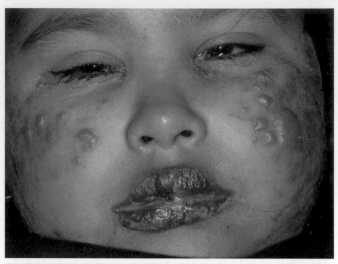

Figure 15.9 Stevens–Johnson syndrome. Purpuric macules became bullous. Note the inflammation of the conjunctivae and lips. (Reproduced with permission from Paller, A. S., & Mancini, A. J. (2021). *Paller and Mancini – Hurwitz clinical pediatric dermatology: A textbook of skin disorders of childhood & adolescence* (6th ed.). Elsevier – Health Sciences Division.)

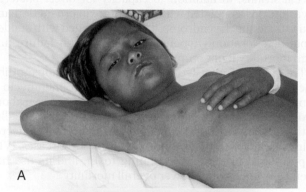

A

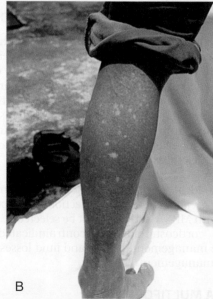

B

Figure 15.10 Characteristic skin manifestations in convalescent dengue A, Early convalescent macular diffuse rash occurring in the first week after recovery. B, Typical convalescent rash with "islands of white in a sea of red." (Reproduced with permission from Vincent JL et al (2011) Textbook of critical care, ed 6, Philadelphia, Saunders.)

Prolonged Unexplained Fever

This is defined as a fever over 38°C daily for 14 days with no diagnosis after an initial evaluation. The great majority have an infectious cause, but a minority may have a rheumatological cause (systemic juvenile idiopathic arthritis (JIA), rheumatic fever or systemic lupus erythematosus (SLE)) or a malignant cause (leukaemia, lymphoma, or neuroblastoma). Kawasaki disease should always be considered in any fever lasting over 5 days. A detailed history and examination are required. Always enquire about foreign travel.

The pattern of fever is important. A sustained fever remains elevated with little variation throughout the day and is characteristic of typhoid fever. Intermittent fever is where the temperature drops to normal at least once a day and is characteristic of tuberculosis, abscesses, lymphoma, systemic JIA and some forms of malaria.

With relapsing fever, the child is afebrile between febrile episodes. Relapsing fever is seen in malaria, brucellosis, sub-acute bacterial endocarditis and lymphoma. Weight loss is important and is associated with chronic diseases such as inflammatory bowel disease, tuberculosis and lymphoma. Investigations should be tailored to the history (particularly foreign travel), examination findings and pattern of fever.

Depending on the geographic region, considerations include malaria (chills, high fevers with rigors, and headaches), hepatitis A, typhoid fever (persistent fever, anorexia and rose spots), tuberculosis and amoebic liver abscess (fever, weight loss and right upper quadrant pain).

Prolonged fever can also occur with subacute bacterial endocarditis (requires echocardiography and serial blood cultures to diagnose), pyelonephritis, abscesses (especially pelvic and perinephric), osteomyelitis (MRI is the imaging modality of choice) and rheumatic fever (must satisfy Jones criteria).

KAWASAKI DISEASE

Ask any student (undergraduate or postgraduate) about prolonged unexplained fever in childhood, and it is very likely Kawasaki disease (KD) will be mentioned. This once rare and exotic condition is poorly understood and was first described in Japan by Dr. Tomisaku Kawasaki in 1967 and is now increasingly identified in Europe, North America and Australia. Debate continues as to whether it is caused by a yet unidentified pathogen, or if it is a superantigen response that can be triggered in genetically susceptible individuals by a variety of viral and bacterial pathogens.

During the recent SARS-CoV-2 pandemic, a number of cases of a Kawasaki-like syndrome, the paediatric inflammatory multisystem disorder temporally associated with SARS-CoV-2 (PIMS-TS) and also referred to as multisystem inflammatory syndrome in children (MIS-C), were noted, sparking a potential association with severe acute respiratory syndrome coronavirus 2 (SARS-CoV-2) infection.

KD is, however, the second most common form of vasculitis in childhood (after Henoch-Schonlein purpura (HSP)) and the most common cause of acquired heart disease in children. The great majority (80 per cent) of cases are in children less than 5 years of age.

Clinical Features

The diagnostic criteria have not changed – a fever for at least 5 days and **at least four** of the following:

- polymorphous skin exanthem (Fig. 15.11)
- bilateral conjunctival injection without exudate (Fig. 15.12)
- changes in lips and oral cavity (erythema, lip cracking, strawberry tongue) (Figs. 15.13 and 15.14)
- cervical lymphadenopathy (usually unilateral and over 1.5 cm in diameter) (Fig. 15.15)
- extremity changes (erythema of the palms and soles with peeling of fingers and toes after 2 to 3 weeks) (Fig. 15.16,15.17)

There is also a condition called incomplete KD, where just three of the criteria are met. Fever is an essential feature of KD and is most often of sudden onset and swinging, going above 40°C. The child with KD is very irritable and

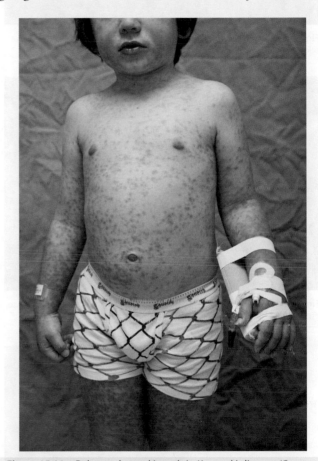

Figure 15.11   Polymorphous skin rash in Kawasaki disease. (Courtesy Kawasaki Disease Foundation.)

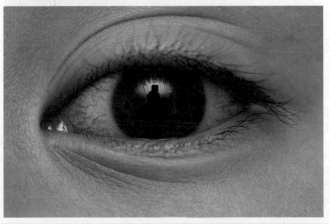

Figure 15.12   Non-purulent conjunctivitis in Kawasaki disease. (Courtesy Kawasaki Disease Foundation.)

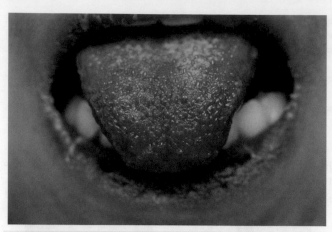

Figure 15.13   Strawberry tongue in Kawasaki disease. (Courtesy Kawasaki Disease Foundation.)

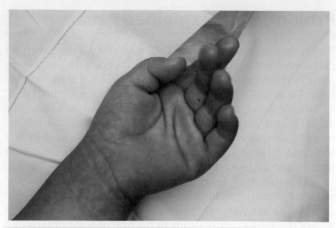

Figure 15.16   Rash on hand with swollen fingers in Kawasaki disease. (Courtesy Kawasaki Disease Foundation.)

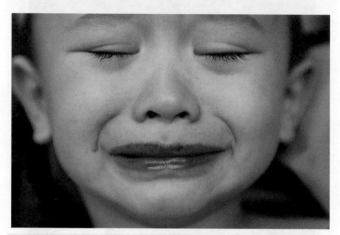

Figure 15.14   Red Lips in an Irritable Child with Kawasaki Disease (Courtesy of Kawasaki Disease Foundation.)

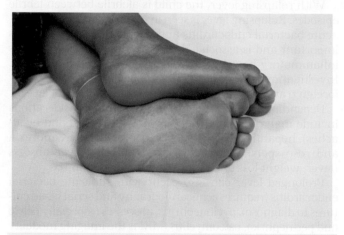

Figure 15.17   Swollen feet in Kawasaki disease. (Courtesy Kawasaki Disease Foundation.)

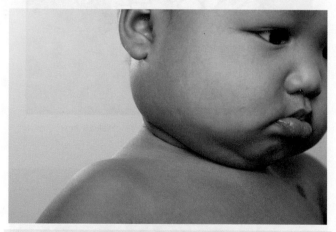

Figure 15.15   Cervical Lymphadenitis in Kawasaki Disease (Courtesy of Kawasaki Disease Foundation.)

inconsolable and may have erythema and induration at the BCG immunization site.

Scarlet fever is quite similar in terms of the rash and oral and peripheral changes. However, conjunctivitis is not seen in scarlet fever, and the fever only lasts 5 to 6 days in total. Scarlet fever responds readily to penicillin treatment. Measles, roseola infantum and infectious mononucleosis are other differential diagnoses in suspected KD.

In terms of investigations in KD, an initial raised white cell count, elevated ESR, sterile pyuria and thrombocytosis by day 14 of the illness are typically seen. A mild rise in transaminases and aseptic meningitis are also common features. Echocardiography is essential to detect coronary artery dilatation or aneurysm.

Management consists of a single dose of intravenous immunoglobulin (IVIG) with either high or moderate doses of aspirin in divided doses. When the fever has settled, low-dose aspirin should be given once daily for 6 weeks. IVIG reduces the risk of developing coronary artery aneurysms to less than 5 per cent. Additional treatment with either a single dose of steroids or infliximab has not shown important benefit in terms of preventing coronary artery abnormalities. A trial in Japan of an extended course of steroids in addition to IVIG for those predicted to be nonresponders (the RAISE study) showed benefit in terms of better response and reduced coronary artery abnormalities. An extended course of steroids (tapered over 2 to 3 weeks) may also be considered as adjunctive initial therapy for those patients predicted to be at high risk for coronary artery involvement (e.g. infants less than 12 months of age, or those with platelets $\leq 30 \times 10^9$/L, albumin ≤ 30 g/L or coronary artery anomalies at presentation).

Therefore, current practice is that if there is no defervescence within 48 hours or disease recrudescence, a repeat dose of IVIG is usually given with or without adjunctive steroids.

Other options for those children refractory to primary treatment include infliximab as a single infusion or the addition of ciclosporin. Ciclosporin has been found to have a modest effect in reducing coronary abnormalities in a study also conducted in Japan. Robust clinical trial data to guide choice of therapy for those children refractory to initial therapy is lacking. Those with documented coronary artery aneurysms require ongoing cardiology review and low-dose aspirin.

(Box 15.1)
(Box 15.2)
(Box 15.3)
(Box 15.4)

Box 15.1   Key Points

The great majority of feverish illnesses in young children are due to self-limiting viral illnesses, but among this large group are a small number with serious bacterial illness.

First, look for any life-threatening features such as a decreased level of consciousness, shock with delayed capillary refill time, tachycardia and cold peripheries or airway compromise.

The recognition and prompt management of sepsis has been helped by the introduction of paediatric early warning system (PEWS) scores, greater situational awareness, improved communication and the Sepsis 6 algorithm.

When clinical observations are converted to a score and combined with the concerns of nurses or family at the bedside, this information is used to help clinicians recognize, intervene and rescue a sick child before they deteriorate. The total PEWS score should never replace clinical judgement.

For acute otitis media, there is a very high rate of spontaneous resolution, and therefore a period of observation (up to 48 hours) with adequate analgesia is preferable to the immediate commencement of antibiotics.

Otitis externa can present with ear pain with discharge, where manipulating the tragus and pinna causes severe discomfort and pain.

While the great majority of children with varicella have a relatively mild illness, complications such as secondary bacterial infection (cellulitis, lymphadenitis),

varicella pneumonia, hepatitis, encephalitis and so-called haemorrhagic chickenpox can occur.

The rash of scarlet fever has a texture like sandpaper and blanches on pressure.

For invasive meningococcal disease, characteristic features are of a sick child with fever and a spreading petechial or purpuric rash. These features can be late. Initial symptoms are remarkably similar to those of a viral illness. Attention should be paid to the sick child with nonspecific rash, leg pains, and cool peripheries, as these may be evident before the characteristic rash emerges.

Some group A streptococcal strains, in addition to capacity for direct bacterial invasion, are associated with virulent toxin production and cause a toxic shock syndrome.

Staphylococcal scalded skin is an exfoliative dermatitis caused by staphylococcal exfoliative toxins and is generally seen in children under 5 years of age.

Erythema multiforme is a hypersensitivity eruption which may follow herpes simplex or other viral infection, mycoplasma or medications.

Severe dengue fever is associated with a marked thrombocytopenia, severe haemorrhage, organ impairment with shock and respiratory distress due to pulmonary oedema.

Kawasaki disease is the second most common form of vasculitis in childhood (after HSP) and the most common cause of acquired heart disease in children.

Box 15.2   A Febrile 4-Week-Old Infant

A 4-week-old male infant presents with a 24-hour history of excessive crying, low-grade fever and poor feeding. He was born by lower segment caesarean section weighing 3.5 kg and was admitted to the special care unit for a short period due to transient tachypnoea. His chest x-ray at the time suggested transient tachypnoea of the newborn. He has been breast-fed from birth, but his milk intake had dropped off over the previous 12 hours, and his mother stated that he was not anxious to feed. He was admitted to hospital for observations and investigation. Subsequent cultures confirmed late-onset *Group B Streptococcus* (GBS) disease.

Clinical Pearls

The risk of serious bacterial infection in infants under 2 months presenting with fever is as high as <u>12 to 14 per cent</u>. Clinical examination alone is a poor predictor of serious bacterial infection in young infants.

Early onset sepsis occurs within 48 hours of birth and may be associated with a rapid onset of fulminant multisystem disease. Pneumonia is a prominent feature and over 75 per cent are associated with maternal risk factors for infection. These risk factors include

prolonged rupture of the membranes, maternal pyrexia in labour, foul-smelling liquor, GBS carriage or bacteriuria or a history of GBS in prior delivery. GBS infections are classified as early onset (from birth to 6 days) or late onset (from 7 days to 3 or 4 months).

Symptoms are often nonspecific and may be insidious. They may present with a high or low temperature, poor feeding, irritability or lethargy, and occasionally with circulatory collapse.

The laboratory evaluation in the emergency department should <u>not</u> be based solely on the presence or absence of fever on presentation.

Interpretation of Investigations

First line investigations include urinalysis and urine culture, stool culture (if diarrhoea), blood cultures, C-reactive protein (CRP), and full blood count. Lumbar puncture should be performed if the infant is unwell or if under 2 months of age and intravenous broad-spectrum antibiotics are empirically started while awaiting cultures.

Bacterial culture positivity, especially in blood cultures, is dependent on the volume of blood and may be related to the timing of the sample collection in relation to the degree and duration of fever

Continued

Box 15.2   A Febrile 4-Week-Old Infant—cont'd

Pitfalls to Avoid

Always be wary of a young infant under 2 months of age with a history of fever or documented fever on arrival. Be wary of lateonset GBS sepsis in particular.

Suspect sepsis if an infant has a poor colour, prolonged capillary refill time, tachycardia (over 160 per minute), a drop in BP (under 30 mmHg if preterm), apnoea or tachypnoea (over 60 breaths per minute).

Prescribe them, **Get** them, and **Give** them with the goal that the infant should receive broad-spectrum intravenous antibiotics within **1 hour** of first contact or admission. The choice of antibiotics should reflect local antimicrobial resistance patterns and target common neonatal pathogens.

For preterm infants still in the neonatal nursery, late onset sepsis does occur, and Coagulase Negative Staphylococcus (CONS) is the predominant pathogen with hand hygiene a key factor in prevention. In this setting, the antibiotics selected should take into account the potential exposure and the addition of an antibiotic with activity against CONS may be required (e.g. vancomycin).

Box 15.3   A Sick 1-Year-Old With a Petechial Rash

A 1-year-old female presents with a short history of fever and an evolving petechial rash. Her past and perinatal history are unremarkable. Her parents have been very reluctant to immunise her, and thus she has not received her scheduled 2-, 4-, or 6-month immunisations. Her examination revealed a high temperature, marked pallor, a capillary refill time of 4 seconds and a tachycardia of 180 per minute. She had several nonblanching spots over her chest and abdomen.

Clinical Pearls

The epidemiology of bacterial meningitis in the UK and Europe has changed dramatically in the past two decades, following the introduction of vaccines to control *Haemophilus influenzae* type b, serogroups B and C meningococcus and some types of pneumococci.

The overall incidence of invasive meningococcal disease (IMD) in England has dropped to one per 100,000. As IMD is now so rarely seen that it may be difficult to recognise, especially in the early stages.

The highest rates of IMD are in children under 5, with the peak incidence under 12 months of age. There is a second, smaller peak in incidence in young people aged 15 to 19 years.

Meningococcal disease can present as bacterial meningitis, as septicaemia or as a combination of the two.

Classical signs of meningitis are often absent in infancy. Infants, children and young people with bacterial meningitis commonly present with non-specific symptoms and signs, including fever, vomiting, irritability and upper respiratory tract symptoms.

Treat suspected meningococcal disease without delay using intravenous ceftriaxone or cefotaxime.

If there are signs of shock, give an immediate fluid bolus by intravenous or intraosseous route and reassess the child immediately afterwards.

If the signs of shock persist, immediately give a second bolus. If still in shock after the first 40 mL/kg, transfer to a paediatric intensive care unit (PICU) and mechanical ventilation are required. In confirmed meningococcal disease, treat with intravenous ceftriaxone for 7 days in total.

Interpretation of Investigations

Real-time polymerase chain reaction testing (PCR) for *Neisseria meningitidis* confirms a diagnosis of meningococcal disease in most cases.

Blood tests to be performed include a full blood count, C-reactive protein (CRP), coagulation screen, blood culture, whole-blood polymerase chain reaction (PCR) for *N. meningitidis,* blood glucose and blood gas.

Pitfalls to Avoid

Timing of LP

Contraindications to performing an LP include signs suggesting raised intracranial pressure, shock, extensive or spreading purpura, respiratory insufficiency, coagulation results outside the normal range or a platelet count below 100 by 10^9/L.

Use clinical judgement and not cranial computed tomography (CT) to decide whether it is safe to perform a lumbar puncture. CT is unreliable for identifying raised intracranial pressure.

Signs of septic shock include a capillary refill time above 2 seconds, tachycardia (age-dependent but over 180 per minute is significant), and later, hypotension, cold hands and feet, an altered mental state with decreased conscious level, and poor urinary output.

Children and young people with recurrent episodes of meningococcal disease should be assessed for complement deficiency by a specialist in infectious disease or immunology.

Box 15.4   A 10-Month-Old With a Prolonged Fever

A 10-month-old male presents with marked irritability, high intermittent fevers and a macular rash over a 5-day period. He has no prior illness, a normal perinatal history and no history of recent foreign travel. He is strikingly irritable on examination. His temperature is 39°C and his heart rate is 170 beats per minute. He has a widespread macular rash and mild conjunctival injection. He is admitted for further assessment and investigation. His blood and Cerebrospinal fluid (CSF) cultures are clear, and his urinalysis shows sterile pyuria. Despite antipyretic measures, his temperature fails to settle while in hospital over the next 48 hours.

Clinical Pearls

The six principal diagnostic criteria in Kawasaki disease (KD) are fever persisting over 5 days (or previous defervescence in response to treatment), bilateral conjunctival injection, oral mucosal changes, polymorphous skin rash, peripheral extremity changes and cervical lymphadenopathy. Five of these criteria must be met to diagnose KD. Atypical KD is when just four criteria are met.

Intravenous immunoglobulin (IVIG) reduces the risk of developing coronary artery aneurysms to less than 5 per cent.

Box 15.4   A 10-Month-Old With a Prolonged Fever—cont'd

Current practice is that if no disease defervescence within 48 hours or disease recrudescence, a repeat dose of IVIG is given with or without adjunctive steroids.

In children presenting with a Kawasaki-like syndrome, consideration should also be given to the possibility of PIMS-TS/MIS-C. History of potential SARS-CoV-2 infection in them or in a family member should be sought, and PCR and antibody testing for SARS-CoV-2 carried out.

In unwell infants and children with a febrile illness associated with anaemia, neutropenia or thrombocytopenia and multi-organ involvement, a diagnosis of haemophagocytic lymphohistiocytosis (HLH) should be considered. HLH is a life-threatening syndrome of excessive inflammation and uncontrolled immune activation. HLH may be secondary to another condition, such as rheumatoid disorders (called macrophage activation syndrome), infections and malignancies. The diagnosis of HLH is based on criteria, which include clinical features (fever, splenomegaly) and markers of excessive inflammation.

Interpretation of Investigations

In KD, an initial raised white cell count, an elevated ESR, thrombocytosis by day 14 of the illness are typically seen and a sterile pyuria, mild increase in transaminases and aseptic meningitis are other features commonly seen. Echocardiography is essential to detect coronary artery dilatation or aneurysm.

Pitfalls to Avoid

If a child has a history of recent foreign travel, consider malaria, and request thick and thin malaria films. *Plasmodium falciparum* accounts for the majority of cases of malaria notified in the UK and is treated with artemether-lumefantrine (Riamet.®) or atovaquone-proguanil (Malarone®/Malarone Paed®). Children with *P. falciparum* malaria can deteriorate quickly. Where facilities permit, those with *P.falciparum* infection should be monitored in hospital. Any child with severe malaria should be admitted to hospital.

During the recent coronavirus pandemic, a potentially new illness termed paediatric multisystem inflammatory syndrome temporally associated with COVID-19 (PIMS) has been described with presenting clinical manifestations of persistent fever, gastrointestinal symptoms (abdominal pain and diarrhoea), vomiting, conjunctivitis and an erythematous rash. PIMS was found to cluster more in certain ethnic groups than others, with reports noting that children of African American, Afro-Caribbean and Hispanic descent were more affected and had a more severe course than those of European descent.

Manifestations of KD and PIMS may overlap in certain aspects but marked differences can also be seen. Unlike KD, PIMS cases present with predominant gastrointestinal respiratory symptoms and meningeal manifestations. Shock was also seen more frequently in PIMS than KD. Cardiac involvement is present in both diseases. However, higher rates of myocarditis and left ventricular dysfunction have been reported in PIMS.

Key References

Chapman, S. M., & Maconochie, I. K. (2019). Early warning scores in paediatrics: An overview. *Archives of Disease in Childhood, 104*(4), 395–399.

Fleischmann-Struzek, C., Goldfarb, D. M., Schlattmann, P., Schlapbach, L. J., Reinhart, K., & Kissoon, N. (2018). The global burden of paediatric and neonatal sepsis: A systematic review. *The Lancet. Respiratory Medicine, 6*(3), 223–230.

Gray, H., & Cornish, J. (2019). Kawasaki disease: A need for earlier diagnosis and treatment. *Archives of Disease in Childhood, 104*(7), 615–616.

Holland, K. E., & Soung, P. J. (2018). Acquired rashes in the older child. In R. M. Kliegman, P. S. Lye, B. Bordini, H. Toth, & D. Basel (Eds.), *Nelson pediatric symptom-based diagnosis* (pp. 866–896). Elsevier.

Harwood R, Allin B, Jones CE, et al. A national consensus management pathway for paediatric inflammatory multisystem syndrome temporally associated with COVID-19 (PIMS-TS): results of a national Delphi process [published correction appears in Lancet Child Adolesc Health. 2021 Feb;5(2):e5]. Lancet Child Adolesc Health. 2021;5(2):133-141.

Kobayashi T, Saji T, Otani T, et al. Efficacy of immunoglobulin plus prednisolone for prevention of coronary artery abnormalities in severe Kawasaki disease (RAISE study): a randomised, open-label, blinded-endpoints trial. Lancet. 2012;379(9826):1613-1620.

Lye, P. S., & Densmore, E. M. (2018). Fever In R. M. Kliegman, P. S. Lye, B. Bordini, H. Toth, & D. Basel (Eds.), *Nelson pediatric symptom-based diagnosis* (pp. 701–725). Elsevier.

McCrindle, B. W., & Rowley, A. H. (2019). Improving coronary artery outcomes for children with Kawasaki disease. *Lancet, 393*(10176), 1077–1078.

National Institute for Health and Care Excellence. (2015, February 1). Meningitis (bacterial) and meningococcal septicaemia in under 16s: Recognition, diagnosis and management. NICE guideline [CG102]. https://www.nice.org.uk/guidance/cg102.

National Institute for Health and Care Excellence. (2017, September 13). Sepsis: Recognition, diagnosis and early management. NICE guideline [NG51]. https://www.nice.org.uk/guidance/ng51.

Nutbeam T, Daniels R on behalf of the UK Sepsis Trust, Available at sepsis-trust.org/professional-resources/clinical/.

National Institute for Health and Care Excellence. (November 7, 2019), *Fever in under 5s: Assessment and initial management*. NICE guideline [NG143]. https://www.nice.org.uk/guidance/ng143.

Player, B. (2018). Earache. In R. M. Kliegman, P. S. Lye, B. Bordini, H. Toth, & D. Basel (Eds.), *Nelson pediatric symptom-based diagnosis* (pp. 61–74). Elsevier.

Ramasamy, R., Willis, L., Kadambari, S., Kelly, D. F., Heath, P. T., Nadel, S., et al. (2018). Management of suspected paediatric meningitis: A multicentre prospective cohort study. *Archives of Disease in Childhood, 103*(12), 1114–1118.

Ramgopal, S., Janofsky, S., Zuckerbraun, N. S., Ramilo, O., Mahajan, P., Kuppermann, N., & Vitale, M. A. (2019). Risk of serious bacterial infection in infants aged ≤60 days presenting to emergency departments with a history of fever only. *The Journal of Pediatrics, 204*, 191–195.

Tracy, A., & Waterfield, T. (2020). How to use clinical signs of meningitis. *Archives of Disease in Childhood. Education and Practice, 105*(1), 46–49.

Waterfield, T., Lyttle, M. D., Munday, C., Foster, S., McNulty, M., Platt, R., et al. (2021). Validating clinical practice guidelines for the management of febrile infants presenting to the emergency department in the UK and Ireland. Archives of Disease in Childhood. *Archdischild*. https://doi.org/10.1136/archdischild-2021-322586. 2021-322586.

Wilder-Smith, A., Lindsay, S. W., Scott, T. W., Ooi, E. E., Gubler, D. J., & Das, P. (2020). The Lancet Commission on dengue and other Aedes-transmitted viral diseases. *Lancet, 395*(10241), 1890–1891.

Online References

Defeating Meningitis by 2030 documents. https://cdn.who.int/media/docs/default-source/immunization/meningitis/defeating--meningitis-by-2030-brochure-rev.pdf?sfvrsn=b5b33f9f_5.

16 Food Allergies in Children

JONATHAN HOURIHANE

A wide range of common foodstuffs can precipitate adverse reactions, but it is reassuring that just a handful of foods account for over 90 per cent of reactions. Milk, eggs, peanuts and tree nuts account for most allergic reactions in European children. Most food-induced allergic reactions occur after first known oral exposure. Milk and egg allergies are the most common food allergies seen and typically resolve in 60 per cent of children by 5 years of age and in 75 per cent of children by 7 years of age. In contrast, allergies to peanut, tree nuts, fish and shellfish are infrequently outgrown. There is no single feature of the clinical history or of the commonly used tests described below that can accurately identify food-allergic children at risk of severe reactions. All must be cautious about accidental exposure (despite well-established thresholds that show very small doses are usually tolerated). Many need to always have adrenaline kits available. Widely implemented school and workplace food allergen bans have no evidence to support their role in preventing food-allergic reactions or deaths, but they are embedded in school cultures in many countries. Oral and other routes of immunotherapy are under investigation at present, with one peanut product now licensed in the US.

The Allergy Focused History

The key to making the diagnosis is the recognition of a strong temporal relationship between exposure to a foodstuff and the onset of very stereotyped allergic symptoms. It is a little like the work of a good detective, and the following questions are helpful.

WHICH FOOD IS THOUGHT TO BE RESPONSIBLE?

The most common offenders in Europe are cow's milk, eggs, peanuts, tree nuts (almonds, brazils, cashews, hazel, walnuts), fish and shellfish (prawns, mussels, crab). Soya and wheat are very unusual allergies even in infancy and usually resolve quicker than other allergies.

Exposure is usually through ingestion, and if symptoms are immediate and florid, there is little difficulty in recognising the cause and effect. Skin contact and exposure to airborne fumes very rarely cause serious allergic reactions (so air travel is much safer than is generally feared). One may have to keep a food diary highlighting when symptoms occur in less clear-cut cases.

WHAT WAS THE STATE OF THE FOOD INGESTED?

The allergic potential of food may differ depending on whether it is raw, lightly cooked or baked. For example, an egg baked in a sponge cake and cooked at a high temperature for a relatively long period may be tolerated, but a raw egg may cause symptoms. Roasted peanut is more allergenic than boiled peanut.

HOW MUCH FOOD WAS INGESTED?

Some children will react to minute amounts of food, whereas others will only react once a large amount is given. It is reassuring for families to know that most low dose exposures result in mild reactions unless other factors are involved, such as physiological stress by exercise or viral illness, alcohol or medications such as beta-blockers and ACE inhibitors, which can all augment reaction severity.

WHAT SYMPTOMS ARE THERE AND DOES THE FOOD CAUSE SYMPTOMS ON EVERY OCCASION?

Mild IgE mediated allergic reactions involve hives like nettle stings and skin swelling that usually settle quickly and do not routinely need medical attention. More significant reactions can include severe breathing difficulty and collapse due to low blood pressure. This is called anaphylaxis, which always needs medical assessment and treatment. Children who can tolerate yoghurt, ice cream, and cheese made from cow's milk are unlikely to have severe or long-lasting cow's milk allergies.

167

HOW LONG IS IT SINCE THE PREVIOUS EXPOSURE?

The natural history of the most common food allergies in childhood is to improve with time. If a child has an acute reaction to a food at 6 months of age and avoids that food for several years, there is a high chance that the child will have outgrown the food allergy. Notable exceptions are peanut, tree nut and shellfish allergies, which tend to be lifelong.

WHAT IS THE FAMILY HISTORY?

The presence of atopy (asthma, eczema, hay fever) or a food allergy in first-degree relatives makes food allergies more likely. Food allergy is slightly more common in boys than girls, but this switches completely in adulthood. Onset is usually in the first year of life, and family size (low) and birth order (first-born) are important factors as viral exposure and gut microbiome diversity are thought to be important protective factors.

Diagnostic Tests

Tests include skin prick tests (SPT) and spIgE blood tests, which may confirm the presence of an IgE-mediated reaction to a particular food, but they do have limitations. As a screening tool when there is no history of reactions, the pretest probability of a true positive SPT is low, and the false positive rate can be as high as 50 per cent. A negative skin prick test is always useful as it is correct 95 per cent of the time. In children seen in allergy clinics with a history of reactions (for whom the pre-test probability of a true positive is much higher), SPT performs much better with a false positive rate of only 20 to 25 per cent and a true negative rate of 95 per cent. SPT should only be done for relevant foods, not in wide-ranging fishing expeditions!

SKIN PRICK TESTS

The basis of these tests is that a drop of purified allergen or occasionally the native food if a commercial solution is not available is inoculated into the skin, usually on the forearm, or the back in young babies, along with positive (histamine) and negative (saline) controls. The presence of antibodies to a food allergen results in the stimulation of mast cells in the skin with the development of a wheal and flare response.

The size of the wheal and flare response relates to the age and sex of the child, the quality of the allergen extract (which may vary greatly) and whether the child is on medications such as antihistamines or topical steroids. Antihistamines must be discontinued a week before testing as they may suppress skin reactivity to skin prick tests for over a week.

IgE SPECIFIC TESTS

The serum specific IgE test measures circulating allergen-specific IgE-antibody levels (which are zero in nonallergic people). IgE tests and skin prick tests usually give similar results, so negative IgE specific tests mean food allergy is very unlikely (95 per cent) and positive tests properly ordered – in a child with symptoms – can be interpreted confidently.

FOOD CHALLENGES

Food challenges are the gold standard diagnostic test but should only be performed by those with expertise. Food challenges do help confirm the parent's story of food allergy and to see if the child has grown out of it.

Food challenges need to be performed in closely monitored situations as there is always a risk of a severe anaphylactic reaction. There are a few points worth remembering. If there is a history of recent anaphylaxis, a food challenge is not indicated. However, over time, if SPT and IgE levels are falling, even children who have had anaphylaxis can pass a food challenge. As in all things in life, timing is everything.

Food challenges may be helpful in cow's milk protein intolerance in infancy where the diagnosis cannot be based on SPT and IgE levels, but rather on a therapeutic trial of improvement with the elimination of cow's milk protein and recurrence of symptoms if cow's milk protein is reintroduced.

Cow's milk protein intolerance (CMPI)

Cow's milk protein intolerance is common and affects 2 to 7 per cent of infants, and the mainstay of treatment is to remove cow's milk protein from the diet while ensuring the nutritional adequacy of any alternative.

CMPI is not IgE mediated, so it does not present with the rapid symptoms mentioned above. CMPI reactions are more delayed, and presentation is with severe infant distress around the time of feeds, feed aversion or refusal, treatment-resistant gastroesophageal reflux, constipation, faltering growth and blood or mucus in the stools. Exclusively breast-fed infants can also develop CMPI because of protein in the maternal diet transferring through breast milk. An emerging form of food allergy is presumed to be an immune-mediated reaction that can occasionally cause a severe reaction with acute gastrointestinal symptoms that mimic sepsis. This is termed food protein-induced enterocolitis syndrome (mercifully shortened to FPIES), without hives and resistant to adrenaline treatment (because it is not IgE and mast cell-mediated) but is very responsive to IV fluid resuscitation.

HISTORY IN CMPI

The history should elicit the symptoms and how quickly they occur after the ingestion of cow's milk protein (usually several hours later), how long they last (GI upset can last several hours, eczema flares a few days later, especially with continuing exposure), their non-life-threatening acute severity (no airway or circulatory problems), which treatments were implemented (dairy exclusion is the only option) and their effects (CMPI may take several days or even a week to settle down on an exclusion diet). It is important to distinguish, by history, those with non-IgE mediated CMPI from those with gastro-oesophageal reflux. Clinical clues lie in the severity of gastrointestinal symptoms and resistance to treatment with proton pump inhibitors.

Investigations of CMPI

Skin prick tests and specific IgE measurements are **_not_** indicated if non-IgE CMPI is suspected, as IgE is not the mediating molecule. The only reliable diagnostic test is a strict, dietitian supervised, elimination diet. If symptoms do not improve within 2 weeks of rigorous dairy exclusion, then non-IgE mediated CMPI is unlikely and milk should be reintroduced. If symptoms do improve during elimination, then milk must still be reintroduced after 6 to 8 weeks as spontaneous resolution can occur very quickly. This prevents persistence with

THE iMAP MILK LADDER

To be used only in children with Mild to Moderate Non-IgE Cow's Milk Allergy
Under the supervision of a healthcare professional
PLEASE SEE THE ACCOMPANYING RECIPE INFORMATION

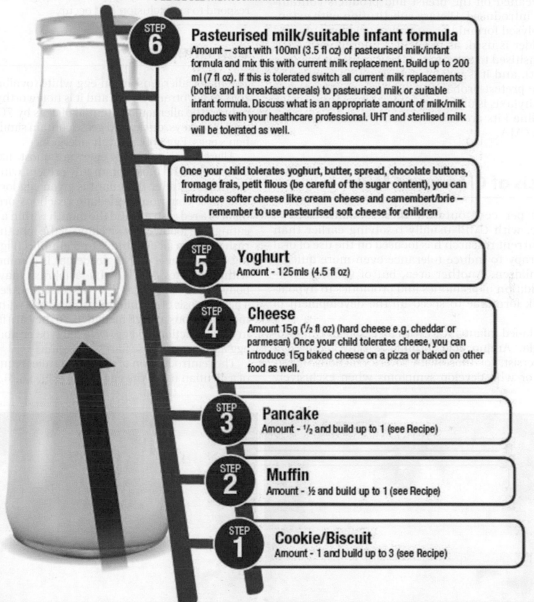

STEP 6 Pasteurised milk/suitable infant formula
Amount – start with 100ml (3.5 fl oz) of pasteurised milk/infant formula and mix this with current milk replacement. Build up to 200 ml (7 fl oz). If this is tolerated switch all current milk replacements (bottle and in breakfast cereals) to pasteurised milk or suitable infant formula. Discuss what is an appropriate amount of milk/milk products with your healthcare professional. UHT and sterilised milk will be tolerated as well.

Once your child tolerates yoghurt, butter, spread, chocolate buttons, fromage frais, petit filous (be careful of the sugar content), you can introduce softer cheese like cream cheese and camembert/brie – remember to use pasteurised soft cheese for children

STEP 5 Yoghurt
Amount - 125mls (4.5 fl oz)

STEP 4 Cheese
Amount 15g (½ fl oz) (hard cheese e.g. cheddar or parmesan) Once your child tolerates cheese, you can introduce 15g baked cheese on a pizza or baked on other food as well.

STEP 3 Pancake
Amount - ½ and build up to 1 (see Recipe)

STEP 2 Muffin
Amount - ½ and build up to 1 (see Recipe)

STEP 1 Cookie/Biscuit
Amount - 1 and build up to 3 (see Recipe)

iMAP GUIDELINE

Figure 16.1   iMAP milk ladder. (Courtesy Dr Carina Venter.)

difficult and expensive diets. If problems recur on reintroduction, then avoidance is restarted for 6 months.

No evidence whatsoever supports the use of serum IgG testing, Vega testing, kinesiology or hair analysis, as they have no scientific basis and are both misleading and a waste of money.

Management of CMPI

For non-IgE mediated CMPI, the diagnostic test and management are the same: cow's milk should be removed from the infant's diet. For exclusively breast-fed infants, the mother should have milk temporarily excluded from her diet, under the supervision of a dietitian. In formula-fed infants, a change to an extensively hydrolysed formula (EHF

tolerated by 90 per cent of infants with CMPI) or amino acid formula (if not tolerating EHF or has had genuine anaphylaxis, but the latter is not a feature of CMPI but of cow's milk allergy,) should be commenced.

Most symptoms will usually resolve within 1 to 4 weeks of an elimination diet. The input of a paediatric dietitian is essential to supervise the reintroductions, eliminations and later reintroduction of milk and other foods into the diet.

Goat's milk or sheep milk must not be used as cow's milk substitutes due to high inter-species cross reactivity (up to 85 per cent between goats and cow's milk). To reintroduce milk, follow guidance in relation to the MAP milk ladder (Fig. 16.1).

Cow's Milk Allergy (CMA)

This condition is mediated by IgE related mast cell degranulation, so its symptoms are the typical hives, itch and swelling. It can present in breast-fed infants, but this is unusual. It often presents when breast-fed children are being weaned off the breast and products containing milk are introduced. Dietary substitution with extensively hydrolysed formula or an amino acid formula and the milk ladder is used, as in CMPI. Children with CMA are often sensitised to egg (up to 60 per cent) and peanut (40 per cent), and it is worth screening this population (because the pretest probability of a true positive test is high). Anaphylaxis is uncommon in any individual case, and adrenaline kits are not commonly needed for most infants with CMA.

Prognosis of CMA and CMPI

At least 60 per cent outgrow these conditions by 5 years of age, with CMPI usually resolving earlier than CMA, and current research has focused on the use of oral immunotherapy to induce tolerance even more quickly in young children. Another area, but of waning interest, is the addition of prebiotics and probiotics to hypoallergenic milk formulae to speed up the development of tolerance.

For formula-fed infants, start with an extensively hydrolysed formula. Amino acid formula is only required if symptoms persist, for those with severe reactions, faltering growth or who develop symptoms when exclusively breast-fed. Soya milk can be tried after 6 months of age, but only 50 per cent of CMPI children tolerate it. Goat's milk is never suitable as an alternative to cow's milk due to cross-reactivity.

Referral to a specialist allergy clinic is needed if multiple food allergies, severe allergic reactions of type one immediate hypersensitivity type, faltering growth or failure to respond to an exclusion diet occur.

Egg Allergy

The major allergens are in egg white (ovalbumin, ovomucoid and ovotransferrin), and it is noteworthy that cooking reduces the allergenic potential of eggs by 70 per cent. The eggs of turkeys, ducks and geese contain similar allergens to hen's eggs. Egg yolk is rarely allergenic.

Allergic reactions to eggs are most likely in under 1-year-olds and most commonly present with a rapid onset of symptoms after the infant is given egg for the first time. The most common immediate reactions are the development of a red rash around the mouth within a few seconds of eating egg, followed by swelling of the mouth and a blotchy rash over the face within 1 to 5 minutes (Fig. 16.2). Swelling around the eyes (angioedema) is common and occurs within minutes. The blotchy facial rash may spread to the body and the infant may get associated wheeze and stridor. The diagnosis of egg allergy usually rests with the history as most reactions are IgE mediated, so they are florid and rapid in onset reactions to egg. Delayed type or non IgE mediated egg allergy can cause flares of eczema.

The reintroduction of egg into the diet requires the advice of a dietitian using the egg ladder (Fig. 16.3).

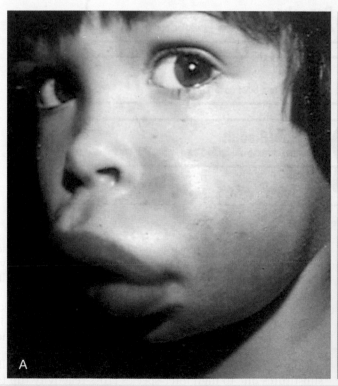 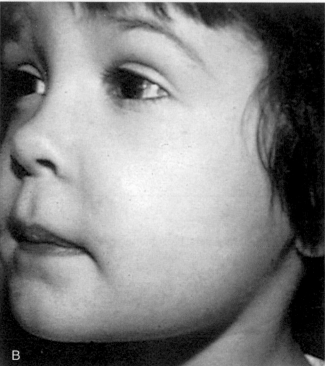

Figure 16.2 Angioedema. (A) Onset was sudden. (B) Resolution was complete within 24 hours. (Reproduced with permission from Zitelli, B. J., McIntire, S. C., & Nowalk, A. J. (2012). *Zitelli and Davis' atlas of pediatric physical diagnosis* (6th ed.). Saunders.)

Egg ladder

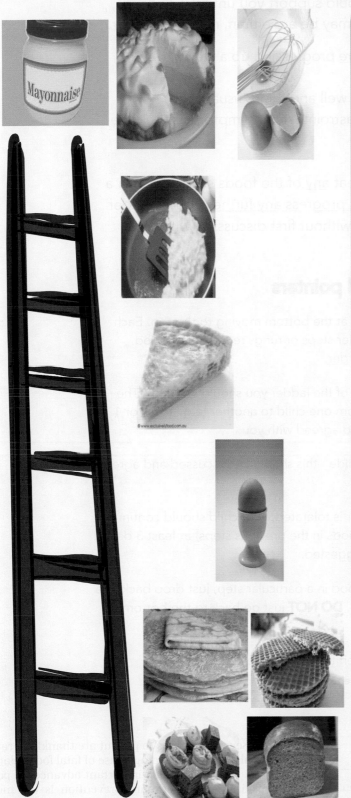

Cracked eggshell	
Utensils with raw cake mixture or raw egg	
Processed meat/burger/sausage	↑
Teacakes™ Milky Way™ Mars™ Snickers™	↑
Crème Egg™ Chewits™	↑
Hollandaise, Horseradish & Tartar sauces	↑
Royal™ icing	↑
Sorbet & Mousse	↑
Mayonnaise/salad cream	↑
Marshmallow-with egg (check label)	↑
Meringue/fresh ice-cream	↑
Crème caramel & Crème Brulé	↑
Scrambled egg	↑
STEP 3 ALMOST RAW	

Omelette	↑
French Toast	↑
Quiche	↑
Yorkshire pudding-with egg (check label)	↑
Fried/hardboiled egg	↑
Cooked batter/tempura/breadcrumb	↑
Fresh egg pasta & fresh egg noodle	↑
STEP 2 LIGHTLY COOKED	

Pancake	↑
Dried egg pasta	↑
Waffle biscuit	↑
Boudoir™ & Lady's finger™ biscuits	↑
Baked sponge/muffin/cake/biscuit	↑
STEP 1 WELL COOKED	

Figure 16.3   Egg ladder. (Courtesy IFAN (Irish Food Allergy Network).)

Continued

Egg ladder

A health care professional (HCP) should support you until the Ladder has been successfully climbed. This may be a dieititan, nurse or doctor.

Before starting this ladder and **_before_** progressing up a step:

1. Please ensure that your child is well and their "usual self".
Any asthma, eczema and /or gastrointestinal symptoms should be settled.

2. If your child cannot or will not eat <u>any</u> of the foods suggested on a particular step 1, 2 or 3, <u>do not progress any further</u> up the ladder from step 1-2 or from step 2-3 without first discussing with your HCP.

Practical pointers

• The ladder has 3 big steps, starting at the bottom moving to the top. Each big step contains a number of smaller steps or rungs representing food examples to be taken <u>in a certain order.</u>

• You need to be advised which step of the ladder you should start on. The time spent on each step will vary from one child to another (e.g. 1 day or 1 month) and should be discussed and agreed with you.

• There are no amounts given as a guide - this should be discussed and agreed with your HCP.

• If the food on any step of the ladder is tolerated, your child should continue to consume this (as well as all the foods in the previous steps) at least 3 days a week and then try the next food suggested.

• If your child does not tolerate the food in a particular step, just drop back one small step/rung to the previous one. **DO NOT** just go back to the bottom of the ladder.

• Contact your HCP for advice on when to retry the next step again.

Figure 16.3, cont'd

Peanut Allergy

Peanut allergy affects around 2 per cent of the population. Fatal anaphylaxis due to peanuts is rare but does occur. Peanut allergy has a considerable negative impact on the quality of life of the child (or adult), and their family and all need to avoid peanuts and the child should carry self-injectable adrenaline. Severe reactions to peanut are thankfully rare, but peanut allergy is the leading cause of fatal food-related anaphylaxis. There have been important advances in peanut desensitisation but primary prevention is the most attractive strategy to address this issue. The early introduction of peanut products into the infant diet prevents most cases of peanut allergy. Oral immunotherapy of established cases does appear to reduce the likelihood of reacting to peanuts in a controlled clinic setting. Epicutaneous immunotherapy which remains a research-based option at present, as it is not yet licensed, has a better safety profile than oral immunotherapy.

Peanut allergy frequently co-exists in infants with severe eczema and egg allergy or both. It remains controversial whether such infants should have skin prick testing or specific IgE testing before peanut is offered either at home or under supervision in clinic or possibly in a formal food challenge. This is not cost-effective and yields a larger number of false positive than true positive tests. All other infants, with no eczema or mild to moderate eczema and no egg allergy, should have age-appropriate peanut-containing foods and other allergenic foods introduced between 4 and 6 months of age. When peanut is tolerated in an infant's diet, it must remain in the diet and be eaten regularly rather than sporadically.

Peanut allergy differs in prevalence and severity in different regions of the world due to its relative prevalence in the local diet (high in North America, low in Southern Europe, for example) and depends on whether the form of peanut eaten is boiled (less allergenic, most common in African, Chinese and Asian diets) or roasted (more allergenic, more common in northern European and North American diets). Between 30 and 60 per cent of peanut-allergic children will have positive skin or blood tests for tree nuts. However, if a full series of supervised feeds with these nuts can be undertaken (huge resources are needed), many can tolerate the nuts, thus demonstrating the difference between sensitisation and clinical allergy. Peanut is a legume, but allergy to other legumes is very unusual alongside peanut allergy; therefore, most peanut-allergic children and adults can and should eat any legume they wish.

Soya Milk Allergy

Although much less common than widely thought, the features of soya milk allergy are very similar to those of cow's milk allergy. Soya protein allergy is most often discovered in children with cow's milk protein allergy. As always, diagnosis rests on a clinical suspicion followed by a trial of withdrawal of and later reintroduction of soya protein. Parents may not be aware that soya protein is a constituent of many flours and is therefore in most breads. The management is to avoid all foods that contain soya flour. However, soya lecithin does not need to be avoided, because it is not thought to be allergenic and is thus found in many packaged and tinned foods.

Fish and Shellfish Allergy

Similar to peanut allergy, fish and shellfish allergies can be expected to persist into adulthood. White fish allergy is most common (cod, haddock and plaice in particular). Most white fish-allergic children can tolerate tuna, and some can tolerate other oily fish like salmon and mackerel. Shellfish allergy (prawn/shrimp, crab, lobster and mussel) may cause rapid onset reactions which are occasionally very severe. Children with fish allergy do not automatically have

to avoid shellfish – and vice versa – as they are phylogenetically distinct.

Anaphylaxis

The incidence of anaphylaxis is rising, and early recognition and the immediate use of intramuscular adrenaline remain the mainstays of treatment. Anaphylaxis is a severe, life-threatening, systemic hypersensitivity reaction due to a rapid release of inflammatory mediators.

Food is the most common trigger in children, followed by drugs and venom. Fatal reactions to food are more common in those who have comorbid asthma.

RECOGNITION OF ANAPHYLAXIS

Anaphylaxis is characterised by the presence of respiratory or cardiovascular symptoms as part of an allergic reaction. Skin or mucosal changes alone are not a sign of an anaphylactic reaction.

Anaphylaxis is a clinical diagnosis. The most common trigger in children and young people is food, with symptoms typically presenting within 15 to 30 minutes of exposure. Anaphylaxis is likely when there is an acute onset of illness with flushing, urticaria and angioedema in tandem with the life-threatening features of lower airway or circulation compromise.

Circulatory compromise causes pallor, clamminess, hypotension and, finally, cardiac arrest. Most paediatric anaphylaxis is primarily respiratory with cardiac arrest finally occurring due to severe acidosis and is therefore very difficult to reverse. In contrast, cardiovascular compromise is more common in older children and adults. In infants under 1 year, anaphylaxis does not always have associated signs of urticaria and angioedema, and it may just present with pallor and collapse. Again, history is the key!

The most common food trigger for fatal anaphylaxis in children in the UK is milk, followed by peanut and tree nuts. Allergy skin prick tests and allergen-specific IgE blood tests do not predict reaction severity, and anaphylaxis can occur in patients with high, low and even negative tests.

Laboratory tests (such as mast cell tryptase (MCT)) are not specific for anaphylaxis nor are results available quickly enough to impact on acute management.

Anaphylaxis can be life-threatening, but most reactions do not result in severe outcomes. Anaphylaxis has a case fatality rate under 0.001 per cent. Severe reactions may mimic more mild anaphylaxis reactions in the first instance. Delay in appropriate treatment almost certainly contributes to fatalities.

In older children, the evolution of non-specific allergic reactions into anaphylaxis makes it hard to distinguish from differential diagnoses, including septic shock, a breath-holding episode, a vasovagal episode or a panic attack. Infants can have cardiovascular compromise and anaphylaxis without cutaneous signs, but this is less common in older children.

Children, young people and their families need to be taught how to use their autoinjector in the event of any respiratory symptoms of which anaphylaxis may be the cause, irrespective of severity.

TREATMENT OF ANAPHYLAXIS

As the diagnosis of anaphylaxis is not always obvious, the systematic ABCDE approach to life-threatening illness is adopted.

Intramuscular adrenaline is the first line of treatment. Adrenaline is an alpha receptor agonist, and thus reverses peripheral vasodilatation and reduces oedema. Its beta-1 agonist effects increase cardiac contractility and heart rate, and its beta-2 agonist effects reverse bronchoconstriction. Intramuscular injection of adrenaline should be given in the anterolateral aspect of the thigh, which has better absorption than either the deltoid muscle or the buttock. The same dose should be repeated after 5 to 10 minutes if there is an inadequate response. Auto-injectors are the preferred method of administration. Nothing should delay the administration of adrenaline as the outcome is superior with early injection. Concurrent high flow oxygen and rapid fluid resuscitation should be given to restore intravascular volume. Bronchospasm should be treated in the same way as life-threatening asthma. Antihistamines are not effective against anaphylaxis.

A recent systematic review and meta-analysis has demonstrated that oral corticosteroids do not reduce the likelihood of a late biphasic reaction.

After treatment and resolution of symptoms, the child should be observed for several hours until biphasic recurrence (5 to 10 per cent) is unlikely. All will require referral to a specialist allergy clinic, and a prescription for a few auto-injectors (no more than two to four) with clear instructions and training for their use in an emergency. An individualised management plan for the family should focus on education, allergen avoidance, knowledge of first aid and the optimal management of comorbidities such as asthma.

(Box16.1)

(Box16.2)

Box 16.1   Key Points

The key to making a diagnosis of food allergy is the recognition of a strong temporal relationship between the exposure to a foodstuff and the onset of very stereotyped allergic symptoms.

Specialist allergy clinic referral is needed if a doctor suspects multiple food allergy, severe allergic reactions of type one immediate hypersensitivity type, faltering growth, or if a child fails to respond to a properly supervised and implemented exclusion diet.

Milk allergy affects 2 to 7 per cent of infants. Most often it is non-IgE mediated and the history is essential in reaching a diagnosis and resolution of symptoms within 1 to 3 weeks of milk protein exclusion is confirmatory. There are no in vitro tests for CMPI.

Unjustified and unsupervised exclusions can significantly affect a child's nutrition, growth and dietary preferences later in life. Most outgrow it (average of 3 years of age if non-IgE mediated and 5 years of age if IgE mediated).

Allergic reactions to eggs are most likely in under 1-year-olds and most commonly present with a rapid onset of symptoms after the infant is given egg for the first time.

The prevalence of peanut allergy in the USA, UK and Australia is about 1 in 25 to 1 in 50 and is rising. Severe reactions to peanut are thankfully rare, but peanut allergy is one of the leading causes of fatal food-related anaphylaxis.

Soya protein allergy is much less common than is thought and is most often discovered in children already identified to have a cow's milk protein allergy.

Shellfish allergy (prawn/shrimp, crab, lobster and mussel) may cause rapid onset reactions, which are occasionally very severe.

Anaphylaxis is likely when there is an acute onset of illness, with flushing, urticaria and angioedema in tandem, with the life-threatening features of lower airway or circulation compromise. Intramuscular adrenaline is the first line treatment for anaphylaxis.

Box 16.2   10-Month-Old With Lip Swelling

A 10-month-old develops significant lip swelling, a perioral rash and mild wheeze after trying scrambled egg for the first time. He has a background history of troublesome atopic dermatitis and has been attending a paediatrician. His parents are very concerned about the possibility of multiple food allergies and have requested referral to a specialist allergy clinic.

Clinical Pearls

Infants with severe atopic dermatitis from an early age (less than 6 months of age) are more likely to develop immediate food allergy than those with normal skin. Extensive allergy testing to foods already tolerated in their diet is **not** recommended.

Foods such as tomato, citrus and berry fruits are very rarely allergenic but do act as irritants when they contact with the face of infants, especially those with facial atopic dermatitis.

Allergic reactions to eggs are most likely in under 1-year-olds and most commonly present with a rapid onset of symptoms (as in this case) after the infant is given egg for the first time. This strong temporal relationship between first egg exposure and the onset of symptoms is key. Delayed type or non-IgE mediated egg allergy can cause flares of eczema.

Box 16.2   10-Month-Old With Lip Swelling—cont'd

Most infants (over 85 per cent) with proven egg allergy can tolerate egg in baked foods such as cake, scones, pancake and egg pasta. If an infant is already tolerating any of these, then they should be kept in their diet because this will help them grow out of the allergy.

Major international studies have shown that delaying the introduction of allergic foods into infant's diets _**increases**_ their risk of developing food allergy, especially if they have atopic dermatitis. This means that infants must eat foods to build a tolerance to them.

Introducing peanuts regularly (three times a week) into an infant's diet as soon as they begin to wean will significantly reduce their risk of developing peanut allergy. Infants with severe atopic dermatitis may need allergy testing before giving them peanut.

Interpretation of Tests

The diagnosis of food allergy usually rests with the history as most reactions are IgE mediated, so they are florid and rapid in onset reactions to a typical food.

IgE tests and skin prick tests usually give similar results, so negative IgE-specific tests mean food allergy is very unlikely (95 per cent) and positive tests properly ordered (a crucial point in a child with symptoms) should be interpreted with confidence.

For skin prick tests, the size of the wheal and flare response relates to the age and sex of the child, the quality of the allergen extract (which may vary greatly) and whether the child is on medications such as antihistamines or topical steroids.

Food challenges are the gold standard, but need to be performed in closely monitored situations as there is always a risk of a severe anaphylactic reaction.

Potential Pitfalls

An allergy-focussed history is crucial, and one needs to avoid performing allergy tests as a 'fishing expedition', as this will pick up sensitisation.

Unjustified and unsupervised dietary exclusions can significantly affect a child's nutrition, growth and dietary preferences later in life. Most food allergy is outgrown (average of 3 years of age if non-IgE mediated and 5 years of age if IgE mediated).

Anaphylaxis is _**characterised by the presence of respiratory or cardiovascular symptoms**_ as part of an allergic reaction. Skin or mucosal changes alone are not a sign of an anaphylactic reaction. Intramuscular adrenaline is the first line of treatment for anaphylaxis.

The most common food trigger for fatal anaphylaxis in children in the UK is milk, followed by peanut and tree nuts. Allergy skin prick tests and allergen-specific IgE blood tests do _**not**_ predict reaction severity, and anaphylaxis can occur in patients with high, low and even negative tests.

In older children, the usual evolution of nonspecific allergic reactions into anaphylaxis makes it hard to distinguish from differential diagnoses, including septic shock, a breath holding episode, a vasovagal episode or a panic attack.

All those who have had anaphylaxis require referral to a specialist allergy clinic and a prescription for a few auto-injectors (two to four) with clear instructions and training in their use in an emergency.

Anaphylaxis can be life-threatening, but most reactions do not result in severe outcomes. In up to 20 per cent of cases, no trigger is identified. Adrenaline is always the first-line treatment, and corticosteroids do not prevent delayed reactions. Autoinjectors are still underused to treat anaphylaxis in the community. Egg allergy (even if prior anaphylaxis) is _**not**_ a contraindication to influenza or MMR vaccination.

Key References

Anagnostou, K., & Turner, P. J. (2019). Myths, facts and controversies in the diagnosis and management of anaphylaxis. *Archives of Disease in Childhood, 104*(1), 83–90.

Chu, D. K., Wood, R. A., French, S., Fiocchi, A., Jordana, M., Waserman, S., et al. (2019). Oral immunotherapy for peanut allergy (PACE): A systematic review and meta-analysis of efficacy and safety. *Lancet, 393*(10187), 2222–2232.

IFAN – Irish Food Allergy Network. (n.d.). Welcome to the Irish Food Allergy Network. www.ifan.ie.

Ludman, S., Shah, N., & Fox, A. T. (2013). Managing cows' milk allergy in children. *BMJ, 347*, f5424.

Roberts, G., & Angier, E. (2019). Peanut oral immunotherapy: Balancing benefits and risks for individuals. *Lancet, 393*(10187), 2180–2181.

Tse, Y., & Rylance, G. (2009). Emergency management of anaphylaxis in children and young people: new guidance from the Resuscitation Council (UK) [published correction appears in Archives of Disease in Childhood. Education and Practice Edition, 95(12), 1071]. *Archives of Disease in Childhood. Education and Practice Edition, 94*(4), 97–101.

17 The Child With Frequent Infections

RONAN LEAHY, AISLING FLINN and KARINA BUTLER

Infants and children with frequent infections commonly present to doctors in both primary and secondary care. In most cases, there is a benign explanation for the recurrent infections, and parents can be reassured.

However, among the many referred, there exists a significant minority of children with an inborn error of immunity (IEI). These children are more susceptible to severe and unusual infection, malignancy, autoimmunity, atopic disease and dysregulated inflammation. Learning to recognise these patients is a crucial skill that can improve outcomes for both children with IEI and their families.

The Immune Response

The human immune system can be thought of as having three lines of defence. The first line of defence is a physical barrier provided by the skin and mucous membranes. It also includes elements such as mucociliary clearance mechanisms in the respiratory tract, a low gastric pH and bacteriolytic lysosomes in tears and saliva.

Conditions that damage the skin (e.g. eczema, burns, wounds), impair the mucociliary escalator (e.g. cystic fibrosis), or damage the oral and gastric mucosa (e.g. chemotherapy, radiation therapy) can therefore lead to increased susceptibility to infection.

The next defensive layer is the innate immune system. The innate system, as its name suggests, is present from birth and produces inflammation. The innate response is fast, but non-specific. The innate immune system has cellular and humoral components. Cellular components include tissue-based macrophages, monocytes and dendritic cells that recognise structures on pathogens (pathogen associated molecular patterns; PAMPs) using pattern recognition receptors (PRRs).

Other innate immune cells include natural killer (NK) cells that can detect stress signals on infected host cells and kill these cells to prevent infection, and neutrophils that phagocytose pathogens and cellular debris. Humoral components of the innate immune system include complement proteins that label bacteria and cellular debris for phagocytosis and lyse bacterial cells themselves by perforating the bacterial cellular membrane.

The third defensive layer is the adaptive immune response, generated by a specific population of blood cells known as lymphocytes. The adaptive immune system is designed to generate a response particular to the pathogen identified (specificity) and protect against subsequent re-infection by the same organism (memory). Lymphocytes are divided into subsets based on cell surface markers. T-lymphocytes coordinate the adaptive immune response and identify and kill cells infected with intracellular pathogens. B-lymphocytes recognise foreign antigen and produce antibodies that can label and neutralise foreign antigen in extracellular spaces. Therefore, activating the adaptive immune response leads to a pathogen-specific immune response that is both intracellular (T cells) and extracellular (B cells). The adaptive immune response also produces memory T cells and memory B cells that remain in the circulation to allow an earlier, more elegant and effective immune response the next time the pathogen is encountered.

The body's response to vaccination is a good example of the adaptive response. The basic principle of vaccination is to generate an adaptive immune response using either a weakened form of the bacteria or virus that is not pathogenic (e.g. BCG/rotavirus/MMR vaccine) or using antigen from the bacteria/virus (e.g. tetanus/diphtheria toxoid) to stimulate production of memory cells and antibody. Children with IEIs that affect the adaptive immune system are often unable to mount a good response to vaccination. Measuring a child's antibody titres after vaccination can therefore be a very useful tool in assessing their adaptive immune system.

The five domains of clinical presentation seen in children with IEI can be classified as shown in Table 17.1.

Table 17.1   Five Domains of Clinical Presentation of Inborn Error of Immunity

Infection	Failure of the immune response against an invading pathogen
Allergy	Inappropriate activation of the immune response to harmless foreign antigen (e.g. peanut)
Autoimmunity	Inappropriate activation of the adaptive immune response to self-antigen (e.g. type 1 diabetes)
Malignancy	Failure of normal tumour surveillance
Autoinflammation	Dysregulated activation of the innate immune response in the absence of infection

The Genetic Basis of Inborn Errors of Immunity

IEIs occur due to mutations in genes encoding proteins (e.g. enzymes, receptors, signalling molecules) that are crucial for normal functioning of the immune system. To date, mutations in over 400 genes have been linked to IEIs. Not all children with IEIs will have an easily identifiable genetic explanation for their illness. For example, only approximately 20 to 25 per cent of children with antibody deficiencies have an identifiable 'monogenic' basis of disease using current diagnostic strategies. With advances in genetic diagnostics, this number of distinct IEIs and the proportion of patients with an identifiable genetic basis is increasing rapidly. These advances have seen the estimated prevalence of IEIs increase to between one in 1000 and one in 5000, an estimate that may well increase in years to come.

Maturation of the Immune System

The immune system, like other organ systems, takes time to mature. Immaturity of the immune system accounts for increased susceptibility to infection early in life, particularly in infancy. For example, newborn infants are more susceptible to infection with *Candida albicans*, a yeast that is not typically pathogenic in older children. Infants and young children are also more susceptible to infection from viruses and *Mycobacterium tuberculosis*. Children under 2 years of age are at increased risk of infection by polysaccharide-encapsulated organisms such as *Streptococcus pneumoniae*, *Haemophilus influenzae* and *Neisseria meningitidis* because of an inability to produce T-cell immune responses to polysaccharide antigens. Vaccination, particularly with protein-conjugated vaccines, is therefore crucial in infancy and early childhood to protect from severe infection.

Transfer of maternal immunoglobulin (IgG) across the placenta affords the newborn protection, particularly in the first 6 months of life. After maternal immunoglobulin IgG has declined, a proportion of infants and young children have hypogammaglobulinaemia for a period of time (transient hypogammaglobulinaemia of infancy) before their immune system fully matures to make up the deficit. Over time, the serum immunoglobulin levels increase to adult ranges. Frequent infections are not uncommon in this age group and discriminating a healthy child from a child with an IEI can be difficult. A period of observation is sometimes needed to allow the immune system to mature or to allow clinical or laboratory features of an IEI to become more apparent before a definitive intervention can be considered.

Secondary Immunodeficiency

Non-immunological host factors and environmental factors can have a negative impact on the functioning of the immune system, leading to 'secondary immunodeficiency'. More recently, the evolution of sophisticated immunotherapies of the immune response (particularly monoclonal antibodies that target components such as cytokines, receptors and cells) has led to an increased number of and complexity in patients with iatrogenic secondary immunodeficiency.

Factors that can cause secondary immune dysfunction are listed in Table 17.2.

Key Points in the History

INFECTION HISTORY

Discriminating the healthy child from a child with an IEI is sometimes difficult since recurrent infection is not unusual, particularly early in childhood. For example, normal children can have up to 11 respiratory infections per year in infancy, 8 per year during preschool and 4 per year in at school-age children. These figures are higher in infants and toddlers attending creche or day care.

A detailed infection history should consider the type, number, and severity of infections, unusual infections (e.g. paronychia due to Pseudomonas (Fig. 17.1)), age at onset, any complications (e.g. empyemas, parapneumonic effusion), need for hospital admission, need for antibiotics (intravenous or oral) and any organisms identified.

Infections in children with IEI tend to be:

Serious (e.g. meningitis, bacteraemia, pneumonia), involving normally sterile sites and requiring inpatient treatment with intravenous antibiotics

Persistent: not responding to standard treatment strategies

Unusual: unusual pathogen (e.g. *Pneumocystis jirovecii* causing pneumonia) or pathogens occurring in unusual circumstances (e.g. oral candidiasis beyond the neonatal period)

Recurrent infections or infections that 'Run in the family'.

This **SPUR** mnemonic can be a useful tool in practice to raise the suspicion of an underlying IEI.

Another tool developed to help identify children with IEI is the list of '10 warning signs' developed by the Jeffrey Modell Foundation (Fig. 17.2).

Of the 10 warning signs, positive family history, use of intravenous antibiotics, and failure to thrive were found to be most strongly associated with a diagnosis of IEI.

Other Medical History

A full systems review may provide information about co-existing immune dysfunction or dysregulation as follows:

- Enteropathy – prolonged or recurrent diarrhoea, with or without blood
- Autoimmunity – including autoimmune cytopaenias, arthritis, type one diabetes, hepatitis, thyroid dysfunction, adrenal insufficiency, hypoparathyroidism
- Autoinflammation – unexplained fevers, rash, arthralgia, arthritis
- Malignancy – lymphoma in childhood, myelodysplasia
- Bone marrow failure

Table 17.2 Causes of Secondary Immunodeficiency

Condition	Secondary Immunological Defect
Protein-Losing states Nephrotic syndrome Severe burns Intestinal lymphangiectasia Protein-losing enteropathy Malnutrition	Loss of immunoglobulins
Premature Birth	Reduced placental transfer of maternal IgG, reduced innate and adaptive immune responses
Breach of Physical Barriers Burns Severe eczema Indwelling catheter or other foreign material Mechanical ventilation	Direct entry of pathogens increasing the risk of bacterial infections particularly staphylococcal and pseudomonal infections
Absent or Reduced Splenic Function Splenectomy Hyposplenism (e.g. haemaglobinopathies) Congenital asplenia or polysplenia	Reduced or absent splenic phagocytic clearance of infected cells and bacteria and production of antibodies that protect against encapsulated bacteria
Medications Corticosteroids Chemotherapy Immunosuppressive medications (e.g. ciclosporin, tacrolimus) Biological therapies (e.g. anti-TNF/IL-6/IL-1 mAbs)	Variable effects on the immune system
HIV	Depletion of CD4 T cells
Haematological Malignancy Leukaemia Lymphoma	Infiltration of bone marrow and lymphoid tissues

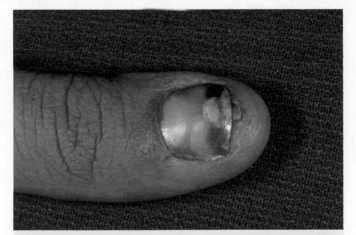

Figure 17.1 Pseudomonas paronychia. Note the green discolouration. (Reproduced with permission from Paller, A. S., & Mancini, A. J. (2021). *Paller and Mancini – Hurwitz clinical pediatric dermatology: A textbook of skin disorders of childhood & adolescence* (6th ed.). Elsevier – Health Sciences Division.)

- Granulomata
- Allergy
- Extensive skin rashes or lesions (e.g. verruca vulgaris (Fig. 17.3))
- History of haemophagocytic lymphohistiocytosis (HLH)

A thorough systems review can also provide clues such as a congenital heart defects (especially conotruncal defects), developmental delay, and feeding difficulties seen in DiGeorge syndrome. Ataxia, telangiectasia and developmental delay are features seen in ataxia-telangiectasia. Petechiae, easy bleeding and eczema are seen in Wiskott-Aldrich syndrome.

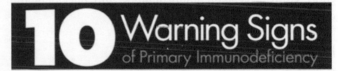

10 Warning Signs of Primary Immunodeficiency

Primary Immunodeficiency (PI) causes children and adults to have infections that come back frequently or are unusually hard to cure. 1:500 persons are affected by one of the known Primary Immunodeficiencies. If you or someone you know is affected by two or more of the following Warning Signs, speak to a physician about the possible presence of an underlying Primary Immunodeficiency.

1 Four or more new ear infections within 1 year.

2 Two or more serious sinus infections within 1 year.

3 Two or more months on antibiotics with little effect.

4 Two or more pneumonias within 1 year.

5 Failure of an infant to gain weight or grow normally.

6 Recurrent, deep skin or organ abscesses.

7 Persistent thrush in mouth or fungal infection on skin.

8 Need for intravenous antibiotics to clear infections.

9 Two or more deep-seated infections including septicemia.

10 A family history of PI.

Figure 17.2 10 Warning signs of primary Immunodeficiency – Jeffrey Modell Foundation. (Reproduced with permission from Jeffrey Modell Foundation. These warning signs were developed by the Jeffrey Modell Foundation Medical Advisory Board. Consultation with Primary Immunodeficiency experts is strongly suggested. © 2016 Jeffrey Modell Foundation.)

BIRTH

Important considerations include gestation, birth weight and maternal illness (e.g. HIV infection). Delayed detachment of

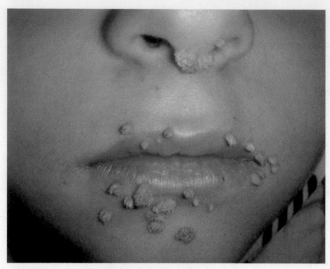

Figure 17.3 Verruca vulgaris warty nodules on the face. (Reproduced with permission from Klatt, E. C. (2020). *Robbins and Cotran Atlas of Pathology* (4th ed.). Elsevier – Health Sciences Division.)

Table 17.3 Features of Inborn Errors of Immunity on Physical Examination

System	Abnormality
General appearance and growth	Failure to thrive
	Short stature
	Microcephaly
	Syndromic features
Ear, nose and throat	Perforated tympanic membranes
	Discharging ears
Mouth	Candidiasis
	Poor or abnormal dentition
	Gingivostomatitis
	Ulcers
Respiratory	Signs of respiratory infection
	Clubbing
Lymphoid tissues	Lymphadenopathy
	Absence of lymphoid tissues, tonsils
	Organomegaly (hepatosplenomegaly)
Skin	Eczema
	Severe warts or molluscum contagiosum
	Albinism
	Telangiectasia

the umbilical cord beyond 30 days is suggestive of a leukocyte adhesion defect.

GROWTH AND DEVELOPMENT

Weight, height and head circumference should be plotted and followed over time.

Failure to thrive is an important potential indicator of an underlying IEI or other chronic disease. Microcephaly, short stature, skeletal abnormalities and developmental delay are associated with certain IEIs.

IMMUNISATION HISTORY

Knowledge of the immunisation history is important to enable interpretation of vaccine responses in the evaluation of antibody function. Live attenuated vaccines can pose a significant risk to children with certain underlying IEI conditions or in immunosuppressed individuals as they can develop into progressive infection.

MEDICATIONS

Current and past medications, durations and dosages should be recorded, particularly any immunosuppressive agents such as corticosteroids and monoclonal antibody therapies.

FAMILY HISTORY

The presence of family members with recurrent infections, similar symptoms or unexplained early death suggests the possibility of a genetic disease. Multiple family members with autoimmune disease or haematological malignancy may also be significant. Enquiring about consanguinity is important in the consideration of autosomal recessive disorders.

EXAMINATION

Physical examination can provide important clues to the presence of an IEI as shown in Table 17.3.

Interpretation of Investigations

Laboratory testing should be tailored according to the findings from a detailed history and examination.

First line investigations typically include:

- full blood count (FBC) with white cell differential
- lymphocyte subset immunophenotyping
- serum immunoglobulins (IgG, IgA, IgM) and serum albumin
- vaccine-specific antibody titres

FULL BLOOD COUNT (FBC)

Neutropenia is defined as an absolute neutrophil count of less than 1.5×10^9/L and is deemed severe if the neutrophil count is less than 0.5×10^9/L. Most neutropenia is transient and post-viral. Neutropenia is not unusual during acute infection, but typically resolves quickly when the patient recovers. A persistently low neutrophil count can indicate either an IEI or can be secondary to medications or autoimmunity.

The normal range for lymphocytes is age dependent. The normal lymphocyte count in a young infant is over 2.7×10^9/L, whereas the normal count in an adult is over 1.0×10^9/L. A persistently lymphocyte count (under 2.0×10^9/L) in an infant should prompt consideration of severe combined immunodeficiency (SCID).

LYMPHOCYTE SUBSET ANALYSIS

Lymphocyte subset analysis by flow cytometry can help to discriminate IEIs from lymphopaenia due to intercurrent infection or secondary causes. Using correct age reference ranges is crucial. In addition to absolute numbers, the ratios of cell subsets are also helpful.

A useful rule of thumb for interpretation of lymphocyte subsets is as follows:

- There should be more T cells than B cells.
- There should be more T_{Helper} cells (CD4) than $T_{cytotoxic}$ cells (CD8).
- There should be more B cells than NK cells.

Cell-mediated immunity is mediated by thymus-derived T_{Helper} and $T_{Cytotoxic}$ lymphocytes. CD4 T cells are necessary for optimal B cell function and express cytokines that activate phagocytes to clear intracellular pathogens. CD8 T cells lyse virally infected cells. Therefore, lymphocyte subsets assess CD3 (total T cells), CD4 (T_{Helper} cells), and CD8 ($T_{Cytotoxic}$ cells).

While it is not unusual for a child to have cell counts that are marginally outside the normal range, persistently severely low or absent cell subset counts merits more careful and urgent evaluation. Normal lymphocyte subpopulations do not rule out IEIs, and results should be discussed with an immunologist if there are any concerns.

SERUM IMMUNOGLOBULINS

Measurement of immunoglobulins (IgA, IgG and IgM) is particularly important if there is a suspicion of B-cell or antibody deficiency. IgG levels are difficult to interpret in early infancy due to the presence of maternal IgG and in early childhood due to immaturity of immune system. Measurement of IgE is also useful in atopy and an elevated serum IgE is a hallmark of some IEIs (e.g. hyper IgE syndrome). In secondary antibody deficiency, hypogammaglobulinaemia is accompanied by loss of other serum proteins such as albumin and alpha$_1$-antitrypsin. While antibody titres can often be outside the normal reference range, complete agammaglobulinaemia or persistently severely low immunoglobulin levels (particularly IgG) merits urgent immunological evaluation.

VACCINE-SPECIFIC ANTIBODY TITRES

Measuring the specific antibody response to previous vaccination is a valuable tool in detection of IEIs involving the adaptive immune system. Measurements of antibody titres to tetanus, diphtheria, H. influenzae type b and protein-conjugated pneumococcal vaccines are frequently used to assess response to protein antigens. In children over the age of 2 years, antibody response to polysaccharide antigens, such as pneumococcal polysaccharide vaccines, can also be measured.

Further investigations are tailored towards the suspected underlying IEI. Diagnostic guidelines for non-immunologists have been developed by the European Society for Immunodeficiencies (ESID) to inform what investigations to carry out depending on the clinical presentation. If an IEI is suspected, early discussion with a paediatric immunologist is recommended.

COMPLEMENT LEVELS AND FUNCTION (CH50/AH50 TESTS)

Complement deficiencies increase susceptibility to encapsulated organisms such as N. meningitidis or pneumococcus and may present as apparent vaccine failures.

HIV Disease in Infants and Children

Globally, 1.8 million children under the age of 14 years were living with HIV in 2019, most in sub-Saharan Africa. The major route of infection is mother-to-child transmission, that can occur during pregnancy, at delivery, or via breast milk. Mother-to-infant transmission has dramatically declined in Europe (now under 0.5 per cent) due to the introduction of routine antenatal screening enabling identification and antiretroviral treatment of HIV-infected women. Studies have shown the earlier treatment is initiated in pregnancy, the lower the risk of transmission. For women on treatment prior to conception who remain fully virally suppressed throughout pregnancy, the risk of transmission approaches zero. Women who are on treatment and virally suppressed can anticipate a normal delivery. Where viral suppression is not achieved by time of delivery (non-adherence to therapy or late presentations), obstetrical management is focused on the avoidance of prolonged rupture of the membranes. Planned caesarean section may be indicated depending on the HIV viral load. Postnatally, in high-income countries formula feeding remains the safest option for infants born to women with HIV. In low- and middle-income countries where this is not feasible, breastfeeding can be made considerably safer if antiretroviral therapy (ART) is given to both the mother and infant.

Untreated, 15 to 20 per cent of HIV-infected infants follow a rapidly progressive course characterised by early onset of opportunistic infections (Pneumocystis jirovecii pneumonia (PJP/PCP), cytomegalovirus (CMV)), progressive encephalopathy, severe and persistent candida infection, failure to thrive and death within the first years of life. Most infants follow a more slowly progressive course. They can remain asymptomatic for months or even years. These children typically present with lymphadenopathy, hepatosplenomegaly, parotid enlargement and frequent infections. In the children with mild to moderate immune compromise, the infections commonly seen are those caused by the usual childhood pathogens, albeit occurring at increased frequency and severity. Bacteraemia with S. pneumoniae, Staphylococcus aureus, H. influenzae type b and Salmonella spp. and focal infections (e.g. recurrent pneumonia, otitis, mastoiditis, lymphadenitis, cellulitis) were common prior to effective ART. Disseminated Varicella-Zoster (Fig. 17.4), recurrent herpes zoster, chronic herpes simplex (HSV), prolonged Cryptosporidium infection, and superficial and mucosal candidiasis can all be problematic for the HIV-infected child. As immunologic decline progresses bacterial pathogens typically associated with immune deficiency such as Pseudomonas spp. and opportunistic infections such as PJP, CMV, disseminated atypical mycobacterial infection are seen.

Any child undergoing evaluation for unexplained recurrent or persisting infection deserves an HIV test, particularly if these occur in association with lymphopenia, hyper- or hypogammaglobulinaemia.

DIAGNOSIS

In the first months of life, all infants born to HIV positive mothers will have a positive HIV antibody test. This reflects the normal transplacental transfer of maternal antibodies.

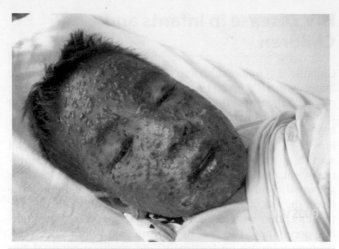

Figure 17.4   Severe Varicella in a child with HIV infection. (Reproduced with permission from Kliegman, R. M. (Ed.). (2015). *Nelson textbook of pediatrics: First South Asia edition, 3 volume set.* Elsevier.)

A positive HIV antibody test in an infant reflects the maternal status and confirms exposure.

The median time to seroreversion (loss of the maternal HIV antibodies) is 10 months and most uninfected infants will test negative by 18 months of age. However, some residual antibodies can persist even up to 24 months of age and give rise to an equivocal test result. Antibody testing should not be used for diagnosis in perinatally exposed infants until they are 24 months of age.

Virologic assays (HIV RNA or DNA PCR (polymerase chain reaction) testing) directly detect HIV and can diagnose infection in more than 95 per cent of infants by 6 weeks of age. Conversely, infection can be excluded in non-breast-feeding infants by 4 months of age if they have two

negative HIV PCR tests taken after neonatal antiretroviral therapy is stopped, and the infants is at least 4 months old at time of the second test. A positive HIV PCR test within 72 hours of birth indicates intrauterine transmission. Infants who have been breast-fed should be tested at 4 to 6 weeks, then 3 and 6 months after cessation of breast-feeding to exclude infection.

IMMUNISATION

All standard childhood vaccinations may be given to HIV-infected or exposed children, although certain live viral vaccines (such as live attenuated influenza virus, varicella, MMR) should be avoided in those who arc severely immunosuppressed (CD4 count under 200 cells/µL and under 15 per cent T cells). HIV-infected infants and children should not receive BCG vaccination. Both MenACWY and meningococcal B vaccination are recommended in HIV-infected infants and children. HIV-infected children should also receive age appropriate COVID-19 vaccination in accordance with the local protocol.

Inactivated vaccines can be given to all HIV-infected children, even if immunocompromised. However, as responses may be suboptimal, repeat vaccination after recovery of immune function is recommended. If antiretroviral treatment is being initiated, delay vaccination until the child's CD4 count is above 15 per cent to optimise the vaccine response.

(Box 17.1)
(Box 17.2)
(Box 17.3)
(Box 17.4)
(Box 17.5)
(Box 17.6)

Box 17.1   Key Points

Inborn errors of immunity are rarely seen but important to diagnose.

The adaptive immune system is designed to provide a specific defence and protect against subsequent re-infection by the same organism by the development of a memory response.

Measuring a child's antibody titres after vaccination is a very useful tool in assessing their adaptive immune system.

Transfer of maternal immunoglobulin (IgG) across the placenta affords the newborn protection, particularly in the first 6 months of life.

Serious infections, **persistent** infections, **unusual** infections (e.g. *Burkholderia cepacian*) or **recurrent** infections are all characteristic of inborn errors of immunity.

First line investigations for immunodeficiency include a full blood count (FBC) with white cell differential, serum immunoglobulins (IgG, IgA, IgM) and serum albumin, lymphocyte subset immunophenotyping and vaccine-specific antibody titres.

HIV transmission during pregnancy has dramatically declined in the developed world (now below 1 per cent) due

to the introduction of routine antenatal screening enabling identification and antiretroviral treatment of HIV-infected women.

HIV-infected infants may present like infants with SCID with chronic diarrhoea, failure to thrive, recurrent bacterial infections and severe candidiasis.

Diagnosis of SCID is a medical emergency and early recognition is essential to improve the outcome. SCID is characterised by the absence of functioning T cells.

Always check IgA levels when performing a coeliac screen. If the IgA is low and coeliac disease is suspected, then test the anti-endomysial IgG antibodies or refer for duodenal biopsy.

Complement deficiencies increase susceptibility to encapsulated organisms such as *N. meningitidis* or pneumococcus and may present as apparent vaccine failures.

The hallmark of transient hypogammaglobulinaemia of infancy (THI) is low IgG (measured on at least two occasions), with normal or low levels of IgA and IgM, and normal antibody responses to vaccinations.

Box 17.2   Severe Failure to Thrive in Early Infancy

A 3-month-old female infant presents with severe failure to thrive (weight on the 0.4th centile), prolonged bronchiolitis and intractable diarrhoea (Fig. 17.5). She has a rash over her abdomen and trunk and an ulcer is noticed in the arm where BCG was given at birth (Fig. 17.6). She is very pale and unwell and has ongoing tachypnoea with persistent infiltrates and an absent thymic shadow on a chest x-ray. Her stool is positive for rotavirus, and initial blood investigations show an absolute lymphocyte count of 0.2 x 10⁹/L. The parents are second cousins and have one other child who is well.

Clinical Pearls

The likely diagnosis is severe combined immunodeficiency (SCID), which is fatal in the first year of life if untreated. The incidence of SCID is approximately one in 50,000, although higher in cultures where consanguineous marriage is common. Diagnosis of SCID is a medical emergency and early recognition is key to improving outcome. SCID is characterised by the absence of functioning T cells. Common early clinical findings include failure to thrive, chronic diarrhoea, persistent mucocutaneous candidiasis, persistent infections with common viral pathogens (e.g. respiratory syncytial virus (RSV), rotavirus, cytomegalovirus and influenza) and opportunistic infections such as with *Pneumocystis jirovecii*. Administration of live vaccines such as rotavirus or BCG can cause disseminated or fatal infection. The thymus gland is small and not visible on a chest x-ray. Any infant with persistent lymphopaenia (less than 2.0 x 10⁹/L), especially if under 6 months of age, should always be investigated to exclude SCID.

Further immunological evaluation must be performed as soon as possible to establish a definite diagnosis, followed by curative treatment with stem cell transplantation. Gene therapy is another therapeutic option for certain forms of SCID.

Potential Pitfalls

Early diagnosis is an issue (as SCID is quite rare) and close attention to the absolute lymphocyte count is vital.

Although the total lymphocyte count is usually low in patients with SCID, it can be normal (e.g. due to normal or elevated numbers of B cells). Further investigation and consultation with a paediatric immunologist are necessary if there is a high index of suspicion for SCID despite a normal lymphocyte count.

In this clinical scenario, the differential diagnosis would include HIV infection, extreme malnutrition, or other types of combined immune deficiency (such as complete DiGeorge syndrome, hyper IgM syndrome, or Wiskott-Aldrich syndrome).

Initial management of a patient with SCID includes keeping the infant in protective isolation with supportive management such as treatment of infections and nutritional optimisation. Prophylaxis with antifungal, antiviral and antimicrobial therapies should be commenced. Live vaccines must be avoided. If any blood products are needed, they must be irradiated, leuko-depleted and cytomegalovirus negative.

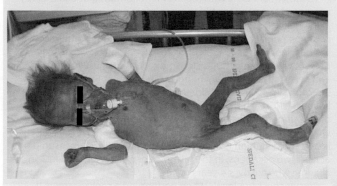

Figure 17.5   Typical appearance of an infant with severe combined immunodeficiency (SCID). Note severe growth failure and respiratory distress. (Reproduced with permission from Leung, D. Y. M., Szefler, S. J., Akdis, C. A., Sampson, H., & Bonilla, F. A. (Eds.). (2021). *Pediatric allergy: Principles and practice* (4th ed.). Elsevier.)

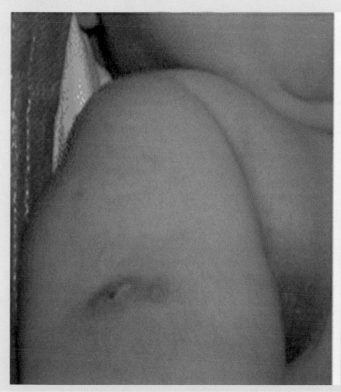
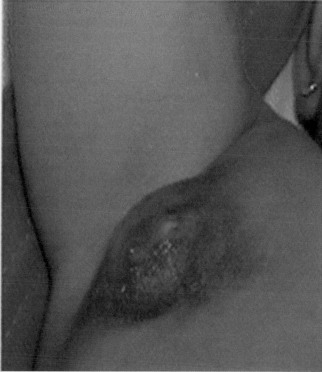

Figure 17.6   Side effect to bacilli Calmette-Guérin vaccine in a severe combined immunodeficiency patient. (CREDIT Reproduced with permission from Aghamohammadi, A., Abolhassani, H., Rezaei, N., & Yazdani, R. (Eds.). (2021). *Inborn errors of immunity: A practical guide.* Academic Press.)

Box 17.3   Repeated Illness in a Toddler

A 12-month-old boy presents with recurrent fevers and episodes of otitis media. He has had six courses of antibiotics to date and his parents are naturally very concerned. He is otherwise thriving and has a normal examination. He was born at term with a normal birth weight. He attends day care and has a 3-year-old brother who is well. There is no significant family history, and the family are non-consanguineous. His serum IgG is low (1.5 g/L), and the remainder of his investigations are normal, including IgA and IgM levels, T and B cells, and vaccine responses to *Haemophilus influenzae type b*, tetanus and pneumococcus.

Clinical Pearls

This boy may have a diagnosis of transient hypogammaglobulinaemia of infancy (THI). Newborn immunoglobulins are mostly derived from maternal transfer of IgG in utero. After birth, as the infant's immunoglobulin production increases, maternal IgG is gradually cleared, resulting in a typical nadir of serum IgG at approximately 6 months of age leading to a transient period of increased vulnerability to infection. This is more pronounced in preterm infants as the majority of maternal IgG is transferred in the third trimester. Prolongation of this normal physiological nadir of immunoglobulin levels occurs in THI. The pathogenesis underlying this disorder is not understood.

Management of most children with suspected THI is as-needed observation and treatment of infections. Children with more frequent or severe infections can be treated with antibiotic prophylaxis.

Interpretation of Investigations

The hallmark of THI is low IgG (measured on at least two occasions), with normal or low levels of IgA and IgM with most children having normal antibody responses to vaccinations. There are normal numbers of B cells and normal T cell-mediated immunity. Toddlers most commonly present with recurrent respiratory tract and ear infections.

Pitfalls to Avoid

THI is a diagnosis of exclusion and can only be made in retrospect because immunoglobulin levels will normalise during childhood (usually by 4 years of age). In a child presenting with recurrent infections and low immunoglobulins, other causes of hypogammaglobulinaemia must be excluded such as X-linked agammaglobulinaemia (XLA) which is characterised by low or absent B cells with normal T cells. Children with XLA may present with recurrent respiratory tract infections, diarrhoea due to *Giardia* species or enterovirus meningoencephalitis.

Although some affected children are asymptomatic until 2 years of age, most show symptoms by 6 to 9 months of age. The diagnosis should be considered if there are very low IgG, IgA and IgM levels (less than 5 per cent of normal values) but preserved T cell function.

Treatment of XLA is with replacement immunoglobulin therapy and aggressive use of antibiotics for infections.

IgA deficiency affects one in 500 children and is by far the most common primary immunodeficiency. Most children with selective IgA deficiency (over 85 per cent) are asymptomatic. Some may present with ear infections, sinusitis, recurrent chest infections and persistent diarrhoea. Antibody replacement therapy is not indicated. IgA-deficient children and adults may be prone to anaphylactic reaction upon administration of blood products. The diagnosis of selective IgA deficiency can only be made once the child reaches 4 years of age, when IgA levels should reach adult levels. The definition is an IgA level less than 0.07 g/L measured on at least two occasions, in the presence of normal IgM and IgG, in children who are over 4 years of age.

Always check IgA levels when performing a coeliac screen. If the IgA is low and coeliac disease is suspected, then test the anti-endomysial IgG antibodies and consider referring the patient for a small intestinal biopsy.

Box 17.4   Recurrent Meningococcal Disease

An 18-month-old girl presents to the emergency department with fever, irritability and vomiting. Cerebrospinal fluid (CSF) analysis demonstrates a white cell count of 800 cells/mm^3, predominantly neutrophils, and the culture subsequently grows *Neisseria meningitidis*. In the history, she was born at full term, with no neonatal complications, and she received all her routine vaccinations. She had a previous episode of meningitis also caused by *N. meningitidis* when she was 6 months old, from which she made a full recovery. There is no family history of note.

Clinical Pearls

Recurrent infection with *N. meningitidis*, raises suspicion of a defect within the complement system.

The complement system can be divided into three pathways: the classical, alternative and lectin pathways. Each pathway has distinct triggers, but all three pathways result in promotion of inflammation, formation of C3 (an important opsonin which helps to facilitate phagocytosis) and the membrane attack complex which disrupts the membranes of target cells causing cell lysis and death.

Management of a child with complement deficiency includes vigilance for early signs of infection, seeking timely medical attention and vaccination (especially against pneumococcus and meningococcus organisms). Antibiotic prophylaxis is often recommended depending on the nature of the deficit and the age of the patient.

Interpretation of Results

In this child, investigation of the complement system revealed absent function of the classical complement pathway using the CH50 test, a reliable method to screen for deficiency of one of the complement components C1-C9. Function of the alternative complement pathway (called the AH50 test) was also absent. The AH50 test also measures C3 and C5-C9, but includes additional complement components specific to the alternative pathway (properdin, factors B and D) and regulatory factors H and I. Further investigation revealed that this child has absent C5, a component of the C5-C9 membrane attack complex.

Potential Pitfalls

Inherited disorders of complete deficiencies of complement components are rare causes of bacterial infections (most encapsulated bacteria) and systemic lupus erythematosus (SLE). SLE is associated with deficiencies in early complement components of the classical pathway such as C2 or C1. Increased consumption of complement proteins can be seen in inflammatory and autoimmune conditions, or during acute infection. Therefore, it is best to delay measurement of CH50/AP50, if possible, until the patient is clinically well.

Box 17.5 Recurrent Pneumonias

An 11-year-old boy had three hospital admissions over the previous 6 months with radiologically proven pneumonias all requiring intravenous antibiotics. He has a persistent wet fruity cough. A sweat test was normal. A CT thorax shows significant bronchiectasis, and an ultrasound abdomen identifies splenomegaly.

Clinical Pearls

His diagnosis is common variable immune deficiency (CVID), which has a typical clinical presentation as outlined above.

Children with CVID are susceptible to frequent respiratory tract infections due to *Streptococcus pneumoniae, Haemophilus influenzae* type b and *Mycoplasma*. Bronchiectasis is a frequent complication in CVID. Gastrointestinal infections with giardia, salmonella, campylobacter and enteroviruses are common. Treatment of CVID is with antibiotic prophylaxis, prompt treatment of infections and immunoglobulin replacement therapy.

Interpretation of Investigations

Serum IgA, IgM, IgG levels will be low and specific antibody response to primary vaccinations (Hib, tetanus, pneumococcus) will be suboptimal. B cell numbers may be normal or reduced, and there may be differences in B cell subpopulations. T cell numbers may be normal or slightly reduced. The ratio of CD4:CD8 positive T cells is sometimes reversed.

Potential Pitfalls

Children with CVID may have enlarged tonsils, lymphadenopathy and splenomegaly. Autoimmune thrombocytopenia and autoimmune haemolytic anaemia occur commonly in CVID. Up to 30 per cent may have non-caseating granulomas in the liver, spleen and lungs. An enteropathy may cause chronic diarrhoea, protein loss, and poor weight gain, and children with CVID are more prone to inflammatory bowel disease.

Box 17.6 Recurrent Skin Abscesses With Recurrent Cervical Lymphadenitis

A 4-year-old boy has a history of recurrent bacterial cervical lymphadenitis. Three episodes required incision and drainage, and *Staphylococcus aureus* was identified on each occasion. He also had pneumonia requiring treatment with intravenous antibiotics at 2 years of age. His growth is on the 2nd centile for height and weight, and he also has a history of diarrhoea and abdominal pain. In the family history, his mother's brother had a history of frequent infections and died as a young child although the cause was not known. Investigations demonstrate anaemia, a mildly elevated C-reactive protein (CRP) and ESR, normal immunoglobulins and normal lymphocyte subsets. A neutrophil oxidative burst assay is abnormal.

Clinical Pearls

The diagnosis is chronic granulomatous disease (CGD), and definitive treatment is with HLA-matched haematopoietic stem cell transplantation.

Neutrophils in CGD are unable to produce reactive oxidative species needed to kill bacteria and fungi engulfed following phagocytosis. Most cases of CGD are X-linked, but, rarely, they can be autosomal recessive. Children present with recurrent bacterial and fungal infections, particularly caused by *S. aureus* and *Aspergillus* species.

Affected children with chronic granulomatous disease may present with recurrent lymphadenitis, bacterial hepatic abscess, lung abscess or osteomyelitis. Examination may reveal anaemia, significant failure to thrive, superficial skin abscesses, hepatosplenomegaly and dermatitis.

Interpretation of Investigations

The diagnostic test is the neutrophil oxidative burst test (a test of the nicotinamide adenine dinucleotide phosphate (NAPDH) respiratory burst system in neutrophils) and is defective in patients with chronic granulomatous disease leading to excessive inflammation and increased susceptibility to infections.

Potential Pitfalls

Children with CGD are prone to the formations of granulomas, which most commonly affect the gastrointestinal and genitourinary tracts. Colitis and growth retardation are common manifestations. Patients with CGD are often initially diagnosed with inflammatory bowel disease.

Key References and Further Reading

Geha, R.S., & Notarangelo, L. (2016). *Case studies in immunology: A clinical companion* (7th ed.). Garland Publishing.

HSE National Immunisation Office. (2021). Chapter 3: Immunisation of immunocompromised persons. *Immunisation guidelines*. Updated 24 September 2021. https://www.hse.ie/eng/health/immunisation/hcpinfo/guidelines/chapter3.pdf.

Jyothi, S., Lissauer, S., Welch, S., & Hackett, S. (2013). Immune deficiencies in children: An overview. *Postgraduate Medical Journal, 89*(1058), 698–708.

Milioglou, I., Kalaitzidou, I., & Ladomenou, F. (2019). Interpretation of lymphocyte subset counts by the general pediatrician. *Pediatrics International: Official Journal of the Japan Pediatric Society, 61*(1), 16–22.

Subbarayan, A., Colarusso, G., Hughes, S. M., Gennery, A. R., Slatter, M., Cant, A. J., & Arkwright, P. D. (2011). Clinical features that identify children with primary immunodeficiency diseases. *Pediatrics, 127*(5), 810–816.

Tangye, S. G., Al-Herz, W., & Bousfiha, A. (2020). Human inborn errors of Immunity: 2019 Update on the classification from the International Union of Immunological Societies Expert Committee [published correction appears in *J Clin Immunol*. 2020, February 22.]. *Journal of Clinical Immunology, 40*(1), 24–64.

Verbsky, J. W., & Routes, J. R. (2018). Recurrent fever, infections, immune disorders, and autoinflammatory diseases. In R. M. Kliegman, P. S. Lye, B. Bordini, H. Toth, & D. Basel (Eds.), *Nelson pediatric symptom-based diagnosis* (pp. 746–773). Elsevier.

de Vries, E., & European Society for Immunodeficiencies (ESID) members. (2012). Patient-centred screening for primary immunodeficiency, a multi-stage diagnostic protocol designed for non-immunologists: 2011 Update: Patient-centred screening for PIDs; 2011 update. *Clinical and Experimental Immunology, 167*(1), 108–119.

Online References

United Kingdom Primary Immunodeficiency Network (UKPIN) further reading. https://www.ukpin.org.uk/.

18 The Child With Headaches

BRYAN LYNCH

Headaches are very common in childhood and adolescence and can be classified as either primary or secondary. Primary headaches include tension headaches and migraine and are not related to underlying disease or structural problems. Secondary headaches, on the other hand, are due to an underlying condition such as an infection, tumour, vascular disorder or intracranial haemorrhage.

The great majority of headaches in childhood are primary headaches, which may be diagnosed by history and a detailed physical examination.

Key Points in the History

The headache description is important and in taking the history focus on:

- the location and laterality of the headache
- the headache timing and frequency
- the duration, quality and severity of the headache
- whether any associated features are present and any aggravating or relieving factors are evident
- The recent pattern of headaches is a key question and should focus on whether a crescendo pattern of headache frequency is present or not.
- Offer a young child the opportunity to describe the headache episode to the best of their ability.
- Try to categorise the pattern of headache to see whether it is acute, acute recurrent, chronic non-progressive or chronic progressive in type.
- Quite often, the headache severity bears no relationship to the seriousness of the aetiology. For instance, tension headaches may be quite distressing, whereas headaches due to a brain tumour may initially be mild.
- Ask about worrisome features such as focal weakness, ataxia, diplopia, visual loss, seizures, confusion, mood changes and sensory symptoms, as all are important and warrant consideration of an underlying neurological condition or complex migraine.
- Ask whether the headache causes the child to awaken from sleep, if it is worse on awakening, or if it worsens when the child is recumbent – these symptoms may indicate raised intracranial pressure.
- Potential triggers (trauma, certain foods or exercise) should be explored.

- A thorough medication history is essential to diagnose analgesia overusage headaches (yes, it does happen!).
- Keeping a headache diary should be encouraged as it will demonstrate headache patterns and is helpful to determine the degree of disability due to the headaches.
- In females, the relationship of the headaches to menses should be established, if present.
- A detailed family and social history should be obtained looking for family stressors and a family history of primary headaches (migraines in particular).

Physical Examination

Firstly, check the key vital signs (heart rate, blood pressure and temperature). Growth parameters (height, weight and head circumference) should be obtained. Obesity should alert one to ask about potential obstructive sleep apnoea or to consider idiopathic intracranial hypertension. Growth failure may be a sign of a lesion affecting the pituitary. Check for classical skin features of neurocutaneous syndromes such as neurofibromatosis and tuberous sclerosis.

A full neurological examination, including cranial nerves and fundoscopy as well as a formal gait assessment, should be performed bearing in mind that the majority of brain tumours in children are infratentorial, potentially impacting balance and coordination. Cerebellar signs may include unsteady gait, difficulties in fine motor tasks (finger-nose test with past-pointing, nystagmus, difficulty in repetitive hand movements (dysdiadokinesis) or dysarthric speech.

Cranial Nerve Examination

The examination of the cranial nerves in a child is far less daunting than you may think and is very similar to the cranial nerve examination in adults. Observation is key, and you should look for an obvious strabismus, ptosis or facial nerve palsy. Examine the cranial nerves in sequence. See further details in chapter 3 (Systems and Developmental examination).

Neuroimaging

Most often neuroimaging for headaches only is not required. Neuroimaging (either CT or preferably MRI scan) may be indicated in several circumstances:

- if abnormal neurological findings are evident, such as a localised weakness or a cranial nerve palsy
- headaches with an early morning pattern or that awake the child from sleep
- any signs of raised intracranial pressure
- crescendo pattern suggestive of a chronic progressive headache on headache diary
- presence of a ventriculoperitoneal shunt

Follow-up assessment is required even if there is a single normal neurological examination with no 'red flag' symptoms. Parents should be advised to reattend if there are progressive symptoms.

Tension Headaches

Tension headaches are the most frequently seen primary headaches. The typical pattern seen is that the child feels well early in the day and the headache appears gradually and tends to get worse as the day progresses. The pain is often described as being constant, squeezing, non-pulsatile and band-like. Photophobia and phonophobia are rarely seen in tension headaches and the child is still able to participate in normal daily activities. These headaches may disturb sleep, lead to lost school days, and the chronic use of analgesics. A detailed psychosocial history and profile is needed.

Migraine

Migraine is a frequently seen and quite disabling headache in children and adolescents. In school-aged children, migraine comes after conduct disorder and anxiety in terms of disease burden.

Migraine is generally diagnosed on history. In childhood migraine, headaches tend to be less frequent, do not last as long and respond better to treatment. Vomiting and abdominal pain are more prominent features. The headache is usually bilateral in children and is more common in pre-pubertal boys and post-pubertal girls. A family history is quite frequently seen.

Cyclical vomiting, benign paroxysmal torticollis or benign paroxysmal vertigo may all precede the onset of migraine in children.

The pattern of migraine headaches in children is quite variable. The most common migraine triggers in children are dietary with chocolate, cheeses and onions being the foods most often responsible. Other triggers include menses, sleep deprivation, stress, hot weather and excessive exertion.

Migraine in the absence of an aura is the most common type seen in childhood. The headaches last from 2 to 72 hours and the headache typically has a slow onset and is dull and constant. The headache typically increases in severity over time and becomes throbbing in character. Intense nausea with occasional vomiting occurs and the child tends to retire to a quiet and dark place and falls asleep. The child awakens hours later and feels tired but is pain free.

In migraine with aura, the headache is preceded by an aura, including visual symptoms such as blurring of vision, scintillating scotomas and hemianopia. Sensory auras such as numbness or tingling are much less common.

Migraine with an aura localisable to the posterior fossa (formerly termed basilar artery migraine) may include symptoms of dysarthria and ataxia. Hemiplegic migraine is associated with transient motor weakness on one side with also symptoms of impairment of speech or vision. There is an autosomal dominant familial hemiplegic migraine syndrome where a clear family history will be evident and genetic testing is possible.

Two rare migraine variants are confusional migraine and *Alice in Wonderland* syndrome. Confusional migraine occurs in children over 5 years old and tends to evolve into typical migraine as the child gets older. The aura in *Alice in Wonderland* syndrome is characteristically associated with changes in senses of proportion and distance.

Ibuprofen and paracetamol are recommended as analgesics in children, and triptans are recommended for children over 12 years of age.

In terms of preventing further episodes of migraine, the evidence base for reducing the frequency and severity of attacks is far less robust with the benefits of preventive medications and generally no better than placebo in most trials to date. Topiramate is the only US Food and Drug Administration (FDA)-approved medication for migraine prevention in children over 12 years old. A US multicentre study of migraine preventive agents in children failed to show benefit for topiramate or amitriptyline in comparison to placebo.

Behavioural and lifestyle interventions that appear to work include increased physical activity, better quality sleep, avoiding skipped meals and reduced exposure to caffeine. The success of these interventions is largely unproven.

Cluster Headaches

In cluster headaches, episodes of pain are followed by long periods of remission. The pain tends to be one-sided and periorbital in position, of sudden onset and quickly gets much worse. The headaches tend to occur at night and may last anywhere from 15 minutes to 3 hours in duration. Associated symptoms include excess tearing, rhinorrhoea, increased sweating and nasal stuffiness. Children become agitated and very restless during cluster headache episodes.

Identifying Brain Tumours

Proper identification of brain tumours in children and adolescents is challenging. A very helpful website, www.headsmart.org.uk, provides guidance on the identification of brain tumours and focuses on how brain tumours present at different ages (Fig. 18.1).

Preschool children may present with persistent or recurrent vomiting, abnormal eye movements, significant behavioural change with lethargy in particular, problems with balance and walking, seizures, head tilt or a progressively increasing head circumference.

Primary school children (5 to 12 years old) tend to present with a crescendo headache pattern, recurrent vomiting, abnormal eye movements, blurred vision, diplopia, behavioural change or seizures.

Secondary school children and adolescents (ages 12 to 19 years) present with a crescendo headache pattern, persistent vomiting without nausea, abnormal eye movements, delayed or arrested puberty and seizures.

THE DIAGNOSIS OF BRAIN TUMOURS IN CHILDREN: A GUIDELINE FOR HEALTHCARE PROFESSIONALS

HEAD SMART
EARLY DIAGNOSIS OF BRAIN TUMOURS

headsmart.org.uk

HeadSmart is funded and promoted by The Brain Tumour Charity and run in partnership with the Children's Brain Tumour Research Centre (CBTRC) and the Royal College of Paediatrics and Child Health RCPCH. The Brain Tumour Charity Registered Charity No. 1150054 (England and Wales) SC045081 (Scotland). CBTRC Charitable Status Inland Revenue No. X15294. RCPCH Registered Charity No. 1057744 (England and Wales) SC038299 (Scotland). © 2016 The Brain Tumour Charity, CETRC and RCPCH.

Referral from primary care
- High risk of tumour – SAME DAY referral to secondary care
- Lower 'risk' – specialist assessment within 2 weeks

Imaging
- High risk of tumour – URGENT CNS imaging
- Lower risk – CNS imaging within 4 weeks

Lower risk = CNS tumour in differential diagnosis, low index of suspicion

Consider a brain tumour in any child presenting with
- Headache
- Nausea and/or vomiting
- Visual symptoms and signs:
  reduced visual acuity and/or fields
  abnormal eye movements
  abnormal fundoscopy
- Motor symptoms and signs:
  abnormal gait
  abnormal co-ordination
  focal motor weakness
- Growth and endocrine symptoms:
  growth failure (weight/height)
  delayed, arrested or precocious puberty
  galactorrhoea
  primary/secondary amenorrhea
  Increasing head circumference
- Behavioural change
- Diabetes insipidus
- Seizures (see www.nice.org.uk/guidance/qs27)
- Altered consciousness (see www.nottingham.ac.uk/paediatric-guideline/Guideline&dg-ithm.pdf)

Assess these children with
- History: associated symptoms, any predisposing factors
- Examination of:
  visual system
  motor system
  height and weight
  head circumference(<2yrs)
  pubertal status

IF TWO OR MORE SYMPTOMS – SCAN

Ask about common predisposing factors
- Personal or FH of brain tumour, sarcoma, leukaemia or early onset breast cancer
- Neurofibromatosis
- Tuberous sclerosis
- Other familial genetic syndromes

Assessment pitfalls
- Initial symptoms of brain tumour can mimic other common illnesses
- Symptoms frequently fluctuate – resolution then recurrence does not exclude a brain tumour
- A normal neurological examination does not exclude a brain tumour
- Language difficulties – use interpreter

This guideline has the support of the RCPCH following a rigorous assessment of the guideline development methodology and a full endorsement is expected upon completion of a full stakeholder consultation.

Headaches
- Consider a brain tumour in any child with a new, persistent* headache
- Headache in isolation, unlikely to be a brain tumour
- Brain tumour headaches occur at any time of day
- Children aged younger than 4 years may not be able to describe a headache – observe behaviour

CNS imaging required with
- Persistent headache that wakes a child from sleep
- Persistent headache that occurs on waking
- Persistent headache in a child under 4
- Confusion or disorientation with a headache
- Persistent headache with 1 or more other symptoms

Common pitfalls
- Failure to reassess a child with a migraine or tension headache when the headache character changes

Persistent = continuous or recurrent headache present for more than 4 weeks

Nausea and vomiting
- Consider a brain tumour in any child with persistent* nausea and/or vomiting
- Head circumference should be measured and plotted in children under 2 with persistent vomiting

CNS imaging required with
- Persistent vomiting on waking (NB: exclude pregnancy where appropriate)
- Persistent nausea/vomiting with 1 or more other symptom

Common pitfalls
- Failing to consider a CNS cause for persistent nausea and vomiting

Persistent = nausea and/or vomiting present for more than 2 weeks

Visual signs and symptoms
- Consider a brain tumour in any child with persistent* visual abnormality
- Visual assessment requires assessment of:
  visual acuity
  eye movements
  pupil responses
  optic disc appearance
  visual fields (>/ 5 yrs)
- Pre-school and unco-operative children should be assessed by hospital eye service within 2 weeks of referral
- Parent concern alone warrants referral for visual assessment

CNS imaging required with
- Papilloedema
- Optic atrophy
- New onset nystagmus
- Reduction in visual acuity not due to refractive error
- Visual field reduction
- Proptosis
- New onset paralytic squint
- Visual symptom with 1 or more other symptom

Common pitfalls
- Failure to fully assess vision – REFER IF NECESSARY
- Failure of communication between community optometry and primary and secondary care

Persistent = visual abnormality present for more than 2 weeks

Head circumference
- Consider a brain tumour in any child under two years with an increasing head circumference outside the normal range in comparison to their height and weight
- Careful assessment of other signs and symptoms of a brain tumour should be undertaken in these babies

CNS imaging required with
- Rapid rate of head circumference growth crossing centiles
- Increasing head circumference with any other associated symptoms

Common pitfalls
- Failing to measure and monitor head circumference in a baby or young child with persistent vomiting

Motor symptoms and signs
- Consider a brain tumour in any child with persisting motor abnormality
- Motor assessment requires history or observation of:
  sitting and crawling in infants
  walking and running
  handwriting in school age children
  handling of small objects
- Brain tumours can cause a loss or a change in motor skills and this can be subtle e.g. ability to play computer games

CNS imaging required with
- Regression in motor skills
- Focal motor weakness
- Abnormal gait/co-ordination (unless local cause)
- Bells palsy with NO improvement within 4 weeks
- Swallowing difficulties (unless local cause)
- Head tilt/torticollis (unless local cause)
- Motor symptom with 1 or more other symptom

Common pitfalls
- Attributing abnormal gait/balance to middle ear disease with no corroborating findings
- Failure to identify swallowing difficulties and aspiration as a cause of recurrent chest infections

Persistent = motor abnormality present for more than 2 weeks

Growth and endocrine
- Consider a brain tumour in any child with any combination of growth failure, delayed/arrested puberty and polyuria/polydipsia
- Early specialist assessment if required for:
  precocious puberty/delayed or arrested puberty
  growth failure
  galactorrhoea
  primary or secondary amenorrhoea

CNS imaging required with
- Growth or endocrine symptom with 1 or more other symptoms

Common pitfalls
- Failure to consider a CNS cause in children with weight loss and vomiting
- Failure to consider diabetes insipidus in children with polyuria and polydipsia

Behaviour
- Consider a brain tumour in any child with new onset lethargy, mood disturbance, withdrawal or disinhibition

Common pitfalls
- Failing to consider a physical cause for behavioural symptoms

Figure 18.1 HeadSmart infographic re-worrying features of headache. (Reproduced with permission of HeadSmart. HeadSmart is funded and promoted by The Brain Tumour Charity and run in partnership with the Children's Brain Tumour Research Centre (CBTRC) and the Royal College of Paediatrics and Child Health (RCPCH). The Brain Tumour Charity Registered Charity No. 1150054 (England and Wales) SC045081 (Scotland), CBTRC Charitable Status Inland Revenue No. X15294, RCPCH Registered Charity No. 1057744 (England and Wales) SC038299 (Scotland).)

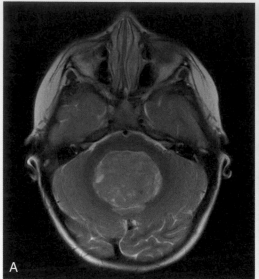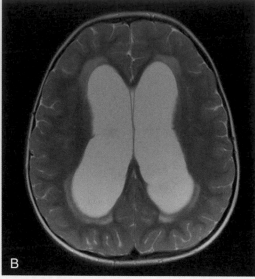

Figure 18.2 Medulloblastoma with hydrocephalus. A 3-year-old boy with vomiting and headache. AxiaT2 Images: (A) through posterior fossa shows a large midline cerebellar tumour;. (B) shows dilated lateral ventricles with periventricular oedema indicating that the hydrocephalus is acute and under pressure. (Courtesy Prof. Stephanie Ryan.)

Children who present with raised intracranial pressure require urgent imaging (Fig. 18.2).

BRAIN TUMOURS

Although 70 per cent of children and adolescents now survive a brain tumour, it is still the leading cause of death due to cancer in childhood. The diagnosis of a brain tumour poses unique challenges. Low-grade gliomas tend to be associated with prolonged symptoms and consequent delayed diagnosis, whereas high-grade gliomas tend to have a rapid onset of symptoms. Tumours located in the cerebellum and brain stem, such as medulloblastoma, tend to have a shorter duration of symptoms as opposed to supratentorial tumours which may present with seizures, papilloedema and other features of raised intracranial pressure. Symptoms at presentation relate primarily to the location of the tumour. Craniopharyngioma, low-grade glioma, optic nerve glioma and germ cell tumours often have a delayed presentation. Posterior fossa tumours, such as cerebellar astrocytoma, medulloblastoma and ependymoma, may present with hydrocephalus due to outlet obstruction of the fourth ventricle.

Idiopathic Intracranial Hypertension (IIH)

Headaches seen in IIH may be intermittent or constant. The characteristic features are headaches, papilloedema, normal neuroimaging and raised intracranial pressure. Idiopathic intracranial hypertension is more frequent in teenage females and is often associated with obesity. Other conditions associated with intracranial hypertension include excess vitamin A consumption, withdrawal of corticosteroids, hypoadrenalism or Cushing's syndrome, hypoparathyroidism, rapid catch-up growth, regain of weight following malnutrition or use of oral contraceptives.

In addition to headache with papilloedema, a sixth or seventh cranial nerve palsy or visual field defect may be evident. The cerebrospinal fluid (CSF) profile is normal apart from an elevated opening pressure. Treatment is with acetazolamide to reduce the risk of permanent visual loss. Rarely, other measures to reduce intracranial pressure, such as shunting, are indicated.

(Box 18.1)
(Box 18.2)

Box 18.1   Key Points

The great majority of headaches in childhood are primary headaches and may be diagnosed by history and a detailed physical examination.

A detailed history of the headache pattern and maintenance of a headache diary are key elements of the assessment.

Neuroimaging is rarely required.

In comparison to adult migraines, childhood migraine episodes tend to be less frequent, of shorter duration, and more responsive to treatment.

The most common migraine triggers in children are chocolate, cheeses, and onions. Other triggers include menses, sleep deprivation, stress, hot weather and excessive exertion.

Ibuprofen and paracetamol are recommended during a migraine episode in children and adolescents. Triptans can be used for pain relief if over 12 years of age. In most trials

to date, the evidence for preventive medications has not demonstrated a marked additional benefit over placebo.

Preschool children with a brain tumour may present with persistent or recurrent vomiting, abnormal eye movements, significant behavioural change with lethargy in particular, problems with balance and walking, seizures, head tilt, or a progressively increasing head circumference.

In school-going children and adolescents, a crescendo pattern of headaches is a key symptom that should prompt request for neuroimaging.

The characteristic features of idiopathic intracranial hypertension include headaches, papilloedema, normal neuroimaging and raised intracranial pressure. Idiopathic intracranial hypertension is most frequent in teenage females and is associated with obesity.

Box 18.2   A 10-Year-Old With a Changing Pattern of Headaches

A 10-year-old girl presents with a 12-month history of headaches occurring once every 4 weeks. She experiences a right-sided frontal dull ache behind the eye that starts after breakfast and progressively worsens over the next few hours to a severity of 9 out of 10. Paracetamol causes some temporary improvement. The headaches are associated with nausea and then uncontrollable vomiting. There is severe photophobia, and she must lie down in a darkened room with a vomit bowl. She then sleeps for several hours and when she wakes up the headache has gone. Her mother has a diagnosis of migraine. Clinical examination is normal.

Her parents have become more concerned as over the past 6 weeks as the headaches have progressively worsened. She now has a dull occipital pain which is worse immediately after wakening but improves later in the day. She feels nausea in the mornings and has vomited the last four mornings. He has taken paracetamol with little effect. Coughing makes the pain worse. Her parents report that she is more irritable, and her teacher has noted her school performance has worsened significantly. She also appears to be somewhat unsteady on her feet.

Clinical Pearls

For the past year, the description of headaches above is characteristic of migraine, and the frequency of once per month obviates the need for migraine prophylaxis.

Migraine affects approximately **7 per cent** of children, and yet there is a remarkable lack of high-quality evidence supporting the effectiveness of preventive therapy in both children and adolescents.

Children with migraine exhibit a shorter duration of headache attacks, an equal frequency in both males and females prior to puberty and may be preceded by periodic syndromes such as cyclical vomiting or abdominal migraine.

The most common migraine triggers in children are chocolate, cheeses, onions, yeast and beans. Other triggers include menses, sleep deprivation, stress, hot weather and excessive exertion. Ibuprofen and paracetamol are used during an attack in children and adolescents. Triptans can be used for pain relief if over 12 years of age.

The key element of this history is that for the past 6 weeks, the pattern of headaches has changed considerably and is no longer typical of migraine. Looking for this crescendo pattern of headaches with an ever-increasing frequency and severity of headaches, should prompt consideration of raised intracranial pressure and the urgent requirement for neuroimaging.

Children between 5 and 12 years old may also present with recurrent vomiting, abnormal eye movements, blurred vision or diplopia, behavioural change or seizures.

Interpretation of Investigations

In this instance, an urgent magnetic resonance imaging (MRI) scan was requested and showed a large posterior fossa tumour with secondary hydrocephalus.

Pitfalls to Avoid

Tension headaches and migraine are by far the commonest reasons for frequent headaches in childhood and adolescence. By contrast brain tumours are rare but, as in this instance, both can co-exist. Migraine was the correct initial diagnosis in this case, but the pattern of headaches did change quite dramatically, and this should always prompt a re-think for an alternative diagnosis.

The headache description, frequency and pattern are key, and one should ask the family to keep a headache diary and review this diary and re-examine the child after 6 to 8 weeks.

The characteristic features of idiopathic intracranial hypertension include headaches, papilloedema, normal neuroimaging and raised intracranial pressure.

 Video on the topic The child with headaches is available online at Elsevier eBooks+.

Key References

Abu-Arafeh, I., Razak, S., Sivaraman, B., & Graham, C. (2010). Prevalence of headache and migraine in children and adolescents: A systematic review of population-based studies. *Developmental Medicine and Child Neurology, 52*(12), 1088–1097.

Dao, J. M., & Qubty, W. (2018). Headache diagnosis in children and adolescents. *Current Pain and Headache Reports, 22*(3), 17.

Friedman, D. I. (2020). Guideline update: Pharmacologic prevention of pediatric migraine. *The Journal of Pediatrics, 216,* 242–245.

HeadSmart. (n.d.). HeadSmart – Early Diagnosis of Brain Tumours. https://www.headsmart.org.uk/

HeadSmart. (n.d.). Healthcare Resources. https://www.headsmart.org.uk/clinical/healthcare-resources/

Oskoui, M., Pringsheim, T., Billinghurst, L., Potrebic, S., Gersz, E. M., Gloss, D., et al. (2019). Practice guideline update summary: Pharmacologic treatment for pediatric migraine prevention: Report of the Guideline Development, Dissemination, and Implementation Subcommittee of the American Academy of Neurology and the American Headache Society. *Neurology, 93*(11), 500–509. https://doi.org/10.1212/wnl.0000000000008105.

Oskoui, M., Pringsheim, T., Holler-Managan, Y., Potrebic, S., Billinghurst, L., Gloss, D., et al. (2019). Practice guideline update summary: Acute treatment of migraine in children and adolescents: Report of the Guideline Development, Dissemination, and Implementation Subcommittee of the American Academy of Neurology and the American Headache Society. *Neurology, 93*(11), 487–499. https://doi.org/10.1212/wnl.0000000000008095.

Papetti, L., Ursitti, F., Moavero, R., Ferilli, M. A. N., Sforza, G., Tarantino, S., et al. (2019). Prophylactic treatment of pediatric migraine: Is there anything new in the last decade? *Frontiers in Neurology, 10,* 771.

Raucci, U., Della Vecchia, N., Ossella, C., Paolino, M. C., Villa, M. P., Reale, A., & Parisi, P. (2019). Management of childhood headache in the emergency department. Review of the literature. *Frontiers in Neurology, 10,* 886.

Shanmugavadivel, D., Liu, J.-F., Murphy, L., Wilne, S., Walker, D., & HeadSmart (2020). Accelerating diagnosis for childhood brain tumours: An analysis of the HeadSmart UK population data. *Archives of Disease in Childhood, 105*(4), 355–362.

The Lancet. (2019). Better evidence needed for preventing paediatric migraine. *Lancet (London, England), 394*(10199), 612.

19 Inborn Errors of Metabolism

ELLEN CRUSHELL

Inborn errors of metabolism (IEM) are inherited, usually resulting from a single gene defect affecting an enzyme in a metabolic pathway. This leads to an accumulation of toxic metabolites (the substrate), a deficiency of essential metabolites (the product) or both. Hundreds of different inborn errors of metabolism have been described and, while individually rare, they collectively account for a significant burden of disease in children.

Newborn bloodspot screening is performed via the neonatal heel prick test (previously known as the Guthrie test after the clinician who first described a bloodspot technique in screening for phenylketonuria) within the first days of life, after feeding has been established. The disorders included in a country's screening programme vary throughout the developed world. Screening for phenylketonuria, classical homocystinuria, maple syrup urine disease, classical galactosemia, medium chain acyl-CoA dehydrogenase deficiency (MCADD), glutaric aciduria type 1, congenital hypothyroidism and cystic fibrosis is routine in Ireland. Established newborn screening programmes are successful in detecting these conditions in most children, but it is essential to remember that these are screening tools rather than diagnostic tests. Positive newborn screens need timely second tier confirmatory testing. Also, if a child subsequently presents with symptoms (for example, those of phenylketonuria (PKU) or homocystinuria), they must undergo targeted tests to rule out these disorders (e.g. by analysis of plasma phenylalanine and homocysteine level) irrespective of their newborn screen result.

A family history of metabolic disease, or consanguinity is notable as most inborn errors of metabolism (IEM) are autosomal recessively inherited. A family history of unexpected infant death is also relevant.

Collectively, all inborn errors of metabolism have an incidence of approximately one in 1000, but this incidence is much higher amongst populations with a culture of consanguinity.

Neonatal Presentations

Metabolic disorders may present at any age; however, there are periods of life when the presentation of IEM is more likely. These include the neonatal period, at weaning due to an increase in protein intake, in the second 6 months of life when infants often acquire their first febrile illness that causes metabolic stress, and at puberty.

Symptoms of IEMs in the neonate are non-specific and mimic other disorders such as sepsis and congenital heart defects. It is particularly important to consider basic metabolic investigations in the work-up of any sick neonate to ensure timely diagnosis and treatment.

INTOXICATION

During the neonatal period, the classical presentation of IEM is one of intoxication following an initial symptom-free period. As a toxic metabolite accumulates when feeds are established, the newborn becomes increasingly drowsy with reduced feeding before full decompensation. Organic acidaemias and urea cycle defects classically present in this way.

ENCEPHALOPATHY DUE TO HIGH AMMONIA LEVELS

Ammonia levels over 120 µmol/L in sick preterm infants, over 100 µmol/L in term newborns, and over 50 µmol/L in older infants and children warrant further assessment and investigation. Ammonia should be measured from a free-flowing venous sample and should arrive at the laboratory within 15 minutes, ideally on ice. Survival and neurological outcome are both related to the duration and degree of hyperammonaemia; therefore, timely diagnosis and treatment are essential to improve the clinical outcome.

Urea cycle disorders cause hyperammonaemia. Ammonia converts into urea in the liver via the urea cycle. A deficiency in any of the enzymes of the urea cycle leads to an elevated ammonia level. Ammonia stimulates respiration centrally, initially leading to respiratory alkalosis – this is an important clue, and the finding of respiratory alkalosis should prompt the immediate measurement of serum ammonia. A high ammonia level with a respiratory alkalosis is characteristic of a urea cycle disorder. A high ammonia level in association with a metabolic acidosis and an increased anion gap is strongly suggestive of an organic acidaemia in which secondary inhibition of the urea cycle may occur.

Although hyperammonaemia is a relatively rare cause of neonatal encephalopathy, it should not be missed given that it is treatable.

In infants and older children with urea cycle disorders, a common clue in the history is a self-restricted diet with the avoidance of high protein foods such as meat, cheese and fish. Testing for ammonia should be considered in all infants and children with unexplained or unusual neurological symptoms, especially in newborns whose clinical history does not match the severity of their illness.

NEONATAL SEIZURES

IEM should always be considered in unexplained refractory neonatal seizures and differential diagnoses include conditions such as pyridoxine-dependent seizures, biotinidase deficiency and non-ketotic hyperglycinaemia. Hiccoughs with subsequent development of apnoeas are seen in non-ketotic hyperglycinaemia. The key diagnostic marker for pyridoxine-dependent seizures is urine for alpha-amino adipic semialdehyde (AASA) and a trial of pyridoxine (or pyridoxal phosphate) is empirically given, and may be effective in terminating the seizures.

Intractable seizures in early infancy may be caused by a deficiency in glucose transporter 1 (GLUT 1) with a characteristically low cerebrospinal fluid (CSF) glucose in association with normal serum glucose concentrations. In GLUT 1 deficiency, the CSF to blood glucose ratio is less than 0.5 (normal being over 0.6), and the blood glucose must be measured simultaneously (preferably just before rather than after the lumbar puncture (LP) procedure) with the CSF for accuracy. Seizures may begin in the neonatal period and respond poorly to antiepileptic drugs with microcephaly and developmental delay if untreated. Treatment for GLUT 1 deficiency is with a ketogenic diet.

Although these disorders are rare, many are treatable, so it is important to consider IEM in the work-up of a neonate with seizures to ensure timely treatment.

Key Investigations of IEM in the neonatal period

Acute intoxication – consider organic acidaemias (for example, methylmalonic acidaemia, propionic aciademia, isovaleric acidaemia), maple syrup urine disease, urea cycle disorders and fatty acid oxidation defects.

Key investigations: (**Basic metabolic panel** – glucose, liver function tests (LFT), blood gas, creatine kinase (CK), lactate, ketones, plasma ammonia, urine organic acids, plasma amino acids, bloodspot acylcarnitine profile.

Encephalopathy + seizures – consider non-ketotic hyperglycinaemia, pyridoxine-dependent seizures, molybdenum cofactor deficiency, urea cycle disorders, congenital lactic acidosis caused by mitochondrial disease and fatty acid oxidation defects.

Key investigations: Basic metabolic panel as above and paired with blood and CSF amino acids and glucose, CSF lactate, plasma urate (low in molybdenum cofactor deficiency), and urine AASA. Sequential trial of response to vitamins (pyridoxine, pyridoxal phosphate, folinic acid).

Neonatal liver disease – consider galactosemia, tyrosinemia, neonatal haemachromatosis, mitochondrial disorders and lysosomal storage disorders. Liver disease may also appear in urea cycle disorders and fatty acid oxidation disorders. Galactosemia is due to an absence of galactose-1-phosphate uridyl transferase and generally presents in the neonatal period or during infancy with vomiting, jaundice and failure to thrive. Affected infants are at risk of *Escherichia coli* sepsis, severe coagulopathy and hepatic failure. In many countries, screening for galactosemia occurs during the neonatal period as early diagnosis and exclusion of galactose from the infant's diet will lead to clinical improvement.

Key investigations: Basic metabolic panel as above + Beutler assay for GALT activity + ferritin

Neurological deterioration – consider peroxisomal disorders (may be associated dysmorphism), sterol disorders such as Smith–Lemli–Opitz syndrome (SLO, there may be dysmorphism and ambiguous genitalia) and mitochondrial disease.

Key investigations: Discuss with metabolic team.

EXAMINATION

Most IEMs do not have specific features requiring identification on examination. Coarse facial features develop progressively in the mucopolysaccharidoses, such as Hurler syndrome (Fig. 19.1). These features may be clear to the experienced eye during the neonatal period in some severe storage disorders, such as I-cell disease (gum hypertrophy is a clue to this disorder). Neonatal dysmorphism may be associated with congenital disorders of glycosylation, peroxisomal disorders, and sterol disorders, such as Smith–Lemli–Opitz (SLO) syndrome. Therefore, transferrin isoforms, very long chain fatty acid (VLCFA) analysis, and 7-dehydrocholesterol testing should be performed if these disorders are thought possible.

Many disorders display eye signs, emphasising the importance of ophthalmology assessment. Oil drop cataracts may be present in galactosemia. In time, sphingolipidoses such as Tay–Sachs and Niemann–Pick disease develop a cherry red spot on the retina (Fig. 19.2). Corneal clouding develops gradually in some mucopolysaccharidoses, such as Hurler syndrome.

Presentations Beyond the Neonatal Period

PROMINENT HEPATOMEGALY OR LIVER FAILURE

A child presenting with marked hepatomegaly in the absence of splenomegaly should prompt consideration of

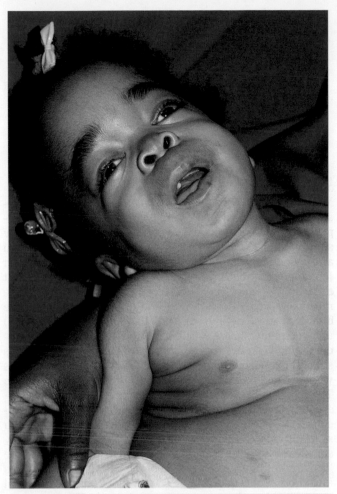

Figure 19.1 Hurler syndrome. Coarse facial features, macrocephaly, scaphocephalic skull, short neck, chest deformity and protuberant abdomen in a girl with Hurler syndrome (MPS1). (Reproduced with permission from Paller, A., & Mancini, A. J. (2021). *Paller and Mancini – Hurwitz clinical pediatric dermatology: A textbook of skin disorders of childhood & adolescence* (6th ed.). Elsevier – Health Sciences Division.)

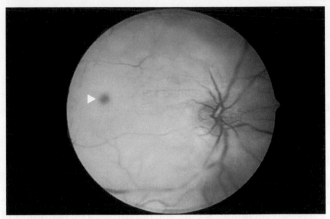

Figure 19.2 Tay–Sachs disease, fundoscopy. Note paleness of the retina, with extensive opacification more characteristic for Tay–Sachs disease, but retinal artery occlusion produces a similar appearance. Tay–Sachs disease results from a deficiency in hexosaminidase A enzyme with accumulation of GM2 trihexosylceramide in retinal ganglion cells, producing the pale appearance that obscures the vascularity. The greatest density of ganglion cells in the macular area leads to greater opacification, except in the foveal pit, which is devoid of ganglion cells, so that a solitary "cherry red" spot (►) can be seen here at the left of the image. The lipids accumulating in retinal ganglion cells lead to ganglion cell hypertrophy followed by cell death and eventual gliosis and blindness. (Reproduced with permission from Klatt, E. (2020). *Robbins and Cotran atlas of pathology* (4th ed.). Elsevier – Health Sciences Division.)

the diagnosis of glycogen storage disease (GSD), which may be associated with pre-feed hypoglycaemia. GSDs are diagnosed through enzyme and genetic testing, making liver biopsy rarely needed.

Coarse facial features developing over time in association with hepatosplenomegaly suggests a storage disorder such as a mucopolysaccharidosis. Urine for glycosaminoglycans (which are mucopolysaccharides and accumulate in these conditions) should be requested along with white cell lysosomal enzyme analysis. Some lysosomal storage disorders that cause hepatosplenomegaly do not have any associated coarsening of features or dysmorphism (e.g. Gaucher disease or Niemann–Pick disease).

Treatable causes of liver failure include galactosemia, tyrosinaemia, hereditary fructose intolerance and urea cycle disorders (in which hyperammonaemia will be a prominent feature). There are many other rarer and recently described IEMs that may present with liver failure, particularly in the setting of fever. Metabolic consultation can be helpful to guide investigations.

Hereditary fructose intolerance is due to a deficiency of hepatic aldolase B. Affected children cannot metabolise fructose (the sugar in fruit) or sucrose (table sugar). This rare condition causes children to avoid sweet food and characteristically have caries-free teeth into adulthood. Babies are asymptomatic until weaning, when the introduction of these sugars in the diet causes liver dysfunction, hypoglycaemia and vomiting. A weaning history is key to arriving at the diagnosis, which may then be confirmed by genetic testing.

ACIDOSIS

The presence of metabolic acidosis with a normal anion gap should be considered as an indicator for bicarbonate loss (either gut or renal) rather than the presence of excess acid. Ketosis and acidosis with a high anion gap in childhood may indicate an organic acidaemia. The ketoacidosis may be similar to that seen in diabetic ketoacidosis (DKA), where there is also a high anion gap (as ketones are acids that accumulate in DKA and organic acidaemias); however, DKA can be immediately detected by the presence of an abnormally high blood glucose level. In fact, hypoglycaemia is more common in IEMs. The key test to diagnose these disorders of protein metabolism is organic acid analysis of the urine at a specialist metabolic laboratory.

Raised Lactate

A raised serum lactate is common and is most often due to hypoperfusion relating to sepsis or hypoxia, but a persistently elevated lactate may indicate a mitochondrial disorder.

Be aware that lactate may be artefactually high due to sampling difficulties (e.g. a struggling child or due to tourniquet effect) and repeated samples may be required to clarify.

Lactate is a weak acid and at levels under 5 mmol/L (i.e. twice the upper normal limit), it is unlikely to significantly contribute to acidosis.

Calculating the anion gap

Anion gap = $[(Na+Na^+) + (K+K^+)] - [(Cl-CL^-) + (HCO_3^-)]$
Normally it is 10 to 18 mmol/L

Acidosis with a normal anion gap suggests bicarbonate loss while acidosis with a high anion gap points to the presence of excess acid in the system and should prompt metabolic investigations.

HYPOGLYCAEMIA

Hypoglycaemia is common in infants and young children, and it is essential to take a critical blood sample at the time of hypoglycaemia to secure the diagnosis. The definition of hypoglycaemia is generally accepted as a blood glucose of or less than 2.6 mmol/L.

The next essential investigation is assessing the hypoglycaemia is documenting the presence or absence of ketones in the urine or on bloodspot point-of-care (POC) testing. If ketones are absent or inappropriately low at the time of hypoglycaemia, the differential diagnosis narrows down to hyperinsulinism (where lipolysis is suppressed), fatty acid oxidation disorders (FAOD) (where lipolysis and ketone production is defective), or liver failure (where the liver is unable to make ketones). Hyperinsulinism usually presents in the neonatal period with a persistent increased requirement for glucose usually in excess of 10 mg/kg/min and can be much higher. Attempts at reducing the level of glucose support results in a prompt recurrence of hypoglycaemia.

Blocks in fat oxidation as seen in fatty acid oxidation disorders (FAOD) lead to hypoketotic hypoglycaemia due to the failure of ketone production despite mobilisation of fat in response to fasting. Rare situations in which ketones cannot be produced (e.g. disorders of ketone synthesis) will require specialist metabolic investigations.

A hypoglycaemia screen should be performed at the time and includes the following:

- glucose
- point of care blood ketones and/or urinary ketones
- insulin and c-peptide
- growth hormone and cortisol
- free fatty acids (FFA), 3 hydroxy butyrate (a ketone)
- acylcarnitine profile
- urine for organic acids

Note: If possible, perform at presentation while hypoglycaemic. Interpretation – particularly of the hormone assays – is difficult if normoglycaemic at the time of sampling. If the opportunity has been missed and the child has already been treated, the metabolic tests are still worth performing, as an IEM such as an FAOD should be diagnosable even when well.

DEVELOPMENTAL REGRESSION

Developmental regression at any age is a significant red flag in paediatrics warranting urgent and often extensive investigation. An early brain MRI is especially useful and may be diagnostic in some leukodystrophies or guide further investigations in others (e.g. as in Leigh disease) (Table 19.1).

Table 19.1   Key Metabolic Investigation in a Child With Developmental Regression

Basic metabolic panel (glucose, LFTs, blood gas, CK, lactate, ketones, plasma ammonia, urine organic acids, plasma amino acids, bloodspot acylcarnitine profile)
+ urine for GAGs, white cell lysosomal enzyme analysis, very long chain fatty acid (VLCFA) analysis, brain MRI, and early discussion with metabolic team if Niemann–Pick C or mitochondrial disease is suspected.

Lysosomal Storage Disorders

Most IEMs do not have dysmorphic features, but the lysosomal storage disorders are a notable exception. The coarsening of features occurs slowly over time. Eye examination may show corneal clouding (classically seen in Hurler syndrome) and abdominal examination may show hepatosplenomegaly. Joints may be stiff and hair coarse in texture. Beware that there may be no or very subtle coarse features in some of the mucopolysaccharidoses (MPS) and other lysosomal storage disorders, most notably in MPS III (San filippo syndrome) and the sphingolipidoses (such as Tay–Sachs disease or metachromatic leukodystrophy); therefore, further investigations should be performed early and routinely when a child presents with regression and behavioural and/or sleep disturbance. The diagnosis of these conditions is often delayed.

A key investigation for MPS is urine for glycosaminoglycans (GAGs), along with lysosomal enzymes (analysed at a specialist supra regional laboratory). Skeletal survey may show dysostosis multiplex, features of which may include 'beaking' of one or more vertebral bodies, dysplastic hips and short phalanges (Fig. 19.3). A blood film may reveal vacuolated lymphocytes to an experienced eye.

Other lysosomal storage disorders include the sphingolipidoses such as Tay–Sachs and Niemann–Pick C disease are associated with a cherry red spot on the retina and significant regression in early or mid-childhood. Splenomegaly and a history of neonatal liver disease or prolonged jaundice may be present in Niemann–Pick C disease.

While there are no cures for these conditions, some may be ameliorated., Significant advances in treatment are being made with enzyme replacement therapies, substrate reduction therapies, haematopoietic stem cell transplant and gene therapy. Timely diagnosis, onward referral and genetic counselling are all essential. Diagnosis of many of these disorders, particularly of Niemann–Pick C, is specialised and should be discussed with the metabolic service.

Peroxisomal Disorders

Peroxisomal disorders such as Zellweger spectrum disorders are associated with dysmorphic features early in life including a large anterior fontanelle, bulbous forehead, ptosis and profound hypotonia (which is a differential for Down syndrome but is quite distinctive). Very long chain fatty acids are metabolised in the peroxisome; therefore, diagnosis of Zellweger and other peroxisomal disorders are usually made through the analysis of very long chain fatty acids (VLCFAs) at a specialist laboratory. VLCFAs should be performed on any child with regression.

Another peroxisomal disorder called X-linked adrenal leukodystrophy (X-ALD) presents very differently. The

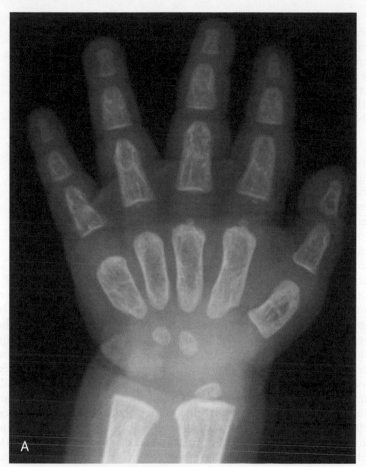

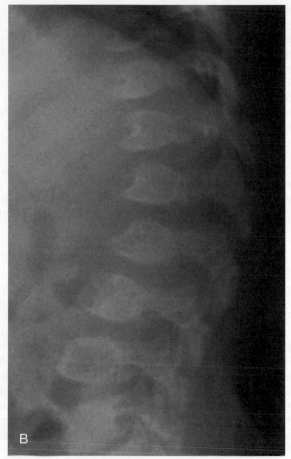

Figure 19.3 Mucopolysaccharidosis type I (Hurler syndrome). (A) X-ray of the hand shows widening of the marrow cavity and thinning of the cortex with all the bones and characteristic pointing of proximal ends of the second to fourth metacarpals. (B) Lateral view of the spine in the same child shows some angulation at the thoracolumbar junction – a gibbus and anteroinferior vertebral body breaking of some of the vertebrae. (Courtesy Prof. Stephanie Ryan.)

symptoms usually begin in previously well boys between the ages of 8 and 12 years with new onset behavioural problems, cognitive difficulties and regression of skills and visual inattention. X-ALD has classic MRI findings of white matter disease (leukodystrophy). If detected early or presymptomatically, the neurological deterioration may be halted with haematopoietic stem cell transplant (HSCT) or gene therapy. Adrenal insufficiency is often also present and a tanned appearance of the skin is common at diagnosis. Some affected boys do not get neurological symptoms, meaning that it is essential to screen family members and monitor known cases with serial brain MRIs to determine if and when HSCT should optimally be performed.

Mitochondrial Disease

It is often said that mitochondrial disease may present at any age and in any organ. Leigh disease is the term given to the appearance of the abnormal symmetrical appearance of T2 hyperintensity of the basal ganglia and brain stem on MRI. It can be caused by many different mitochondrial disorders. Leigh disease may present at any age with neurological regression, which is typically stepwise and classically occurs in infants or toddlers. It may be associated with nystagmus, external ophthalmoplegia and abnormal movements. Elevated brain or CSF lactate may be seen on MR Spectroscopy or can be determined

through biochemical CSF analysis. Until recently, tissue sampling (e.g. muscle or liver biopsy) was necessary to make the diagnosis of mitochondrial disease. With the advent of next generation genetic sequencing techniques, tissue sampling is often no longer necessary. Achieving an underlying genetic diagnosis requires specialist input and may be challenging.

SEVERE HYPOTONIA IN AN INFANT

Hypotonia often accompanies other symptoms of IEMs, but isolated early hypotonia is rarely caused by an IEM, and is more commonly caused by neuromuscular disorders or Prader–Willi syndrome. A notable exception is Pompe disease, in which babies have a frog leg posture and cardiomyopathy. Enzyme replacement therapy is available for this condition.

DEVELOPMENTAL DELAY AND LEARNING DISABILITY

Isolated developmental delay and learning disability is rarely caused by IEMs. When caused by an IEM, it is seen more often seen alongside other features such as abnormal head size, epilepsy and other neurological problems (Table 19.2). A history of regression is a red flag that warrants urgent investigation. Phenylketonuria is the most common IEM in which, without dietary interventions, the natural history is one of developmental delay, acquired microcephaly and severe learning disability. Neonatal detection via newborn screening and early specialist dietary treatment (phenylalanine restriction) allows a normal outcome for these children. Recently, PKU has been detected in several migrant children with developmental delay who were born in countries without newborn screening or where treatment was not available due to conflict.

Isolated speech delay has been reported in disorders of creatine synthesis, which may be detected on MR spectroscopy as the brain creatine peak is reduced. These disorders are exceedingly rare and usually associated with global delay and seizures. Diagnosis is via analysis of urine creatine and related metabolites at a specialised lab. Treatment is available for some forms.

A workup of isolated developmental delay without regression includes a detailed history (look for a family history of consanguinity) and examination, which may give clues. For example, the presence of scoliosis or severe myopia may suggest homocystinuria. As many IEMs are amenable to treatment, metabolic investigations should be considered in cases of unexplained developmental delay despite low diagnostic yield in countries where newborn bloodspot screening is available. When developmental delay is isolated with no associated abnormalities found on examination, the following minimum investigations should be considered: thyroid function tests (including T3 in boys), LFTs, CK, urate, ammonia, blood gas, lactate, amino acids (including phenylalanine and homocysteine), urine GAGs and urine organic acids. Genetic studies including CGH microarray should be done in parallel.

Consider urine creatine studies (discuss with lab) for severe associated speech delay, especially if seizures are present. Consider lysosomal storage disorders and arrange testing for white cell lysosomal enzymes.

Table 19.2 Developmental Delay – Key Symptoms or Signs of IEM

Macrocephaly – glutaric aciduria type 1, lysosomal storage disorders, Canavan disease
Seizures – creatine disorders, methylene tetrahydrofolate reductase deficiency (MHTFR) deficiency, purine/pyrimidine disorders, biotinidase deficiency, vitamin disorders, GLUT 1 deficiency
Dystonia – movement disorders, oculogyric crises, hypersalivation- neurotransmitter disorders
Odd or kinky hair – Menke's syndrome, argininosuccinase (ASA) deficiency
Tight ankles and toe walking – mucopolysaccharidoses and other lysosomal storage disorders
Multisystem involvement – mitochondrial disorders, congenital disorders of glycosylation, peroxisomal disorders
Dysmorphic features – congenital disorders of glycosylation, Smith–Lemli–Opitz, homocystinuria

UNEXPECTED INFANT OR CHILD DEATH

Sadly, children still die of undiagnosed metabolic disease. In the event of an unexplained and unexpected child death, metabolic disease should be considered; especially if the death was preceded by a febrile illness, vomiting or fasting. When possible, pre- or post-mortem samples of blood (serum, plasma and bloodspot card), urine and CSF should be saved for biochemical analysis. Tissue sample for biochemical analysis such as mitochondrial studies are time sensitive but can sometimes be useful. Further investigation can be discussed with a metabolic specialist. It is essential to ensure that DNA (3 mLs of blood in EDTA) is saved for possible genetic investigation as with improvements in genetic techniques, this is the most promising route to a post-mortem diagnosis of an IEM or another genetic condition now and into the future.

(Box 19.1)
(Box 19.2)
(Box 19.3)

Box 19.1 **Key Points**

Consider an inborn error of metabolism (IEM) in all neonates with unexplained or progressive disease, especially after a normal pregnancy and delivery, and in all children with acute physiological deterioration and/or reduced level of consciousness, especially when preceded by an intercurrent illness or fasting, and in all children with metabolic acidosis or hypoglycaemia.

A family history of metabolic disease is critical, as is a history of consanguinity or a family history of unexpected infant death. In the neonatal period, the classical presentation of IEM is one of intoxication following an initial symptom-free period.

Essential first line investigations for an acute presentation of an IEM include a blood glucose, LFTS, CK, U&E, venous blood gas, ketones, ammonia, lactate. Second line investigations include plasma amino acids, bloodspot acylcarnitine profile (filter paper), and urine for organic acids.

Although hyperammonaemia is an uncommon cause of neonatal encephalopathy, it should not be overlooked given that it is treatable. Respiratory alkalosis is an important

clue. Intractable seizures in infancy (and childhood) may be caused by a deficiency in glucose transporter 1 (GLUT 1) with a characteristic low CSF glucose in association with normal serum glucose concentrations.

If ketones are absent or inappropriately low at the time of hypoglycaemia, the differential diagnosis essentially narrows down to hyperinsulinism, fatty acid oxidation disorders (FAOD) or liver failure (when the liver is unable to make ketones).

Immediate management if an IEM is suspected is to start intravenous dextrose 10 per cent with 0.9 per cent saline and appropriate electrolytes pending investigations and discussion with metabolic service. The treatment will be tailored according to results following metabolic consultation.

Metabolic disease should be considered in the event of an unexplained and unexpected child death, especially if the death was preceded by a febrile illness, vomiting or fasting.

Always discuss with the metabolic clinicians and laboratory if an IEM is suspected.

Box 19.2   5-Day-Old With Marked Acidosis

A 5-day-old infant, exclusively breast-fed, is rushed to hospital with pallor, mottling and drowsiness. He is tachypnoeic (52 breaths per minute), floppy and has cold peripheries. His parents are second cousins, and his birth history was normal. Blood results show pH 7.07, bicarbonate 7, base excess -15.0 mmol/L, PO2 – 3.85 kPa and PCO2 – 4.35 and blood glucose was 2.2 mmol, with normal urea and electrolytes.

Results in this case showed urine +4 for ketones, an elevated anion gap of 33 and normal ammonia and lactate. This elevated anion gap indicates the presence of excess acid. Urine for organic acids showed a large peak of methylmalonic acid (MMA) and the acylcarnitine profile showed an elevated C3 (proprionylcarnitine) in keeping with the final diagnosis of methylmalonic acidaemia (MMA), which is a recessively inherited organic acidaemia.

Clinical Pearls

The main clinical differentials in a sick and mottled 5-day-old are sepsis, cardiac defect (in particular left ventricular (LV) outflow obstruction) and inborn errors of metabolism (IEM). Basic biochemical screen done early in tandem with septic workup may alert to an IEM and prompt further tests and appropriate treatment. In this case, the finding of an elevated anion gap and the presence of ketosis were both important in signposting towards an IEM. This degree of ketone production is very unusual in a neonate but common in organic acidurias or maple syrup urine disease.

Look out for red flags that might point towards an IEM – consanguinity, well period before deterioration, raised anion gap metabolic acidosis, ketosis, hypoglycaemia and unusual odours (which classically include the odour of burnt sugar in maple syrup urine disease or the odour of sweaty feet reported in isovaleric acidaemia).

Long-term treatment of MMA involves a specialised low protein diet and vitamin B12, with illness plans in place to prevent further decompensations, which are usually prompted by intercurrent illness.

Key Investigations

Ask for serum ammonia, urine or bloodspot ketones (the presence of ketones in newborns is unusual and prompts investigation for IEMs), and serum lactate, glucose, a venous or capillary blood gas, creatine kinase (CK) and liver function tests as first line investigations.

Second line investigations (following discussion with the metabolic team) include plasma amino acids, bloodspot acylcarnitine profile and urine for organic acids. These tests will take more time but appropriate treatment can be initiated in the interim when an IEM is suspected.

Pitfalls to Avoid

Suspect an inborn error of metabolism if a metabolic acidosis with a raised anion gap is present in a sick newborn infant. Seek advice from the metabolic team.

Initial Management is to stop feeds temporarily and give intravenous 10 per cent dextrose to correct hypoglycaemia and stop catabolism. Lipid should be avoided until diagnosis is known, as it is contraindicated in the management of fatty acid oxidation disorders. Insulin may also be used if hyperglycaemia develops and is useful for its anabolic effect.

Remove toxins via stimulation of the alternative pathway or scavenger drugs (e.g. sodium benzoate, if high ammonia) or dialysis may be necessary.

Box 19.3   Hypoglycaemia in a 10-Month-Old

A 10-month-old female infant presents to hospital with 2-day history of being off feeds with vomiting and diarrhoea. On admission she looks quite unwell with striking lethargy. A 3 cm liver edge was noted on examination. Blood sugar was 0.8 mmol/L on arrival. Her urine is negative for ketones. Critical samples were taken immediately.

Results showed that the CK, AST, and ALT levels were all significantly elevated, and the FFA was elevated with low 3 hydroxybutyrate (a ketone). The serum insulin was appropriately undetectable. Urine for organic acids showed suberyl- and hexanoyl-glycine, and the acylcarnitine profile showed elevated medium chain acylcarnitines at C8 and C10.

Clinical Pearls

FAOD such as MCADD is the most likely diagnosis in this setting of hypoketotic hypoglycaemia and can be diagnosed by typical findings on acylcarnitine profile and on organic acids. Elevated CK and LFTs are usually found acutely (this acute constellation of features of liver dysfunction and encephalopathy was previously called 'Reye syndrome').

Hyperinsulinism (over 10 mg/kg/min dextrose needed to maintain normoglycaemia) is unusual in this age group but also causes non-ketotic hypoglycaemia. In this case, the insulin was appropriately suppressed, thus ruling out hyperinsulinism.

Idiopathic ketotic hypoglycaemia ('starvation hypoglycaemia') is relatively common in infants and toddlers in the setting of gastroenteritis; however, glucose is very rarely as low as 0.8 mmol/L

and is excluded here by the lack of significant ketosis (beware that trace or small amounts of ketones can be misleading and is not reassuring).

Other possibilities for consideration include glycogen storage disorders (may be ketotic and massive hepatomegaly often present) and hepatic failure.

Thus, given the characteristic findings on organic acids and acylcarnitine profile, a diagnosis of Medium Chain Co-acyl A Dehydrogenase Deficiency (MCADD) was made. MCADD is now part of many neonatal bloodspot screening programmes via the detection of abnormal levels of C8 and C10. Genetic confirmation is made via mutation analysis of the ACADM gene. Treatment principles include a normal diet with strict avoidance of fasting, especially if sick.

Pitfalls to Avoid

Think MCADD or hyperinsulinism if both hypoglycaemia and urine negative for ketones are present (beware a 'trace' or small number of ketones are not reassuring when hypoglycaemia is present).

MCADD is an autosomal recessive disorder and the most common fatty acid oxidation disorder. Clinical features arise during fasting or intercurrent illness and include drowsiness, lethargy or encephalopathy and hypoketotic hypoglycaemia.

While the condition is associated with a high mortality rate on first clinical presentation, the prognosis is excellent after diagnosis has been made. Siblings must also be screened on diagnosis of an index case, as affected children may be asymptomatic.

Key References

Ashrafi, M. R., & Tavasoli, A. R. (2017). Childhood leukodystrophies: A literature review of updates on new definitions, classification, diagnostic approach and management. *Brain & Development, 39*(5), 369–385.

Broomfield, A., & Grunewald, S. (2012). How to use serum ammonia. *Archives of Disease in Childhood Education and Practice Edition, 97*(2), 72–80.

Champion, M. P. (2010). An approach to the diagnosis of inherited metabolic disease. *Archives of Disease in Childhood Education and Practice Edition, 95*(2), 40–46.

Fukao, T., & Nakamura, K. (2019). Advances in inborn errors of metabolism. *Journal of Human Genetics, 64*(2), 65.

Kansra, A. R. (2018). Hypoglycaemia. in R. M. Kliegman, P. S. Lye, B. Bordini, H. Toth, & D. Basel (Eds.), *Nelson Pediatric Symptom-Based Diagnosis* (pp. 811–823). Elsevier.

Saudubray, J. M., & Garcia-Cazorla, À. (2018). Inborn errors of metabolism overview: Pathophysiology, manifestations, evaluation, and management. *Pediatric Clinics of North America, 65*(2), 179–208.

20 Joint Pains in Childhood

CLODAGH LOWRY

Musculoskeletal disorders are relatively frequent in childhood, and most are minor and self-limiting. A detailed history and examination are key to making a diagnosis. The critical issue in the history is to establish whether the child has non-inflammatory or inflammatory joint pain.

Non-Inflammatory or Inflammatory Joint Pain

Our first consideration should be to differentiate inflammatory from non-inflammatory joint pain. Non-inflammatory causes (often hypermobility or minor trauma) are widespread, and activity usually precipitates the pain. If due to a non-inflammatory cause, symptoms in a child with arthralgia (a painful joint) can be variable, intermittent or constant. There is no significant early morning stiffness or swelling – or, if present, swelling is short-lived and the pain experienced is constant or improves with rest. There is no warmth or swelling of the joint, no systemic symptoms and a normal range of movement on examination.

In inflammatory causes of joint pain, on the other hand, symptoms are consistent and tend to be present all or most of the time regardless of activity level. There is morning stiffness for more than 15 minutes following an overnight rest. The joint is warm with prominent swelling and a limited range of movement. Causes of inflammatory joint pain or arthritis in children include reactive arthritis, Henoch–Schonlein purpura arthritis, septic arthritis, juvenile idiopathic arthritis (JIA) and haemarthrosis associated with haemophilia.

Reactive arthritis is defined as sterile synovitis associated with infection elsewhere in the body and is the most frequent cause of acute arthritis in childhood. Reactive arthritis most often follows a viral upper respiratory tract infection. *Shigella*, *Salmonella*, *Campylobacter* and *Yersinia enterocolitica* infections can all be associated with reactive arthritis. Many viruses are also implicated as causes of reactive arthritis, including rubella (which typically affects small joints of the hand), herpes simplex, cytomegalovirus, varicella (usually pauciarticular) and mumps (large joint arthritis).

History and Examination

A clear description of the pain experienced is required, including whether present daily or not. Seek a detailed description of the pain in terms of its site, duration, frequency and precipitating or relieving factors. Stiffness (over 15 minutes), especially in the morning, is key as significant stiffness may point to an inflammatory cause. Pain related to activity and improved by rest is more likely to relate to overuse injury or joint hypermobility.

Enquire about any systemic symptoms such as fever (try to establish if a pattern is evident), fatigue, poor appetite or weight loss.

Nocturnal pain may be seen in benign bone tumours such as osteoid osteoma or leukaemia but is most often related to joint hypermobility and is sometimes described as 'growing pains'.

If the onset of joint pain is sudden and severe, consider septic arthritis, osteomyelitis or trauma with or without a fracture.

Limping (especially in the mornings) and difficulty running and jumping may indicate trauma or arthritis affecting joints of the lower limbs.

Conditions such as inflammatory bowel disease, psoriasis and sickle cell anaemia are associated with joint or bone pain.

Family history is especially relevant with inflammatory bowel disease and lupus-related or psoriatic arthritis.

Travel history can be important, as *Borrelia burgdorferi* is more prevalent in certain states or countries. Lyme arthritis most commonly affects the knee.

Some skin changes may be evident and are helpful. These include the salmon pink evanescent rash of JIA, the classical malar rash of systemic lupus, the purple heliotrope rash of dermatomyositis and the erythema migrans rash seen in Lyme disease. A formal joint examination should take place (see Chapter 3: Systems and Developmental examination).

Laboratory and Radiology Studies

An elevated white cell count may be a feature seen in both septic arthritis and osteomyelitis but must be considered in context. ESR elevation can be helpful if the physical examination is inconclusive. While the antinuclear antibody test (ANA) is relatively non-specific, the anti-double-stranded DNA test is highly sensitive (up to 80 per cent) and specific for systemic lupus erythematosus (SLE). Just 5 per cent of JIA patients have a positive rheumatoid factor, whereas 30 per cent of SLE patients are positive.

Plain x-rays are helpful in the diagnosis of trauma or solid bone tumours. Bone scans may help to diagnose osteomyelitis and osteoid osteoma. Hip ultrasound helps pick up a joint effusion that points to synovitis. MRI is a very sensitive investigation to diagnose conditions such as bone tumours, osteomyelitis and avascular necrosis.

Joint aspiration is helpful to confirm or exclude septic arthritis and haemarthrosis. Fluid aspirated should be for bacterial culture. Also, check a polymerase chain reaction for *Kingella kingae*, a relatively common cause of septic arthritis in young children.

Joint Hypermobility Syndrome

Joint hypermobility is very common (10–20 per cent of children have it) and is one of the most frequent causes of non-inflammatory joint pain in children. It is frequently associated with sporting activities and tends to improve upon resting.

Common clues suggesting the possibility of joint hypermobility in childhood include a prior history of developmental dysplasia of the hip, a history of delayed walking with bottom shuffling, recurrent ankle sprains, tiring easily when compared to peers, joint dislocations, poor catching and handwriting skills, and so-called 'growing pains' with leg pains associated with nocturnal awakening.

The Beighton score (maximum score of nine) enables assessment for joint hypermobility by performing the following manoeuvre with one point for each side if positive:

- passive dorsiflexion of the fifth metacarpophalangeal joint to 90 degrees
- opposition of the thumb to the volar aspect of the ipsilateral forearm
- hyperextension of the elbow to 10 degrees
- hyperextension of the knee to 10 degrees
- placing the hands flat on the floor without bending the knees

The diagnosis of joint hypermobility is entirely clinical and may be diagnosed based on two major criteria (Beighton score of four or over and arthralgia in at least four joints for 3 months or more), one major and two minor criteria (Beighton score under four, arthralgia in under three joints,

joint dislocation, soft tissue lesions, skin hyperextensibility, or striae or Marfanoid habitus), or four minor criteria as per Beighton.

The physiotherapist plays a key role in managing joint hypermobility with general and core fitness training.

Ligamentous laxity is also a feature consistent with variants of Ehlers–Danlos syndrome (EDS), where the useful Gorlin sign (the ability to touch the nasal tip with the tongue) is a feature in many cases of EDS. Other features of EDS include blue sclerae, skin hyperextensibility, easy bruisability, scarring disproportionate to the degree of trauma and joint dislocation. There is often a history of delayed early motor milestones in EDS but with normal intelligence. Kyphoscoliosis is a feature of EDS type 6, as is the absence of the normal three crease pattern of the fingers.

Juvenile Idiopathic Arthritis (JIA)

Categories of JIA include systemic, oligoarticular (less than four joints), extended oligoarticular, polyarticular (both rheumatoid factor positive and negative), enthesitis-related and psoriatic.

Oligoarticular

Oligoarticular JIA typically presents as monoarticular arthritis of the knee (Fig. 20.1). Key symptoms include early morning stiffness and an affected warm and swollen joint in an otherwise systemically well child.

Polyarticular

Rheumatoid positive polyarticular JIA closely resembles adult-onset rheumatoid arthritis (RA) and associated symptoms of fatigue and a poor appetite. Typically, the child has symmetrical arthritis affecting both small and large joints with small joint involvement of the hands, feet and wrists.

Enthesitis-Related

Common features include predominance in males, arthritis of the axial skeleton and peripheral arthritis in less than four joints. Acute symptomatic anterior uveitis is not uncommon, and they are often HLA-B27 positive (Fig. 20.2).

Psoriatic

An early-onset form (peaks at 2 to 3 years of age) with associated dactylitis affects girls more than boys. The late-onset form (10–12 years of age) is more common in boys and manifests as axial arthritis. Arthritis may rarely precede the onset of the rash. A diagnosis of psoriatic arthritis is made if there are signs of dactylitis or nail pitting and a history of psoriasis in the child or a first-degree relative

Systemic

A characteristic fever pattern with one or two high fever spikes per day with a rapid return to normal is typical. Usually, a pink, macular rash coincides with the fever and disappears when the fever settles (Fig. 20.3). Commonly

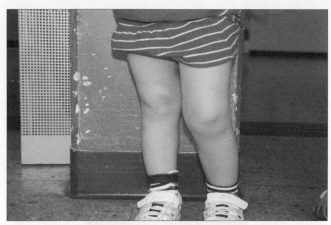

Figure 20.1 Oligoarticular juvenile idiopathic arthritis in a 2-year-old girl with arthritis in her left knee. (Reproduced with permission from Hochberg, M. C., Gravallese, E. M., Silman, A. J., Smolen, J. S., Weinblatt, M. E., & Weisman, M. H. (2018). *Rheumatology, 2-volume set* (7th ed.). Elsevier – Health Sciences.)

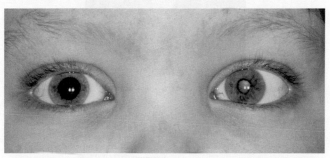

Figure 20.2 Idiopathic chronic anterior uveitis in white eyes presenting with left cataract in a 4-year-old. Juvenile idiopathic arthritis developed 7 years later. (Reproduced with permission from Lyons, C. J., & Lambert, S. R. (2017). *Taylor & Hoyt's pediatric ophthalmology and strabismus* (5th ed.). Elsevier.)

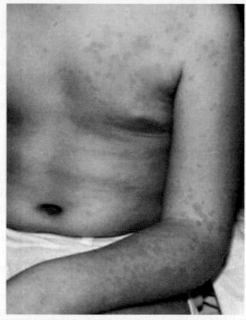

Figure 20.3 Typical rash of systemic juvenile idiopathic arthritis (sJIA) in a 3-year-old boy. The rash is salmon coloured, macular and nonpruritic. Individual lesions are transient, occur in crops over the trunk and extremities, and may occur in a linear distribution (Koebner phenomenon) after minor trauma such as scratching. (Reproduced with permission from Petty, R. E., Laxer, R., Lindsley, C., Wedderburn, L., Fuhlbrigge, R. C., & Mellins, E. D. (2021). *Textbook of pediatric rheumatology* (8th ed.). Elsevier – Health Sciences.)

associated symptoms include striking fatigue, a poor appetite and consequent weight loss. Hepatosplenomegaly and generalised lymphadenopathy are often evident. Uveitis is very rarely seen in systemic JIA.

MANAGING JIA

Non-steroidal anti-inflammatory (NSAID) drugs may be used before diagnosis. These relieve pain but do not alter the disease course. Intra-articular corticosteroids and NSAIDs are used for oligoarticular JIA, with triamcinolone increasingly being used with good effect.

In both polyarticular JIA and oligoarticular JIA refractory to intra-articular steroids, disease-modifying drugs such as methotrexate are widely used. Methotrexate is given orally once a week or by subcutaneous injection. Common side effects are anorexia, nausea and vomiting, and – less frequently – transient rises in transaminases and bone marrow effects, including neutropaenia. Folic acid is indicated after starting methotrexate to reduce gastrointestinal and hepatic side effects.

Tumour necrosis factors, interleukins 1 and 6, are important cytokines inhibited by drugs such as etanercept, adalimumab and abatacept. Others include infliximab, anakinra and tocilizumab, and the improvements seen in disease activity are very significant.

Physiotherapy is important and employs heat or cold treatments, therapeutic exercise, massage and splints. All help to promote a return to normal activity levels.

Evaluating Acute Limp in Childhood

In evaluating acute limp in childhood, the diagnostic challenge is to distinguish a benign and self-limiting diagnosis (such as transient synovitis) from conditions that require rapid diagnosis and treatment (such as septic arthritis or leukaemia) or generally painless conditions with a long-standing limp (such as Perthes disease).

Most limping in children relates to minor trauma, so a limp without a history of trauma requires careful consideration to reach a diagnosis. Age is important in terms of differential diagnoses of a limp. Clinical confusion may be due to referral of pain from the hip to the knee.

TRANSIENT SYNOVITIS

Transient synovitis generally affects the hip, largely affects children aged 4 to 8, and is seen more often in boys. Typical features are hip pain and mild restriction of hip movement, particularly hip abduction and internal rotation. Hip ultrasound will confirm the presence of hip effusion, but other potential causes require exclusion. Laboratory tests and x-rays are generally normal.

TODDLER'S FRACTURE

An undisplaced spiral fracture of the tibia is termed a toddler's fracture. Tenderness over the tibial shaft is generally absent. Diagnosis is by x-ray or, in some instances, bone scan (Fig. 20.4). The history, which may be vague, may include seemingly innocuous trauma such as tripping while walking or falling from a low height such as a couch.

SEPTIC ARTHRITIS AND OSTEOMYELITIS

Bone and joint infections are important causes of limp in children. Septic arthritis reflects infection confined to the joint space whereas, in osteomyelitis, the focus of infection is within the bone. Septic arthritis tends to affect weight-bearing joints such as the hip, knee or ankle. Acute osteomyelitis is most frequently seen in the neck of the femur, the distal femoral metaphysis or the proximal tibial metaphysis. Early diagnosis is essential in both conditions.

In osteomyelitis, point tenderness is seen over the involved site and can become more diffuse as the infection progresses. Plain x-rays are generally unhelpful in the diagnosis of acute osteomyelitis with MRI (or alternative bone scanning) being the preferred test for diagnosis (Fig. 20.5).

Staphylococcus aureus is the most frequent cause of septic arthritis in children, with group B *Streptococcus* being the most common cause in neonates. Children with background sickle cell disease can develop osteomyelitis either due to pneumococcal infections or *Salmonella*.

Septic arthritis typically presents with fever, a limp and refusal to weight bear. In infancy, the presentation may be that the affected limb is not moved. If septic arthritis of the hip is suspected, an ultrasound may be helpful to demonstrate an effusion. If an effusion is present, fluid aspiration is recommended, with aspirated fluid sent for culture and sensitivity. Be aware that *Kingella kingae* PCR testing should be requested in children under 5. Septic arthritis is most frequently seen in infants, toddlers and preschool children. Orthopaedic input is required, and treatment is joint aspiration and intravenous antibiotics. Delays in diagnosis and treatment can damage the growth plate or cause avascular necrosis.

PERTHES DISEASE

Perthes disease has a peak age of 4 to 8 years, is more common in boys and is due to avascular necrosis of the developing femoral head (Fig. 20.6). The cause is unknown, and it is bilateral in 20 per cent of cases. Children often present with a persistent painless limp with associated discomfort in the anterior thigh or knee. Bed rest and containing the hip within the acetabulum is the basis of treatment in Perthes disease.

SLIPPED CAPITAL FEMORAL EPIPHYSIS (SCFE)

Slipped capital femoral epiphysis is a hip disorder often seen in adolescence (Fig. 20.7). It is an important diagnosis not to miss. It can either occur in adolescents who are overweight or obese or in tall, thin adolescents who have had a recent growth spurt.

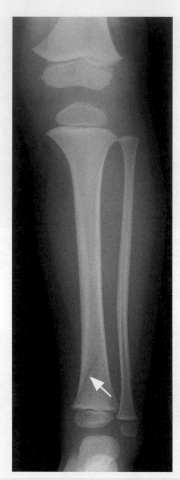

Figure 20.4   Toddler fracture. An 18-month-old toddler, not weight-bearing on his left leg for 1 day. X-ray shows an oblique fracture (arrow) in the distal tibia. (Courtesy Prof. Stephanie Ryan.)

Common Variants in the Legs Causing Parental Concern

Common variants include habitual toe walking, knock knees, pes planus, metatarsus varus and tibial bowing. Most are evident in the early toddler years and cause significant parental concern.

Habitual toe walking is when a young child (usually a toddler) walks on their toes voluntarily. It tends to be intermittent, and the toddler tends to rest with their feet flat on the floor when they stop walking. This is in stark contrast to a child with spastic diplegia, where lower limb tone is high and deep tendon reflexes are brisk.

Toe walking can be a normal finding up to 3 years of age. The physical examination, not least the tone and deep tendon reflexes in the lower limbs and back examination, is normal. Therefore, habitual toe walking is a diagnosis of exclusion with other differentials, including spinal cord tethering and proximal myopathy due to muscular dystrophy.

Many healthy children develop **knock knees** after 2 years of age, which may cause frequent falls when they run. It usually resolves by 8 years of age. If tibial bowing increases progressively, conditions such as Blount disease, rickets or metaphyseal dysplasia need to be considered.

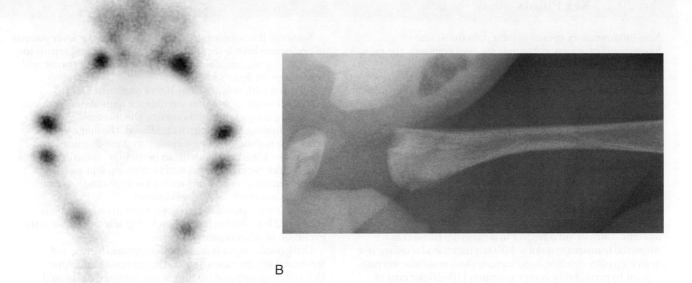

Figure 20.5 Osteomyelitis. Three-week-old baby not moving her left leg. (A) Bone scan shows normal high activity in all the growth plates but increased activity adjacent to the left proximal femoral physis. (B) X-ray shows a small lucent area in the metaphysis of the left proximal femur consistent with osteomyelitis. (Courtesy Prof. Stephanie Ryan.)

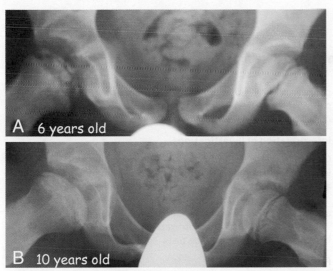

Figure 20.6 Perthes disease. X-rays of hips (A) in a 6-year-old boy with pain in his right hip. There is advanced Perthes disease with fragmentation and sclerosis of the right femoral head and widening of the femoral neck. (B) At 10 years old, the femoral head has reformed and is smooth but flattened. The femoral neck remains widened – coxa magna. (Courtesy Prof. Stephanie Ryan)

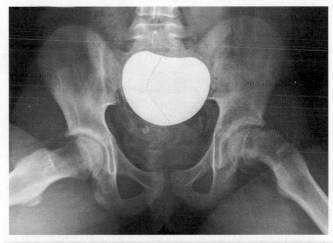

Figure 20.7 Slipped femoral capital epiphysis. A 13-year-old boy with a 2-week history of pain in his left hip. There is significant displacement of the left femoral head. (Courtesy Prof. Stephanie Ryan.)

Knock knees may also develop in markedly obese children and children with renal osteodystrophy.

Pes planus is common in toddlers and tends to improve by age 6. In older children, pes planus is helped by arch supports. When a toddler with pes planus sits on a couch, the arch reappears as the feet are suspended in space!

Internal tibial torsion frequently leads to in-toeing in children under 2 years of age and usually resolves by 5 years. With internal tibial torsion, the patellae turn toward each other.

Metatarsus varus is a very common congenital foot abnormality, and up to one in 10 have associated developmental dysplasia of the hip. The forefoot is adducted, while the midfoot and hindfoot are normal. Ankle movements are also normal. Mild to moderate metatarsus varus usually corrects itself as it is a result of in-utero positioning.

Positional talipes equinovarus is a common condition wherein the foot is held in an equinovarus position but is flexible on newborn examination. Positional talipes resolves with passive stretching.

(Box 20.1)
(Box 20.2)
(Box 20.3)
(Box 20.4)

Box 20.1   **Key Points**

Non-inflammatory causes of joint pain (most often hypermobility or minor trauma) are very common, the pain of which is precipitated by activity.

In inflammatory joint pain, morning stiffness will be evident for more than 15 min following an overnight rest. The joint is warm with prominent swelling and a limited range of movement. Causes of inflammatory joint pain or arthritis in children include reactive arthritis, Henoch–Schonlein purpura arthritis, septic arthritis, juvenile idiopathic arthritis (JIA) and haemarthrosis associated with haemophilia.

Shigella, Salmonella, Campylobacter and *Yersinia enterocolitica* infections can all be associated with reactive arthritis.

If the onset of joint pain is sudden and severe, consider septic arthritis, osteomyelitis or trauma with or without a fracture.

Bone scans may help to diagnose osteomyelitis and osteoid osteoma. Ultrasound is helpful to pick up hip effusion in suspected transient synovitis. MRI is a useful and sensitive test to pick up osteomyelitis, bone tumours and avascular necrosis.

Joint hypermobility is very common (10–20 per cent of children have it) and is one of the most frequent causes of non-inflammatory joint pain in children.

The physiotherapist plays a key role in managing joint hypermobility with general and core fitness training.

Categories of JIA include systemic, oligoarticular (less than four joints), extended oligoarticular, polyarticular (both rheumatoid factor positive and negative), enthesitis-related and psoriatic.

Systemic JIA is associated with a characteristic fever pattern of one or two high fever spikes per day with a rapid return to normal. A pink, macular rash coincides with fever onset and resolves as the fever settles.

Children with polyarticular JIA or oligoarticular JIA refractory to intra-articular steroids are candidates for disease-modifying drugs, with methotrexate the most widely used.

In evaluating acute limp in childhood, the diagnostic challenge is distinguishing a benign and self-limiting diagnosis – transient synovitis in particular – from conditions that require rapid diagnosis and treatment (septic arthritis or leukaemia) or conditions with a longstanding, generally painless limp (such as Perthes disease).

Definitive diagnosis of transient synovitis is based on a confirmed hip effusion (picked up by hip ultrasound) and the exclusion of other potential causes.

Orthopaedic input is required for septic arthritis, and treatment is joint aspiration and intravenous antibiotics. Delayed diagnosis and treatment can damage the growth plate or cause avascular necrosis.

Perthes disease typically presents in boys ages 4 to 8.

Slipped capital femoral epiphysis tends to occur in obese adolescents or those with a recent growth spurt.

Common normal variants seen include habitual toe walking, knock knees, pes planus, metatarsus varus and tibial bowing. Most are evident in the early toddler years and cause significant parental concern.

Box 20.2   **A 4-Year-Old With Early Morning Stiffness and Knee Swelling**

A 4-year-old girl presents with a 6-week history of intermittent limp and stiffness, especially noted in the mornings. On examination, her right knee is swollen and warm to the touch and is held in flexion. Her investigations show a positive antinuclear factor (ANF) and negative rheumatoid factor.

Clinical Pearls

Juvenile idiopathic arthritis (JIA) is one of the most common chronic diseases of childhood, with an estimated prevalence of one per 1000 children. All forms of JIA may persist into adulthood, causing ongoing significant morbidity and impaired quality of life.

A diagnosis of JIA requires symptoms and signs of inflammatory arthritis persisting for <u>at least 6 weeks</u> and beginning before 16 years of age.

Refer to a paediatric rheumatologist if suspected or confirmed JIA is present. A general practitioner (GP) should prescribe a non-steroidal anti-inflammatory drug to relieve symptoms.

Prompt initiation of appropriate therapy is critical in preventing permanent damage and improving outcomes.

The principal treatments for JIA are non-steroidal anti-inflammatory drugs (NSAIDs), systemic and intra-articular corticosteroids, and nonbiologic and biologic disease-modifying antirheumatic drugs (DMARDs).

Etanercept is useful for polyarticular JIA, is not so effective in managing uveitis, and has an excellent side effect profile. Adalimumab has proven to be very effective for joint symptoms and uveitis in JIA.

Anakinra is an interleukin 1 receptor antagonist useful in systemic-onset JIA. The child may not have psoriasis with

psoriatic arthritis, but there should be a family history in a first-degree relative. The severity of skin psoriasis and arthritis are not correlated.

Interpretation of Investigations

Characteristic laboratory findings in systemic JIA include leucocytosis, thrombocytosis and anaemia. Rheumatoid factor and antinuclear antibody (ANA) are invariably negative.

Children with pauciarticular JIA may have a positive ANA test and are at high risk (20 per cent) for developing anterior uveitis.

The child with JIA on methotrexate should undergo regular full blood count and liver function tests.

Pitfalls to Avoid

One of the key elements to follow up on is uveitis screening, as the screening and management of uveitis are of great importance. Sight may be lost if screening is inadequate. <u>Regular formal ophthalmology review is essential.</u>

Children with systemic JIA are at risk for macrophage activation syndrome (MAS), resulting in disseminated intravascular coagulation, which may be life-threatening. MAS manifests through disseminated intravascular coagulation, hepatosplenomegaly and multiorgan dysfunction.

Laboratory investigations in MAS tend to show an elevated C-reactive protein, markedly elevated ferritin, low fibrinogen and a low platelet count. High-dose intravenous corticosteroids are required for therapy.

Box 20.3 An 18-Month-Old With a Painful Hip Now Refusing to Walk

An 18-month-old boy presents with a 3-day history of a painful left hip and refusal to walk. He had a recent upper respiratory tract infection and is now pyrexial (39 °C) and looks unwell. His left hip is painful at rest, and he resists any hip movement on that side. All blood inflammatory markers are raised (Full blood count (FBC), C-reactive protein (CRP), and ESR). Blood cultures are requested, and an orthopaedic opinion regarding joint aspiration is sought.

Clinical Pearls

Septic arthritis typically presents as pain in a single joint with associated swelling and pain on palpation and movement.
    Early diagnosis of septic arthritis is essential to avoid joint destruction. Differential diagnoses include transient synovitis, osteomyelitis, reactive arthritis, Lyme arthritis and haemarthrosis due to Haemophilia A or B.
    If septic arthritis of the hip, the affected hip is held in flexion, abduction and external rotation, and the child will greatly resist passive movement of the affected hip.
    Kocher's criteria, such as fever over 38.5 degrees, refusal to weight bear, ESR over 40 and a white cell count over 12, help distinguish septic arthritis from transient synovitis.
    Acute osteomyelitis is a key differential; the distinguishing features include involvement of the femoral neck, the distal femoral metaphysis or proximal tibial metaphysis. Point tenderness over the site of osteomyelitis is typical.

Interpretation of Investigations

Ultrasound demonstrates the presence of joint fluid and joint aspiration is required to diagnose septic arthritis.
    Staphylococcus aureus is the most frequent microorganism cultured in septic arthritis, but *Kingella kingae* is a frequent reason in children under five.
    Magnetic resonance imaging (MRI) is now the preferred imaging method for diagnosing osteomyelitis as x-rays are normal for the first 7 to 10 days. X-rays may show periosteal elevation after 10 to 14 days of active infection in cases of osteomyelitis.

Pitfalls to Avoid

In septic arthritis, early diagnosis and treatment are key to avoid complications of avascular necrosis or damage to the growth plate. Rapid joint destruction occurs within days if septic arthritis is not adequately treated.
    Multifocal osteomyelitis in children with sickle cell disease may be hard to distinguish from a vaso-occlusive crisis. Children with chronic granulomatous disease may develop septic arthritis or osteomyelitis caused by uncommon bacteria or fungi.

Box 20.4 A 12-Year-Old With a 4-Week History of Groin Pain

A 12-year-old obese boy presents with a 4-week history of groin pain and difficulty walking. There is no history of trauma or fever. Clinical examination shows apparent shortening of the right leg, which is held in external rotation. Blood is normal, and a hip x-ray is requested.

Clinical Pearls

Slipped capital femoral epiphysis (SCFE) is the displacement of the capital femoral epiphysis through the physis from the metaphysis. In stable SCFE, the young person can walk with or without assistance, and in unstable SCFE, there is an inability to walk with or without aid. Obesity is a key risk factor for SCFE.
    SCFE is more common in boys, is bilateral in 20 per cent, and requires a high index of suspicion in an adolescent presenting with hip or knee pain, as early diagnosis is critical.
    Although SCFE has been associated with hypothyroidism, growth hormone use, and prior radiation exposure to the area, it normally occurs in young people with no risk factors other than obesity.
    In an unstable or acute slipped capital femoral epiphysis, the capital femoral epiphysis is separated from the femoral neck. It is very painful with an inability to stand or bear weight.
    The stable slipped capital femoral epiphysis is more common with a more chronic and slower slip, and the capital femoral epiphysis and femoral neck are in continuity. The affected hip shows limited internal rotation and an increase in external rotation.
    Surgery is needed to stabilise and thereby prevent further displacement. A single cannulated screw fixation achieves this under image intensifier control. Severe displacement may necessitate femoral neck osteotomy.

Interpretation of Investigations

Diagnosis is by anteroposterior or frog-leg x-rays of the pelvis. The so-called Klein line is drawn along the superior border of the femoral neck and should cross at least a portion of the femoral epiphysis.

Pitfalls to Avoid

Not all SCFE adolescents are obese.
    Children without obesity have been found to have a greater risk of severe, unstable SCFEs compared with children with obesity, and this may contribute to a delayed diagnosis. Non-obese young people are more likely to present with a severe slip, regardless of age or sex.
    Always consider SCFE in obese and non-obese children and adolescents presenting with hip, groin, thigh or knee pain.

Key References

Fehr, S. D. (2018). Gait disturbances. In R. M. Kleigman, P. S. Lye, B. Bordini, H. Toth, & D. Basel (Eds.), *Nelson pediatric symptom-based diagnosis* (pp. 614–632). Elsevier.

Mooney, J. F., 3rd, & Murphy, R. F. (2019). Septic arthritis of the pediatric hip: update on diagnosis and treatment. *Current Opinion in Pediatrics, 31*(1), 79–85.

Nocton, J., & Co, D. (2018). Arthritis. In R. M. Kleigman, P. S. Lye, B. Bordini, H. Toth, & D. Basel (Eds.), *Nelson pediatric symptom-based diagnosis* (pp. 594–613). Elsevier.

Obana, K. K., Siddiqui, A. A., Broom, A. M., Barrett, K., Andras, L. M., Millis, M. B., et al. (2020). Slipped capital femoral epiphysis in children without obesity. *The Journal of Pediatrics, 218*, 192–197.e1.

Prince, F. H., Otten, M. H., & van Suijlekom-Smit, L. W. (2010). Diagnosis and management of juvenile idiopathic arthritis. *BMJ (Clinical Research Ed.), 341*, c6434.

Ringold, S., Angeles-Han, S. T., Beukelman, T., Lovell, D., Cuello, C. A., Becker, M. L., et al. (2019). 2019 American College of Rheumatology/Arthritis Foundation Guideline for the Treatment of Juvenile Idiopathic Arthritis: therapeutic approaches for non–systemic polyarthritis, sacroiliitis, and enthesitis. *Arthritis Care & Research, 71*(6), 717–734.

Smits-Engelsman, B., Klerks, M., & Kirby, A. (2011). Beighton score: a valid measure for generalized hypermobility in children. *The Journal of Pediatrics, 158*(1), 119–123, 123.e1–4.

21 Problems Relating to the Kidneys

MICHAEL RIORDAN

The most common kidney problem seen in infants and children by far is a urinary tract infection. Children may also present with significant proteinuria or haematuria, which require a logical approach to diagnosis and management.

Urinary Tract Infections

Fever without an obvious source is a common symptom in young children under 2 years of age, and as such, a sample of urine should be collected to rule out urinary tract infection. Over 90 per cent of urinary tract infections in infants under 1 year of age are due to *Escherichia coli*. The most widely used threshold for the diagnosis of UTI is greater than 100,000 colony-forming units per mL for a voided urine specimen or any growth of a urinary pathogen from a suprapubic sample. UTI is more common in uncircumcised males, but it would be necessary to circumcise 100 to 200 boys to prevent a single UTI. Febrile infants have a 5 per cent chance of having a UTI, making a urine culture the investigation with the highest yield in this age group. The most frequent symptoms of UTI in children under 2 years old are vomiting, poor feeding, diarrhoea and irritability.

OBTAINING A URINE SAMPLE

The optimal method of collection is a clean catch midstream sample. Firstly, lay the infant down with the nappy open, offer a feed and clean the perineum. Ask the parent to hold an open sample jar and to catch a midstream sample as urine is being passed. This requires concentration on the part of the parent, as a momentary lapse can lead to a missed opportunity.

Do not delay treatment in a sick child if a urine sample cannot be obtained quickly. Urine may also be obtained via suprapubic aspiration under ultrasound guidance.

Bag specimens may be used to exclude urinary tract infections but are prone to sample contamination.

URINALYSIS

Urine microscopy may show white cells or bacteria under the microscope. Indirect measurement of white cells is possible with dipstick assessment of leucocyte esterase, but the presence of white cells is not specific for UTI. Dipsticks can also provide an indirect measurement of bacteriuria through the nitrite test, which is virtually always negative in children without UTI. Unfortunately, the sensitivity is just 50 per cent.

The choice of empiric antibiotic will depend on age and the local bacterial resistance patterns in the community. If under 6 months old or presenting with symptoms of acute pyelonephritis (high fever, chills, rigours, renal angle tenderness), the infant should be admitted for intravenous antibiotics.

Treatment and Age-Related Investigations

BIRTH TO 6 MONTHS

In infants under 6 months old, symptoms may be quite subtle and include low-grade fever, jaundice, poor feeding and faltering growth. Infants may not have a fever despite being critically unwell, thus requiring a high index of suspicion in under 3-month-old infants. Obtain urine by means of a clean-catch sample.

Continue intravenous antibiotics for at least 48 hours and confirm culture results before discharge. Antibiotic prophylaxis is indicated pending follow-up investigations.

KEY INVESTIGATIONS

Renal Ultrasound

A renal ultrasound scan should be performed on all children admitted with UTI, ideally within 72 hours of admission, to exclude any underlying anatomical abnormality that may increase the risk of UTI. Children with a poor urinary stream, oliguria or a palpable mass need an immediate ultrasound, as a urinary obstruction in the presence of infection is a surgical emergency. A repeat ultrasound should be performed 6 months later to look for possible evolving scarring.

Micturating Cystourethrogram (MCUG)

MCUG outlines the bladder structure and demonstrates vesicoureteric reflux (VUR) (Fig. 21.1). The disadvantages of MCUG are discomfort relating to catheterisation and radiation exposure. Experienced staff, use of an image intensifier and follow-up isotope cystography may help to mitigate the disadvantages of MCUG.

Obtain a negative urine culture prior to the MCUG (ideally obtained between 2 and 7 days prior to the test). Avoid requesting an MCUG in children over 1 year of age without specialist advice.

Tc-99m Dimercaptosuccinic Acid (DMSA)

DMSA scan provides a functional assessment of the renal parenchyma based on proximal tubular uptake of the isotope and measures the relative percentage of total function provided by each kidney (Fig. 21.2).

MAG3 Renogram

The MAG3 renogram provides an evaluation of the differential perfusion and excretion of the kidneys and indicates whether an obstruction is present (Fig. 21.3).

SIX MONTHS TO 2 YEARS OF AGE AND SYSTEMICALLY WELL

Renal ultrasound should be performed six months post-UTI unless concerns arise regarding the possibility of underlying renal obstruction (e.g. a poor urinary stream, previously

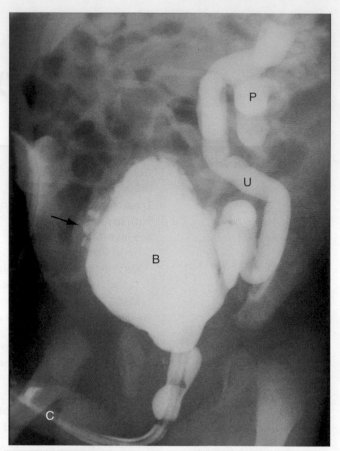

Figure 21.1 Vesicoureteric Reflux. Micturating cystourethrogram in a child with recurrent urinary tract infections. The bladder (B) is trabeculated (diverticula arrowed). On voiding, the left ureter (U) and pelvicalyceal system (P) filled with contrast as a result of severe dilating vesicoureteric reflux. This is defined as grade V reflux. The urethral catheter (C) is used to instil contrast into the bladder. (Reproduced with permission from Quick, C. R. G., Biers, S., & Arulampalam, T. (Eds.). (2020). *Essential surgery: Problems, diagnosis and management* (6th ed.). Elsevier Ltd.)

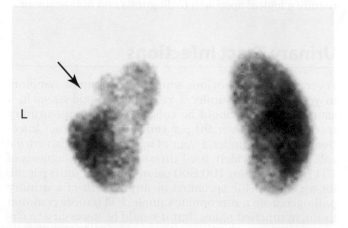

Figure 21.2 Pyelonephritis. The posterior planar image from a 99mTc-dimercaptosuccinic acid (DMSA) scan in a young child shows cortical defects in the upper pole of the left kidney (arrow). (Reproduced with permission from Mettler, F. A., Jr, & Guiberteau, M. J. (2012). *Essentials of nuclear medicine imaging: Expert consult* (6th ed.). W B Saunders.)

abnormal antenatal imaging and a palpable bladder or mass). DMSA is an alternative, but renal ultrasound alone is likely to be sufficient.

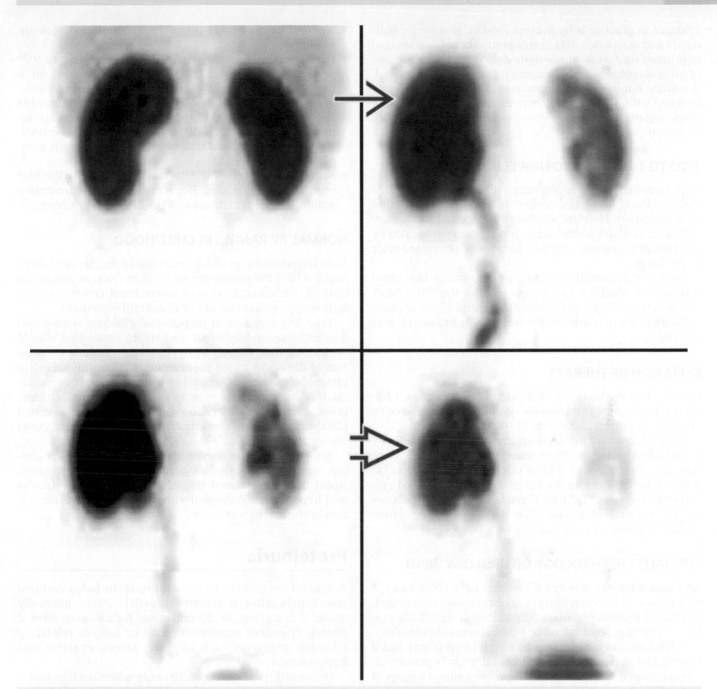

Figure 21.3 Tc-99m MAG3 renogram in a 6-week-old infant with left hydronephrosis shows retention of radiotracer despite furosemide administration. This study is positive for left pelvic-ureteric junction obstruction. (Reproduced with permission from Bennett, P. A. (2020). *Diagnostic imaging: Nuclear medicine* (3rd ed.). Elsevier – Health Sciences Division.)

Consider prophylactic antibiotics pending the results of imaging in children less than 1 year of age. Always check antibiotic sensitivities. No further follow up is required if the ultrasound is normal 6 months later.

SIX MONTHS TO 2 YEARS AND UNWELL

Hospital admission is required with intravenous co-amoxiclav and gentamicin (guided by local sensitivities). A renal ultrasound is required prior to discharge. Discuss any concerns about obstruction with the specialist

paediatric urology team. Renal ultrasound should be repeated 6 months after the UTI to pick up any renal scarring. Prescribe prophylactic antibiotics (based on sensitivities) for children under 1 year of age pending the result of follow-up scans.

TWO TO 16 YEARS AND SYSTEMICALLY WELL

A diagnosis of UTI in this age group can be made by means of a single midstream clean-catch sample with a significant white cell count in the absence of epithelial cells. Presumptive evidence in practice is by a urine dipstick positive for both nitrite and leucocytes. UTI in this group should be managed in primary care with an adequate dose of oral co-amoxiclav or an oral cephalosporin. Imaging is generally not required. A routine outpatient renal ultrasound should be requested in a boy with a UTI where there is significant growth of a single organism and no evidence of balanitis or if UTIs are recurrent.

TWO TO 16 YEARS AND UNWELL

Symptoms at this age are of acute pyelonephritis and include rigours, fever, loin pain, tachycardia, polyuria, vomiting or dehydration. Hospital admission is required for therapy with intravenous co-amoxiclav and gentamicin (guided by local sensitivities) and a request for a renal ultrasound prior to discharge.

Look for potential scarring by repeating the renal ultrasound, ideally 6 to 12 months after the UTI. DMSA is a potential alternative, but ultrasound alone is often sufficient, particularly if the original ultrasound was normal.

DURATION OF THERAPY

Oral antibiotics should be continued for 5 to 7 days. Children who require intravenous antibiotics should receive antibiotic treatment for a total of 10 days.

After 48 hours of intravenous antibiotics, the child may be switched to oral antibiotics and discharged home once they are clinically well with a normal temperature for at least 24 hours. Prior to discharge, confirm that blood cultures are negative and that there is no significant abnormality on renal ultrasound. The choice of oral antibiotic should be based on urine culture sensitivities.

SPECIALIST NEPHROLOGY OR UROLOGY INPUT

Specialist advice is required if imaging for a child under 2 years of age with recurrent UTI suggests urinary obstruction, significant hydronephrosis, single kidney or significant unilateral scarring, renal calculi or bilateral renal abnormality.

Advice should also be sought for children of any age if the bladder is palpable, an abdominal mass is present on examination or the child is not improving after 48 hours of IV treatment.

Hypertension in Childhood

MEASURING BP

In practical terms, correct cuff size equates to a cuff containing a bladder that completely encircles the forearm. By tradition, the BP is measured in the child's right arm while they are relaxed and seated.

The gold standard is BP measurement by auscultation in preference to automated devices. If a high BP is found by an automated device, then always repeat by auscultation.

BP is classified by systolic BP (SBP) and diastolic BP (DBP). Percentiles for age, sex and height are available (see NHIBI online references). If the SBP or DBP is above the 90th percentile, the advice is to repeat twice in the same visit using a manual measurement.

- **Normal BP:** SBP and DBP <90th percentile. Recheck annually.
- **Prehypertension:** SBP or DBP 90th percentile to 95th percentile or BP over 120/80 mmHg. Recheck in 6 months. Start a weight management plan if overweight.
- **Stage 1 Hypertension:** SBP and/or DBP 95th percentile to 99th percentile plus 5 mmHg. Recheck the measurement in 1 to 2 weeks. If BP remains the same at recheck, start investigation and treatment including weight management if overweight.
- **Stage 2 Hypertension:** SBP and/or DBP above the 99th percentile plus 5 mmHg. Begin evaluation and treatment within 1 week or right away if the child has symptoms.

NORMAL BP RANGES IN CHILDHOOD

Most hypertension in childhood is due to the circumstances under which the measurement is taken (pain or emotional distress, for instance) or to measurement errors, particularly inappropriate cuff size or site of cuff placement.

True hypertension in prepubertal children is rare and frequently secondary to an underlying cause that should be investigated. Causes of hypertension include coarctation of the aorta, acute postinfectious glomerulonephritis, phaeochromocytoma, neuroblastoma, renal artery stenosis, Cushing syndrome or exogenous steroids, and chronic renal scarring secondary to reflux nephropathy. Elevated blood pressure may also complicate diabetes, obesity and chronic renal disease.

Symptomatic hypertension is always of concern. Presenting symptoms include headache, vomiting and seizures. Apart from an elevated BP, left ventricular hypertrophy and hypertensive retinopathy may be found on examination in chronic hypertension.

Proteinuria

A spot urine protein to creatinine ratio helps confirm proteinuria after a positive dipstick (ratio normally under 0.2 mg/mg, or 20 mg/mmol for children over 2 years). Transient proteinuria may be seen in relatively common scenarios such as fever, stress, exercise and hypovolemia.

Orthostatic proteinuria occurs only when upright and is suggested by the absence of protein in the first voided urine in the morning. On the other hand, persistent proteinuria is an important indicator of significant renal pathology and requires an in-depth evaluation to find a cause.

ASSESSING PERSISTENT PROTEINURIA

In the history, ask about respiratory problems preceding the proteinuria, coincident haematuria, family history of renal disease or deafness, and whether oedema is present.

Findings of oedema, hypertension and red cell casts in the urine are all significant. Pyuria and bacteriuria point to a urinary tract infection.

Renal ultrasound will out rule dysplastic or cystic kidney disease.

Blood investigations should include a full blood count; renal, liver and bone biochemistry profiles; and cholesterol and thyroid function tests. More specific tests may include complement (C3 and C4) levels, antinuclear, and ANCA and dsDNA antibody studies.

NEPHROTIC SYNDROME

Almost all cases of nephrotic syndrome in children are due to minimal change disease. Focal segmental glomerulosclerosis and membranous glomerulonephritis are rarely seen. Nephrotic syndrome can also occur in association with conditions that more commonly cause nephritis – for example, Henoch–Schonlein purpura or systemic lupus erythematosus (SLE).

Presentation is with periorbital puffiness on waking in the morning (Fig. 21.4), an increased abdominal girth due to ascites, pitting oedema of the feet or scrotal oedema.

Treatment is with high dose oral prednisolone for 4 to 6 weeks followed by a lower dose on alternate days for another 6 weeks. A complete resolution of proteinuria is expected within 10 to 21 days. About 80 per cent of children with minimal change disease will relapse and are defined as having frequent relapses if they suffer more than two relapses over a 6-month period.

Second-line therapy is often needed for those with frequent relapses. Options include cyclophosphamide, cyclosporin, tacrolimus, mycophenolate, levamisole or rituximab.

A lack of response to prednisolone may be the first indication of focal segmental sclerosis as the cause of nephrotic syndrome, and a biopsy is indicated. The prognosis of focal segmental sclerosis is poor with up to one-third noted to be in chronic renal failure within 10 years.

Membranous glomerulonephritis may be primary or secondary to hepatitis B, systemic lupus erythematosus or a number of drugs (such as penicillamine).

Congenital nephrotic syndrome is inherited in an autosomal recessive fashion. Massive proteinuria leading to both ascites and peripheral oedema is usually evident in the first few weeks of life. Initial treatment includes a high-calorie and high-protein formula usually given via nasogastric tube feeds. Subsequently, peritoneal dialysis and nephrectomy are required, with most also requiring renal transplantation.

Haematuria

To parents, haematuria is an alarming symptom. Any child who presents with visible or microscopic haematuria with symptoms or signs such as hypertension, oedema, sinusitis, epistaxis, poor growth or a fever requires a thorough evaluation. The more difficult issue is the investigative approach to a perfectly well child with isolated microscopic haematuria. A cause of haematuria requiring specific treatment is unlikely if no other symptoms are present, the physical examination is normal (including blood pressure), and there is no family history of renal disease.

HISTORY

Pain with haematuria is usually indicative of a lower urinary tract source. Urinary tract infection is a very common cause of gross haematuria. Colicky flank pain should raise concern regarding renal calculi.

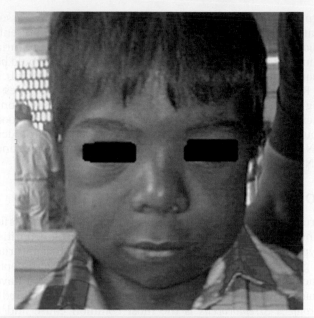

Figure 21.4 A child with nephrotic syndrome. (Reproduced with permission from Thirunavukkarasu AB. (2017). *Pediatrics for Medical Graduates*. Elsevier, a division of RELX India, Pvt. Ltd.)

Recurrent painless gross haematuria is seen with IgA nephropathy and often coincides with an upper respiratory tract illness. Sinusitis, epistaxis or haemoptysis can be associated with anti-neutrophil cytoplasmic antibody (ANCA) associated disease and urgent specialist assessment is required.

Sickle cell disease can be associated with gross haematuria relating to renal papillary necrosis. Cyclophosphamide therapy has a rare side effect of haemorrhagic cystitis.

A family history of kidney disease in male relatives that leads to end-stage renal failure could suggest Alport's syndrome. Alport's syndrome may cause gross haematuria in childhood during an intercurrent viral illness or present with persistent microscopic haematuria. Hearing loss is frequently seen in Alport's syndrome.

Benign familial haematuria is where there is persistent isolated haematuria without any progression to significant renal disease.

Gross haematuria, which is isolated to the beginning or the end of the urinary stream, is local in origin, beginning either in the bladder or the urethra. Gynaecological causes of apparent haematuria should be considered, particularly when drops of blood are observed. Rarely, dyes or food colourings can give the appearance of haematuria.

EXAMINATION

Check and plot the child's growth and accurately measure the blood pressure. Examine for rashes (for instance, the rash of HSP) and palpate the abdomen for masses while considering Wilms tumour, hydronephrosis or polycystic kidney disease as potential causes.

INVESTIGATIONS

Possible indications of a glomerular cause include RBC casts in the urine and if the urine dipstick is +2 or more for protein. Always request a urine culture, especially if associated flank pain, fever or bladder symptoms are present. Idiopathic hypercalciuria is another cause of haematuria and thus a spot urine calcium to creatinine ratio should be requested (over 0.7 mmol/mmol is considered abnormal).

Renal and bladder ultrasounds are helpful in assessing children with gross haematuria. Blood investigations include urea and electrolytes, serum creatinine, a full blood count, C3 and C4 complement levels, anti-double-stranded DNA, anti-glomerular basement membrane antibodies and ANCA antibodies.

POSTINFECTIOUS GLOMERULONEPHRITIS

Gross haematuria evident 2 to 4 weeks following a febrile illness is suggestive of postinfectious glomerulonephritis. Typically, a school-aged child presents with haematuria, oliguria, hypertension and renal insufficiency. Microscopic haematuria is very often seen and about 30 per cent have macroscopic haematuria (often described as cola coloured). *Group A Streptococcus* is the most common cause and a recent throat swab confirming its presence is helpful. In most cases, C3 complement levels are typically low at presentation and later return to normal. If the C3 level does not return to normal after 3 months, other causes of glomerulonephritis must be considered. Complete recovery is expected in over 95 per cent of children with postinfectious glomerulonephritis. The main acute complication is hypertension, which may be severe and require diuretic treatment. Microscopic haematuria can persist for up to a year following an episode of postinfectious glomerulonephritis. In the absence of proteinuria or hypertension, further aggressive investigation would not be indicated in this period.

IgA NEPHROPATHY

The most frequent presentation of IgA nephropathy is with recurrent episodes of painless, gross haematuria associated with intercurrent viral illnesses. Underlying IgA can be readily differentiated from postinfectious glomerular nephritis by the timing of the haematuria in relation to infection, as haematuria in IgA nephritis occurs **with** infection; haematuria with postinfectious GN occurs **after** the infection has resolved. Serum C3 complement levels are normal. IgA nephropathy is a benign condition with recurrent episodes of gross haematuria during viral illnesses followed by a complete resolution within a few days. Renal biopsy can confirm the diagnosis with typical features being immune deposits of IgA in the mesangium of the glomeruli. Renal biopsy is indicated if features such as hypertension, abnormal renal function, nephrotic syndrome or proteinuria persist once the bleeding has stopped.

Persistent Microscopic Haematuria as an Incidental Finding

Microscopic haematuria is a frequent incidental finding, either in association with acute illness or on screening. In the absence of hypertension, abnormal renal function, an abdominal mass or associated proteinuria, microscopic haematuria is very rarely associated with significant renal

pathology requiring urgent treatment. In the first instance, the urine should be checked again following recovery from acute illness or within 4 to 6 weeks. If microscopic haematuria persists in a well child over a period of 12 months, then further investigation may be indicated at that stage. Asymptomatic intermittent microscopic haematuria does not require investigation.

Management of Antenatal Diagnosed Hydronephrosis (ANH)

The classification and definition of ANH are based on the measurement of the anteroposterior diameter (APD) of the renal pelvis with an APD above 15 mm representing significant hydronephrosis.

POSTNATAL MANAGEMENT

Infants with unilateral hydronephrosis will have a spontaneous resolution in over 90 per cent of cases. Intervention may be required if bilateral hydronephrosis, pelvic dilatation over 15 mm or bladder wall thickening is present. Unilateral renal agenesis is not uncommon – however, if the remaining kidney is hydronephrotic, then specialist renal advice should be sought prior to neonatal discharge.

ANTIBIOTIC PROPHYLAXIS

Prophylactic antibiotics are recommended if further evaluation is planned as we know the risk of UTI is highest during the first year of life.

INVESTIGATIONS

Ultrasound Scan

For those with mild dilatation, renal ultrasound may be the only imaging required for long-term follow up with emphasis on the size of the renal pelvis.

Micturating Cystourethrogram (MCUG)

If there are concerns about bladder outlet obstruction (as in posterior urethral valves), urgent MCUG prior to hospital discharge is advised (Fig. 21.5).

Functional Imaging

Functional kidney assessment with either 99mTc MAG3 (mercaptoacetyltriglycine) or 99mTc DMSA (dimercaptosuccinic acid) is not indicated for children with mild dilatation.

A MAG3 study is recommended if significant upper tract dilatation is present. If the renal pelvis is between 15 and 20 mm in the absence of significant calyceal dilatation, a MAG3 study should be performed at 3 to 4 months of age.

(Box 21.1)
(Box 21.2)
(Box 21.3)
(Box 21.4)
(Box 21.5)

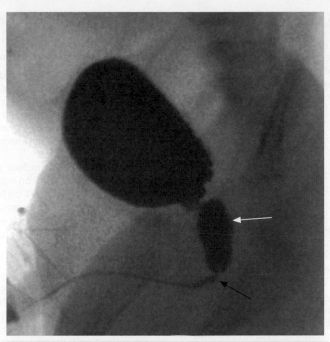

Figure 21.5 Micturating cystogram in a 3-month-old boy with a UTI. The image during voiding shows a dilated posterior urethra (white arrow) and a sudden change in calibre at the black arrow to normal calibre anterior urethra. (Courtesy Prof. Stephanie Ryan.)

Box 21.1   Key Points

Fever without an obvious source is a common symptom in young children under 2 years of age, and thus a sample of urine should be collected to rule out urinary tract infection (UTI). A clean-catch sample is the preferred method of urine collection.

Infants with a suspected UTI require hospital admission with those under 2 months receiving intravenous cefotaxime, amoxycillin and gentamicin and those 2 to 6 months of age receiving co-amoxiclav and gentamicin (guided by local bacterial sensitivities).

Infants with a poor urinary stream, oliguria or a palpable mass need an immediate ultrasound as urinary obstruction in the presence of infection is a surgical emergency.

Micturating cystourethrogram (MCUG) outlines the bladder structure and demonstrates vesico-ureteric reflux (VUR).

The MAG3 renogram provides an evaluation of the differential perfusion of the kidneys and indicates if obstruction is present. It is especially useful in the evaluation of pelvi-ureteric junction (PUJ) obstruction diagnosed antenatally.

Specialist nephro-urology advice is required if under 2 years of age with recurrent UTI, urinary obstruction is suggested or hydronephrosis, renal calculi, a single kidney or significant unilateral scarring is evident.

To measure blood pressure in children, correct cuff size equates to a cuff containing a bladder which completely encircles the forearm. BP normal ranges for children are available online.

Most hypertension in childhood is due to the circumstances under which the measurement is taken (for instance, pain or distress) or due to measurement errors, in particular inappropriate cuff size or site of cuff placement.

True hypertension in pre-pubertal children is rare and frequently secondary to an underlying cause which should be sought.

Transient proteinuria may be due to fever, stress, exercise and hypovolaemia. Persistent proteinuria is an important indicator of significant renal pathology and requires an in-depth evaluation to find a cause.

Proteinuria, hypoalbuminemia, oedema and hyperlipidemia are the key features of nephrotic syndrome. Over 90 per cent respond to oral prednisolone. About 80 per cent of children with minimal change disease will relapse, and if they have more than two relapses over a 6-month period, it is regarded as frequent relapses.

Urinary tract infection is the most common identifiable cause of gross haematuria. Recurrent painless gross haematuria is often seen with IgA nephropathy and a concurrent upper respiratory illness.

Haematuria in IgA nephritis occurs **_with_** infection, and haematuria with postinfectious GN occurs **_after_** the infection has resolved. The findings of red blood cells (RBC) casts in the urine and whether the urine dipstick is +2 or more for protein both point to a glomerular cause.

Gross haematuria appearing 2 to 4 weeks after a febrile illness is suggestive of postinfectious glomerulonephritis. Typically, a school-aged child presents with haematuria, oliguria, hypertension and renal insufficiency.

In terms of antenatal hydronephrosis, an urgent neonatal referral is indicated if there is evidence of severe bilateral antenatal hydronephrosis, no urine is passed within 12 h of birth or if the bladder is palpable at birth (possibly posterior urethral valves), or if there is a maternal history of oligohydramnios.

Box 21.2   Urinary Tract Infection

A 3-month-old presents with poor feeding, irritability and low-grade fever. There is nothing of note on clinical examination, but a clean-catch urine sample shows significant pyuria, and the culture reveals pure growth of *Escherichia coli*. He is admitted for intravenous antibiotics for 48 h. His fever settles within that time, and he is discharged home on oral antibiotics. His renal ultrasound is normal, and he is booked for a micturating cystourethrogram.

Clinical Pearls

The above scenario is very frequent as urinary tract infection (UTI) has a prevalence of 5 per cent among febrile children from birth to 24 months of age.

Collecting urine from infants and young children is often challenging. Recent studies have demonstrated that voiding stimulation techniques performed for 5 min, such as bladder–lumbar manoeuvres, can expedite clean-catch collection.

The most practical strategy in a general practice setting is to obtain a urine specimen in children with unexplained fever and to initiate antibiotic treatment in those who have a positive leucocyte esterase or nitrite test pending the return of urine culture results.

Infants under 6 months of age with a suspected UTI require hospital admission. Those under 2 months receiving intravenous cefotaxime, amoxycillin and gentamicin, and those 2 to 6 months of age receiving co-amoxiclav and gentamicin, according to local bacterial sensitivities.

Those in the age group of 6 months to 2 years who are systemically well can be safely managed at home on an adequate dose of oral co-amoxiclav or an appropriate cephalosporin determined by local sensitivities.

Children 2 to 12 years of age should be managed in primary care with an adequate dose of oral co-amoxiclav or an oral cephalosporin. Imaging is generally not required for this age group.

Interpretation of Investigations

All infants and children admitted with UTI should have a renal ultrasound performed during admission. MCUG is recommended in infants under 6 months of age.

Age under 3 months at presentation, male gender, recurrent infection, strong family history of reflux nephropathy or known abnormalities of antenatal imaging suggestive of reflux are all indications for MCUG.

Indications for DMSA include pyelonephritis or significant anatomical abnormalities on initial ultrasound, renal size discrepancy of more than 1 cm between left and right kidneys, or the suspicion of evolving renal scarring on a follow-up renal ultrasound. MAG3 renogram is especially useful in the evaluation of pelvic-ureteric junction (PUJ) obstruction diagnosed antenatally.

Pitfalls to Avoid

Ask specifically about the urine stream in males. Consider posterior urethral valves if a history of a poor stream is given. Posterior urethral valves may present with UTI, acute renal failure and severe biochemical disturbance with hyponatraemia and hyperkalaemia.

Obtaining a clean-catch urine sample is the optimal method of urine collection; bag specimens should be avoided.

Due to the risk of procedurally induced urosepsis, MCUG should be scheduled for when the infant is over 3 months of age unless there are concerns about obstruction (such as posterior urethral valves). MCUG should not be performed in children under 3 months of age without IV antibiotic prophylaxis.

MCUG should not be performed in a child over 3 months without oral antibiotic cover at treatment dose for 48 h following the procedure.

Box 21.3   Nephrotic Syndrome in a Toddler

A 3-year-old boy presents with a 5-day history of puffiness around his eyes most notable in the morning. He was seen by his family doctor, and an antihistamine was prescribed as it was initially thought to be an allergic reaction. He reattended 4 days later with the same symptom in addition to scrotal swelling and abdominal distension. His examination showed him to have significant periorbital oedema, marked ascites and bilateral scrotal oedema. His urinalysis was +4 for protein and, following admission, his serum albumin was noted to be markedly low and his urinary output dropped to less than 0.5 mL/kg/24 h postadmission.

He was commenced on oral prednisolone, which helped resolve his proteinuria within 3 weeks. However, he had a recurrence of similar symptoms 3 months later wherein urinalysis for protein was +3 for 3 consecutive days.

Clinical Pearls

In the early stages, periorbital puffiness can make confusion with an allergic reaction quite possible. Always check the urine for protein Proteinuria is usually detected by means of a dipstick test and may be transient, orthostatic or persistent.

The defining features of nephrotic syndrome are proteinuria, hypoalbuminemia, oedema and hyperlipidemia. The hallmark of minimal change disease is the total clearing of proteinuria with oral prednisolone therapy, usually within 10 to 21 days.

About 80 per cent of children with minimal change disease will relapse and are defined as having frequent relapse if they suffer more than two relapses over a 6-month period. For those

with frequent relapses, second-line therapy is often needed; options include cyclophosphamide, cyclosporin, tacrolimus, mycophenolate, levamisole and rituximab.

Interpretation of Investigations

Urinalysis will show +3 or +4 proteinuria. Microscopic haematuria may be present but no red cell casts are seen. Serum albumin levels are low, and serum cholesterol levels are elevated. Renal biopsy is rarely indicated as over 90 per cent respond to oral prednisolone.

Pitfalls to Avoid

Complications of nephrotic syndrome include infection (such as spontaneous bacterial peritonitis), thrombosis (both arterial and venous) and hypovolaemia with acute renal impairment and associated oliguria (as in the case scenario above). Spontaneous bacterial peritonitis occurs in those who have significant ascites and is most often due to *Streptococcus pneumoniae*.

Frequent relapses requiring further courses of prednisolone are common. Therefore, a nephrology referral with a view to disease-modifying agents is required to avoid the toxic effects of frequent steroid courses.

Avoid diuretic therapy, instead opting for intravenous salt-poor albumin treatment. Marked oedema, cold peripheries and oliguria all indicate hypovolaemia and may lead to acute renal impairment with a poor urinary output.

Box 21.4   Haematuria

A 7-year-old presents with a recent sore throat and now has painless macroscopic haematuria. He has had no previous episodes of haematuria. There is no family history of either deafness or renal disease. His examination shows that he is well grown and that his chest and abdominal examinations are normal. His blood pressure is elevated at 140/90. His urine is described as cola-coloured, and his urinalysis shows evidence of red blood cell casts. C3 complement levels are tested and found to be reduced.

Clinical Pearls

Painful haematuria is indicative of a source in the lower urinary tract with urinary tract infection being most likely.

Painless gross haematuria is seen with IgA nephropathy and linked to a concurrent upper respiratory illness. Recurrent episodes of gross haematuria during an intercurrent viral illness followed by a complete resolution within a few days are typically seen in IgA nephropathy. Renal biopsy will demonstrate IgA immune deposits in the mesangium of the glomeruli.

Haematuria with postinfectious glomerulonephritis (GN) occurs **after** the infection has resolved, as in this case.

A school-aged child with postinfectious GN typically presents with haematuria, oliguria, hypertension and acute renal insufficiency. Postinfectious GN is most likely due to *Group A Streptococcus.*

Treatment is geared at treating hypertension. Most acute complications of postinfectious GN relate to hypertension and may include hypertensive encephalopathy, seizures and left heart failure. Overall, over 95 per cent of children with postinfectious GN make a complete recovery.

Interpretation of Investigations

Evidence of recent streptococcal infection (a positive throat swab for group A streptococcal (GAS) is helpful but anti streptolysin O titre (ASOT) titres can give variable results.

In almost all cases, the C3 complement is low at presentation and returns to normal 6 to 12 weeks later.

Pitfalls to Avoid

The key differential diagnosis is IgA nephropathy where the C3 complement will be normal.

A low C3 complement (returning to normal after 6 to 12 weeks) and the presence of red blood cell casts are the key findings in postinfectious GN. ASOT titres may be variable.

The C3 complement remains low in lupus nephritis or membranoproliferative GN. C3 and C4 complement levels both remain low in lupus nephritis, whereas the C3 remains low and C4 is normal in membranoproliferative GN.

Alport's syndrome is suggested by a family history of renal disease progressing to chronic renal failure with associated deafness and restriction to males. Female carriers may just have microscopic haematuria. Renal biopsy provides the definitive diagnosis in Alport's syndrome.

Box 21.5   Acute Kidney Injury Following an Episode of Gastroenteritis

A 4-year-old boy presents with a 3-day history of bloody diarrhoea and abdominal cramps. The history given was that he had been at a barbeque and consumed a hamburger and sausages several days prior to his presentation. He has a noticeable pallor and looks quite unwell with obvious bruising. He is referred to a hospital where a stool culture is performed and is found positive for *Escherichia coli* O157:H7. Blood tests including a full blood count, blood film, and urea and creatinine are also requested.

Clinical Pearls

Acute kidney injury (AKI) is an acute decline in renal function characterised by an increase in blood urea and creatinine values, often with accompanying hyperkalaemia, metabolic acidosis and hypertension. AKI may be prerenal (as in septic shock or severe gastroenteritis with dehydration), intrinsic (as in haemolytic uraemic syndrome) and postrenal (best exemplified by posterior urethral valves in newborns).

The classical triad for haemolytic uremic syndrome (HUS) is microangiopathic haemolytic anaemia, thrombocytopaenia and acute kidney injury (AKI). HUS is the leading cause of intrinsic AKI in children with a peak incidence occurring before 5 years of age.

E. coli O157:H7 infection can be acquired by eating undercooked contaminated minced beef. Other possible sources include drinking contaminated water, eating contaminated vegetables or having direct contact with infected animals. Just 10 to 15 per cent of *E. coli* O157:H7 infected children develop HUS.

Three to 5 per cent of children with acute HUS die and up to one-third of survivors may have long-term morbidity.

In children with confirmed *E. coli* O157:H7 infection, simple measures such as maintenance of adequate hydration and the avoidance of drugs such as antibiotics, non-steroidal anti-inflammatory drugs (NSAIDs) and anti-diarrhoeal agents can have a positive effect.

Atypical HUS needs to be considered if there had been no preceding bloody diarrhoea or if prior pneumococcal disease has occurred.

Intravenous furosemide is helpful in inducing diuresis in HUS. Try to maintain a neutral fluid balance by replacing both insensible losses and measured losses. Consult with your regional nephrology service for consideration of dialysis. Red cell and platelet transfusions may be required in the acute phase.

About 50 per cent of children require either haemodialysis or peritoneal dialysis. Current evidence suggests that neither modality is superior to the other.

Interpretation of Investigations

A full blood count may show anaemia with leucocytosis and thrombocytopaenia. A blood film will show red blood cells fragments (Fig. 21.6).

A significantly raised serum creatinine and urea will be seen.

A raised unconjugated bilirubin, raised lactate dehydrogenase (LDH), and low haptoglobins all point to haemolytic anaemia.

Continued

Box 21.5 Acute Kidney Injury Following an Episode of Gastroenteritis – cont'd

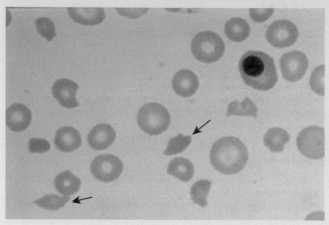

Figure 21.6 Peripheral blood film. Note the absence of platelets and the presence of nucleated erythrocyte and schistocytes (arrows) consistent with a microangiopathic process. (Reproduced with permission from Schneidewend, R., Epperla, N., & Friedman, K. D. (2018). Thrombotic thrombocytopenic purpura and the hemolytic uremic syndromes. In R. Hoffman, E. J. Benz, H. Heslop, Silberstein, L. E., Weitz, J., & Anastasi, J. (Eds.), *Hematology: Basic principles and practice* (7th ed., pp. 1984–2000). Elsevier.)

A stool culture may *show E. coli* O157:H7 (responsible for 80 per cent of cases in the UK), other Shiga toxin-producing *E. coli* serotypes or *Shigella dysenteriae*.

Pitfalls to Avoid

Avoid antibiotics and anti-diarrhoeal agents in children with gastroenteritis who have a positive stool culture for *E. coli* O157:H7. Nonsteroidal anti-inflammatory agents should likewise be avoided.

Atypical HUS, which is much less common (10 per cent of cases of HUS), has no preceding bloody diarrhoea, a poor prognosis with death or dialysis-dependent renal failure in up to 50 per cent of cases. Plasma exchange is recommended but many suffer a relapse. Eculizumab is a humanised monoclonal antibody against C5 complement and shows both efficacy and a good safety profile in atypical HUS.

▶ **Video on the topic Urinary tract infection is available online at Elsevier eBooks+.**

Key References

Kaufman, J., Knight, A. J., Bryant, P. A., Babl, F. E., & Dalziel, K. (2020). Liquid gold: the cost-effectiveness of urine sample collection methods for young precontinent children. *Archives of Disease in Childhood, 105*(3), 253–259. https://doi.org/10.1136/archdischild-2019-317561.

Lande, M.B., & Batisky, D.L. (2019). New American Academy of Pediatrics Hypertension Guideline. *Hypertension. 73*(1), 31–32. https://doi.org/10.1161/HYPERTENSIONAHA.118.11819.

Platt, C., Larcombe, J., Dudley, J., McNulty, C., Banerjee, J., Gyoffry, G., et al. (2015). Implementation of NICE guidance on urinary tract infections in children in primary and secondary care. *Acta Paediatrica (Oslo, Norway: 1992), 104*(6), 630–637. https://doi.org/10.1111/apa.12979.

Ronco, C., Bellomo, R., & Kellum, J. A. (2019). Acute kidney injury. *Lancet, 394*(10212), 1949–1964. https://doi.org/10.1016/S0140-6736(19)32563-2.

Singh, C., Jones, H., Copeman, H., & Sinha, M. D. (2017). Fifteen-minute consultation: the child with systemic arterial hypertension. *Archives of Disease in Childhood. Education and Practice Edition, 102*(1), 2–7. https://doi.org/10.1136/archdischild-2014-306487.

Sreedharan, R. (2018). Proteinuria. In R. M. Kleigman, P. S. Lye, B. Bordini, H. Toth, & D. Basel (Eds.), *Nelson pediatric symptom-based diagnosis* (pp. 312–320). Elsevier.

Walsh, P. R., & Johnson, S. (2018). Treatment and management of children with haemolytic uraemic syndrome. *Archives of Disease in Childhood, 103*(3), 285–291. https://doi.org/10.1136/archdischild-2016-311377.

Online References

Durnin, S., & Children's Health Ireland (2016, July). *Vulvovaginitis: Diagnosis and management in prepubertal girls (Reference: VDMPG-07-2016-SDGCSHCBGORNOSEB-V1)*. Department of Emergency Medicine. https://www.olchc.ie/healthcare-professionals/clinical-guidelines/vulvovaginitis.pdf.

Gobin, A., Blackburn, C., & Children's Health Ireland (2018), November). *Haematuria: diagnosis and management in the ED (Document Reference: H-10-2018-CBMSTBRM-V2)*. Department of Emergency Medicine. https://www.olchc.ie/healthcare-professionals/clinical-guidelines/haematuria.pdf.

National Heart, Lung, and Blood Institute. (2007, May). *A pocket guide to blood pressure measurement in children – From the National High Blood Pressure Education Program Working Group on High Blood Pressure in Children and Adolescents (NIH Publication No. 07-5268)*. U.S. Department of Health and Human Services, National Institutes of Health. https://www.nhlbi.nih.gov/files/docs/bp_child_pocket.pdf.

National Heart, Lung, and Blood Institute. (n.d.). *Blood pressure levels for boys and girls by age and height percentile*. U.S. Department of Health and Human Services, National Institutes of Health. https://www.nhlbi.nih.gov/files/docs/guidelines/child_tbl.pdf

National High Blood Pressure Education Program. (2005, May). The *Fourth report on the diagnosis, evaluation, and treatment of high blood pressure in children and adolescents (NIH Publication No. 05-5267)*. U.S. Department of Health and Human Services, National Institutes of Health, National Heart, Lung, and Blood Institute. https://www.nhlbi.nih.gov/files/docs/resources/heart/hbp_ped.pdf.

National Institute for Health and Care Excellence. (2018, October 31). *Urinary tract infection in under 16s: diagnosis and management*. Clinical guideline [CG54] https://www.nice.org.uk/guidance/cg54.

RCPCH Hypertension. https://www.olchc.ie/healthcare-professionals/clinical-guidelines/haematuria.pdf

22 *Neurodisability*

LOUISE BAKER and KEVIN DUNNE

In this chapter, we will address the major conditions causing neurodisability and their management, including the use of multidisciplinary teams. The most common cause of childhood-onset lifelong physical disability is cerebral palsy, which will be discussed alongside important but less frequently seen conditions.

Cerebral Palsy

The most widely used definition of cerebral palsy (CP) is that of Rosenbaum et al. (2007), which describes a group of permanent disorders of the development of <u>movement and posture</u> causing activity limitation attributed to <u>non-progressive</u> disturbances that occurred in the <u>developing foetal or infant brain</u>. As Rosenbaum points out 10 years later, cerebral palsy remains a concept rather than a disease entity.

Motor disorders of cerebral palsy may be accompanied by disturbances of sensation, cognition, communication and behaviour. Epilepsy and secondary musculoskeletal problems may also occur.

The diagnosis of CP is clinical with a delay in motor milestones associated with either the presence of abnormal movements or high or low muscle tone, leading to excessive stiffness (termed spasticity) or floppiness.

CP has an incidence of 1.44 to 1.77 per 1000 live births (recent figures from the Australian CP Register) and has diminished over time from previous rates of two to three per 1000 live births reflecting improved perinatal care. Preterms and infants of very low birth weight are at greater risk as opposed to term infants.

Most CP cases are prenatal and are due to an insult or injury to the developing brain in utero, with just 10 per cent being attributed to perinatal asphyxia. Postnatal therapeutic hypothermia can lessen the adverse neurodevelopmental outcome. Postnatal causes of CP include neonatal meningitis and abusive head trauma during the first 2 years of life.

It is important to actively screen for visual, hearing and cognitive impairments and behavioural issues in CP. One should also treat spasticity and other movement disorders. Active surveillance for orthopaedic deformities such as hip migration and scoliosis is also recommended. A proportion of children with CP have exceptional healthcare needs (Gross Motor Function Classification System *GMFCS* 4 and 5).

Diagnosis of Cerebral Palsy

Delayed motor milestones associated with alterations in muscle tone is characteristically seen. The diagnosis is a clinical one following a detailed antenatal and perinatal history, a full developmental assessment and a full neurological examination. Key points arousing concern include poor head control at 6 months of age, an infant being unable to sit unsupported by 9 months of age, a child not walking by 18 months and an obvious hand preference before 18 months. While the insult or injury to the brain is static, the clinical signs and tone abnormalities evolve over time. Once the diagnosis is being considered, a detailed multidisciplinary assessment via the early intervention team should be coordinated, and an MRI brain scan ordered.

Physical Examination

The relevant examination includes measurement of the head circumference and a full neurological examination to

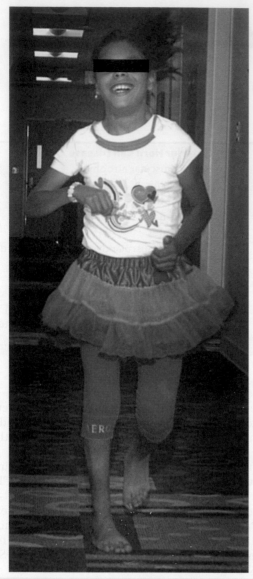

Figure 22.1   Child with spastic hemiplegia. (Reproduced with permission from Niedzwecki, C. M., Thomas, S. P., & Schwabe, A. L. (2021). Cerebral palsy. In D. X. Cifu (Ed.), *Braddom's physical medicine and rehabilitation* (6th ed., pp. 1006–1026.e2). Elsevier – Health Sciences Division.)

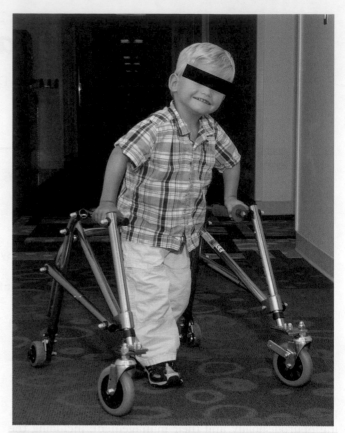

Figure 22.2   Child with spastic diplegia. (Reproduced with permission from Niedzwecki, C. M., Thomas, S. P., & Schwabe, A. L. (2021). Cerebral palsy. In D. X. Cifu (Ed.), *Braddom's physical medicine and rehabilitation* (6th ed., pp. 1006–1026.e2). Elsevier – Health Sciences Division.)

check central and peripheral tone, reflexes, plantar reflexes and cerebellar signs. Check for leg length discrepancy and examine the back to see if scoliosis is present.

GAIT ASSESSMENT

Observe the child walking and note characteristic patterns. Assessment of gait (if able to mobilise) is important to look for a hemiplegic gait (Fig. 22.1) or scissoring of the lower limbs due to spastic diplegia (Fig. 22.2).

Ask the child to walk firstly on their toes and then their heels.

Always observe the upper limb posture during gait as this may be abnormal.

Ask the child to walk on the outsides of their feet (the Fog test) to bring out signs of subtle hemiplegia if present.

Ask the child to hop on one foot and then the other.

Always examine the lower back and inspect feet for evidence of pes cavus.

Tone

Check central truncal tone. Check the limb tone by passive movements of the upper and lower limbs at each joint. The lower limb tone may also be assessed by rapid movements of both lower limbs called 'log-rolling', dropping the legs and ankle plantar and dorsiflexion.

Deep Tendon Reflexes. Check upper and lower limb reflexes with reinforcement if necessary. Relax the muscles and remove gravity, then use a swinging motion of the patellar hammer to obtain the reflexes. If hyperreflexia is obtained, then clonus may be present.

Plantar Reflexes/Babinski Reflexes. Check the plantar reflexes noting that the plantar responses may normally be upgoing up until 18 months of age. Use a wooden spatula or thumb and move up the lateral side of the foot and then below the toes. Never use the pointed end of a patellar tendon hammer in children to obtain the plantar reflex, as this may cut the skin.

Cerebellar signs

Check speech for dysarthria (phrases like British constitution), eyes for nystagmus, limb coordination (upper limb check finger–nose test and past-pointing, lower limb

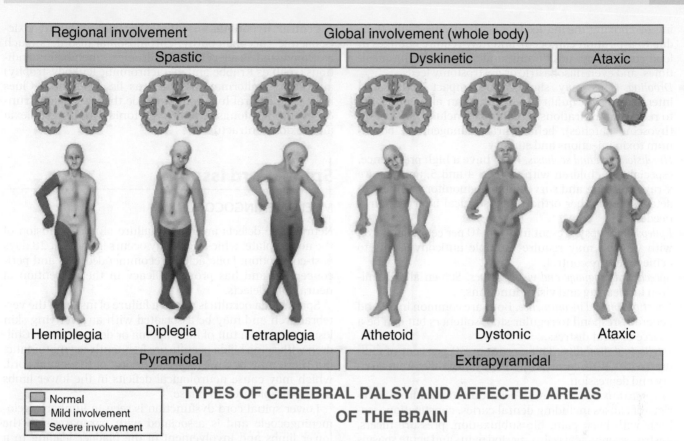

Regional involvement	Global involvement (whole body)	
Spastic	Dyskinetic	Ataxic

Hemiplegia   Diplegia   Tetraplegia   Athetoid   Dystonic   Ataxic

Pyramidal	Extrapyramidal

☐ Normal
☐ Mild involvement
■ Severe involvement

TYPES OF CEREBRAL PALSY AND AFFECTED AREAS OF THE BRAIN

Figure 22.3 Classification of cerebral palsy. (Reproduced with permission. Redrawn from Pellegrino, L. (1997). Cerebral palsy. In M.L. Batshaw (Ed.), *Children with disabilities* (4th ed.). Brookes Publishing.)

heel–shin test and foot-tapping), unsteady gait and dysdiadokinesis (rapid alternating movements of pronation and supination at the wrist).

CLASSIFICATION OF CEREBRAL PALSY

The Surveillance of Cerebral Palsy in Europe Collaboration describes CP as being either unilateral (as seen in hemiplegic CP) or bilateral (both spastic diplegia or quadriplegia). In spastic diplegia, all four limbs may be affected, but the legs are much more severely affected than the arms. All four limbs are severely affected in spastic quadriplegia.

The four main types of CP include spastic, dyskinetic, ataxic or mixed (Fig. 22.3).

In the spastic type, there is an upper motor pattern in the affected limbs with hypertonia, hyperreflexia and an upgoing plantar response. There may be clasp knife rigidity where increased tone suddenly 'gives' on movement.

In the dyskinetic type, there are uncontrolled and involuntary movements with either dystonia or choreoathetosis where uncontrolled writhing and jerky movements are seen.

In the ataxic type, there is overall hypotonia with a lack of control over movements.

In the mixed type, a combination of the above is seen.

The Gross Motor Function Classification System (GMFCS) divides children with CP into one of **five levels** based

on ability to mobilise and reflects the severity of motor impairment:

- Level 1 – walks without limitations
- Level 2 – limitations in walking long distances, using stairs and balancing
- Level 3 – walks using a hand-held mobility device
- Level 4 – limited self-mobility requiring a wheelchair
- Level 5 – only mobilises using a wheelchair and has poor head control

MANAGING CP

Cerebral palsy management should focus on increasing activity, and management programmes should be individualised. Management of spasticity should facilitate alleviating pain and controlling spasms as well as improving mobility.

Features of CP and recommended treatment strategies:

- *Reducing spasticity and preventing contractures.* Consider physiotherapy, ankle–foot orthoses (AFOs) and/or oral baclofen. Botulinum neurotoxin type A may be helpful for localised spasticity, especially in the lower limbs. Selective dorsal rhizotomy (SDR) and surgery with tendon releases may relieve severe spasticity in selected cases. Intrathecal baclofen may be indicated for severe movement disorder management.
- *Feeding issues.* Feeding difficulties relate to GMFCS level – especially in levels 4 and 5 – and may present with cough-

ing or choking during feeds. Recurrent chest infections due to aspiration can occur and may require changes in food consistency, positioning and support during mealtimes, and even nasogastric or gastrostomy feeds.

■ *Drooling.* This may significantly impact both social interactions and quality of life and can also contribute to recurrent aspirations. Treatments include medication (hyoscine patches), behavioural management, botulinum toxin injections and surgery.

■ *Hip dislocation and scoliosis.* Both have a high prevalence, especially in children with GMFCS 4 and 5, and require x-ray screening and surveillance to monitor both and to determine whether orthopaedic surgical intervention is needed.

■ *Epilepsy.* Epilepsy present in 30 to 40 per cent of children with CP and may require multiple anticonvulsants to achieve seizure control.

■ *Speech and language and visual issues.* Screen all CP children for hearing and vision functions.

■ *Constipation and incontinence.* Both are common in CP and generally respond to regular stool softeners but can be a source of great distress.

■ *Intellectual disability.* This occurs in 30 per cent of children with CP. Children with CP may also suffer from anxiety and depression.

■ *Sleep disturbance.* This may arise due to pain from a variety of causes including dental caries, constipation, scoliosis with back pain, hip subluxation, pressure ulcers, gastro-oesophageal reflux, period pains and acute spasms relating to spasticity.

Assessment of the Floppy Infant

Tone is defined as the passive resistance to stretch and is divided into both truncal and peripheral tone. Tone varies in the sense that infants are often quite hypotonic during sleep, meaning that the optimal time to assess tone is about 30 minutes prior to the next feed. Tone is also affected by head position; the infant's head should therefore be in the midline during a tone assessment.

Truncal tone is assessed by examining for head lag in vertical suspension and in ventral suspension. Head lag should disappear by 4 months of age. Perform vertical suspension to assess both general and shoulder girdle tone.

Peripheral tone is examined in upper and lower limbs. In the upper limbs, assess peripheral tone by abducting the shoulders, flexing and extending the elbows, and pronation and supination at the wrists. In the lower limbs, assess tone by abducting the hips, flexion and extension of the knees, and dorsiflexion and plantarflexion at the ankles. Low tone or hypotonia is best subdivided into central and peripheral types with 80 to 90 per cent of hypotonia in infants being central in origin.

Peripheral hypotonia is caused by problems in the spinal cord, anterior horn cell, peripheral nerve and neuromuscular junction. The key distinguishing features are the presence of weakness, marked hypotonia and reduced or absent deep tendon reflexes. The affected infant has diminished spontaneous movements, a frog-like posture and fasciculations may be evident.

Central hypotonia in infants is caused by hypoxic-ischaemic encephalopathy, chromosomal disorders (such as Down and Prader–Willi syndromes), metabolic conditions (such as Krabbe and metachromatic leukodystrophy) and brain malformations (such as lissencephaly). Clues indicating central hypotonia include the presence of truncal hypotonia alongside limb hypertonia with hyperreflexia and flexion contractures.

Spinal Cord Issues

MYELOMENINGOCOELE

Neural tube defects are due to failure of normal fusion of the neural plate, which normally occurs in the first 28 days post-conception. Folic acid is recommended pre- and peri-conception and has proven efficacy in the prevention of neural tube defects.

Spina bifida occulta is due to a failure of fusion of the vertebral arch and may be associated with an overlying skin lesion (such as a tuft of hair, lipoma or dermal sinus). Children with spina bifida occulta are frequently asymptomatic, but there may be underlying tethering of the spinal cord, which may cause neurological deficits in the lower limbs during a rapid growth phase.

Lower spinal cord dysfunction is seen in lumbar myelomeningocoele and is associated with paraparesis of the lower limbs and involvement of the bladder leading to a neurogenic bladder and a patulous anus if S2, S3 and S4 nerve roots are affected. The affected lower limbs will show a lower motor neurone pattern with hypotonia, hyporeflexia and plantar reflexes either reduced or absent. Variable weakness also occurs.

Myelomeningocoele affects about one in 1000 pregnancies and is often picked up antenatally. The spinal defect is obvious at birth (Fig. 22.4) and the associated presence of the Arnold–Chiari malformation leads to associated hydrocephalous in most cases. Management of myelomeningocoele requires a multidisciplinary approach with a paediatric neurosurgeon (closure of the defect soon after birth and insertion of a ventriculoperitoneal shunt if required), a paediatric urologist, a paediatrician with expertise in managing spina bifida, a paediatric orthopaedic surgeon (if associated talipes, hip dislocation or scoliosis are present) and a team of health and social care professionals.

The back lesion in myelomeningocoele is usually closed soon after birth but many have significant neurological deficits in the lower limbs. These deficits necessitate physiotherapy input and splints, and many will also require a walking aid or wheelchair for mobility. The neurogenic bladder is managed by intermittent catheterisation with regular urology review for renal function, hypertension and infection. Constipation is frequently seen and requires laxatives and the intermittent use of suppositories as instructed.

Children with a spinal lesion above L3 are unlikely to walk, often develop scoliosis, have associated hydrocephalous requiring a shunt, and have issues relating to a neurogenic bladder.

A specialist multidisciplinary team best delivers care for all children with myelomeningocoele.

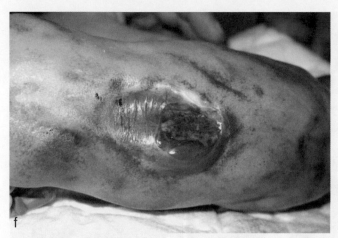

Figure 22.4 Myelomeningocoele, gross neural tube defect (NTDs) result from improper embryonic neural tube closure. (Reproduced with permission from Bourgeot, P., Houfflin-Debarge, V., Robert, Y., Ardaens, Y., Bigot, J., Coulon, C., et al. (2021). In V. Robin-Prevallee (Ed.), *Echographie en pratique obstetricale* (6th ed.). Elsevier Masson.)

TRANSVERSE MYELITIS

Transverse myelitis is rare and is associated with both acute weakness and hypotonia. Key characteristics include impairment of bowel and bladder function and of a definite sensory level. Initially, deep tendon reflexes are reduced, and they later become exaggerated with clonus. Diagnosis is by MRI and lumbar puncture (mild pleocytosis and elevated CSF protein).

Anterior Horn Cell Disease

SPINAL MUSCULAR ATROPHY

Spinal muscle atrophy (SMA) types 0 to 4 are characterised by degeneration in the anterior horn cells (Fig. 22.5). SMA is inherited in an autosomal recessive fashion. Type 1 SMA presents very early in life and signs include marked hypotonia with weakness and a flaccid posture with an alert face accompanied by tongue and muscle fasciculations. Over 95 per cent have homozygous deletion of *survival motor neurone 1 (SMN1)* gene, which is now the preferred diagnostic test. Nusinersen is a new therapy to improve weakness in SMA with promising results in clinical trials.

POLIOMYELITIS

Poliomyelitis is a contagious disease caused by poliovirus. A small proportion of affected individuals will develop an asymmetric flaccid paralysis, typically in the lower limbs caused by involvement of the anterior horn cells followed by muscle atrophy. Thankfully, vaccination programmes are effective in eradicating poliomyelitis.

Neuropathies

GUILLAIN–BARRE SYNDROME (GBS)

GBS is an acute demyelinating polyneuropathy that follows an acute viral illness or gastroenteritis. Typical features include symmetrical ascending weakness with areflexia and subsequent weakness of the respiratory muscles leading to respiratory compromise. Common presentations of GBS include acute difficulty in walking, rising from the floor, climbing stairs or a refusal to weight bear. The rare Miller Fisher variant of GBS has presenting features of ophthalmoplegia, areflexia and ataxia without overt weakness.

After day 7 of the illness, CSF analysis shows a high protein. MRI of the spine (with Gadolinium) demonstrates nerve root and peripheral nerve enhancement in over 90 per cent of cases. The most effective treatment in children is immune modulation using intravenous gamma globulin.

Myopathies

DUCHENNE MUSCULAR DYSTROPHY (DMD) AND BECKER'S MUSCULAR DYSTROPHY (BMD)

DMD and BMD are both due to mutations in the *dystrophin* gene. Both are inherited in an X-linked recessive fashion. In DMD, an absence of dystrophin in muscle is seen. Most boys with DMD come to medical attention with a history of being slower in walking or running than their peers. Consider DMD in any boy who is not walking by 18 months of age, or having trouble climbing stairs. The classical clinical signs are the Gower sign (difficulty rising from the floor), which is typically evident by 3 years of age, and calf pseudohypertrophy (due to proliferation of fat and collagen) (Fig. 22.6). Many also experience language delay and cognitive issues.

With the use of oral steroids, wheelchair dependence may be delayed until 9 to 14 years of age. Cardiomyopathy, kyphoscoliosis and respiratory muscle failure all contribute to cardiopulmonary insufficiency. Becker's is a milder form and has a variable age of onset. Calf pseudohypertrophy and proximal muscle weakness are other features in Becker's, and those affected may also eventually exhibit a positive Gower sign. Both forms of muscular dystrophy show markedly elevated CPK levels (up to 30,000 IU/l) with mutations in the *dystrophin* gene. Muscle biopsy is now rarely required for diagnosis.

CONGENITAL MYOTONIC DYSTROPHY

Congenital myotonic dystrophy is rare and presents with marked hypotonia and weakness at birth, facial weakness, a carp-like mouth, congenital joint contractures and feeding issues. There is often a history of polyhydramnios in utero. Genetic testing shows the trinucleotide repeat expansion of the *DMPK* gene.

NEUROMUSCULAR JUNCTION

Myasthenia gravis is a disorder of neuromuscular transmission (Fig. 22.7) that leads to fatigue of skeletal muscles and fluctuating weakness. Transplacental transfer of acetylcholine receptor antibodies from a mother with myasthenia gravis to their infant leads to transient neonatal myasthenia. These infants are often strikingly hypotonic soon after birth with associated feeding issues. Complete

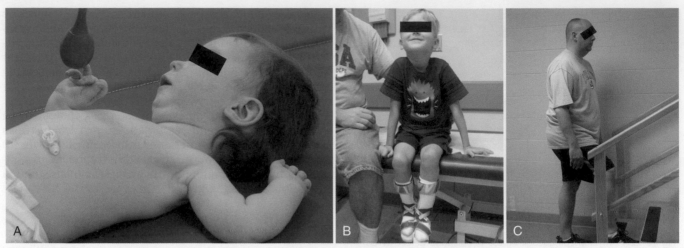

Figure 22.5 Subtypes of proximal spinal muscular atrophy (SMA) related to *SMN1* deletion. (A) SMA type 1, the most usual form, has onset before 6 months of age and the ability to sit upright is never achieved. (B) SMA type 2 has onset between 6 and 18 months and the ability to sit independently, but not stand, is achieved. SMA type 3 is associated with onset after 18 months and patients can stand or walk at least temporarily. (C) SMA type 4 is the mildest subtype with onset after 30 years of age. Type 0 with onset before birth is not shown. (Reproduced with permission from Cifu, D. X. (2021). *Braddom's physical medicine and rehabilitation* (6th ed.). Elsevier – Health Sciences Division.)

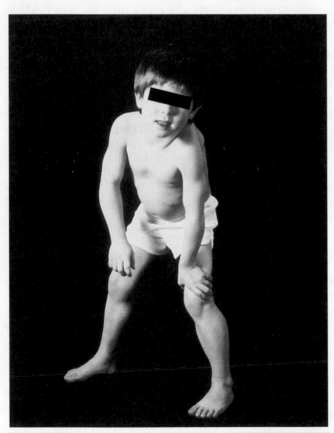

Figure 22.6 Duchenne muscular dystrophy (*Xp21* dystrophy). There is pseudohypertrophy of the weak muscles (e.g. the calves and deltoids). The child is 'climbing up himself' with legs widely placed as he gets up from the sitting position to the standing position. This is Gowers' sign. (Reproduced with permission from Glynn, M., & Drake, W. M. (2012). *Hutchison's Clinical methods: An integrated Approach to clinical practice* (23rd ed.). Elsevier.)

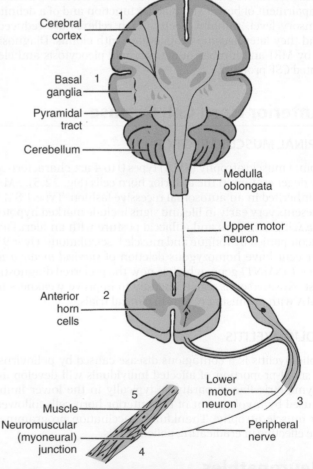

Figure 22.7 Site of origin for neuromuscular disorders. 1, Cerebral palsy; 2, poliomyelitis, spinal muscular atrophy; 3, mononeuropathies, polyneuropathies; 4, myasthenia gravis, neurotoxic disorders; 5, muscular dystrophies. (Reproduced with permission from Hockenberry, M. J., & Wilson, D. (2019). *Wong's nursing care of infants and children* (11th ed.). Elsevier.)

recovery takes place within 4 to 6 weeks. The other forms of myasthenia gravis in children (congenital myasthenic syndromes and juvenile myasthenia gravis) are incredibly rare and present a diagnostic challenge.

Infant botulism presents include poor sucking, constipation, a weak cry, hypotonia, ptosis, mydriasis and bladder atony. Presentation is between 2 to 6 months of age. First symptoms are apparent in the face and bulbar region. *Clostridium botulinum* is found in honey, corn syrup, terrapins and soil.

Roles of Multidisciplinary Team (MDT) Members in the Provision of Services to Children With Neurodisability

The MDT includes a paediatrician, clinical nurse specialist, physiotherapist, occupational therapist, speech and language therapist, psychologist, social worker, dietician and administrative staff. If required, child and adolescent mental health services (CAMHS) should be available to support children and families where there are mental health issues in a shared care model.

The paediatrician plays a key role in the initial assessment and in the holistic palliative care of the child or adolescent with a life-limiting condition. The clinical nurse specialist supports the family in navigating the system and helps managing acute medical concerns in the community.

Physiotherapy is vital and includes neurodevelopmental therapy, strengthening, assisted mobilisation, hydrotherapy, sensory integration, 24-hour postural management, equipment management, balance and gait re-education, fitness and endurance intervention. The role of the occupational therapist (OT) is to support specific fine motor skill development and, with the physiotherapist, postural management. The OT is also responsible for the provision of aids to help with activities of daily living. The speech and language therapist is skilled in the assessment and treatment of communication or feeding and swallowing difficulties with the aim of maximising oral intake whenever possible while minimising the risk of aspiration. The psychologist assesses the child's abilities and identifies the appropriate strategies to optimise progress. The dietician also plays a significant role. Issues that may arise include both undernutrition and overnutrition, inefficient or unsafe oral feeding, dependence on enteral or parenteral nutrition, and common symptoms such as reflux and constipation. Social workers play a vital role in supporting families and carers in the face of day-to-day challenges, including access to respite services. A central administrative support provider is a point of contact for children, families, teachers and other healthcare professionals, and is essential to all children's network disability teams.

(Box 22.1)
(Box 22.2)
(Box 22.3)
(Box 22.4)

Box 22.1 **Key Points**

Cerebral palsy (CP) is a non-progressive disorder of posture and movement attributed to disturbances in the developing brain that causes limitations in activity. Screening for visual, hearing and cognitive impairments and behavioural issues in CP is important, as is the treatment of spasticity and other movement disorders.

CP should be suspected if poor head control at 6 months of age, inability to sit unsupported by 9 months of age or to walk by 18 months or an obvious hand preference before 18 months.

The Gross Motor Function Classification System (GMFCS) divides children with CP into one of **five levels** based on ability to mobilise and reflects the severity of motor impairment.

Low tone or hypotonia is best sub-divided into central and peripheral types with 80 to 90 per cent of hypotonia in infants being central in origin. Peripheral hypotonia is caused by problems in the spinal cord, anterior horn cell, peripheral nerve and neuromuscular junction.

Neural tube defects are due to failure of normal fusion of the neural plate. This normally occurs in the first 28 days following conception.

Periconceptual folic acid is recommended and is proven to be effective in preventing neural tube defects.

Myelomeningocoele affects about one in 1000 pregnancies and is often picked up antenatally. The spinal defect is obvious at birth and presence of the Arnold–Chiari malformation leads to associated hydrocephalous in most cases. Care is best managed by a specialist multidisciplinary team for all children with myelomeningocoele.

A clear sensory level and impairment of bowel and bladder function are key characteristics in transverse myelitis.

In spinal muscular atrophy, over 95 per cent have a homozygous deletion of *survival motor neurone 1 (SMN1)* gene, which is now the preferred diagnostic test.

Guillain–Barre syndrome is characterised by symmetrical ascending weakness with areflexia and may cause respiratory compromise due to weakness of the respiratory muscles.

Most boys with Duchenne muscular dystrophy (DMD) come to attention with a history of being slower in walking or running than their peers and difficulties in rising from the floor or climbing stairs.

Congenital myotonic dystrophy is rare and presents with marked hypotonia and weakness at birth, facial weakness, a carp-like mouth, congenital joint contractures and feeding issues.

Infant botulism presents between 2 and 6 months of age with poor sucking and swallowing, constipation, a weak cry, hypotonia, ptosis, mydriasis and bladder atony.

Box 22.2   An Ex-Preterm 2-Year-Old With Spastic Diplegia

A male infant is born at 25 weeks' gestation weighing 800 g at birth. He had a 4-month stay in neonatal intensive care and has subsequent follow-up from a neurodevelopmental perspective. He did not walk until 21 months and is noted by his parents to be walking on his tiptoes at 2 years of age. Examination reveals significant hypertonia of both lower limbs with brisk deep tendon reflexes, upgoing plantars and bilateral tightening of the Achilles tendon. His brain MRI shows features consistent with periventricular leukomalacia.

Clinical Pearls

The overall prevalence of cerebral palsy (CP) in developed countries in premature infants (under 28 weeks' gestation) is 10 per cent.

The Gross Motor Functional Classification System (GMFCS) is a helpful indicator of motor function.

The aim of current multidisciplinary management of CP is to minimise the impact of secondary musculoskeletal complications.

Bilateral lower limb spasticity is usually associated with lesions in the periventricular white matter and is typically seen in ex-preterms. Most importantly, cognition is often well preserved, and epilepsy is unlikely.

In a case of spastic diplegia (such as this) the child requires orthotics, botulinum toxin injections and potentially later bilateral release of the Achilles tendon to relieve tightening.

The goals of physiotherapy, occupational therapy and speech therapy are to help the child reach their developmental potential. Therapists work through parent-delivered interventions, so support must be given to training parents and other caregivers. Therapists also provide equipment and advice for home and school to allow the child to fully participate in these settings.

Baclofen is the most used drug to tackle hypertonia. It has difficulty crossing the blood–brain barrier, and therefore may require high doses of oral medicine.

Careful clinical assessment should precede treatment with botulinum toxin.

Both preventative surgical intervention for hip subluxation and early identification of scoliosis are main objectives for the orthopaedic team.

Intrathecal baclofen pump insertion, selective dorsal rhizotomy and deep brain stimulation are only performed on selected children in specialist centres.

Other frequent co-morbidities are poor salivary control, gastro-oesophageal reflux, severe constipation and recurrent aspiration pneumonia.

Interpretation of Investigations

Brain MRI is often performed in the neonatal period but repeat imaging at 2 years of age is more dependable in predicting prognosis. Additional metabolic and genetic investigations should be pursued if the diagnosis is uncertain. Otherwise, only a brain MRI is required.

Pitfalls to Avoid

As CP is a clinical diagnosis, it is important to clearly outline your concerns to the parents and to emphasise the varied presentations and functional outcomes.

Supporting children and their families through adolescence into adulthood is essential.

The intrathecal baclofen pump is used for CP GMFCS IV–V and requires frequent refills. A sudden withdrawal, either due to pump failure or leakage from the catheter, may lead to status dystonicus. Infection at the site of insertion is another complication.

Selective dorsal rhizotomy is irreversible and long-term mobility may not be improved.

Box 22.3   A 3-Year-Old Who Has Trouble Climbing Stairs

A 3-year-old boy is referred for specialist opinion as he appears to have significant difficulties climbing stairs. His past and perinatal history is unremarkable, and he is the first born in the family. There is no family history of muscular disorders. On examination, he has prominence of both calves, normal deep tendon reflexes and a positive Gower's sign. His creatine phosphokinase (CPK) is measured and is markedly elevated at 20,000 IU/L.

Clinical Pearls

Duchenne muscular dystrophy (DMD) is a progressive and life-limiting X-linked recessive disorder due to mutations in the DMD gene resulting in reduced or absent dystrophin production. The absence of dystrophin leads to muscle fibrosis and fatty replacement of muscles with typical pseudohypertrophy.

DMD is the most frequently seen form of muscular dystrophy in children with an annual incidence of about one in 5000 live males.

Classical symptoms of DMD include frequent falls and difficulty running and climbing stairs. Boys with DMD have trouble getting up from the floor, requiring the help of their hands to push on the knees and provide sufficient momentum to get upright. This is the classical Gower's sign.

Up to 50 per cent of boys with DMD have speech delay, and intellectual disability, autism spectrum disorder and attention deficit disorder are frequent co-morbidities.

In 10 to 15 per cent of boys with DMD, an underlying nonsense mutation in the DMD gene is found, which could potentially benefit from treatment with a new agent called ataluren.

Interpretation of Investigations

In both DMD and Becker's muscular dystrophy, markedly elevated CPK levels (up to 30,000 IU/L) and mutations in the dystrophin gene are key findings in testing, and muscle biopsy is now rarely required for diagnosis.

The site of the DMD gene mutation also determines how many brain dystrophin isoforms are affected and helps explain the variability in observed brain involvement.

Pitfalls to Avoid

DMD remains relatively stable until the age of about 7 years, at which time more rapid progression becomes apparent. Most have lost independent ambulation by the age of 12 years, with a mean age of 9.5 years. Other issues include scoliosis, loss of upper limb function, respiratory insufficiency and cardiomyopathy.

Most boys with DMD previously survived into their late teens. With multidisciplinary care and the use of corticosteroids, ambulation is now maintained until a mean age of 13 to 14 years, and the mean age of survival is now the late 20s.

Progressive dilated cardiomyopathy is now a leading cause of mortality in DMD.

Box 22.4   A 2-Month-Old With a Lower Back Lesion and a Rapidly Increasing Head Circumference

A female infant is born by spontaneous vertex delivery at term to a 19-year-old primigravid mother following an unplanned pregnancy. An antenatal scan suggested a myelomeningocoele and soon after birth she was referred to a specialist paediatric neurosurgery service. She had operative closure of her L4/L5 lower back lesion on day 2 of life. Subsequently she was noted to have dribbling of urine, a patulous anus and limited movement of both lower limbs. Her head circumference was rising by over 2 cm/week, and an MRI scan showed hydrocephalous. She had a ventriculoperitoneal shunt inserted, and an uneventful postoperative recovery. She now attends for multidisciplinary review and her mother is anxious to know what the future holds.

Clinical Pearls

Up to 70 per cent of neural tube defects can be prevented by maternal periconceptional folic acid supplementation. An increase in incidence is also associated with in-utero exposure to valproic acid or carbamazepine alone, or in combination with each other or other anticonvulsants. Other risk factors include a family history of neural tube defects and maternal diabetes mellitus.

Most cases of myelomeningocoele are diagnosed antenatally and, in primigravids, elective lower segment caesarean section is the delivery method of choice.

Outcomes for myelomeningocoele have improved in terms of neurosurgical management with the advent of microsurgical techniques and the rise of a multidisciplinary team approach in a specialist service.

Surgical closure should take place in the first 48 hours of life, as delay significantly increases the risk of infection and affects neurogenic bladder prognosis.

In children with myelomeningocoele, specific cognitive disabilities and language difficulties are common and can adversely affect educational and occupational achievements and the ability to live independently.

The level of the myelomeningocoele is one of the most crucial factors that influences walking ability. Most have a good prognosis if at the level of L4 and below with a walking rate of up to 90 per cent.

On the other hand, infants with high lesions L3 and above often have a poor functional outcome and, in this group, prenatal surgery may be indicated.

About two-thirds will be able to walk, often with orthotic supports, and the remainder will require a wheelchair for mobility. Orthopaedic problems include talipes equinovarus and evolving scoliosis.

Bowel and bladder management focus on maintaining normal renal function and promoting continence to give children a good quality of life with normal attendance at school and independence in both urinary and faecal elimination. Many will require intermittent self-catheterisation and intensive treatment of constipation.

Coincident central nervous system (CNS) malformations such as Chiari II malformation, Dandy–Walker complex, and encephalocoele may lead to hydrocephalous, and thus monitoring of head growth is essential.

In infancy, hydrocephalous presents with a rapidly increasing head circumference (over 2 cm/week), irritability, vomiting, a bulging anterior fontanelle, and splaying of the sutures.

The most common type of shunt that diverts CSF from the ventricles to the peritoneal cavity is a ventriculoperitoneal shunt.

Interpretation of Investigations

Cranial ultrasound is helpful in infants with an open fontanelle, but an MRI brain scan helps elucidate the anatomy and cause of hydrocephalous. A Chiari II malformation is typically seen in myelomeningocoele.

Renal and bladder ultrasound and urodynamic studies should be done at intervals to assess the status of the urinary tract and provide a baseline for continuing assessment.

A shunt series of x-rays and an urgent CT scan should be performed if shunt malfunction is suspected.

Pitfalls to Avoid

If a myelomeningocoele is below L3, the balance of risks for both the foetus and the mother are strongly in favour of postnatal surgery ahead of foetal surgery.

Shunt malfunction, usually due to mechanical obstruction, occurs in 40 per cent of children within the first 2 years after original placement with continued risk thereafter. Suspect shunt malfunction if symptoms of irritability, headaches or vomiting occur, especially if there is no fever or contact with infection. Anticipated signs in infants include increasing head growth away from the previous centiles and a bulging anterior fontanelle. Signs in children may include upper motor neurone limb signs, papilloedema and a decreasing level of consciousness with bradycardia and hypertension. Diagnosis is by confirming increased ventricular size compared to baseline.

Shunt malfunction requires increased vigilance in parents and professionals.

The rate of shunt infection is about 5 to 9 per cent and mostly occurs within 3 months of surgery with presenting symptoms of fever, irritability, wound erythema and symptoms of shunt malfunction.

Shunt over-drainage can present acutely with the so-called slit-ventricle syndrome, in which the ventricle size is exceedingly small (slit-like) and typically presents with frequent headaches or intermittent symptoms of shunt obstruction.

Headaches are reported to some degree in most children with shunted hydrocephalous and are severe in 10 to 20 per cent.

Key References

Adzick, N. S., Thom, E. A., Spong, C. Y., Brock, J. W., 3rd, Burrows, P. K., Johnson, M. P., et al. (2011). A randomised trial of prenatal versus postnatal repair of myelomeningocele. *The New England Journal of Medicine*, 364(11), 993–1004.

Australian Cerebral Palsy Register. (2017, May 16). *AusACPDM*. https://www.ausacpdm.org.au/resources/australian-cerebral-palsy-register/.

Beuriat, P.-A., Poirot, I., Hameury, F., Szathmari, A., Rousselle, C., Sabatier, I., et al. (2018). Postnatal management of myelomeningocele: outcome with a multidisciplinary team experience. *World Neurosurgery*, 110, e24–e31.

Cadwgan, J., Goodwin, J., & Fairhurst, C. (2019). Fifteen-minute consultation: modern-day art and science of managing cerebral palsy. *Archives of Disease in Childhood Education and Practice Edition*, 104(2), 66–73.

CanChild. (n.d.). GMFCS – E&R – Gross Motor Function Classification System – Expanded & Revised. https://canchild.ca/en/resources/42-gross-motor-function-classification-system-expanded-revised-gmfcs-e-r.

Graham, H. K., Rosenbaum, P., Paneth, N., Dan, B., Lin, J.-P., Damiano, D. L., et al. (2016). Cerebral palsy. *Natural Review Disease Primers*, 2, 15082.

Kahle, K. T., Kulkarni, A. V., Limbrick, D. D., Jr., & Warf, B. C. (2016). Hydrocephalus in children. *Lancet*, 387(10020), 788–799.

Mercuri, E., Bönnemann, C. G., & Muntoni, F. (2019). Muscular dystrophies. *Lancet*, 394(10213), 2025–2038.

Mitchell, L. E., Adzick, N. S., Melchionne, J., Pasquariello, P. S., Sutton, L. N., & Whitehead, A. S. (2004). Spina bifida. *Lancet*, 364(9448), 1885–1895.

National Clinical Programme for Paediatrics and Neonatology. (2015). A National Model of Care for Paediatric Healthcare Services in Ireland. Chapter 33: Neurodisability. *Clinical Strategy and Programmes Division, Health Service Executive, Royal College of Physicians of Ireland.* https://www.hse.ie/eng/services/publications/clinical-strategy-and-programmes/paediatric-neurodisabilty.pdf.

National Institute for Health and Care Excellence. (2017, January 25). *Cerebral palsy in under 25s: assessment and management (NICE guideline NG62).* https://www.nice.org.uk/guidance/ng62.

Palisano, R., Rosenbaum, P., Walter, S., Russell, D., Wood, E., & Galuppi, B. (1997). Development and reliability of a system to classify gross motor function in children with cerebral palsy. *Developmental Medicine & Child Neurology, 39*(4), 214–223.

Peragallo, J. H. (2017). Pediatric Myasthenia Gravis. *Seminars in Pediatric Neurology, 24*(2), 116–121.

Prevalence and characteristics of children with cerebral palsy in Europe. Developmental Medicine & Child Neurology, 44(9), 633–640.

Rosenbaum, P., Paneth, N., Leviton, A., Goldstein, M., Bax, M., Damiano, D., et al. (2007). A report: the definition and classification of cerebral palsy April 2006. [published correction appears in *Developmental Medicine & Child Neurology, 49*(6), 480.]. *Developmental Medicine & Child Neurology Supplement, 109,* 8–14.

Rosenbaum, P. (2017). Cerebral palsy: is the concept still viable? *Developmental Medicine & Child Neurology, 59*(6), 564.

Sewell, M. D., Eastwood, D. M., & Wimalasundera, N. (2014). Managing common symptoms of cerebral palsy in children. *BMJ, 349,* g5474.

The Lancet (2019). Muscular dystrophy: new treatments, new hopes. *Lancet, 394*(10213), 1966.

Wood, C. L., & Cheetham, T. (2017). Treatment of Duchenne muscular dystrophy: first small steps. *Lancet, 390*(10101), 1467–1468.

23 The Child With a Rash

FIONA BROWNE

Believe it or not, the skin is the largest organ in the body. It provides many essential functions, including a barrier function, ultraviolet light protection, thermoregulation via sweat glands and vitamin D synthesis, and contains sensory nerve endings detecting touch, pain and temperature changes. The epidermis is the uppermost layer with the dermis and subcutaneous layers lying beneath.

The morphological classification of common skin eruptions in childhood can be subdivided as follows:

- **Macular** – A flat area of skin discolouration. Erythema multiforme and many viral exanthems are typically macular or maculopapular (Fig. 23.1).
- **Papular** – A raised lesion less than 0.5 cm in diameter, elevated above the skin surface such as that seen in acne or molluscum contagiosum (Fig. 23.2).
- **Papulosquamous** – A combination of scaly papules and plaques such as that typically seen in psoriasis (Fig. 23.3).
- **Vesicular** – Raised fluid filled lesions less than 0.5 cm in diameter. Two noted examples of a vesicular eruption include varicella (single vesicles) and herpes simplex (clusters of vesicles) (Fig. 23.4).
- **Bullous** – Large clear fluid-filled lesions such as that seen in staphylococcal scalded skin, bullous impetigo and in many autoimmune and inherited blistering conditions (Fig. 23.5).
- **Petechial** – Small, non-blanching, pinpoint macules such as those seen in Henoch Schonlein purpura and all causes of childhood thrombocytopenia (Fig. 23.6). Larger non-blanching lesions are called purpura.

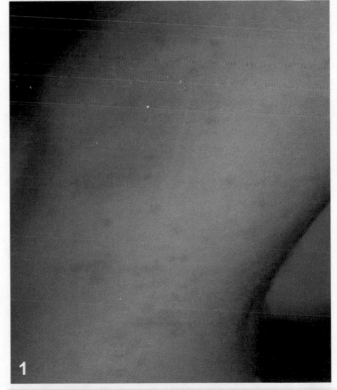

Figure 23.1 Macular rash. (Reproduced with permission from Neri, I., Virdi, A., Baraldi, C., & Annalisa, P. (2015). An uncommon rash: Here is the culprit! *Journal of the American Academy of Dermatology, 72*(6), e139–e140.)

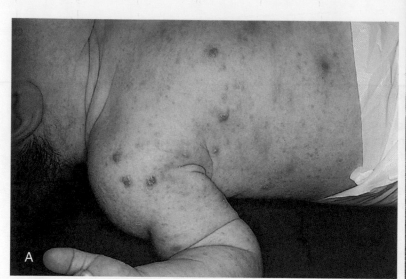

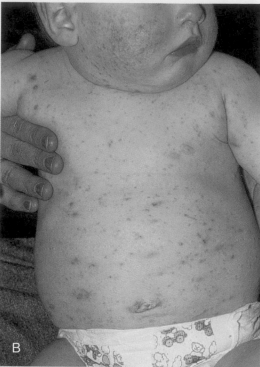

Figure 23.2 Papular rash – scabies. (A) Infant with a diffuse, papular, pruritic rash on the abdomen, chest and axillae. The face is usually spared. (B) Usual distribution. (Reproduced with permission from Lawrence, C. M., & Cox, N. H. (2001). *Physical signs in dermatology* (2nd ed., p. 277). London: Mosby.)

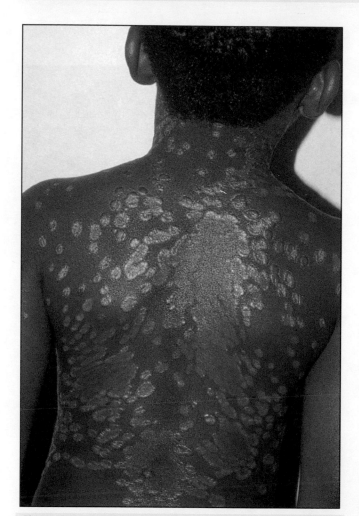

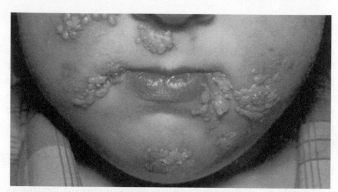

Figure 23.4 Vesicular rash of herpetic gingivostomatitis. (Reproduced with permission from Cohen, B. A. (2013). *Pediatric dermatology* (4th ed.). Saunders/Elsevier.)

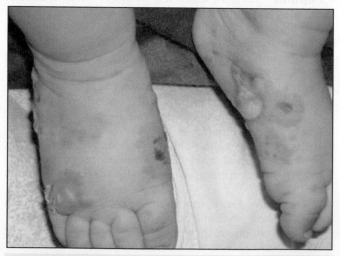

Figure 23.3 Guttate psoriasis. Close-up of back of a patient shows red, scaly, small, teardrop-shaped spots present on dark pigmented skin. (Reproduced with permission from White, G. M., & Cox, N. H. (Eds.). (2006). *Diseases of the skin: A color atlas and text* (2nd ed.). Mosby.)

Figure 23.5 Bullous rash in a 5-month-old girl. (Reproduced with permission from Khaled, A., Kharfi, M., Fazaa, B., & Kamoun, M. R. (2010). Bullous eruption in a five-month-old girl. *Journal de l'Association Medicale Canadienne* [*Canadian Medical Association Journal*], *182*(12), 1325–1327.)

Common Skin Disorders in Paediatric Skin of Colour

It is important to note potential differences in presentation, pathophysiology and treatment modalities in those with richly pigmented skin (Table 23.1).

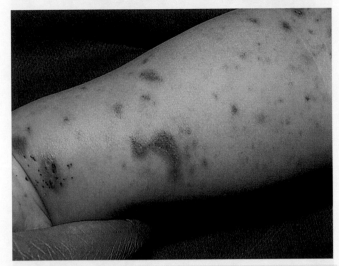

Figure 23.6 Petechial rash. (Reproduced with permission from McMahon, M. C., & Stryjewski, G. R. (2011). *Pediatrics: A competency-based companion.* Philadelphia, PA: Saunders/Elsevier.)

Infantile Haemangioma (IH)

Infantile haemangiomas (or strawberry naevi, as they are affectionately known) are the most frequent benign tumours in childhood, occurring in up to 10 per cent of Caucasian infants. Girls are affected three times more often than boys and the incidence is higher in preterm infants. Lesions typically present by 4 weeks of age and can undergo rapid growth phase between 4 and 12 weeks of age. Eighty per cent reaches maximum size by 12 weeks and most growth has occurred by 5 months of age. Infantile haemangiomas can be superficial, deep or mixed. Deep haemangiomas have a delayed onset of growth, but also have sustained growth when compared to superficial infantile haemangiomas.

Lesions typically regress from the age of 12 months at a rate of 10 per cent a year. While regression can occur up to the age of 10 years, they will typically have undergone most regression by 5 years of age.

COMPLICATIONS OF INFANTILE HAEMANGIOMAS

For most infantile haemangiomas, no treatment is required. Those requiring treatment include those located on or near vital structures such as the periorbital region, lips, nose,

TABLE 23.1   Common Paediatric Skin Disorders in Skin of Colour

Diagnosis	Age of Onset	Clinical Features	Treatment
Acne	Adolescence	Inflammatory papules and pustules, comedones ± cystic lesions Typically located on face ± chest and back	Topical antibiotics (clindamycin erythromycin), topical benzoyl peroxide, topical retinoids, oral tetracyclines Oral contraceptives and spironolactone (females only) Isotretinoin for severe cases
Atopic dermatitis	Varies (infantile atopic dermatitis has onset <2 years of age)	Infantile atopic dermatitis: eczematous dermatitis on cheeks and extensor surfaces Childhood atopic dermatitis: subacute and chronic dermatitis predominantly on flexural areas	Topical steriods, topical calcineurin inhibitors, phosphodiaterase-4 inhibitors, systemic medication or phototherapy for severe disease
Pityriasis alba	3–16 years of age	Poorly defined, hypopigmented macules and patches with minimal scale, typically on face	Emollients, low-potency topical steriods, topical calcineurin inhibitors, sun protection
Tinea versicolor	Adolescence	Hypopigmented, hyperpigmented or erythematous round to oval macules or thin papules that coalesce into patches or thin plaques Typically seen on trunk but can be seen on face/neck in darker-skinned patients	Topical antifungals (ketoconazole), selenium sulfide shampoo Systemic antifungals for severe disease photo-protective measures
Progressive macular hypomelanosis	Adolescence	Nonscaly, hypopigmented macules, typically on the trunk	Benzoyl peroxide, topical antibiotics, oral antibiotics, phototherapy
Traction alopecia	Adolescence/ adulthood	Early stage: mild hair loss (typically on frontal and temporal scalp), no loss of orifices ± perifollicular erythema and scale, ± fringe sign Late stage: alopecia (typically on frontal and temporal scalp) with partial or total loss of orifices ± fringe sign	Discontinuation of tight hairstyles, avoidance of chemical relaxers and heat styling, topical steriods, intralesional steriods, sub-antimicrobial doses of oral antibiotics
Confluent and reticulated papillomatosis	Adolescence	Scaly, brown, thin papules that coalesce into reticulated plaques, often on central chest and back	Oral minocycline (first line) Isotretinoin
Keloids	Adolescence	Skin-colored to hyperpigmented firm plaques that extend beyond wound margins	Topical and intralesional steriods, intralesional injection of interferon or 5-fluorouracil, cryotherapy, surgical excision, laser therapy, silicone gel sheets, pressure application or conbination treatment

Reproduced with permission from Maymone, M. B. C., Watchmaker, J. D., Dubiel, M., Wirya, S. A., Shen, L. Y., & Vashi, N. A. (2019). Common skin disorders in pediatric skin of color. *Journal of Pediatric Health Care, 33*(6), 727–737.

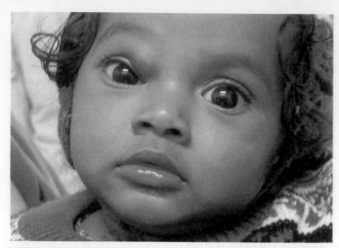

Figure 23.7 Capillary haemangioma. (Reproduced with permission from Tandon, R., & Sihota, R. (2015). *Parsons' diseases of the eye* (22nd ed.). Elsevier Inc.)

genitalia, and lesions that are at risk of ulceration, such as the perianal area or nappy area.

MANAGEMENT OF INFANTILE HAEMANGIOMAS

In 2008, Léauté-Labrèze et al. demonstrated the highly effective treatment of IH with oral propranolol. Side effects may include hypoglycaemia (caution in prolonged vomiting, fasting pre-op and on concurrent steroids), bronchospasm (particularly during concurrent viral infections), a reduction in blood pressure and heart rate, cold extremities and sleep disturbance. Treatment with propanol has revolutionised management of IH and has made the use of long-term systemic steroids largely redundant.

CAPILLARY MALFORMATIONS (PORT WINE STAINS)

Capillary malformations are more commonly called port wine stains (PWS). They are relatively common, present at birth, and most do not have any significant implications (Fig. 23.7). Lesions on the upper face (forehead and eyelids) can be associated with Sturge-Weber syndrome, resulting from somatic activating mutation in the *GNAQ* gene (Fig. 23.8). Consequences of Sturge-Weber include seizures, developmental delay, hemiplegia and glaucoma. Lesions elsewhere can be associated with overgrowth syndromes.

Molluscum Contagiosum

Molluscum contagiosum is a common presentation due to a poxvirus and with an incubation period lasting between 2 and 26 weeks (Fig. 23.9). Incidence peaks at 8 to 12 years of age, with a predilection for the axillary and groin regions. Each lesion may last under 2 months, but the entire eruption can persist for some time. They present as asymptomatic flesh-coloured papules with central umbilication. They may have associated eczematous changes or become inflamed prior to involution. Multiple

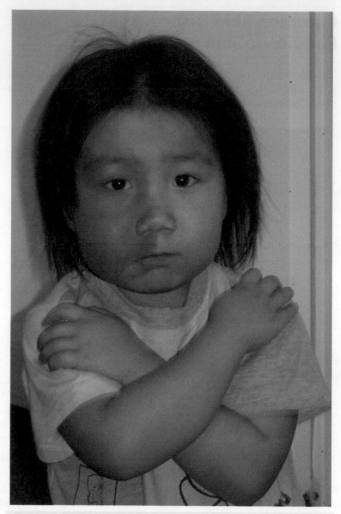

Figure 23.8 Sturge-Weber syndrome. (Reproduced with permission from Davis, P. J., & Cladis, F. P. (Eds.), (2017). *Smith's anesthesia for infants and children* (9th ed.). Elsevier.)

family members can be affected. Extensive lesions should prompt consideration of immunosuppression.

Typically, no treatment is required as molluscum is felt to be benign and self-limiting. Where treatment is indicated, curettage, topical cantharidin, cryotherapy, topical retinoids and 5 per cent potassium hydroxide are options.

Atopic Dermatitis (AD)

Atopic dermatitis affects one in five children and is commonly seen in children with other atopic tendencies such as asthma or hay fever (Fig. 23.10). The filaggrin gene plays a key role in skin barrier function and encodes an essential protein for both epidermal function and skin barrier integrity.

Filaggrin gene (FLG) mutations have been found in both atopic dermatitis and food sensitisation. This skin barrier defect is fundamental in both atopic dermatitis and food allergies. A recent study found that emollient use in infancy sadly does not prevent atopic dermatitis.

AD is a clinical diagnosis (with typical features of itch and skin inflammation) that is responsive to topical steroids and is susceptible to skin infection. Pityriasis alba often coexists with AD atopic dermatitis, especially in dark-skinned children (Fig. 23.11).

Treatment aims include the reduction of symptoms, improvement in life quality, and reduction in both the frequency and severity of flares.

EDUCATION

The primary care management of AD by family doctors involves both patient and parent education, liberal use of emollients, and the use of topical corticosteroids of mild to

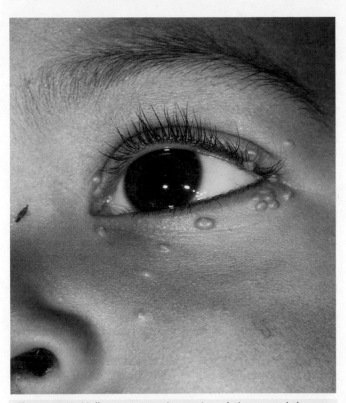

Figure 23.9 Molluscum contagiosum. Inoculation around the eye, a typical presentation for children. (Reproduced with permission from Dinulos, J. G. H. (Ed.). (2021). *Habif's clinical dermatology: A color guide to diagnosis and therapy* (7th ed.). Elsevier.)

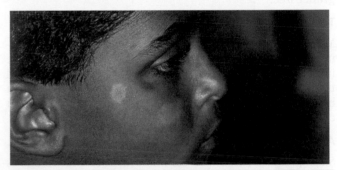

Figure 23.11 Pityriasis alba. Hypopigmented, slightly scaly plaques with indistinct borders on a child's face. (Reproduced with permission from Morelli, J., & Torres-Zegarra, C. (Eds.). (2021). *Pediatric dermatology DDX deck* (3rd ed.). Elsevier.)

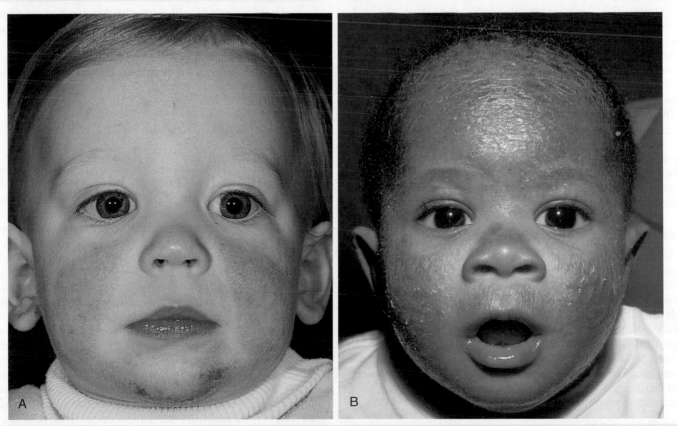

Figure 23.10 (A) A common appearance of atopic dermatitis in children, with erythema and scaling confined to the cheeks, sparing the perioral and paranasal areas. (B) Extensive erythema and crusting in a baby with secondarily infected atopic dermatitis of the face. Eczematous patches may look dark brown, purple, or grey on black or brown skin. (Reproduced with permission from Dinulos, J. G. H. (Ed.). (2021). *Habif's clinical dermatology: A color guide to diagnosis and therapy* (7th ed.). Elsevier.)

moderate potency, which is determined by the patient's age and the site being treated. Patient and parent education is an essential element that improves quality of life and reduces disease severity.

Bathing and Use of Emollients

Daily, liberal use of emollients is a cornerstone of effective treatment for mild eczema. Daily baths and the use of emollient-based soap substitutes to avoid skin irritation are helpful.

Ointments are more effective than creams due to higher lipid concentrations; however, patient preference should be considered when prescribing so as to improve adherence to treatment. Emollients applied to the skin should be fragrance free.

Topical Corticosteroids

Mild to moderate potency topical corticosteroids are recommended in both mild and moderate AD. Potency should be increased for flares and topical corticosteroids continued until skin clearing has taken place. Steroids should then be gradually weaned and used intermittently to maintain control.

Antimicrobial Treatments

Staphylococcus aureus is a common microbe that colonises the skin of patients with eczema and can lead to infection causing a flare of symptoms. Signs may be subtle but include weeping, crusting, pustules and rapid worsening of the eczema.

Combined corticosteroid and antimicrobial ointments (such as hydrocortisone 1 per cent and fusidic acid (Fucidin H) and betamethasone valerate 0.1 per cent and fusidic acid 2 per cent (Fucibet)) can be used for short periods in infected eczema during which there is no systemic upset. More severe infection warrants oral or intravenous antibiotics. Prolonged use of topical antimicrobials should be avoided to reduce the risk of resistance.

In those with moderate to severe AD, there is an increased risk of eczema herpeticum, which may recur. For eczema herpeticum, early diagnosis and treatment with aciclovir is recommended. Parents should be educated to recognise the early signs of recurrence.

Key Principles Managing Infected AD

Always swab the affected areas. Suggest short bleach baths using Milton solution. Ensure the solution is completely diluted in water. Soak in bleach bath for 5 to 7 minutes twice or three times per week. After bathing, pat the skin dry and apply topical steroid. Increase the use of emollients (use new pots) and start Fucibet lipid twice a day (bd) for 10 to 14 days or systemic antibiotic. Flucloxacillin (or erythromycin if penicillin allergic) may be required. Consider empirical acyclovir for 5 days if there are clinical concerns about herpes simplex virus infection whilst awaiting viral skin swab results.

Antihistamines

Contrary to popular myth, quality evidence is lacking for the use of antihistamines in the management of AD. However, in an infant over 6 months of age with an acute flare and associated severe sleep disturbance, a short trial of a sedating antihistamine may be considered.

Specialist referral

Specialist paediatric dermatology referral is recommended if the disease is out of control despite appropriate first line treatments, or if there is severe facial involvement. While most cases are mild, severe AD may pose significant challenges in primary care.

Managing More Severe Atopic Dermatitis

TOPICAL CALCINEURIN INHIBITORS

Topical calcineurin inhibitors, namely tacrolimus or pimecrolimus, inhibit both the production and release of proinflammatory cytokines. Both topical agents are approved for use in managing moderate to severe AD in immunocompetent children over 24 months of age. They are particularly beneficial in areas where steroids should be avoided, such as the periorbital region, the face and neck, and the nappy area.

OCCLUSIVE BANDAGING

Applying occlusive dressings improves skin hydration and reduces scratching, thereby enabling more restful sleep. These dressings aid with the penetration of topical corticosteroids. They should be left on overnight and applied nightly over a period of about 1 week. While they add to the burden of care and can promote infection, they are a helpful short-term measure to induce remission from flares. They should not be used on infected skins.

SYSTEMIC IMMUNOMODULATORY TREATMENTS

Some children with severe disease will require these treatments to achieve better control and improve quality of life. Methotrexate is quickly becoming the most popular first line systemic immunosuppressive agent for severe disease. Methotrexate has an efficacy like that of ciclosporin but has a better safety and side effect profile.

Ciclosporin has both an inhibitory effect on both T cell responses and interleukin 2 production and has a relatively fast action to induce remission. Beware of potential side effects such as acute kidney injury and hypertension, as these tend to preclude long-term treatment.

Azathiporine and mycophenolate mofetil, commonly used in the past, are now largely considered to be third line agents with poor evidence base and safety concerns in childhood.

The relatively new era of biological agents has certainly arrived with the recent approval of the anti-IL-4 receptor alpha antibody dupilumab. Research on additional agents that target type 2 pathways and janus kinases (JAK) inhibitors is ongoing.

Dupilumab acts as a human monoclonal antibody by inhibiting interleukin 4 (IL-4) and has recently been

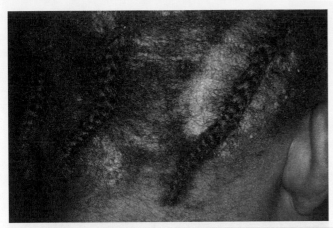

Figure 23.12   Scalp psoriasis. (Reproduced with permission from Paller, A. S., & Mancini, A. J. (Eds.). (2021). *Hurwitz clinical pediatric dermatology: A textbook of skin disorders of childhood and adolescence.* Elsevier.)

licensed as the first biologic agent for use in children with moderate to severe disease from the age of 6 years and up. JAK inhibitors, both topical and oral, are a welcome addition in managing severe AD.

Psoriasis

Characteristic features of psoriasis include erythematous, scaly patches and plaques. Areas of the skin most affected include the scalp, elbows, knees, genitalia, and lumbosacral region. Scaly scalp lesions in childhood are typical due to psoriasis (Fig. 23.12). Nail changes, such as onycholysis and nail pitting, are seen in 25 per cent of children and young people with psoriasis.

The most common variant in childhood is guttate psoriasis (Fig. 23.3) with typical features of round or oval pink scaly patches that arise in crops, especially over the trunk. There may be a history of preceding streptococcal infection 1 to 3 weeks earlier.

Topical therapy with emollients, corticosteroids, vitamin D analogues and tar are first line treatments. However, for more extensive disease, immunosuppressants or phototherapy may be needed.

Alopecia in children

Alopecia, or hair loss, is a distressing symptom and may vary in severity from focal patches of hair loss to diffuse thinning.

Alopecia areata is relatively common and there may be a positive family history. There is typically a localised area of hair loss and exclamation point hairs are characteristic. Hair regrows without intervention in many cases (Fig. 23.13).

Poor prognostic factors in terms of regrowth include sudden extensive hair loss, onset at an early age, nail involvement and an atopic background.

Trichotillomania causes a child to habitually pull, break, and twist hair from the scalp, causing the remaining hairs to be

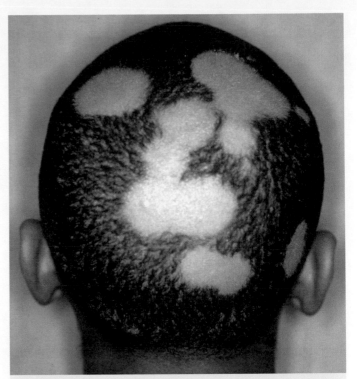

Figure 23.13   Alopecia areata. (Reproduced with permission from James, W. D., Elston, D., Treat, J., Rosenbach, M., & Micheletti, R. G. (2020). *Andrews' diseases of the skin: clinical dermatology* (13th ed.). Elsevier Inc.)

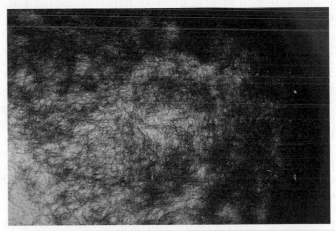

Figure 23.14   Tinea capitis. Diffuse scaling with minimal erythema and patchy alopecia. (Reproduced with permission from Paller, A. S., & Mancini, A. J. (Eds.). (2021). *Hurwitz clinical pediatric dermatology: A textbook of skin disorders of childhood and adolescence.* Elsevier.)

of varying length with bizarre patterns. Treatment is directed towards alleviation of potential stressors and habit reversal.

Tinea capitis is a frequent cause of alopecia in children and may be misdiagnosed as dandruff or psoriasis. Occasionally, a boggy inflammatory plaque called a kerion forms on the scalp (Fig. 23.14). The most common reason for tinea capitis is *Trichophyton tonsurans*, but some are due to *Microsporum canis*.

Request fungal cultures in suspected cases and commence treatment with oral fungicidals (griseofulvin, terbinafine or itraconazole). Fungal cultures from skin

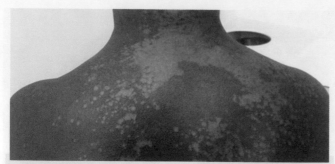

Figure 23.15   Hypopigmented macules of tinea versicolor on the back of a teenager. (Reproduced with permission from Morelli, J., & Torres-Zegarra, C. (Eds.). (2021). *Pediatric dermatology DDX deck* (3rd ed.). Elsevier.)

scrapings or hair plucking help guide treatment choice. Tinea capitis is confirmed by the visualisation of fungal elements using 10 per cent potassium hydroxide or by the isolation of fungi in Saboraud agar. Scalp dermoscopy (magnified visualisation) is a rapid and non-invasive method, which can circumvent the need for laboratory investigation.

Tinea Versicolor

Tinea versicolor is a common fungal infection of the skin particularly affecting teenagers and adolescents. It is characterised by oval hypo- or hyperpigmented macules often on the back, upper chest or arms (Fig. 23.15).

Scabies

Scabies is very common and results in infestation by *Sarcoptes scabiei*. The incubation period is 2 to 6 weeks (or shorter if there has been prior exposure). A burrow is characteristically seen. Scabies is extremely pruritic. Typical sites of involvement in babies are the head, palms and soles (Fig. 23.16). The typical distribution of scabies in older children is somewhat different and affects the wrists, ankles and the interdigital spaces.

If over 2 months of age, topical 5 per cent permethrin is recommended. Apply permethrin over the entire body from the neck down at bedtime and wash off the following morning. Scalp and neck treatment is required for infants with scabies. It is very important to treat all household members and close contacts to prevent reinfestation and to thoroughly wash bedlinens. Treatment should be repeated one week later.

Note that pruritus may last for several weeks after treatment and may be relieved by taking emollients, topical corticosteroids or antihistamines. The burden of scabies is higher among refugees and those living in overcrowded situations with a higher rate of secondary infection. Standard treatment with topical permethrin is unlikely to contain outbreaks in refugee camps and, in this instance, oral ivermectin may be considered. Moxidectin or slow release ivermectin may provide added value to control scabies outbreaks in these settings.

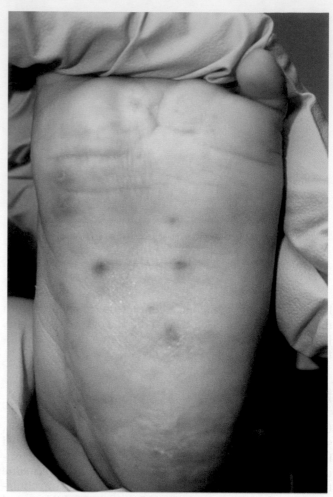

Figure 23.16   Scabies of the sole of the foot.

Henoch-Schonlein Purpura

Henoch-Schonlein purpura (HSP) is the most frequently seen form of vasculitis in childhood. It presents with non-thrombocytopenic, palpable purpura especially of the lower extremities and buttocks (Fig. 23.17). Children frequently have oedema of the hands, feet, face and genitalia. Children with HSP often experience abdominal pain and arthritis (particularly affecting joints of the lower limbs). Colicky abdominal pain can be very severe and mimic an acute abdomen. Rarely, intussusception may occur. Renal involvement manifests as haematuria and proteinuria with or without hypertension. Up to 15 per cent of boys may have orchitis.

HSP is generally a self-limiting illness, but recurrences may arise in up to one-third of children and symptoms may last for several weeks prior to resolution.

The diagnosis of HSP is usually a clinical one, but skin biopsy will confirm the presence of a vasculitis. Steroids may be required for significant gastrointestinal, or renal involvement. HSP has an excellent long-term prognosis. Significant nephritis is most unlikely to develop if both blood pressure and urinalysis are normal 6 months following initial presentation.

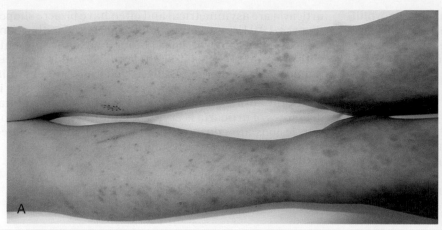
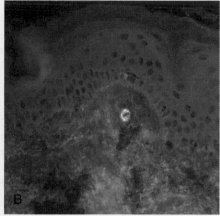

Figure 23.17   (A) A 7-year-old boy presenting to clinic with purpura on the legs, including several areas on the upper legs and ankles of linear purpura (>3 cm in length). (B) A biopsy for haematoxylin and eosin staining displayed leukocytoclastic vasculitis (LCV; not shown), and direct immunofluorescence revealed granular deposition of IgA within superficial dermal blood vessel walls, compatible with IgA-mediated LCV/Henoch-Schönlein purpura (original magnification ×20). (Reproduced with permission from Fernandez, A. P. (2019). *Connective tissue disease: Current concepts.* Elsevier.)

Epidermolysis Bullosa (EB)

Epidermolysis bullosa is an inherited blistering disorder with characteristic spontaneous and posttraumatic bulla formation (Fig. 23.18). Of the many different forms of EB, the mildest is EB simplex, which is mostly autosomal dominant in inheritance. In EB simplex, bullae formation is localised to areas of frequent trauma, such as the hands and feet.

In dystrophic EB, on the other hand, inheritance may be either autosomal recessive or dominant, with the recessive form being far more severe. All forms of dystrophic EB result from mutations in COL7A1. Early blister formations with consequent scarring, poor weight gain and joint contractures are characteristic features in recessive dystrophic EB. There is a heightened risk of squamous cell carcinoma. The dystrophic EB group of dominant inheritance have a more localised disease, and thus a much better prognosis. Skin biopsies and genetic analyses are required to distinguish between variants of EB. For children with severe variants of EB, a multidisciplinary approach is required with an emphasis on avoiding trauma, improving nutrition, excellent wound care, preventing infection and managing long-term complications. Genetic counselling should be offered to all families.

Drug eruptions

Morbilliform drug eruptions are the most frequently seen and consist of fine erythematous papules and macules over the trunk, which may be pruritic. Morbilliform drug eruptions may be quite similar to viral exanthems. Antibiotics, non-steroidal anti-inflammatory drugs, and anticonvulsants such as carbamazepine can all trigger a morbilliform drug reaction. The first step is to stop the medication and treat symptoms with topical steroids, emollients and antihistamines. The rash may last over a week.

Amoxycillin and ampicillin, if prescribed for a child or adolescent with infectious mononucleosis, may be

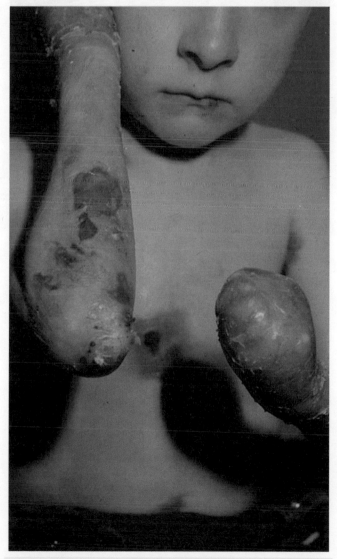

Figure 23.18   Recessive dystrophic epidermolysis bullosa – erosions and 'mitten' deformity of the hand. (Reproduced with permission from Marks, J. G., & Miller, J. J. (2018). *Lookingbill and Marks' principles of dermatology* (6th ed.). Elsevier.)

associated with a widespread and striking morbilliform rash that can take 2 weeks to disappear. Therefore, these antibiotics are best avoided in managing a sore throat in which infectious mononucleosis is a possibility.

Urticaria

Urticaria is associated with transient erythematous and annular wheals and is very common. Acute urticaria (lasting under 6 weeks) may be idiopathic, but also may be associated with viral infection, insect bites, antibiotics or – rarely – foods. The skin lesions of urticaria are asymmetrical and often have bizarre shapes (Fig. 23.19). Urticaria is usually generalised with a continued appearance of new lesions and often presents with associated oedema of the eyelids, hands and feet (angioedema). Allergy testing is generally unhelpful in the assessment of urticaria. Treatment of urticaria is with oral antihistamines. One of the major differential diagnoses of urticaria is erythema multiforme where the skin lesions are constant, round or oval and associated with 'target lesions' (see Chapter 15).

(Box 23.1)
(Box 23.2)
(Box 23.3)
(Box 23.4)

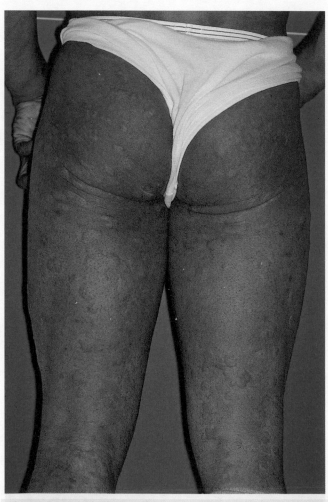

Figure 23.19   Urticaria secondary to hepatitis B. (Reproduced with permission from James, W. D., Elston, D., Treat, J., Rosenbach, M., & Micheletti, R. G. (2021). *Andrews' diseases of the skin: Clinical dermatology* (13th ed.). Elsevier.)

Box 23.1   Key Points

Infantile haemangiomas are very common, affecting one in 10 Caucasian infants.

Infantile haemangiomas (or strawberry naevi) can be superficial, deep or mixed.

Haemangiomas requiring treatment include those located on, or near, vital structures, including the periorbital region, lips, nose, genitalia or lesions at risk of ulceration, such as the perianal area or nappy area.

Port wine stains are relatively common, present at birth, and mostly do not have any significant implications.

Molluscum contagiosum is a viral infection of the skin caused by a large DNA poxvirus.

Mutations in the filaggrin gene (FLG) are associated with both atopic dermatitis (AD) and food sensitisation.

Mild AD can be managed in primary care with parent education, and regular use of emollients with or without topical corticosteroids of mild to moderate potency.

Flares are often due to infection, usually *Staphylococcus aureus*. Signs may be subtle but include weeping, crusting, pustules and rapidly worsening AD.

For eczema herpeticum, early diagnosis and treatment with intravenous aciclovir is recommended.

Psoriasis is characterised by well-demarcated, erythematous, scaly patches and plaques located most often on the scalp, elbows, knees, genitalia and lumbosacral region. Guttate psoriasis is the most common variant in children.

There is typically a localised area of hair loss in alopecia areata and exclamation point hairs are characteristic.

Tinea capitis is treated with oral fungicidals (griseofulvin, terbinafine or itraconazole).

Scabies is very common and results in infestation by *Sarcoptes scabiei*. The incubation period is 2 to 6 weeks but may be shorter if any prior exposure. Scabies is extremely pruritic.

Topical 5 per cent permethrin is the treatment of choice for scabies.

BOX 23.2 An Infant With Troublesome Atopic Dermatitis

A 6-month-old male infant presents with a longstanding itchy rash first noted over the face but now apparent all over the trunk. There is a strong family history of atopy, and his parents are concerned about introducing new foods into his diet.

Clinical Pearls

Atopic dermatitis (AD) is a condition due to defects of the epidermal barrier.

Factors associated with increased prevalence of AD include a strong family history of AD, other atopic tendencies, smaller family size, higher household educational level and living in an urban setting.

Treatment focuses on the restoration of epidermal barrier function best achieved using topical emollients and topical steroids. Emollients should be used at least twice per day all over the body. Non-soap, fragrance-free products are recommended.

Topical corticosteroids remain the first-line treatment in acute flares and topical calcineurin inhibitors (for instance tacrolimus) can help maintain remission.

Low potency corticosteroids are preferred, especially on the face. Tacrolimus is roughly equivalent in potency to a moderately potent topical corticosteroid.

Food allergies affect about 30 per cent of infants and children with early and severe atopic dermatitis, and is much less likely in mild cases.

Topical emollients and corticosteroids need to be applied correctly and consistently. Family education is key.

Address parental concerns regarding topical steroid use.

Consider infection in children who do not respond to first-line therapy.

Refer for specialist opinion those who do not respond to first- or second-line therapy, especially if compliance with treatment is assured.

If failing to respond to first-line treatment, look for infection first and foremost.

Always seek potential triggers such as use of soaps, detergents, fragrances, overheating, aeroallergens (pollens, animal dander, grasses and house dust mites).

Interpretation of Investigations

Taking bacterial and viral swabs from the skin is recommended if infection if suspected.

IgE-specific allergy testing should be reserved for infants with severe atopic dermatitis and needs to be interpreted with caution as sensitisation frequently occurs. Restrictive diets are rarely required.

Pitfalls to Avoid

Be aware of key differentials; diagnoses include scabies (described above), ichthyosis vulgaris (typified by dry skin with fine scaling, especially over the lower abdomen and extensor areas) and Wiskott-Aldrich syndrome (a rash identical to AD with onset usually in first weeks of life in boys also with a low platelet count).

Staphylococcus aureus is the leading cause of bacterial skin infection in children with AD.

Eczema herpeticum is due to herpes simplex virus and occurs in up to 3 per cent of children with AD. Once suspected, start treatment with systemic aciclovir.

BOX 23.3 A 5-Month-Old With a Capillary Haemangioma Over the Eyelid

A 5-month-old presents for specialist opinion, having been referred by his family doctor, with a significant infant haemangioma over the right eyelid which had increased significantly in size and was partially occluding vision from that eye.

Clinical Pearls

Infantile haemangiomas occur in one in 20 infants, are more common in preterms, and typically first proliferate and later involve over time.

Some precursor lesions may be evident at birth or develop within the first 2 months of life with most reaching their final size by 3 months of age. Most completely regress by 4 years of age. Frequently seen complications include pressure effects or ulceration.

Oral propranolol is very effective and leads to regression in approximately 70 per cent of cases.

Propranolol is indicated if periorbital in position causing imminent visual loss, or if obstructing the nose or the external ear, or if significant ulceration occurs.

The most common side effect of propranolol is a disturbance of sleep (20 per cent). The most important side effect is hypoglycaemia. Parents should be educated in the recognition and management of hypoglycaemia. Just 1 per cent of those treated

experience side effects of either bronchospasm or asymptomatic hypotension.

Interpretation of Investigations

Typically, no investigations are required.

For segmental lesions over the lumbosacral area, a pelvic ultrasound should be requested to exclude syndromic anomalies.

Segmental lesions of the face may be associated with PHACES syndrome and should be investigated accordingly (magnetic resonance imaging (MRI) of head and neck, echocardiogram).

Infants with more than five cutaneous haemangiomas should have a liver ultrasound to exclude hepatic/visceral lesions, which may lead to a consumptive hypothyroidism and high output cardiac failure.

Pitfalls to Avoid

Periorbital haemangiomas can lead to permanent amblyopia and frequently require propranolol treatment.

Intratracheal infantile haemangioma may be heralded by haemangiomas around the beard area and can cause life-threatening upper airway obstruction. Large infantile haemangiomas of the neck region may be associated with positional torticollis.

Ulceration is more likely in a haemangioma of the lip, the head and neck area or the nappy area and can be quite troublesome.

BOX 23.4   A 6-Year-Old With a Purpuric Rash Over the Buttocks and Severe Abdominal Pain

A 6-year-old previously well girl presents with a 24-hour history of severe abdominal cramps and is sent to the local hospital for assessment. In the emergency department, she was noted to be apyrexial but quite distressed. Her examination revealed a florid purpuric rash over the extensor surfaces of her legs and swelling of both her ankles. Her urinalysis revealed microscopic haematuria.

Clinical Pearls

Henoch-Schönlein purpura (HSP) is the most common form of childhood vasculitis with a peak age of onset between 4 and 6 years of age. The rash is symmetrical and non-blanching (petechiae and larger purpura), starting on the lower limbs or buttocks.

Gastrointestinal (GI) symptoms are common and may present with abdominal pain (often severe), intussusception or occasionally GI haemorrhage. Severe crampy abdominal pain is an indication for steroids once intussusception has been excluded.

In HSP, arthritis mainly of the knee and ankle joints may occur.

Kidneys will be involved in almost half of cases. Most cases of nephritis are mild with trace proteinuria and/or microscopic or macroscopic haematuria and resolve without treatment. There is no evidence that steroids prevent nephritis in children with HSP.

The parents should be taught to monitor the urine for blood and protein at home for at least 6 months after admission, even if the initial urinalysis in hospital is normal. If urinalysis remains normal, then the renal long-term outcome is excellent.

Interpretation of Investigations

Check urinalysis and blood pressure at regular intervals. If ongoing haematuria or heavy proteinuria, a renal biopsy is required to determine and grade the extent of renal inflammation

Pitfalls to Avoid

Gastrointestinal manifestations (particularly abdominal pain) may precede the skin rash typical of HSP by a few days or a week, thereby causing clinical confusion.

Intussusception can also occur and may be diagnosed on ultrasound.

Epididymo-orchitis is seen in 15 per cent of males with HSP and may present with pain and swelling that is difficult to distinguish from testicular torsion.

HSP nephritis is the most serious long-term manifestation and is the cause of 1 to 2 per cent of all childhood end-stage kidney disease (ESKD).

  Video on the topic Atopic dermatitis in childhood is available online at Elsevier eBooks+.

Key References

Barbarot, S., Auziere, S., Gadkari, A., Girolomoni, G., Puig, L., Simpson, E. L., Margolis, D. J., et al. (2018). Epidemiology of atopic dermatitis in adults: Results from an international survey. *Allergy, 73*(6), 1284–1293.

Engelman, D., Cantey, P. T., Marks, M., Solomon, A. W., Chang, A. Y., Chosidow, O., et al. (2019). The public health control of scabies: Priorities for research and action. *Lancet, 394*(10192), 81–92.

Holland, K. E., & Soung, P. J. (2018). Acquired rashes in the older child. In R. M. Kliegman, P. S. Lye, B. Bordini, H. Toth, & D. Basel (Eds.), volume number. *Nelson pediatric symptom-based diagnosis* (pp. 866–896). location missing Elsevier.

Léauté-Labrèze, C., Dumas de la Roque, E., Hubiche, T., Boralevi, F., Thambo, J. B., & Taïeb, A. (2008). Propranolol for severe hemangiomas of infancy. *The New England Journal of Medicine, 358*(24), 2649–2651.

Léauté-Labrèze, C., Harper, J. I., & Hoeger, P. H. (2017). Infantile haemangioma. *Lancet (London, England), 390*(10089), 85–94.

Leung, A. K. C., Barankin, B., & Leong, K. F. (2020). Henoch-Schhaeman purpura in children: an updated review. *Current Pediatric Reviews, 16*(4), 265–276.

Maymone, M. B. C., Watchmaker, J. D., Dubiel, M., Wirya, S. A., Shen, L. Y., & Vashi, N. A. (2019). Common skin disorders in pediatric skin of color. *Journal of Pediatric Health Care, 33*(6), 727–737.

McAleer, M. A., Flohr, C., & Irvine, A. D. (2012). Management of difficult and severe eczema in childhood. *BMJ, 345*, e4770.

Oni, L., & Sampath, S. (2019). Childhood IgA vasculitis (henoch schonlein purpura) – advances and knowledge gaps. *Frontiers in Pediatrics, 7*, 257.

Panigrahi, A., Sil, A., & Biswas, S. K. (2020). Tinea capitis: bedside diagnosis by dermoscopy. *The Journal of Pediatrics, 222*, 248.

Skjerven, H. O., Rehbinder, E. M., Vettukattil, R., LeBlanc, M., Granum, B., Haugen, G., et al. (2020). Skin emollient and early complementary feeding to prevent infant atopic dermatitis (PreventADALL): A factorial, multicentre, cluster-randomised trial [published correction appears in *Lancet*, 395(10228), e53]. *Lancet, 395*(10228), 951–961.

Weidinger, S., Beck, L. A., Bieber, T., Kabashima, K., & Irvine, A. D. (2018). Atopic dermatitis. *Nature Reviews Disease Primers, 4*(1), 1.

Weidinger, S., & Novak, N. (2016). Atopic dermatitis. *Lancet, 387*(10023), 1109–1122.

24 Safeguarding Infants and Children

SABINE MAGUIRE and LOUISE KYNE

Sadly, child maltreatment is relatively common, occurs in all countries and across all social classes and requires considerable sensitivity, courage and expertise to manage in a highly professional way. Recognition in the community and the emergency department is key, and first responders often have little paediatric training. Knowledge of common childhood injuries and 'red flags' for abusive injuries can aid in correctly identifying the abused child.

Physical Abuse

Physical abuse may involve burning, hitting, poisoning, scalding, shaking, stabbing or throwing, causing physical harm to the child. Physical harm may also be caused when a parent intentionally causes illness in their child or invents symptoms (factitious induced illness). Physical abuse may present with abusive head trauma in infancy, unexplained bruising, fractures, repeated or delayed attendances at emergency departments and unusual patterns of scalds or contact burns. However, training and vigilance of frontline staff are needed to recognise these presentations.

Sexual Abuse

Sexual abuse is where a child or young person is forced or enticed to participate in sexual activities for which they cannot give consent and do not understand. The activities may involve non-penetrative acts such as kissing, stroking or masturbation but may escalate to forced oral sex or penetration. Males, females or older children can commit acts of sexual abuse. It is important to remember that female genital mutilation is still practised in some cultures. If this is suspected clinically, expert gynaecological help should be sought.

Emotional Abuse

Emotional abuse has been defined in many reports as the emotional maltreatment of a child, with consequent negative effects on the child's emotional development. The child may be threatened, silenced, ridiculed and made to feel worthless or unloved. In older children, the parents may be more demanding and show less support and involvement. Emotional abuse may involve witnessing the ill-treatment of another family member. It may also involve serious bullying (including cyberbullying) with the effect that the child is frightened or feels in danger.

Neglect

Neglect has been defined as the persistent failure to meet the child's basic physical and psychological needs resulting in an impairment of the child's healthy development.

Neglect may involve failure by one or both parents where they have the resources to clothe, feed or shelter them. The child may not be appropriately supervised or protected from danger. The parents may fail to obtain suitable medical care or treatment or proper access to education. Neglectful parents of young children may be more aggressive towards them. Emotional neglect includes failure to show love, affection, warmth or acceptance of the child or failure to meet their emotional needs in an age-appropriate way.

In outpatient departments, repeated non-attendance should be viewed as 'was not brought', and if the child has a condition requiring close outpatient review (such as diabetes mellitus), repeated failure to attend with the child can be considered in some instances to constitute neglect.

Online Abuse

One of the most frequent forms of child abuse happens online. Online child abuse is the use of technology and the internet to manipulate, exploit, coerce or intimidate a child (by adults and peers). One form is child sexual abuse in which the child may be forced to watch or take part in sexually inappropriate activities which may be recorded or posted online, sometimes in a coordinated way.

A common form is cyberbullying, which mainly occurs in adolescence but may happen in younger age groups who now have much more regular access to the internet.

Reporting Child Abuse

A core duty and responsibility as a healthcare professional is to both recognise and report suspected abuse to safeguard the child from further abuse. Mandatory reporting is in place in many countries, and thus it is important to follow national guidelines.

All healthcare professionals who work with children must have the appropriate competencies to recognise child maltreatment and its consequences and take effective action as appropriate to their role. Senior doctors are also required to participate in child protection conferences and court proceedings.

Consequences of Child Maltreatment

Adverse childhood experiences incorporate all forms of child abuse, interpersonal violence, incarceration of a family member, drug or alcohol abuse in the home, household severe mental illness and parental separation. Studies from many countries have confirmed that the larger the number of adverse childhood experiences, the greater the risk of adverse future health and wellbeing outcomes.

Risk Factors

Child maltreatment is rarely a one-off event, and the risk factors contributing to persistently abusive environments are as follows:

- *Parental factors*: Young, single or socially isolated parents of low educational attainment in association with alcohol or drug abuse, parental psychiatric illness inclusive of depression and anxiety, prior history of abuse in childhood
- *Child factors*: Low birth weight, prematurity and prolonged stay in neonatal intensive care are all associated with maltreatment, and children with disabilities have at least a threefold increased risk of maltreatment
- *Family factors*: Dysfunctional families and poor family cohesion, unstable living accommodation, insecure attachment and intimate partner violence are all associated with increased risk. Domestic violence is very commonly seen alongside serious child maltreatment.

Prevention of Maltreatment

Protective factors include social support, strong social networks, a supportive family environment, stable parent relationships and a secure parent-child relationship.

Early childhood home interventions (e.g. the Early Start Programme in New Zealand, Healthy Families America, and Nurse Family Partnership) help reduce child maltreatment. Hospital-based interventions with parents of newborn infants, highlighting the importance of not losing control when an infant cries, have had mixed results, with some showing a significant reduction in abusive head trauma.

Many countries have banned smacking. In Sweden, this has improved the social attitude towards physical punishment. For a long time, Sweden has had the lowest childhood mortality from trauma, but the link to a ban on corporal punishment is unclear.

Recognising Child Abuse

Important considerations include whether the injuries sustained are consistent with the history given and whether the story given by the parents can readily explain the injuries. A delay in seeking medical advice, aggressive responses when delicate questions are posed, a negative attitude towards the child, and inconsistencies in the story are all causes for concern.

Key issues to remember:

- Listen very carefully to the child and parents.
- Carefully and accurately record details of the history (particularly details of the injury), the sequence of events, who was present at the time, subsequent symptoms, what action was taken after the trauma, physical findings and investigation results.
- Assess the child's appearance, demeanour and interactions with the parents.
- Consult a senior colleague if you have concerns, and err on the side of caution, with hospitalisation the safest option to allow time for consideration of all the facts.

The Royal College of Paediatrics and Child Health has produced an excellent series of systematic reviews (https://www.rcpch.ac.uk/key-topics/child-protection/evidence-reviews) that identify and critically appraise the evidence behind the recognition and investigation of child abuse and neglect and have produced information derived from the scientific evidence base highlighting the essential features to look out for across various injury types (bruising, burns, fractures, oral injury, head injury and neglect at different ages).

Acting Upon Child Maltreatment Concerns

If a healthcare professional suspects child maltreatment, a referral to the local child protection team is required, and local safeguarding pathways should be followed. The level of immediate risk to the child is key and will inform decisions as to whether to admit to hospital or not.

Suppose there is an immediate risk to the child or other children in the household. In that case, an emergency protection order is sought, and the child should be moved to a place of safety, which may include admission to hospital. A child protection case conference is then convened and involves all the relevant professionals and the family. Information is shared, risks are identified and a child protection plan is developed during this meeting. The child protection plan should clarify the responsibilities of professionals, parents and agencies, including actions to be taken with planned reviews to monitor progress. Healthcare professionals play a key role in developing a child protection plan.

Taking the History in Suspected Child Abuse

The doctor's role is to ascertain whether the history provided is consistent with clinical findings. The doctor responsible is either the most senior on-call doctor or the designated paediatrician with a special interest in child protection. This requires a detailed medical and social history initially and full examination with appropriate investigations. The clinician must not jump to conclusions or be judgmental and should calmly determine whether the injuries sustained and the history provided are consistent.

In particular, the mechanism of injury, the force required to cause the injury, and the child's developmental age should be in keeping with the findings. For instance, a young infant falling from a baby bouncer would not be expected to sustain a significant head injury or present to hospital unconscious or with seizures.

Consider the events leading up to the injury and the parental or caregiver responses post injury. Concerning suspected immersion burns, ask open-ended questions about the child's alleged position at the time of scalding, who was there at the time, and the exact timing involved, if known. Vague, changing or inconsistent injury mechanisms should always lead to additional concern. Performing an investigation at the scene of the injury is very helpful, including the determination of hot water temperature, and is usually coordinated by the community social work team.

Documentation of prior injuries or emergency department attendances is important, as is a detailed review of prior contact with social services. Be sure to contact the general practitioner and health visitor (or public health nurse) with parental consent, seeking a detailed background of professional input prior to this presentation.

Birth and perinatal history should focus on whether single or multiple births (maltreatment is increased in multiple births), whether preterm and admitted to neonatal intensive care, and whether ongoing neurodevelopmental concerns are present (again, a higher risk of maltreatment).

A detailed social history is critical in identifying stressors such as family and others. Some research has shown increased prevalence of physical abuse among immigrant children, asylum seekers, and internationally adopted children.

Physical Examination for Suspected Physical Abuse

Examine the child in an area with good lighting. Pay close attention to how the child and parents interact. The examination involves a full physical assessment of the child and charting on a centile chart for weight, length and head circumference. Ensure the child is fully examined. Document injuries on a body map with measurements and ensure the paperwork is correctly signed and dated.

BRUISES

Bruises are often hidden in areas typically covered by clothing, so the child must be fully undressed to visualise all the skin, especially for bruising. Bruising in unusual places such as the posterior pinna can be highly significant. To the inexperienced eye, bruising may sometimes not be easily differentiated from Mongolian blue spots, café au lait spots or other pigmented birthmarks (see chapter 8 on newborn examination). Bruising may also relate to coagulopathy, which can occur with idiopathic thrombocytopenic purpura, von Willebrands disease or acute leukaemia, and these differentials should always be considered. It may be tempting to attempt to date the bruises seen, however, as bruises cannot be dated with any degree of accuracy, it is best simply to document any pattern or clustering of bruises and measure such bruises with a right-angled measuring device. It is vital to obtain accurate clinical photographs in multiple planes, including a right-angled measuring device in the image for measurement purposes, and to consider the addition of cross-polarised imaging to reduce reflections.

Check the head and neck region for bruising of the face, ear or neck, a torn frenulum, or subconjunctival haemorrhages.

Regular non-worrisome childhood bruises tend to be over the anterior tibial surfaces and the forehead, nose or chin (facial T) and are due to the normal activities of a toddler or young child.

A young child's level of independent mobility strongly influences accidental bruising. Non-mobile infants are very unlikely to sustain accidental bruises, so *any* bruising in this group should arouse concern and prompt a full investigation.

Abusive bruises are predominantly found on the head and neck (ear, neck and cheeks in particular), soft tissue areas such as the inner thigh, upper arm, abdomen or genital areas (Fig. 24.1). However, any part of the body may be bruised due to physical abuse. The presence of petechiae in association with bruising is a strong predictor of abusive injury. Remember that the absence of bruising does not preclude an abusive injury, such as internal abdominal injury. These may include ruptured liver or spleen or a classical pattern of transection or laceration of the third or fourth part of the duodenum in children less than 2 years of age. If the latter is found in the absence of a motor vehicle collision, it should always prompt a full child abuse evaluation.

FRACTURES

Again, children who are not yet walking are far less likely to sustain accidental long bone fractures. Non-supracondylar fractures of the humerus, femoral shaft fractures and metaphyseal fractures all have a higher probability of indicating abuse in non-ambulatory children. Any rib fractures (in the absence of a history of bone disease or major trauma) are highly specific for abuse (Figs 24.2 and 24.3). All

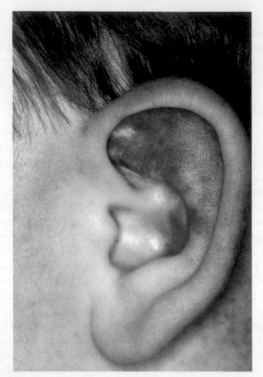

Bruised Pinna
characteristic feature of NAI

Figure 24.1   Non-accidental bruising – bruised pinna.

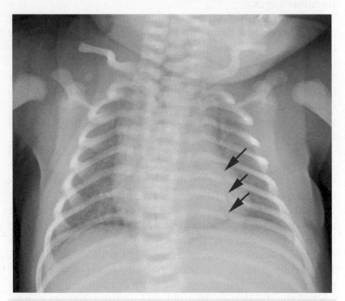

Figure 24.2   Non-accidental injury. Oblique view of the left ribs in a 3-month-old with respiratory infection shows fractures of left sixth, seventh and eighth ribs. (Courtesy Prof Stephanie Ryan.)

children under 2 years of age with suspected physical abuse should have a full skeletal survey, including oblique views of the ribs, performed initially and repeated 2 weeks later (at which time the skull and pelvis x-rays can be omitted).

BURNS

Most intentional scalds are hot water immersion scalds involving the lower limbs or buttocks due to immersion or

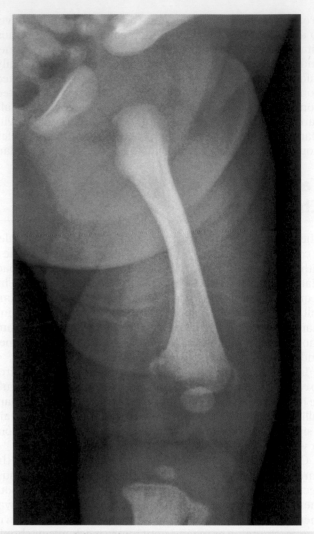

Figure 24.3   Left femur of the same baby shows a bucket handle type of metaphyseal fracture with separation of a thin rim of the distal femoral metaphysis on each side. (Courtesy Prof Stephanie Ryan.)

'glove and stocking' burns to the hands and feet (Fig. 24.4). The severity of the scald depends on the water's temperature and the duration of contact. Deliberate cigarette burns are infrequent, but other contact burns such as hairdryer, iron, cigarette lighter may be seen; a home assessment can often match the implement involved.

Abusive Head Trauma (AHT)

Abusive head trauma (AHT) is not a new condition. In 1860, *Auguste Ambroise Tardieu* (a French pathologist) described injuries in 32 young children resulting from maltreatment. In 1946, Dr *John Caffey* (a radiologist) described skeletal injuries associated with chronic subdural collections, and in 1962, Dr *Henry Kempe* (a paediatrician) used the term 'battered child syndrome'.

In 2011, Professor Carol Jenny observed that 'abusive head trauma begins with intense frustration and anger. In its aftermath lives, relationships, families and futures can be changed forever'. The debate surrounding AHT is legal rather than scientific or medical.

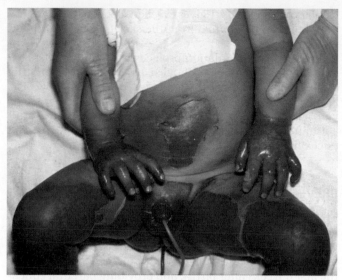

Figure 24.4 Case of non-accidental trauma with immersion pattern scald burns. Note the sharp transverse linear demarcation between the burned and unburned skin. (Reproduced with permission from Herndon, D. N. (2012). *Total Burn Care* (4th ed.). Elsevier Inc.)

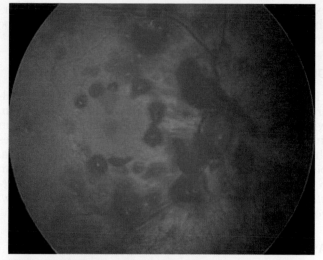

Figure 24.5 Retinal haemorrhages in abusive head trauma (AHT)

AHT is characterised by repetitive acceleration/deceleration forces with or without blunt head impact occurring in infants and resulting in ocular, intracranial and sometimes other injuries. At first, it has a variable presentation with inconsolable crying, seizures, apnoea, vomiting, drowsiness, apparent sepsis and apparent life-threatening events.

In considering AHT, questions that need to be asked include whether the history is consistent with the injuries seen and whether there was an immediate onset of symptoms? Is there evidence of subdural bleeding, with or without hypoxic-ischaemic injury? Are retinal haemorrhages present with or without rib fractures? Are there potential home stressors? Lastly (and most importantly), have other differential diagnoses have been ruled out?

Healthcare professionals must stress that there are difficulties in confronting the issue and that dealing with a case of suspected AHT is very time-consuming and emotionally draining. It is critical to emphasise that not all cases are from high-risk backgrounds. The children who are most likely to have their abuse missed by health professionals are Caucasian (often with higher income), from two-parent families and attending a non-paediatric hospital.

AHT has an estimated prevalence of 16.1 to 38.8 per 100,000 infants per year. Its manifestations can be mild, moderate or life-threatening. Infants may be reinjured after a missed diagnosis or a prior sentinel injury. Sentinel injury is variably defined as a minor injury in a non-mobile child, which precedes a more severe injury. Repeated studies have shown that up to a third of children who go on to be severely abused had a sentinel injury seen by health professionals within the preceding month, the significance of which went unrecognised.

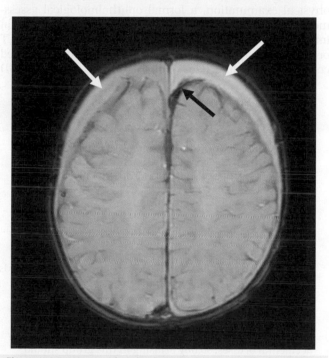

Figure 24.6 Non-accidental injury. A pale and difficult to rouse 3-month-old. Gradient echo sequence MRI shows bilateral frontal subdural collections (white arrows), each with slightly different signals and each extending into the interhemispheric fissure. The left subdural also extends around to the posterior aspect of the parietal lobe and into the posterior aspect of the interhemispheric fissure. The dark signal (black arrow) adjacent to the medial frontal lobe is consistent with blood products in the subarachnoid space. Collections in at least three different spaces, right and left subdural and left subarachnoid spaces, each with different signal characteristics and in the absence of a history of trauma, is highly suggestive of non-accidental injury. (Courtesy Prof Stephanie Ryan.)

KEY FEATURES OF AHT

Key features of AHT, including subdural haemorrhage (SDH), retinal haemorrhages (Fig. 24.5) and encephalopathy are associated with an elevated level of morbidity and mortality. Other intracranial injuries include hypoxic-ischaemic injury, subarachnoid haemorrhage, diffuse axonal injury, and cerebral oedema (Fig. 24.6). The SDH may extend down the spine when posterior subdural haemorrhages are present. Spinal ligamentous injury may also be found if MRI is performed.

DIFFERENTIAL DIAGNOSIS

There are a wide range of differential diagnoses to be considered, including benign extra-axial fluid (BEAF) collection, which may be familial with normal development, and an increased head circumference. Other differential diagnoses that must also be considered are accidental head trauma, birth-related retinal haemorrhages (small and gone by 4 to 6 weeks of age), meningitis with subdural collections (*Haemophilus influenzae type B (Hib) or Neisseria. meningitidis*), coagulopathy or (very rarely) glutaric aciduria type 1.

ASSESSMENT

When AHT is suspected, assessment involves a detailed physical examination, a formal ophthalmological assessment, neuroimaging (MRI is preferred) including spinal images, a formal skeletal survey (possibly also a 3D rib CT or repeat chest x-ray after 10 to 14 days), and a detailed coagulation profile. If a skull fracture is present, a 3D

reconstruction from CT gives excellent detail of the fracture. The skull can be omitted from the skeletal survey if this is performed.

The detailed coagulation profile can be done in a staged manner and involves a detailed assessment of both the extrinsic and intrinsic coagulation pathways (FBC, PT, APTT, Factor 13 assay, intrinsic and extrinsic factor assays, von Willebrand screen, lupus anticoagulant, alpha 2 antiplasmin, blood group and platelet function tests and platelet nucleotides).

PREVENTION

Prevention of AHT involves identifying high-risk families, increasing community recognition, supporting parents who may be suffering exhaustion and frustration or who may have experienced a traumatic childhood (especially in the first 6 weeks after birth), and providing parental education and links with support groups.

(Box 24.1)
(Box 24.2)
(Box 24.3)
(Box 24.4)

Box 24.1   Key Points

Physical abuse may present with abusive head trauma in infancy, unexplained bruising or fractures, repeated or delayed attendances at emergency departments, unusual patterns of scalds or contact burns and requires training and vigilance of frontline staff to recognise.

A core duty and responsibility as a healthcare professional is to both recognise and report suspected abuse to safeguard the child from further abuse.

A delay in seeking medical advice, aggressive responses when delicate questions are posed, a negative attitude towards the child and inconsistencies in the story are all causes for concern.

The immediate risk level to the child is key and will inform decisions as to whether hospital admission is warranted.

Non-mobile infants are very unlikely to sustain accidental bruises, so *any* bruising in this group should arouse concern.

Non-supracondylar fractures of the humerus, femoral shaft fractures and metaphyseal fractures have a higher probability of originating from abuse in non-ambulatory children.

Intentional scalds are hot water immersion scalds involving the lower limbs or buttocks due to immersion or 'glove and stocking' burns to the hands and feet.

Abusive head trauma (AHT) is characterised by repetitive acceleration/deceleration forces with or without blunt head impact occurring in infants and resulting in ocular, intracranial, and sometimes other injuries.

The combination of subdural haemorrhage, retinal haemorrhages and encephalopathy in AHT is associated with elevated morbidity and mortality.

When AHT is suspected, assessment involves a detailed physical examination, a formal ophthalmological assessment, neuroimaging (MRI is preferred) including spinal images, a formal skeletal survey (possibly with a 3D rib CT or repeat chest x-ray after 10 to 14 days) and a detailed coagulation profile.

Box 24.2   A 4-Month-Old Infant Presenting With a Seizure

A female infant was born by lower segment caesarean section at 37 weeks' gestation weighing 2.1 kg at birth. The infant stayed for 5 days in hospital for mild physiological jaundice and some minor feeding issues. Her mother and her mother's partner were both immigrants currently living in a hostel.

Over the first 8 weeks, the infant presented to the local Emergency Department on three occasions with irritability, excess crying and an episode of brief apnoea felt to be a brief resolved unexplained event (BRUE). She was observed for 4 hours and discharged home.

At 4 months of age, the infant had a sudden collapse episode with a 10-minute generalised seizure and was rushed to hospital via ambulance. On assessment, she had a full fontanelle and a

depressed conscious state and was therefore admitted to paediatric intensive care. Subsequent investigations showed bilateral subdural bleeds. Indirect ophthalmoscopy showed multiple bilateral retinal haemorrhages, and a chest CT scan confirmed multiple rib fractures.

A case conference was convened, a diagnosis of abusive head trauma was made, and the infant was subsequently taken into care.

Clinical Pearls

Abusive head trauma (AHT) is a combination of subdural haemorrhage, retinal haemorrhages and encephalopathy, often in combination with other intracranial pathology or additional clinical features, and is associated with elevated morbidity and mortality.

Box 24.2   A 4-Month-Old Infant Presenting With a Seizure – cont'd

Its variable presentation includes inconsolable crying, seizures, apnoea, vomiting, drowsiness, apparent sepsis and apparent life-threatening events.

AHT may easily be missed, and infants may be reinjured after a missed diagnosis or a prior sentinel injury. A sentinel injury is variably defined as a minor injury in a non-mobile child that precedes a more severe injury.

Interpretation of Investigations

Neuroimaging and a formal skeletal survey are advised. If a skull fracture is present, a 3D CT reconstruction shows intricate fracture detail.

The detailed coagulation profile can be done in a staged manner and involves a detailed assessment of both the extrinsic and intrinsic coagulation pathways.

A paediatric ophthalmologist should perform an indirect ophthalmoscopy, which may show multiple retinal haemorrhages with or without associated retinoschisis.

Pitfalls to Avoid

There are a wide range of differential diagnoses to consider, including benign extra-axial fluid (BEAF) collection, which may be familial with normal development, and an increased occipitofrontal circumference (OFC).

Re-presentation on multiple occasions to an emergency department with a young infant should be considered a 'red flag', and a BRUE may indicate a minor shaking incident.

Dealing with AHT is very emotionally draining for the whole team, and one should prioritise the safety of the infant and <u>not</u> become a part-time investigator.

As a trainee, seeking a senior opinion and admitting the infant to hospital are the first steps.

Watch carefully and listen while a senior colleague interviews the parents in a suspected case. A non-accusatory approach and detailed written documentation of discussions are fundamental learning points.

Box 24.3   Repeated Brief Resolved Unexplained Events in a Young Infant

A 4-month-old male infant presented to hospital with a brief resolved unexplained event (BRUE) witnessed at home by his mother. The episode consisted of pallor with cyanosis and possible apnoea occurring 30 minutes following a feed. He had a prior episode at 2 months of age and was admitted for overnight observation at another hospital.

He was admitted for observation and investigation because of family concerns and, while in a single isolation room alone with his mother, he had a repeat episode of cyanosis and limpness, which caused great concern.

The following investigations were performed and found to be normal:
CXR / ECG / Echocardiography
Routine bloods
MRI brain and video EEG
Barium swallow
Urine for organic acids

He remained in hospital for 10 days and was discharged with outpatient follow up and close health visitor support. He was readmitted 8 weeks later for further investigation after another episode of cyanosis and lifelessness, as his mother was most anxious for a diagnosis to be made.

He had a full airway assessment including microlaryngoscopy and bronchoscopy (MLB) which was normal, a detailed metabolic work up, and a further 2-week stay in hospital. He was discharged only to be readmitted just 6 days later with a further BRUE where his mother (who had received basic life support training) gave two rescue breaths. On this occasion, he had a further comprehensive work up with testing of the PHOX 2B gene, a polysomnography study, and a CT scan of the thorax, all of which were negative. A second opinion of an experienced paediatrician was sought.

At this point, his mother was on 'first name terms' with all the team and an adult psychiatry assessment of the mother was coordinated as was a social work referral. After over 90 days in hospital, a case conference of all the relevant parties (including extended family) was convened.

The case conference explored the possibility of factitious induced illness (FII) and was a particularly challenging affair for all concerned. The options of foster care as opposed to maternal grandmother support were considered. Day ward reviews took place twice weekly while the child was with the maternal grandmother, and no further BRUE episodes occurred. The infant was noted to have subsequent mild developmental delay.

Clinical Pearls

Factitious induced illness (FII) is defined as occurring when someone persistently fabricates symptoms on behalf of another, usually a child, causing that person to be regarded as ill, or induces illness in another person, usually a child.

FII may be a perverse fulfilment of the carer's unmet emotional needs for attention and status, or a carer's mistaken beliefs, extreme anxiety and concern about the child's state of health, to the detriment of the child.

These carer behaviours are often accompanied by repeated consultations and 'doctor shopping'.

Clues to a possibility of FII include an unusual, bizarre and recurrent illness with inconsistent histories, observations and tests. The illness begins only when perpetrator present, and the child is inexplicably better away from the perpetrator. The perpetrator tends to be happy in hospital and always appears knowledgeable and calm. Treatment is ineffective and there may be a history of previous unusual illness or deaths in the family. The most common perpetrator is the mother, who may have a history of working in health care.

Although intention to harm the child is not an essential part of FII, the child is harmed in the process. However, some of the harm is inadvertently caused by prolonged admission and extensive invasive investigations, thus earning the term 'medical child abuse' in North America.

Interpretation of Investigations

This will often take a long time and may involve eyewitness accounts.

Continued

Box 24.3   Repeated Brief Resolved Unexplained Events in a Young Infant – cont'd

Always clarify whether episodes ever <u>start</u> with someone else and obtain all general practitioner (GP), hospital and social services records.

Strategies on the ward include 'one-to-one' nursing and covert video surveillance. It is always a diagnosis of exclusion.

In cases where the infant or child presents with hypoglycaemia, the importance of C-peptide testing at the time of hypoglycaemia is emphasised to help identify exogenous insulin administration.

Pitfalls to Avoid

Factitious induced illness, although uncommon, is increasingly being recognised in tertiary care settings. The pattern is that there is increasing risk to the child, or an escalation of the harm the child is subjected to.

Raising a concern about FII is fraught with a need for possibly elusive evidence and the involvement of other safeguarding agencies. Doctors may feel isolated, insecure, and uncertain how to proceed.

It is a diagnosis of exclusion, but one that should be considered when symptoms remain unexplained despite extensive consultation and investigation.

Resolution requires stopping iatrogenic harm to the child by further unnecessary investigations and treatment and restoring the child's daily life to optimal normality.

The calm attitude and behaviour of the mother despite very worrying symptoms is quite characteristic. Explore the family dynamics in detail and access documentation, especially from community sources.

<u>Always seek the advice of a senior colleague.</u>

Box 24.4   A 6-Month-Old With Acute Bronchiolitis and Earlobe Bruising

A 6-month-old male infant presents to the Emergency Department with a 2-day history of cough and respiratory distress and a clinical diagnosis of acute bronchiolitis is made. He is managed with nasal prong oxygen and orogastric feeds. On admission, bruising of the left earlobe is noted and the parents state that he fell out of a baby bouncer 3 days prior to admission. His chest x-ray is consistent with acute bronchiolitis and his coagulation profile is normal. Following a detailed discussion with the parents, a full skeletal survey is ordered that shows evidence of a metaphyseal fracture of the distal humerus. An MRI of the brain and spinal cord is arranged, and the case is reported to social services, resulting in a case conference.

Clinical Pearls

A non-mobile infant is extremely unlikely to sustain accidental bruises or fractures.

Accidental bruising in mobile toddlers usually occurs over the anterior tibial surfaces and in a 'T' shape across the forehead, nose, upper lip and chin. Abusive bruising, on the other hand, occurs on the ear, neck, cheeks or over the trunk or legs or upper arms. The presence of petechiae in association with bruising is predictive of abusive injury.

Accidental fractures may relate to falls, playground or sporting activities, or may be road related. Upper limb fractures are most common. Pre-mobile children are very unlikely to sustain accidental long bone fractures. Any rib fractures in the absence of metabolic bone disease or major trauma are highly specific for abuse.

Interpretation of Investigations

All children less than 2 years with suspected physical abuse should undergo a skeletal survey, which involves 19 images and oblique views of the ribs. Bearing in mind that acute fractures may be missed on a skeletal survey, a bone scan or repeat skeletal survey (omitting skull and pelvis) should be considered if concerns persist. Metaphyseal fractures of the long bones are more likely due to abuse than to other causes.

von Willebrand disease is the most common bleeding disorder to present with bruising. Both von Willebrand disease and idiopathic thrombocytopenic purpura (ITP) are associated with epistaxis, gum bleeding and menorrhagia, and prolonged bleeding following separation of the umbilical cord.

First stage investigations include a full blood count, platelet count and blood film, PT and APTT, factor 8, 9 and 13 assays, and platelet function analyser-100. Large platelets are characteristic of Bernard-Soulier syndrome and small platelets are seen in Wiskott-Aldrich syndrome.

Pitfalls to Avoid

Always consider differential diagnoses not least coagulation disorders (von Willebrand disease has an incidence of one in 100), Mongolian blue spots, and Henoch-Schönlein purpura. It is not possible to date bruises.

Key References

Children in Wales. (n.d.). Safeguarding. https://www.childreninwales.org.uk/safeguarding/.

Davis, P., Murtagh, U., & Glaser, D. (2019). 40 years of fabricated or induced illness (FII): where next for paediatricians? Paper 1: Epidemiology and definition of FII. *Archives of Disease in Childhood, 104*(2), 110–114.

Debelle, G. D., Maguire, S., Watts, P., Nieto-Hernandez, R., Kemp, A. M., Child Protection Standing Committee, & Royal College of Paediatrics and Child Health. (2018). Abusive head trauma and the triad: A critique on behalf of RCPCH of 'Traumatic shaking: the role of the triad in medical investigations of suspected traumatic shaking'. *Archives of Disease in Childhood, 103*(6), 606–610.

Glaser, D., & Davis, P. (2019). Forty years of fabricated or induced illness (FII): Where next for paediatricians? Paper 2: Management of perplexing presentations including FII. *Archives of Disease in Childhood, 104*(1), 7–11, For debate.

Kemp, A. M. (2011). Abusive head trauma: Recognition and the essential investigation. *Archives of Disease in Childhood Education and Practice Edition, 96*(6), 202–208.

Levin, A. V., Christian, C. W., Committee on Child Abuse and Neglect, & Section on Ophthalmology. (2010). The eye examination in the evaluation of child abuse [published correction appears in *Pediatrics, 126*(5):1053. Ellis, G.S., Jr., [added]]. *Pediatrics, 126*(2), 376–380.

Lorenz, D. J., Pierce, M. C., Kaczor, K., Berger, R. P., Bertocci, G., Herman, B. E., et al. (2018). Classifying injuries in young children as abusive or accidental: Reliability and accuracy of an expert panel approach. *The Journal of Pediatrics, 198*, 144–150. e4.

Maguire, S. (2010). Which injuries may indicate child abuse? *Archives of Disease in Childhood Education and Practice Edition, 95*(6), 170–177.

Minford, A. M, & Richards, E. M. (2010). Excluding medical and haematological conditions as a cause of bruising in suspected non-accidental injury. *Archives of Disease in Childhood Education and Practice Edition, 95*(1), 2–8.

National Society for the Prevention of Cruelty to Children. (n.d.). NSPCC Learning Homepage – Safeguarding training and resources. learning.nspcc.org.uk.

Nicholson, A. (n.d.). Recognition and management of Shaken Baby Syndrome. *Irish Medical Journal*. https://imj.ie/recognition-and-management-of-shaken-baby-syndrome/.

Pierce, M. C., Magana, J. N., Kaczor, K., Lorenz, D. J., Meyers, G., Bennett, B. L., & Kanegaye, J. T. (2016). The prevalence of bruising among infants in pediatric emergency departments. *Annals of Emergency Medicine, 67*(1), 1–8.

Royal College of Paediatrics and Child Health. (n.d.). Child protection evidence. https://www.rcpch.ac.uk/key-topics/child-protection/evidence-reviews.

Royal College of Paediatrics and Child Health. (n.d.). RCPCH online learning. www.rcpch.ac.uk/e-learning

Royal College of Paediatrics and Child Health. (n.d.). Safeguarding children and young people – Roles and competencies. www.rcpch.ac.uk/resources/safeguarding-children-young-people-roles-competencies-healthcare-staff.

25 The Child With a Seizure

AMRE SHAHWAN

Background

The key learning outcomes for this chapter include the ability to perform a focussed history and relevant examination in a child with a suspected seizure and to be aware of the many differential diagnoses of seizures and epilepsy in childhood. We would like you to understand the latest classification of seizures and to be able to recognise common epilepsy syndromes. The immediate management and the investigations indicated in seizure assessment will be described, as will the initiation and choice of antiepileptic medications. We will highlight all these principles using five common case scenarios you will likely encounter in clinical practice.

Diagnostic Approach to Assessing a Child With Seizures

A child presenting with an epileptic seizure may declare the onset of epilepsy or merely have an isolated seizure. Some of the most important predictors of recurrence are the presence of an underlying neurological disorder such as intellectual disability, a genetic syndrome, cerebral palsy, history of significant central nervous system (CNS) insult (previous CNS infection, stroke, vascular injury or traumatic brain injury) or noteworthy family history. Genetic factors are

of paramount importance in childhood epilepsy. If one parent has epilepsy, the overall risk of epilepsy in their children is about 4 per cent and rises to 10 per cent if both parents are affected (sometimes more, depending on the nature of underlying genetic abnormality).

An abnormal neurological examination, EEG or MRI abnormalities may all be, individually or collectively, predictors of seizure recurrence and indeed determinants of whether the commencement of antiepileptic drugs (AEDs) is required.

HISTORY

History is the most valuable tool in diagnosing epilepsy or seizure disorders. Ask whether the child had prior episodes and enquire as to the frequency of these episodes. Seek clarity regarding where the episode occurred and what the child was doing at the time.

Ask who witnessed the episode and what action, if any, was taken by those in attendance. Make efforts to contact witnesses to get a complete history.

Enquire about seizure onset, looking for subtle or minimal features seen before a larger seizure. Examples of witnessed minor features might include head or eyes turning to one side, unilateral limb stiffening or jerking before the more obvious seizure. Visual, auditory, sensory, autonomic

251

and gastric symptoms expressed by an older child are particularly important, as they may point to a focal onset of seizures and help classify the seizure more clearly.

Nowadays, we often take videos of events on our smart devices. If there are videos of the seizure taken by witnesses, these are invaluable!

Ask how long the episode lasted and how it ended. For example, if one symptom of seizures is prolonged (loss of contact with surroundings and unresponsiveness beyond a minute or so), this would be much more consistent with a focal impaired awareness seizure (FIAS) rather than an absence seizure, which are usually shorter (between approximately 5 and 20 seconds). The duration of a seizure will undoubtedly influence current and future treatment strategies.

Ask about associated incontinence, tongue biting or injury as the presence of these features supports a definite diagnosis of epileptic seizure.

Ask about the condition of the child in the postictal phase (the period following an epileptic seizure). Several features may be seen during the postictal phase. Examples include postictal confusion, postictal sleep (some may sleep for hours after a prolonged seizure) and temporary postictal unilateral weakness after a focal seizure with or without convulsive seizure activity (Todd's paresis), which can sometimes last for hours.

> **REMEMBER**
>
> Nowadays, video/mobile phone recordings on smart devices are extremely helpful and are often the best diagnostic tool available to confirm or dispute the diagnosis of an epileptic seizure. Such recordings should be encouraged when possible.

CLINICAL EXAMINATION

As much as history is undoubtedly the most useful tool when trying to diagnose or classify a seizure disorder or epilepsy type, a careful clinical examination is also essential.

Perform a systematic examination to identify features of neurological disorders associated with epilepsy. Examples include examining the skin for features of tuberous sclerosis (ash leaf macules in particular), features of neurofibromatosis (café-au-lait spots), dysmorphic facial and somatic features of known genetic syndromes such as trisomy 21, and other, less common genetic syndromes.

Neurological examination should be comprehensive from steps such as measurement of head circumference (microcephaly is associated with many congenital and neurological disorders acquired early in life) to a full neurological examination.

Uncovering focal neurological abnormalities is extremely important in directing your further approach to performing more specific investigations.

Seizure and Epilepsy Classification

An epileptic seizure is a manifestation of excessive and hypersynchronous epileptic activity of neurones in the brain. Epilepsy is defined as a chronic neurological condition characterised by recurrent epileptic seizures, which are often unprovoked.

SEIZURE CLASSIFICATION

Seizures are classified into two main categories: focal and generalised. After considerable discussion, the ILAE (International League Against Epilepsy) developed a new classification system in 2017, as summarised in the corresponding diagram (Fig. 25.1). Seizures are initially categorised based on their clinical characterisation and description taken from history provided by the patient, their family and other health professionals, and then more formally after investigations (particularly the electroencephalogram (EEG)). Note the recurring use of the word 'onset' as this is what counts when classifying a type or category of seizure.

If a child presents with seizures charecterised by unilateral stiffening of one side at onset and maintaining the abilty to speak and contact with surroundings, this seizure is classified as focal onset aware seizure (FAS) motor onset. If the child loses contact with surroundings and becomes unresponsive, then focal onset impaired awareness seizures (FIAS) motor onset is the label! If, on careful history, the child has sensory symptoms (paraesthesiae, for instance) in an arm before it stiffens, then FIAS, non-motor onset is the correct classification, putting the seizure origin more likely in the sensory cortex.

EPILEPSY CLASSIFICATION AND CONCEPT

Classification of epilepsy is different to the classification of seizures. The classification of seizures is to decide whether they originate from a specific area of the brain at onset. Epilepsy classification attempts to understand the underlying cause (or causes), whether congenital or acquired, genetic or with genetic influence, and whether there are structural brain abnormalities or metabolic derangements. Epilepsy classification also considers the accompanying clinical features such as learning problems, movement disorders, family history and other neurological findings. All this information, including all investigatory test results (EEG, metabolic and genetic tests, and MRI) is combined to eventually label the type of epilepsy syndrome (Fig. 25.2).

For example, a girl presenting with seizures described as clonic jerking of the left upper limb and losing contact with surroundings. Seizures are classified as focal onset impaired awareness seizure (FIAS). On clinical examination, she has ash leaf macules on Wood's lamp skin examination, and there is family history of tuberous sclerosis (TS) – thus her provisional epilepsy classification is focal epilepsy caused by TS. When genetic and neuroimaging tests confirm a diagnosis of TS, then the epilepsy classification is confirmed to be focal epilepsy caused by TS.

Indications for Investigations

The purposes of investigations are to establish underlying aetiology, confirm epilepsy diagnosis and further define the epilepsy type.

Investigating for Underlying Aetiology

In recent years, knowledge of underlying causes of paediatric epilepsy has markedly improved with advances in both neuroimaging and molecular genetics.

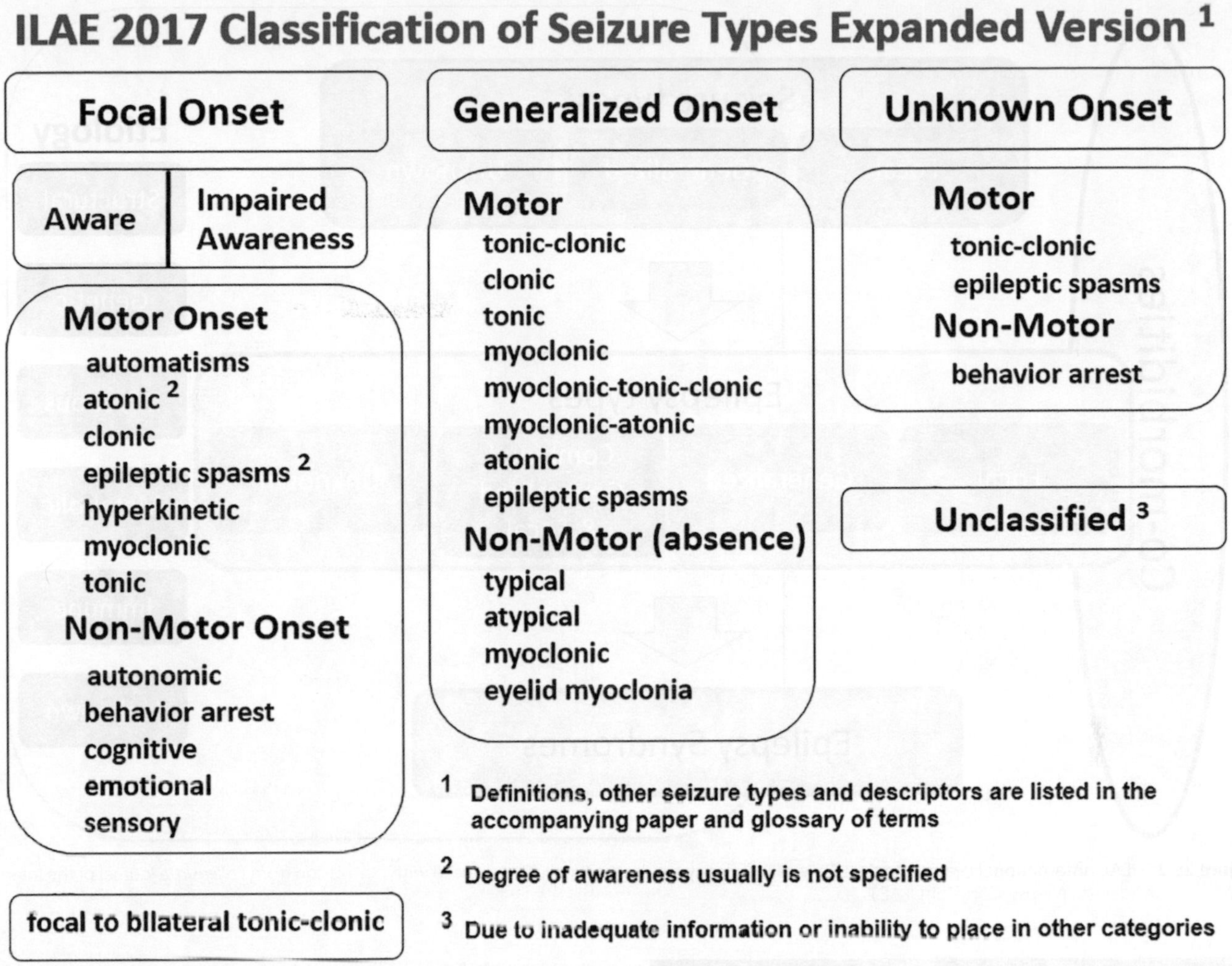

ILAE 2017 Classification of Seizure Types Expanded Version [1]

Focal Onset

Aware	Impaired Awareness

Motor Onset

automatisms
atonic [2]
clonic
epileptic spasms [2]
hyperkinetic
myoclonic
tonic

Non-Motor Onset

autonomic
behavior arrest
cognitive
emotional
sensory

focal to bilateral tonic-clonic

Generalized Onset

Motor
tonic-clonic
clonic
tonic
myoclonic
myoclonic-tonic-clonic
myoclonic-atonic
atonic
epileptic spasms

Non-Motor (absence)
typical
atypical
myoclonic
eyelid myoclonia

Unknown Onset

Motor
tonic-clonic
epileptic spasms

Non-Motor
behavior arrest

Unclassified [3]

[1] Definitions, other seizure types and descriptors are listed in the accompanying paper and glossary of terms

[2] Degree of awareness usually is not specified

[3] Due to inadequate information or inability to place in other categories

Figure 25.1   ILAE (International League Against Epilepsy) 2017 epilepsy classification system. (Reproduced with permission from Fisher, R. S., Cross, J. H., French, J. A., Higurashi, N., Hirsch, E., Jansen, F. E., et al. (2017). Operational classification of seizure types by the International League Against Epilepsy: position paper of the ILAE Commission for Classification and Terminology. *Epilepsia, 58*(4), 522–530.)

GENETIC AND GENETICALLY INFLUENCED EPILEPSIES

These vary from very benign and often age-related epilepsies seen mostly in childhood (e.g. benign focal epilepsy of childhood) to much more serious types of difficult epilepsies seen mostly in early infancy as exemplified by infantile spasms. Inheritance of epilepsy is polygenic in nature, but there are well known and less known single-gene mutations that can cause epilepsy syndromes. Some of these syndromes are easily recognisable and identifiable (for instance, Down syndrome), but many are not easily recognised. Therefore, genetic tests (microarray and whole genome sequencing) have become extremely important and are now almost routine in assessing more complex epilepsy.

STRUCTURAL ABNORMALITIES OF BRAIN DEVELOPMENT

These are common, whether diffuse and generalised such as lissencephaly (smooth brain), involving half of the brain or one hemisphere (hemimegaloencephaly) or the much more common focal cortical dysplasia (FCD) (Fig. 25.3). With advances in neuroimaging resolution and increased experience in interpretation of subtle FCD, FCD is the most expected cause of difficult to treat (refractory) focal epilepsy. Neuroimaging helps to identify a suspected specific focal abnormality guided or prompted by clinical history, examination, and/or EEG.

ACQUIRED LESIONS/CAUSES

Epilepsy can be due to acquired lesions such as those following meningitis or encephalitis, immune-mediated encephalitis, brain tumours or an intracerebral haemorrhage. Significant head injury (particularly if associated with brain haemorrhage) and hypoxic-ischaemic brain injury are other causes, particularly in newborns.

METABOLIC CAUSES

These are also often caused by underlying genetic aetiology and are likely to be revealed with genetic testing, but a baseline metabolic work up is especially important, as some of

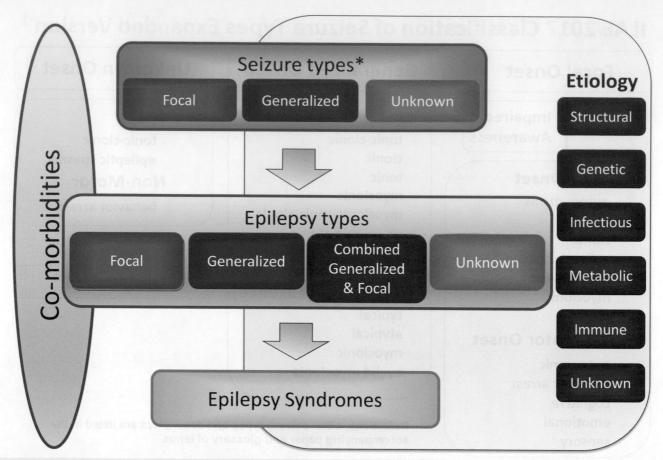

Figure 25.2 ILAE (International League Against Epilepsy) epilepsy syndrome types. (Reproduced with permission from *Epilepsia*, a journal of the International League against Epilepsy. Copyright ILAE.)

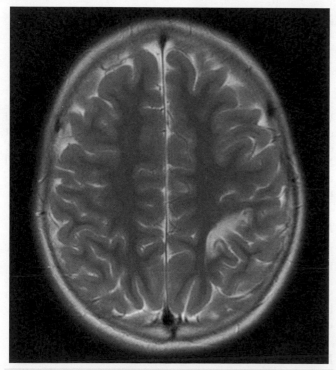

Figure 25.3 Focal cortical dysplasia. An 8-year-old with severe epilepsy. A T2 axial MRI image shows a left posterior parietal area of abnormal signal without mass effect and with some preservation of the gyral pattern within the lesion. (Courtesy Prof. Stephanie Ryan.)

these conditions are treatable (but not necessarily curable). Examples are pyridoxine responsive seizures/epilepsy, mitochondrial disorders, and disorders of glucose transport.

SUBSEQUENT CLINICAL APPROACH

Your approach to investigations into the cause of epilepsy depends on the age of the child, the clinical history and the clinical examination. For example, a child with childhood absence epilepsy or benign focal epilepsy of childhood does not require any genetic or neuroimaging investigations once the diagnosis is made and confirmed with an EEG. However, a young infant presenting with developmental delay and epilepsy will need extensive investigation (including genetic and metabolic studies and MRI of the brain). When investigating for a cause of epilepsy, an MRI of the brain is the neuroimaging modality of choice.

Confirm Epilepsy Diagnosis and Define Epilepsy Type

EEG IS THE NECESSARY AND GOLD STANDARD TEST

When suspecting epilepsy or having made a clinical diagnosis of potential epilepsy, an EEG helps confirm the diagnosis.

EEGs also help to differentiate generalised from focal epilepsy, thus indicating the appropriate choice of antiepileptic drug.

Immediate Management of a Convulsive Seizure

RECOGNITION

Tonic-clonic seizures are the most recognised of epileptic seizures. A sustained contraction of the facial, axial and limb muscles heralds the tonic phase. This phase lasts for seconds to minutes during which time the child may fall suddenly if standing, may become cyanosed, may bite their tongue and may have urinary incontinence. In the clonic phase, tonic contraction is interrupted by periods of momentary relaxation. Generalised jerking takes place and the body relaxes at the end of the clonic phase, at which time the child will have a reduced conscious level (postictal phase), often with deep respirations. The child will be difficult to rouse, appear confused and will wish to go to sleep. Most tonic-clonic seizures last under 5 minutes but occasionally are prolonged and may require immediate management if they last beyond 5 minutes.

FIRST AID MANAGEMENT

When a child is in a convulsive seizure (typically a generalised tonic-clonic seizure or GTCS), try to place them in the recovery position to ensure adequate breathing and patent airway. However, if the child is vigorously jerking and very stiff, do not force them to the recovery position, but instead concentrate on making sure they are safe from injury.

Never place objects in the child's mouth.

Administer rescue medication if a convulsive seizure is prolonged (more than 5 minutes). The most often used rescue medications are either buccal midazolam or, in infants, rectal diazepam.

Conduct a systematic and thorough history and a detailed clinical examination including a neurological examination and rapid checks (for example, an 'Alert', 'Voice', 'Pain', 'Unresponsive' (AVPU) score).

Identify simple and treatable causes (such as hypoglycaemia) and also **serious** but treatable causes for which you can rapidly initiate treatment (meningitis or encephalitis) and identify **serious** causes needing neuroimaging and possible neurosurgical intervention (e.g. stroke, intracranial bleed or tumour).

Management of Status Epilepticus

Status epilepticus is a medical emergency where epileptic seizures are prolonged or occur in rapid succession without recovery between seizures. The definition of status epilepticus is either prolonged seizure activity (over 5 minutes for GTCS) or recurrent seizures without recovery of consciousness.

The goals of therapy for status epilepticus are to maintain normal cardiorespiratory function and cerebral oxygenation, to stop clinical and electrical seizure activity, to identify precipitating factors, and to correct any metabolic disturbances.

The mainstay of management, with the aim of maintaining adequate oxygenation, is rapid ABCDE (airway, breathing, circulation, disability, exposure) assessment with airway management and breathing support where required. This rapid assessment must also quickly look for and treat hypoglycaemia if present; look for signs of shock and reverse if present. Quickly terminate the seizure using anticonvulsants.

Treated according to guidelines, status epilepticus can be expected to resolve in about 70 per cent of patients after first-line treatment with benzodiazepines. In the remaining 30 per cent that do not respond to first-line treatment with benzodiazepines, guidelines recommend treatment with any one of several second-line anticonvulsants with recent clinical trials providing more clarity as to how to proceed.

It is important to also take blood for laboratory glucose, urea and electrolytes, calcium, magnesium, lactic acid, blood gas, full blood count, blood cultures (if pyrexial) and drug levels for antiepileptic medications if on therapy. Check if any rescue medications were administered before presentation to hospital.

If there is any suspicion of a head injury, obtain an urgent CT or MRI brain scan. If meningitis or encephalitis are suspected, begin empirical antibiotics and aciclovir therapy and defer lumbar puncture.

Anticonvulsants Used in Status Epilepticus:

FIRST LINE: BENZODIAZEPINES

Benzodiazepines are the recommended first-line drug treatment of convulsive status epilepticus. Reasonably good scientific evidence based on several randomised controlled trials exists to support their use. Lorazepam given as a slow intravenous push is the preferred benzodiazepine where IV access is available. Buccal midazolam can be administered while obtaining IV access. Rectal diazepam has an equally rapid effect as IV lorazepam but a shorter duration of action and can also be administered while obtaining IV access.

SECOND LINE TREATMENT

Intravenous phenytoin (or fosphenytoin) and levetiracetam are the current recommended second-line drug treatments in status epilepticus in children over 6 months of age. Based on a recent randomised controlled trial, current evidence suggests the sequential use of levetiracetam and phenytoin (in any order) before progressing to third-line management in the intensive care unit (ICU).

THIRD LINE: RAPID SEQUENCE INDUCTION WITH ANAESTHESIA

This involves management in paediatric intensive care with rapid sequence induction with anaesthesia, intubation and a midazolam or propofol/thiopentone infusion to achieve burst suppression. In some institutions, lacosamide or sodium valproate are used prior to rapid sequence induction with anaesthesia, especially if there is any delay in transportation to ICU.

Basic Principles of Antiepileptic Drugs (AEDs)

AEDs work by either decreasing excitation or enhancing inhibition of electrical activity in the brain. Parents and older children should receive written information about the prescribed AED and potential side effects. It is generally advised to start with a low dose and gradually increase up to a maintenance dose of an AED. Aim for seizure control with one AED whenever possible.

The choice of AED is dependent on the type of epilepsy, frequency of seizures and the age of the child or adolescent.

When a decision is being made to initiate AED therapy, the initial duration is for 2 years in straightforward cases. However, with difficult epilepsy and epilepsies caused by known structural abnormalities or genetic abnormalities known to continue into adulthood, AEDs are continued for longer periods of time.

Initiating and weaning AEDs is a gradual process (building up or winding down usually over a period of weeks) with some taking longer than others. AEDs should never be stopped suddenly; this may provoke prolonged seizures or even status epilepticus.

A gradual process of withdrawal of AEDs should take place when a child has been seizure free for 2 years. Most of the time, it is not necessary to perform an EEG before discontinuation. However, in childhood absence epilepsy (CAE) for example, it is important to repeat an EEG with hyperventilation before considering withdrawing AEDs.

There are many AEDs which can be used for several types of epilepsy. However, there are a few instances in which specific drugs are best for specific syndromes. Examples include the use of ethosuximide or sodium valproate for childhood absence epilepsy and the use of steroids and vigabatrin for infantile spasms.

For focal epilepsy, many options exist depending on the epilepsy syndrome. These include levetiracetam, oxcarbazepine, carbamazepine, lacosamide, lamotrigine, zonisamide, topiramate and sodium valproate. For generalised epilepsy, sodium valproate, levetiracetam, lamotrigine, topiramate and zonisamde and others are options. As you can see, some AEDs can be used for both focal and generalised epilepsy syndromes. The choice of AED as detailed above is dependent on the epilepsy syndrome and underlying aetiology.

It is important to remember that carbamazepine and oxcarbazepine can worsen absence epilepsy and myoclonic seizures. Carbamazepine and lamotrigine can be associated with significant skin rashes, including Stevens–Johnson syndrome (lamotrigine) and exfoliative dermatitis (carbamazepine). Both should be introduced slowly and closely monitored.

Despite being an extremely efficacious AED, sodium valproate should be avoided in infants with new onset epilepsy as it may aggravate undiagnosed metabolic conditions, particularly of mitochondrial origin, in girls who have reached puberty, and during childbearing years, due to its proven teratogenicity.

Non-Epileptic Events That Mimic Epileptic Seizures

SYNCOPE AND FAINTS

Syncope of cardiovascular origin may resemble an epileptic seizure. These include structural heart defects and rhythmic disturbances such as *long QT syndrome*. Important clinical features distinguishing syncope from seizures include light-headedness, chest pain, palpitations or low pulse, pallor and sweating. The most frequent form of syncope is vasovagal episodes (simple faints) with a clear trigger, such as after seeing blood or a prolonged period of standing.

BREATH HOLDING SPELLS

Breath holding spells occur in approximately 5 per cent of children below the age of 5 years, and are always provoked. They are preceded by the child vigorously crying due to frustration, anger or pain, followed by the child holding their breath in expiration. The child stops breathing, becomes cyanotic, loses consciousness, becomes limp and may experience a brief convulsion towards the end in more extreme cases. There is quick recovery. Diagnosis is based on the history.

REFLEX ANOXIC SEIZURES

These occur most often in the second year of life and may be precipitated by an unexpected bump to the head or a fall. The child becomes pale, loses muscle tone and consciousness, and may present with body stiffening, limb jerking and eye deviation. The episode usually resolves within a minute.

NIGHT TERRORS

Night terrors are often familial and are most common between 3 and 8 years of age. They usually occur in the first hours of sleep during non-REM sleep. Typically, the child screams while sitting in bed terrified, often crying and wide-eyed (*often described as out of contact with surroundings*). Any attempts to wake the child or bring them out of the episode are ineffective. These episodes can last for minutes, then the child goes back to sleep. These episodes do not cause the child any harm, despite the dramatic and 'scary' situation experienced by those witnessing the child, and the fearful sensation the child may have during the episode. The child has no recollection of the event, which suggests a sleep disorder seen in toddlers and preschool children. Children grow out of these with no long-term consequences.

BENIGN SLEEP MYOCLONUS

This is mostly seen in neonates (quite common and frequent in sleep) but is also seen in infants and sometimes older children. Rhythmical brief jerks of the limbs, whether generalised or focal, occur in brief or prolonged clusters that can last for several minutes. The trunk and the face are usually not involved. The jerks cease on wakening and can be induced by rocking the crib while a baby is asleep. Frequent neonatal sleep myoclonus resolves after a few weeks.

ACUTE PSYCHOGENIC/EPISODES (CONVERSION DISORDER)

These are seen mostly in adolescents but can occur (albeit rarer) in children as young as 5 years old. They can be misjudged as epileptic seizures. Attacks vary from hypermotor/ hyperkinetic erratic movements (thrashing around) and often non-rhythmic jerking (often mimicking frontal lobe seizures or generalised tonic-clonic seizures/convulsions) to more 'quiet/silent' episodes of prolonged unresponsiveness, apparent loss of consciousness or loss of contact with surroundings. These can be tricky to diagnose and video EEG recording may be required. A home video is often sufficient for an experienced paediatric neurologist to diagnose with complete confidence.

TICS, MANNERISMS AND STEREOTYPIES

These are non-epileptic behavioural movements often of the face, mouth, neck or shoulders. A sudden muscle spasm causing contortion of the face and jerk of the neck with stereotypical and repetitive appearance is seen. In more established tic disorders (such as Tourette syndrome), vocal tics such as throat clearing and coprolalia may be very pronounced, making diagnosis much easier.

SELF-GRATIFICATION EPISODES

Self-gratification is commonly observed in infancy and early childhood as episodes of rhythmic contractions of the lower limbs and trunk, usually with adduction of thighs with some posturing, with or without grunting and facial flushing. The child is usually completely occupied with these movements and rarely interested in anything else once the episode takes place. The child is never distressed nor upset. They have a very characteristic appearance and are quite easy to recognise when seen on video. These episodes often occur when the child is in a car seat or highchair and can easily be misjudged to be epileptic in nature to the inexperienced eye. These episodes are purely behavioural and do not have any long-term implications.

Box 25.1   Key Points

One in 20 children will have an epileptic seizure in their lifetime, and one in 200 will have epilepsy.

History is the most valuable tool in diagnosing epilepsy or seizure disorders.

Video mobile phone recordings on smart devices are extremely helpful and are often the best diagnostic tool available to confirm or dispute the diagnosis of an epileptic seizure.

Uncovering focal neurological abnormalities is extremely important in directing your further approach to performing more specific investigations and tests.

Seizure classification helps clarify the type of seizure and origin in the brain (focal or generalised). On the other hand, epilepsy classification attempts to understand the underlying cause (or causes), whether congenital or acquired, genetic or with genetic influence, and whether structural brain abnormalities or metabolic derangements are present.

EEG is the necessary and gold standard test.

Parents and older children should receive written information about the prescribed antiepileptic drug (AED) and potential side effects. In general, start with a low dose and gradually increase up to a maintenance dose of an AED. When possible, aim for seizure control with one AED.

The choice of AED is dependent on the type of epilepsy, the frequency of seizures and the age of the child or adolescent.

Febrile convulsions are common (one in 20), may recur (in at least 30 per cent), are usually short-lived under 5 minutes (but can be prolonged up to 10 or 15 minutes), and are usually generalised.

Febrile seizures (FS) as an entity are a diagnosis of exclusion. Therefore, you must rule out other causes of seizures with fever, particularly meningitis or encephalitis.

Benign focal epilepsy of childhood (BFEC) accounts for 15 per cent of all children presenting with seizures. Symptoms of BFEC include a feeling of tingling on one side of the mouth involving the tongue and lips with unilateral jerking of the face, drooling and numbness of the face and mouth with guttural sounds or speech arrest (symptoms sometimes involve the upper or even lower limb on same side). In most cases, seizures come out of sleep rather than from wakefulness.

In childhood absence epilepsy (CAE), seizures are characterised by sudden (complete or incomplete) loss of contact with surroundings, during which the child stares blankly and is usually unresponsive. The seizures are frequent and brief, lasting 5 to 20 seconds. Hyperventilation is a very efficient precipitant of typical absence seizures and can safely be performed during the EEG.

West syndrome consists of a triad of infantile epileptic spasms, developmental delay, or regression and hypsarrhythmia on EEG. Clustering is the key feature that should draw attention to the possibility of infantile spasm diagnosis.

The key symptom of juvenile myoclonic epilepsy (JME) is early morning myoclonus involving upper limb muscles on awakening. A clustering of myoclonic jerks may be followed by a tonic-clonic seizure. Sodium valproate is the preferred anticonvulsant, but levetiracetam or lamotrigine should be used for adolescent females. Seizures are well controlled in the vast majority, but lifelong treatment is required.

Box 25.2   Common Paediatric Epilepsy Syndromes you should know: Febrile Seizure in an 18-Month-Old

An 18-month-old male presents with an intercurrent viral illness associated with fever. He has no relevant history and has met all developmental milestones. There is a positive family history of childhood febrile seizures in the father.

While in the waiting room to see by his family doctor, he has jerking involving all four limbs. The episode ceases spontaneously after 4 minutes and afterwards he is pale and very sleepy. His temperature is measured to be 39°C.

Clinical Pearls

Febrile seizures are defined as seizures occurring in those between 6 months and 6 years of age associated with a fever above 38.5°C in the absence of CNS infection. Febrile seizures are most often described as a generalised tonic-clonic seizure.

While benign, febrile seizures are terrifying to watch by parents and carers. Thus, significant reassurance from a confident and calm doctor is required.

Febrile convulsions are common (one in 20), may recur (in at least 30 per cent), are usually short-lived under 5 minutes (but can be prolonged up to 10 or 15 minutes), and are usually generalised. Complex febrile seizures are those lasting over 15 minutes, recurring during a single febrile illness, if focal in nature and associated with a transient Todd's paresis.

Risk of recurrence is increased if the child is younger than 12 months of age at first febrile seizure, the initial seizure is focal or prolonged, or if there is prior developmental delay.

The risk of epilepsy, however, is not increased following a febrile seizure (a popular myth debunked).

Interpretation of Investigations in FS

Blood glucose, urinalysis and urine culture are the only mandatory investigations. EEG or neuroimaging are <u>not</u> indicated unless other neurological concerns arise (such as focal neurological signs on examination or significant developmental delay).

Pitfalls to Avoid

Febrile seizures/convulsions as an entity are a <u>diagnosis of exclusion</u>. Therefore, you must rule out other causes of seizures with fever, particularly meningitis or encephalitis.

If very prolonged (for example, beyond 15 minutes or requiring intervention with rescue drugs to stop) or frequently recurrent with minimal temperatures (below 38°C with minimal febrile illnesses), Dravet syndrome should be considered.

Dravet syndrome has a peak presentation between 9 and 18 months of age. Seizures are provoked by warm ambient temperatures, hot baths, fever (often low-grade) or vaccinations. There may be multiple episodes of febrile status epilepticus often with focal features. *SCN1A* or *SCN9A* gene mutations occur in 80 per cent of cases of Dravet syndrome. While some AEDs as valproate, stiripentol and benzodiazepines are useful, fenfluramine is most recently reported to be effective in treating Dravet syndrome seizures.

Box 25.3   A 7-Year-Old With Benign Focal Epilepsy of Childhood (BFEC)

A 7-year-old girl attends with normal development and no significant medical history. Parents report nocturnal episodes of right-sided face twitching with choking sounds and drooling. She is aware of the facial twitching and describes a feeling that her tongue is being pulled to one side. The episodes are infrequent but have caused understandable anxiety.

Clinical Pearls

This history is quite typical of benign focal epilepsy of childhood (BFEC). The peak age of onset is 8 to 9 years with 75 per cent of cases occurring between 7 and 10 years of age. BFEC accounts for 15 per cent of all children presenting with seizures.

Most are nocturnal or 'coming out of sleep' seizures. Symptoms include a feeling of tingling on one side of the mouth involving the tongue and lips with unilateral jerking of the face, drooling, numbness of the face and mouth with guttural sounds, or speech arrest. BFEC can sometimes progress to a bilateral convulsive (tonic-clonic) seizure.

Many cases do very well and may not need AEDs with remission in most before 16 years of age. A few patients develop linguistic abnormalities and learning and behavioural problems.

Interpretation of Investigations

EEG confirms the diagnosis (with centrotemporal spikes). It is necessary to request a sleep-deprived EEG to record sleep EEG where and when most spikes are seen.

Pitfalls to Avoid

You must request a <u>sleep-deprived</u> EEG.

Presuming a seizure is generalised at onset; seizures may occur at night as tonic-clonic seizures with an unwitnessed focal onset and then progression to generalised tonic-clonic seizure.

Confusing with other epileptic or non-epileptic events; differential diagnoses for BFEC include nocturnal frontal lobe seizures. In frontal lobe seizures, bizarre hypermotor behaviours (rolling, yelling and fumbling) are clear and very brief (usually a few seconds).

Only treat BFEC with antiepileptic drugs (AED) if the seizures are too frequent causing disruption of sleep or postictal headaches, significant parental anxiety **or** if seizures habitually progress to bilateral convulsive activity, **or** if seizures start to become diurnal from wakefulness.

Box 25.4   An 8-Year-Old With Absence Seizures

An 8-year-old child presents with a history of recurrent episodes of 'zoning out', 'staring' and unresponsiveness. He is otherwise well and developmentally normal. The episodes were witnessed multiple times per day and all were short-lived, each lasting for less than 10 seconds.

Clinical Pearls

Childhood absence epilepsy (CAE) is a common childhood epilepsy syndrome with onset usually between 4 and 10 years of age and peak incidence around 8 years of age.

Seizures are characterised by sudden onset with (complete or incomplete) loss of contact with surroundings during which the child stares blankly and is usually unresponsive. The seizures are frequent and brief, lasting 5 to 20 seconds.

Typically, multiple seizures occur daily, sometimes tens of seizures daily before treatment. Thus, if events/seizures are long (a minute or more) and infrequent (a few times a week, for example), these are not typical absence seizures.

Oral and hand automatisms may occur, including lip smacking, swallowing movements, lip pursing, hand plucking at cloths or clapping. There is no recollection of the event and no postictal phase.

Children may be aware of a 'lapse' in concentration or losing track of a conversation. Those in the child's company often report this more than the patients themselves. School performance can be adversely affected if CAE is not recognised and treated.

The AED treatment of choice is ethosuximide or sodium valproate, and sometimes a combination of both. Most children respond well to drug treatment and most with typical CAE remit with no further seizures by mid-late teen years, or sometimes earlier.

Interpretation of Investigations

EEG shows characteristic regular 3 Hz generalised spike and wave activity (Fig. 25.4). Hyperventilation is a very efficient precipitant of typical absence seizures and can safely be performed during the EEG.

Pitfalls to Avoid

Infrequent and more prolonged seizures (over 20 seconds) are not typical of CAE.

Carbamazepine and oxcarbazepine are contraindicated in the treatment of absence seizures.

In CAE, it is important to repeat an EEG with hyperventilation before considering withdrawing AEDs.

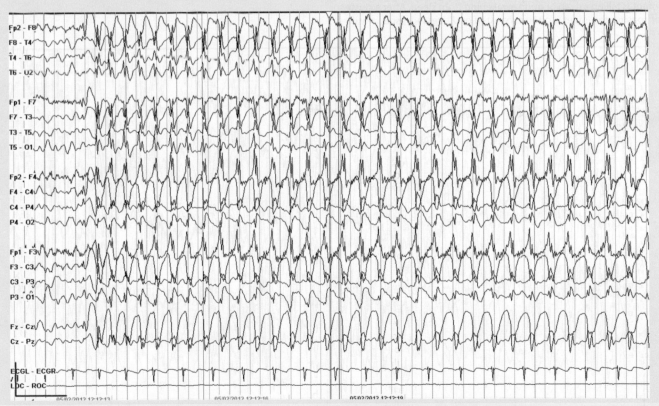

Figure 25.4   Childhood absence epilepsy. An EEG shows characteristic regular 3 Hz generalised spike and wave slow activity.

Box 25.5   An 8-Month-Old With Infantile Spasms

An 8-month-old female infant presents with episodes of clusters of repetitive arm and body jerks described as spasms or jolts by the parents. Her arms extend and then flex repetitively. Her legs sometimes come up to her trunk in the more noticeable spasms. She is developmentally delayed and has poor muscle tone.

Clinical Pearls

West syndrome consists of a triad of infantile epileptic spasms, developmental delay, or regression, and hypsarrhythmia on EEG.

West syndrome is a combination of clinical and EEG findings, not an aetiological diagnosis. In fact, it can be caused by a multitude of disorders and insults (congenital or acquired), affecting the infant brain at a very early age.

Common and familiar causes of infantile spasms include tuberous sclerosis, Down syndrome, other genetic entities, structural brain malformations (which are currently becoming more recognised), HIE (hypoxic-ischaemic encephalopathy), congenital infections, following meningitis or encephalitis, and intracranial vascular insults or strokes.

Infantile spasms usually have onset during the first year of life, typically between four and 12 months of age. Later onset is rare, but the spasms can continue thereafter for variable periods if not treated successfully or if not responsive to treatment.

The key feature that should draw attention to the possibility of an infantile spasm diagnosis is **clustering**. In a cluster, an infant can have spasms one after the other over a brief period of time (usually within 5 to 20 minutes). Clusters may recur several times a day, but may occur only once a day. Spasms are usually seen when the infant is falling asleep or upon awakening from sleep. After a cluster of spasms, the infant is often exhausted or distressed, especially if the spasms are forceful or the clusters are prolonged. They are not painful but can be startling or scary to babies.

Developmental delay or regression is often noted early. The longer the condition remains untreated, the more developmental delay and regression will be seen.

The main drugs used for treatment are corticosteroids and vigabatrin, but seizure control is often difficult to achieve.

It is important to know that infantile spams are, as the name implies, mostly a disease of infancy, which tends to evolve into distinct types of epilepsy in later childhood, including Lennox–Gastaut syndrome (a severe type of childhood epilepsy).

Interpretation of Investigations

An EEG should be performed promptly within a few days. It shows the characteristic pattern of hypsarrhythmia (Fig. 25.5). This term describes a 'chaotic'-appearing EEG with a disorganised background and very frequent high amplitude epileptiform.

Pitfalls to Avoid

Some parents may feel that infantile spasms may be related to feeding because spasm clusters often take place upon falling asleep or awakening. After feeding, the infant may become drowsy or drift into sleep. Thus, spasms relate to drowsiness and arousal rather than a relationship to feeding.

Symptoms such as presumed brief hiccoughs or startle seizures particularly on awakening or falling asleep with an associated developmental regression should prompt a neurology review and prompt EEG (within 3 to 5 days).

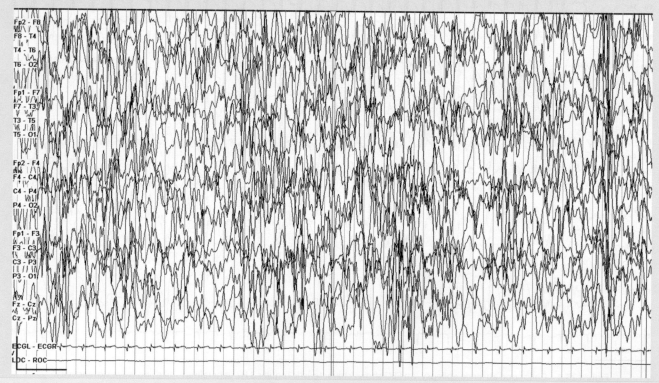

Figure 25.5   An EEG showing hypsarrhythmia.

Box 25.6   A 13-Year-Old Girl With Myoclonic Jerks

A 13-year-old girl presents firstly with episodes in which she tended to spill her cereal bowl in the morning and move clumsily upon awakening. She subsequently developed an early morning tonic-clonic seizure lasting 10 minutes.

Clinical Pearls

The hallmark of juvenile myoclonic epilepsy (JME) is early morning myoclonus involving upper limb muscles with typical episodes on awakening. Tonic-clonic seizures occur in the majority and often begin with a clustering of repeated myoclonic jerks.

Parents often comment that the young person (usually 12 to 18 years of age) has shakiness or clumsiness during the first 2 hours of the morning, sometimes spilling their cereal (the 'flying cornflakes') or dropping their toothbrush. Fatigue, stress, sleep deprivation, and alcohol all exacerbate the seizures.

Interpretation of Investigations

EEGs typically show generalised and often irregular spike and polyspike wave complexes if regular at a faster frequency of 4 to 6 Hz (compare to the slower 3 Hz of CAE). Brain MRIs are typically normal and need not be requested if clinical and EEG diagnosis is clear.

JME is one of the epilepsy syndromes often associated with photic sensitivity (30 per cent of patients). This can be confirmed during EEG testing by flashlight stimulation.

Pitfalls to Avoid

Sodium valproate is the preferred anticonvulsant, but levetiracetam or lamotrigine is more appropriate in adolescent females. Seizures are well controlled in the vast majority, but lifelong treatment is often required. Carbamazepine and oxcarbazepine are contraindicated (as in CAE), as they worsen myoclonic jerks.

▶ **Videos on the topic Seizures in childhood and Common paediatric epilepsy syndromes are available online at Elsevier eBooks+.**

Key References

Appleton, R. E. (2020). Second-line anticonvulsants for paediatric convulsive status epilepticus. *Lancet, 395*(10231), 1172–1173.

Berkovic, S. F. (2019). Epileptic encephalopathies of infancy: welcome advances. *Lancet, 394*(10216), 2203–2204.

Epilepsy Foundation. (n.d.). *Epilepsy Foundation–End Epilepsy Together.* https://www.epilepsy.com/

Howell, K. B., Eggers, S., Dalziel, K., Riseley, J., Mandelstam, S., Myers, C. T., et al. (2018). A population-based cost-effectiveness study of early genetic testing in severe epilepsies of infancy. *Epilepsia, 59*(6), 1177–1187.

International League Against Epilepsy. (n.d.). *Welcome to the International League Against Epilepsy.* https://www.ilae.org/

Kapur, J., Elm, J., Chamberlain, J. M., Barsan, W., Cloyd, J., Lowenstein, D., et al. (2019). Randomised trial of three anticonvulsant medications for status epilepticus. *The New England Journal of Medicine, 381*(22), 2103–2113.

Monrad, P. (2018). Paroxysmal disorders. In R. M. Kliegman, P. S. Lye, B. Bordini, H. Toth, & D. Basel (Eds.), *Nelson pediatric symptom-based diagnosis* (pp. 508–542). Elsevier.

Silbergleit, R., & Elm, J. J. (2019). Levetiracetam no better than phenytoin in children with convulsive status epilepticus. *Lancet, 393*(10186), 2101–2102.

26 *Severe Illness in Infancy and Childhood*

CORMAC BREATHNACH and IKE OFAKOR

Presentations with acute severe illness are thankfully rare but tend to test us the most. Here, key issues regarding the recognition and early management of the severely unwell child will be addressed. Paediatric Acute Life Support (PALS) and Advanced Paediatric Life Support (APLS) course materials are excellent resources. The rapid clinical assessment of the seriously ill child should identify potential airway, respiratory, circulatory or neurological dysfunction and should take less than 1 minute. The child with acute severe illness may present with airway compromise, respiratory distress, shock (covered in the chapter 15 on fever), acute adrenal crisis or signs of direct or secondary brain injury manifesting as impaired consciousness. Alternatively, hospital paediatric teams may be presented with a seriously injured child or surgical emergency (covered in the chapter 27 on surgery). Early recognition of the deteriorating child is key to a successful outcome in all cases.

Rapid Assessment Using the ABCDE Approach

AB (AIRWAY AND BREATHING)

When a child is trying to breathe, listen for signs of airway obstruction or respiratory distress such as stridor, grunting or wheezing. Estimate the work of breathing by counting the respiratory rate and assessing the force the child is generating to inspire. Accessory muscle use and indrawing of the chest wall indicate increased effort in the absence of exhaustion. Cyanosis and/or reduced oxygen saturation on oximetry suggest decompensation of the respiratory system and impending secondary cardiac arrest.

When there is no patient effort to breathe, airway patency cannot be confirmed until positive pressure breaths are applied.

C (CIRCULATION)

Check the heart rate and pulse volume and assess the capillary refill time. To check the capillary refill time, apply blanching pressure on the sternum for 5 seconds and measure the time taken for blush to return. This should be under 2 seconds. Check the child's blood pressure. Cold or mottled skin, reduced urine output and abnormal mentation all suggest insufficient end-organ perfusion.

D (DISABILITY)

Note the level of consciousness using the rapid AVPU scale (as discussed below). Assess posture (which may be hypotonic, decorticate or decerebrate) and check pupil size, symmetry and reactivity. Check for focal or lateralising neurological signs.

E (EXPOSURE)

Check the child's temperature and perform a full head-to-toe examination.

Upper Airway Obstruction

ACUTE SEVERE VIRAL CROUP

Laryngotracheobronchitis or croup is a self-limiting viral infection of the subglottic larynx which can on occasion be quite severe. Croup has a myriad of causes including para-influenza virus types 1 and 3, influenza A, adenovirus and respiratory syncytial virus. Children present with a low-grade fever, barking cough, rhinorrhoea and inspiratory stridor. Stridor tends to be worse when the child is active or upset.

Oral dexamethasone is recommended for viral croup and is preferred to nebulised budesonide. In more severe cases, nebulised racemic adrenaline is used if severe stridor is present at rest or severe retractions. Thereafter observation in hospital for at least 6 hours is necessary. In cases of recurrent croup or an atypical presentation, referral to ENT with a view to laryngoscopy and bronchoscopy is required.

BACTERIAL TRACHEITIS

Bacterial tracheitis is caused by *Staphylococcus aureus*, *Moxarella catarrhalis*, *Streptococcus pneumoniae* and non-typeable *Haemophilus influenzae*. Intravenous antibiotics are required and endotracheal intubation with pulmonary toilet to remove plugs of pus and sloughed tissue is frequently needed.

ACUTE EPIGLOTTITIS

Acute epiglottitis presents as a rapidly progressive illness due to *H. influenzae type b* and is now rarely seen due to immunisation. Children with epiglottitis appear unwell with toxicity, a high fever and drooling. Typically, the child leans forward with a hyperextended head and weight on their hands (tripod position) and is reluctant to lie down (Fig. 26.1). The child should not be disturbed from their position of comfort with blow-by O$_2$ until the airway can be secured in theatre by an experienced anaesthetist with an ENT surgeon on hand in case of tracheostomy – a 'double set-up'. Blood cultures are taken post intubation and intravenous cefotaxime or ceftriaxone is commenced.

RETROPHARYNGEAL ABSCESS

Retropharyngeal abscess represents the extension of infection from the pharynx into the retropharyngeal space. Children under 4 years of age are most often affected. Typical symptoms include fever, dysphagia,

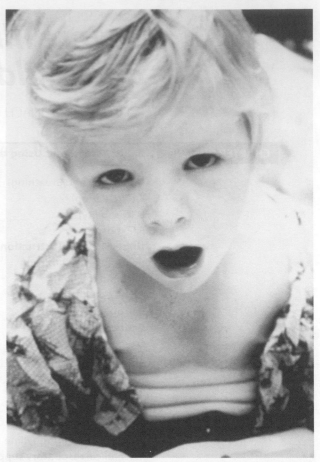

Figure 26.1 Child with epiglottitis. Characteristic posture in a patient with epiglottitis. The child is leaning forward, drooling and the neck is hyperextended. (Reproduced with Permission from Sharma, Anjali, et al. In R. M. Kliegman, P.S. Lye, B. Bordini, H. Toth, & D. Basel (Eds.), *Nelson pediatric symptom-based diagnosis* (pp. 39–60.e1). Elsevier.)

stridor with drooling and reduced neck movement. Treatment is with intravenous antibiotics with a review by the ENT team. For those with severe obstruction, the same approach to airway management used for epiglottitis should be employed.

Acute Severe Asthma

Indicators of life-threatening asthma include oxygen saturation below 90 per cent, inability to talk, altered consciousness, agitation, poor respiratory effort, silent chest, cyanosis, bradycardia and hypotension.

Indications of a severe asthmatic attack include:

- inability to complete sentences
- oxygen saturation under 92 per cent
- peak flow below 50 per cent predicted
- heart rate over 140 (under 5 years) or 125 (over 5 years)
- respiratory rate over 40 (under 5 years) or 30 (over 5 years)
- noticeable recession
- pulsus paradoxus

Pulsus paradoxus (PP) is an objective bedside measurement to assess airway obstruction and response to treatment. Originally described by Adolf Kussmaul in 1873, PP is a decrease in systolic blood pressure of more than 10 mmHg during inspiration.

Pulse oximeters can give a qualitative display of the pulse amplitude of the vascular bed underlying the probe. This pulse oximeter plethysmographic waveform on the cardiac monitor can detect the presence of PP.

If PP is still present after initial bronchodilator therapy, it may be helpful in the evaluation of the severity of acute asthma and thereby guide further management.

The acute management plan for severe asthma includes high flow oxygen via mask or nasal cannula to achieve normal saturations and nebulised salbutamol. If the response is poor, repeat every 20 minutes and add nebulised ipratropium bromide. Give oral prednisolone or intravenous hydrocortisone if unable to tolerate oral medication. Salbutamol may be weaned to one or two hourly, and ipratropium four to six hourly, pending a good clinical response.

OXYGEN

Acute severe asthma leads to hypoxemia and supplementary oxygen is urgently required to maintain SpO_2 above 92 per cent. A raised blood CO_2 level is very significant and should signal the need for anaesthetic assessment and intervention.

BRONCHODILATORS

Inhaled β2-agonists given in high doses act rapidly to relieve bronchospasm with few side effects.

In acute moderate asthma, inhaled β2-agonists should be administered by repeated activations of a metered dose inhaler (MDI) via an appropriate spacer or, less preferably, by nebulisation driven by oxygen.

Oxygen-driven nebulisers are indicated for severe asthma with a flow rate of 6 L/min with frequent nebulisation over the first few hours. Continuous nebulisation of β2-agonists is more effective than bolus nebulisation in life-threatening disease.

GLUCOCORTICOSTEROIDS

Steroids reduce mortality in acute asthma with either oral prednisolone for 3 days or parenteral hydrocortisone in severe asthma.

IPRATROPIUM BROMIDE

The combination of nebulised ipratropium bromide given together with nebulised β2-agonist ensures a synergistic effect than with a β2-agonist alone in moderate-to-severe asthma thereby promoting a speedier recovery.

MAGNESIUM SULPHATE

Magnesium sulphate reduces the need for admission to intensive care in acute severe asthma.

Intravenous magnesium sulphate is used in moderate to severe asthma but requires consultation with senior medical staff.

INTRAVENOUS β2-AGONISTS

Intravenous salbutamol is used in children requiring high dependency or intensive care for asthma.

INTRAVENOUS AMINOPHYLLINE

Some patients with life-threatening asthma may gain additional benefits from intravenous aminophylline. Daily levels should be checked for children on an aminophylline infusion.

MECHANICAL RESPIRATORY SUPPORTS

Humidified high flow oxygen and non-invasive ventilation are both helpful in severe asthma. Ventilation is seen as a last resort in a situation with progressive fatigue, worsening hypoxia or after a respiratory arrest.

The Unconscious Child

The approach to the unconscious child requires a rapid ABCDE assessment ensuring airway patency and that the child is breathing. A rapid neurological assessment using the 'Alert', 'Voice', 'Pain', 'Unresponsive' (AVPU) scale should be performed. Identify and reverse immediately treatable causes such as hypoglycaemia.

Stabilisation

Initial stabilisation follows ABC assessment. Ensure a patent airway. Airway manoeuvres, such as the neutral position for infants and the sniffing position for older children, may be required to relieve obstruction from reduced tone. Intubation is traditionally considered to protect against aspiration when glasgow coma scale (GCS) is less than or equal to eight (P or U on AVPU), albeit supporting evidence is lacking. Check for adequate breathing and provide support with positive pressure if respiratory depression is apparent. Oxygen should be administered if oxygen saturations are 95 per cent or less. Establish vascular access and confirm circulatory sufficiency.

Always request a capillary blood glucose and, if the blood glucose is under 2.6 mmol/L proceed to performing a hypoglycaemia screen and promptly correct the blood glucose level using intravenous dextrose 10 per cent.

Rapid Clinical Assessment

Record the vital signs including the respiratory rate, heart rate, blood pressure and temperature.

Look for focal features on neurological assessment. Check for asymmetry in size or reactivity of the pupils and examine for asymmetrical movement of the limbs or face. The respiratory pattern, corneal reflexes and the oculocephalic and oculovestibular reflexes are all tests of brain stem function. Raised intracranial pressure may give the so-called Cushing triad (hypertension, bradycardia and irregularities of respiration), decerebrate or opisthotonic posturing, or a lateral rectus palsy.

REVERSAL OF IMMEDIATELY TREATABLE CAUSES

Check for hypoglycaemia and correct with 10 per cent dextrose intravenously if blood sugar is below 2.6 mmol/L. Naloxone is given to children with marked depression in consciousness with associated hypoventilation, where opioid ingestion (often inadvertent) is suspected; pinpoint pupils are suggestive. Continue close monitoring. Repeated doses of naloxone may be required due to its relatively short half-life.

If inadequate cerebral perfusion is the apparent cause, reverse shock and treat the underlying cause.

If head trauma is suspected, address the ABCs as above to prevent secondary injury and then obtain an emergency brain CT with prompt referral to the neurosurgical team. Apart from head trauma, consider other causes of raised intracranial pressure such as space-occupying lesions, non-traumatic bleeds and acute hydrocephalus.

PUPILLARY RESPONSES

In metabolic encephalopathy, pupillary responses are preserved, whereas they may be absent if an underlying structural lesion is present in the brain (such as an intracerebral bleed). Drugs including scopolamine or atropine (both with a potent anticholinergic effect) can lead to fixed and dilated pupils. Uncal herniation with pressure on the third cranial nerve can lead to a unilateral fixed dilated pupil.

Finding the Cause

Additional investigations to be considered include a cranial CT or MRI scan, urine toxicology, an electroencephalogram (EEG) and serum electrolytes, lactate and ammonia. A lumbar puncture is generally deferred.

SEPSIS WITH SHOCK

Signs of sepsis include a low or elevated temperature, marked tachycardia, or a non-blanching rash, any or all of which should prompt commencement of broad-spectrum intravenous antibiotics.

HYPERAMMONAEMIA

If the ammonia level is over 100 μmol/L, discuss with a metabolic specialist team as urea cycle defects may present with an impaired level of consciousness.

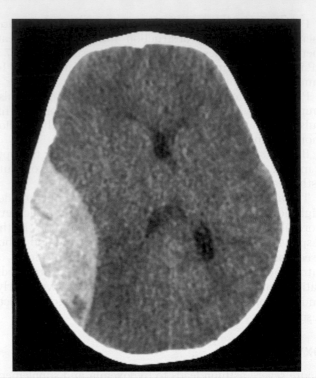

Figure 26.2 A 5-year-old with a head injury. CT shows a large right posterior extradural haematoma with a biconcave shape. It is causing some midline shift. (Courtesy Prof Stephanie Ryan.)

MENINGITIS OR ENCEPHALITIS

Bacterial meningitis is suggested by classical symptoms of neck stiffness, a bulging fontanelle, photophobia or a focal neurological deficit.

If there are focal neurological signs, a conscious level that appears to fluctuate or a history of a prolonged seizure, then herpes simplex encephalitis (HSE) should be considered and intravenous aciclovir commenced.

ELECTROLYTE DISTURBANCE

Seizures may occur if the sodium level drops to below 125 mmol/L, the calcium level is under 1.7 mmol/L, or the plasma magnesium level drops to less than 0.65 mmol/L. If seizures are refractory to treatment, always consider electrolyte disturbance.

INTOXICATION/POISONING

Request an urgent urine sample to be sent for toxicology and call your local regional poisons unit for advice.

TRAUMA

This is usually clear-cut in older children but may not be so in under 1-year-olds with suspected abusive head trauma. CT scan of the brain is urgently required, and neurosurgical intervention is urgently needed if an extradural haemorrhage is present (Fig. 26.2).

HYPERTENSION WITH ENCEPHALOPATHY

Severe hypertension is associated with encephalopathy and requires input from both intensive care and nephrology to slowly reduce the blood pressure to prevent ischaemic injuries. Infusions of short-acting agents with invasive arterial BP monitoring is the safest approach.

INTRACEREBRAL BLEED

A significant intracerebral or subarachnoid bleed can be associated with a reduced level of consciousness often of rapid onset. In the absence of trauma, spontaneous intracranial bleeds are uncommon in children and are often associated with pre-existing aneurysms, AV malformations or severe bleeding disorders. In infants, consider abusive head trauma as a cause.

MALFUNCTION OF A VENTRICULOPERITONEAL SHUNT

Any child who has a ventriculoperitoneal (VP) shunt in situ who has a reduced level of consciousness, perhaps with signs of raised intracranial pressure, should have a shunt series and CT brain scan urgently to rule out shunt malfunction. Discuss with a neurosurgical specialist even in the absence of abnormal neuroimaging if clinical suspicion persists.

Investigations at Presentation

ROUTINE ON PRESENTATION

Capillary blood glucose (as soon as possible) and subsequently a confirmatory laboratory blood glucose, full blood count, blood gases, urea and electrolytes, lactate, liver function tests and plasma ammonia, blood cultures and urinalysis (dipstick at bedside) for ketones, glucose and protein.

Save 10 mL of urine for later analysis and a plasma sample for future toxicology analysis.

AS CLINICALLY INDICATED

Urgent Cranial CT or MRI. Urgent cerebral function monitoring or formal electroencephalogram may be required for some patients.

TIMING OF LUMBAR PUNCTURE (LP)

Defer performing a lumbar puncture if there are clinical features of raised intracranial pressure, a GCS of less than or equal to eight, or a dropping GCS, if focal neurological signs or following a seizure where consciousness remains impaired. Severe meningococcaemia, coagulopathy, thrombocytopenia, or overlying skin infection are other contraindications.

Be aware that a normal CT scan does not exclude raised intracranial pressure. A specialist registrar or consultant should examine the child first before reaching a decision.

The Seriously Injured Child

The child with serious injuries requires a structured approach to ensure these injuries are identified and managed during the primary survey before less serious injuries are managed during the secondary survey. Assume a cervical spine injury and immobilise by holding the neck in the midline neutral position followed by head blocks and straps if necessary. In major trauma, catastrophic haemorrhage requires immediate management. Regional and national trauma networks with appropriate transport are essential to improve survival from major trauma.

For the seriously injured child, follow the ABCDE format as outlined below, and life-threatening problems (such as severe haemorrhage) should be treated as they are identified during the primary survey. Try to stop severe uncontrolled bleeding by applying direct pressure over the site, maintaining the blood pressure, and keeping the haemoglobin above 10 g/dL by the administration of blood if required.

If the child deteriorates further, then return to the primary survey and reassess. For pain relief, morphine is the standard drug used and fentanyl is a useful alternative and may be administered intranasally.

A joint interventional radiology and surgical approach to control arterial bleeding in children is helpful. A formal written process should be used to hand a child over to the next level of care.

The ABCDE Approach to the Severely Injured Child

A: If a severely injured child cannot maintain their airway, use a rapid sequence induction and intubate the child.

B: Consider chest x-ray or ultrasound as first-line imaging (as opposed to CT) to assess chest trauma in children. For children with severe respiratory compromise or haemodynamic instability, needle decompression should precede imaging if a tension pneumothorax is suspected.

C: For children with active bleeding, use packed red cells instead of crystalloid solutions. Use intravenous tranexamic acid as soon as possible in children with suspected or active bleeding. Paediatric haematology advice may be required. Generally, if more than 20 mL/kg of volume replacement is required, then urgent interventional radiology or surgery consultation should be considered. First try peripheral intravenous access and, if unsuccessful, consider intraosseous access.

D: Assess the level of alertness based on the AVPU scale. If traumatic brain injury is suspected, use volume resuscitation to maintain cerebral perfusion. Assess pain early in patients with major trauma using a pain assessment scale and give intravenous morphine as the first-line analgesic to achieve adequate pain relief. Reassess pain regularly using the same pain assessment scale.

E: Encourage the child's family members to stay within eyesight of the child to support the child at the bedside.

Box 26.1   Key Points

The rapid clinical assessment of a seriously ill child should identify potential airway, respiratory, circulatory or neurological dysfunction, taking less than 1 minute to do so.

The child with acute severe illness may present with airway compromise, respiratory distress or signs of direct or secondary brain injury manifesting as impaired consciousness.

Note the level of consciousness using the rapid AVPU scale, assess posture (may be hypotonic, decorticate or decerebrate) and check pupil size, symmetry and reactivity.

If a child with stridor looks systemically unwell, has drooling, or is rapidly deteriorating, acute epiglottitis or bacterial tracheitis should be considered.

For acute epiglottitis, the child should be left undisturbed in their position of comfort with blow-by O_2 until the airway can be secured in theatre by an experienced anaesthetist with an ENT surgeon on hand. Post intubation, blood cultures are taken and intravenous cefotaxime or ceftriaxone is commenced.

Typical symptoms of retropharyngeal abscess include fever, dysphagia, stridor with drooling and reduced neck movement.

Indicators of life-threatening asthma include SpO2 under 90 per cent, inability to talk, altered consciousness, agitation, poor respiratory effort, silent chest, cyanosis, bradycardia and hypotension.

In acute severe asthma, give repeated rapid-acting inhaled β2-agonist bronchodilator, glucocorticosteroids and oxygen.

Magnesium sulphate is effective in reducing the need for intensive care and improves lung function in children with acute severe asthma.

For a child with impaired consciousness, a rapid neurological assessment using the AVPU scale should be performed. Identify and reverse immediately treatable causes such as hypoglycaemia.

In metabolic encephalopathy, pupillary reactions are usually preserved, and confusion, lethargy, and delirium often precede coma.

A normal CT scan does not exclude raised intracranial pressure.

For the seriously injured child, follow the ABCDE format and life-threatening problems (such as severe haemorrhage) should be treated as they are identified during the primary survey. For severe uncontrolled bleeding, try to stop the bleeding by applying direct pressure over the site, maintaining the blood pressure, and keeping the haemoglobin above 10 g/dL by the administration of blood if required.

Regional and national trauma networks with appropriate transport are essential to improve survival from major trauma.

Box 26.2   An Ill 10-Month-Old With Stridor and Severe Respiratory Distress

A 10-month-old male presents with a brief history of fever and audible stridor. His history was unremarkable but, he did not receive his 2-, 4-and 6-month immunisations due to parental vaccine hesitancy. He is noted to be pyrexial, toxic and has obvious drooling. He is quickly transferred to theatre for intubation and thereafter started on intravenous cefotaxime. A red swollen epiglottis was noted at intubation and blood cultures were positive for *Haemophilus influenzae* type b.

Clinical Pearls

Acute epiglottitis or bacterial tracheitis should be considered in acute stridor if an infant or child looks systemically unwell, develops drooling or showed rapidly progressing respiratory distress.

In acute epiglottitis (as above), the tongue is often protruding, the mouth is open, and there is a 'hot potato' voice and drooling of saliva. Mild stridor is evident.

For acute epiglottitis, the child should be left undisturbed in their position of comfort with blow-by oxygen until the airway can be secured in theatre by an experienced anaesthetist with an ENT surgeon on hand. Post intubation, blood cultures are taken and intravenous cefotaxime or ceftriaxone is commenced.

Typical symptoms of retropharyngeal abscess include fever, dysphagia, stridor with drooling and reduced neck movement.

Interpretation of Investigations

Lateral neck x-rays are of limited value in assessing acute stridor where bacterial tracheitis or epiglottitis are being considered.

In contrast, the lateral x-ray of the neck in retropharyngeal abscess may be helpful and may reveal soft tissue swelling with anterior displacement of the airway with confirmation by contrast-enhanced CT.

Blood cultures are helpful in the diagnosis of acute epiglottitis after the airway has been secured.

Pitfalls to Avoid

Acute stridor in children is most often due to viral croup with oral dexamethasone being the treatment of choice.

If epiglottitis is suspected, airway maintenance is key – the child should be quickly transferred to theatre for intubation, blood cultures should be taken and intravenous antibiotics commenced.

Never check the throat with a spatula - you may cause complete airway obstruction.

Acquired subglottic stenosis usually follows prolonged intubation or multiple reintubations and typically presents under 3 months of age. It may, however, be seen after relatively short periods of intubation.

BOX 26.3   A 10-Year-Old With Acute Severe Asthma

A 10-year-old girl has a background history of atopy and has a history of frequent nocturnal and exercise-induced coughing with concomitant wheeze. There is a strong family history of atopy, and both her parents are smokers. She has visited her family doctor on several occasions and received oral steroids and inhaled salbutamol. She was commenced on inhaled steroid prophylaxis 3 months ago but has not been compliant with treatment.

She is very breathless, is unable to complete a sentence, and has marked tachycardia. She is promptly referred to the nearest emergency department where her saturations are noted to have dropped to 86 per cent. She receives face mask oxygen and continuous salbutamol via nebuliser and intravenous hydrocortisone but remains very distressed. The paediatric intensive care team are called.

Clinical Pearls

Compliance is a key issue, as is asthma education; one should only prescribe inhalers aligned to training in the use of the inhaler device. The child should be able to demonstrate satisfactory inhaler technique.

If symptoms are refractory to initial β2-agonist treatment, add ipratropium bromide mixed with the nebulised β2-agonist solution.

In children who respond poorly to first-line treatments, intravenous magnesium sulphate is now the first-line intravenous treatment ahead of intravenous salbutamol or aminophylline.

Written personalised asthma action plans (PAAPs) are key in terms of self-management education.

Telehealth is now an option for supporting self-management for children and young people with chronic asthma.

A partnership approach works best, essentially involving children and young people from the start and encouraging them to take responsibility for managing their asthma. Listen to and address their needs fully and ask about any acute asthma episodes, whether breathless with exercise or not, whether they have needed frequent reliever therapy, and any reasons for non-adherence, if that seems to be an issue.

Interpretation of Investigations

In acute asthma, a chest x-ray is required if subcutaneous emphysema, a pneumothorax, lobar collapse, or consolidation are suspected, or if life-threatening asthma is unresponsive to treatment.

Asthma severity, classified by symptoms and use of medication, correlates poorly with single measurements of forced expiratory volume in 1 second (FEV1) in children over 5 years of age.

Pitfalls to Avoid

A hospital admission with acute asthma (especially severe cases) represents a window of opportunity to review self-management skills.

No child should leave the hospital without a written PAAP. Poor adherence or non-compliance should always be considered when there is poor asthma control.

The dose or duration of inhaled corticosteroids required to place a child at risk of clinical adrenal insufficiency is unknown but is unlikely to occur unless doses exceed 800 micrograms per day over an extended period.

Box 26.4   A Child With Fever, Recurrent Seizures and a Depressed Level of Consciousness

A developmentally appropriate 20-month-old female presented to hospital with a fever-related seizure lasting 10 minutes. There was a family history of febrile seizures and the working diagnosis on admission was that of a simple febrile seizure. Blood glucose, urinalysis and blood cultures were performed on admission.

Her ongoing drowsiness caused significant parental concern. She had a further febrile episode with a 7-minute-long seizure.

Minor inflammatory changes were seen on chest x-ray and thus oral co-amoxiclav was commenced. A focal seizure lasting 45 minutes occurred 3 days after admission and led to further assessment and investigations. A cerebrospinal fluid (CSF) sample was taken, which showed lymphocytosis and a positive polymerase chain reaction (PCR) for herpes simplex DNA.

Clinical Pearls

Consider the possibility of herpes simplex encephalitis (HSE) in a child with a decreased conscious level and focal neurological signs.

If HSE or meningitis are suspected, empirical intravenous cefotaxime and aciclovir treatment should be started, neuroimaging coordinated, and lumbar puncture deferred if contraindications such as raised intracranial pressure are evident.

Encephalitis may result from an infection of the brain (infectious encephalitis) or from autoantibodies that affect the brain (immune-mediated encephalitis), or from both.

Interpretation of Investigations

In a child with unexplained encephalopathy, urgent neuroimaging is recommended, and empirical cefotaxime and acyclovir should be commenced.

In HSE, CSF examination shows an increased number of white cells and red cells and an elevated CSF protein. MRI brain scan and EEG may show a temporal lobe focus.

PCR of CSF for herpes simplex DNA provides a specific diagnosis.

Pitfalls to Avoid

An elevated level of clinical suspicion is required to diagnose herpes encephalitis. Aciclovir should be commenced if the diagnosis is considered. Neurological sequelae occur in up to 60 per cent (including either seizures or developmental delay) with reported complications including severe physical impairment, and behavioural, psychosocial and educational difficulties.

Ornithine transcarbamylase (OTC) deficiency is an x-linked urea cycle disorder that presents with marked hyperammonaemia; therefore, request a serum ammonia in otherwise unexplained encephalopathy.

Finally, always consider poisoning. Poisoning in younger children is usually accidental and may be related to ingestion of medications belonging to household members. In older children and adolescents, also consider recreational substances, especially alcohol.

Video on the topic Recognising the sick child is available online at Elsevier eBooks+.

Key References

Healthcare Improvement Scotland. (2019, July). British guideline on the management of asthma: A national clinical guideline (SIGN158). Scottish Intercollegiate Guidelines Network, British Thoracic Society, NHS Scotland. https://www.sign.ac.uk/media/1773/sign158-updated.pdf.

Hoskison, E., & Grainger, J. (2017). Fifteen-minute consultation: Investigation and management of an infant with stridor. *Archives of Disease in Childhood Education and Practice Edition, 102*(3), 124–126.

Kanani, A. N., & Hartshorn, S. (2017). NICE clinical guideline NG39: Major trauma: assessment and initial management. *Archives of Disease in Childhood Education and Practice Edition, 102*, 20–23.

Krishnan, S. G., Wong, H. C., Ganapathy, S., & Ong, G. Y.-K. (2020). Oximetry-detected pulsus paradoxus predicts for severity in paediatric asthma. *Archives of Disease in Childhood, 105*(6), 533–538.

Kuzminski, J. C. (2018). Altered mental status. In R. M. Kliegman, P. S. Lye, B. Bordini, H. Toth, & D. Basel (Eds.), *Nelson pediatric symptom-based diagnosis* (pp. 543–562). Elsevier.

National Clinic Programme for Asthma. (2013, April). Emergency paediatric asthma guideline. Health Service Executive, Royal College of Physicians of Ireland. https://www.hse.ie/eng/services/publications/clinical-strategy-and-programmes/emergency-paediatric-asthma--guidelines.pdf.

National Institute for Health and Care Excellence. (2016, February 17). Major trauma: Assessment and initial management. NICE guideline [NG39]. https://www.nice.org.uk/guidance/ng39.

Royal College of Paediatrics and Child Health. (2019). The management of children and young people with an acute decrease in conscious level: A nationally developed evidence-based guideline for practitioners. https://www.rcpch.ac.uk/sites/default/files/2019-04/decon_guideline_revised_2019_08.04.19.pdf.

Sims, C., Weber, D., & Johnson, C. (2020). *A Guide to Pediatric Anesthesia.* Springer International Publishing.

Tanz, R. R. (2018). Sore throat. In R. M. Kliegman, P. S. Lye, B. Bordini, H. Toth, & D. Basel (Eds.), *Nelson pediatric symptom-based diagnosis* (pp. 1–14). Elsevier.

Topjian, A. A., Raymond, T. T., Atkins, D., Chan, M., Duff, J. P., Joyner, B. L., Jr., et al, & Pediatric Basic and Advanced Life Support Collaborators. (2020). Part 4: Pediatric basic and advanced life support: 2020 American heart association guidelines for cardiopulmonary resuscitation and emergency cardiovascular care. *Circulation, 142*(16_suppl_2), S469–S523. https://doi.org/10.1161/CIR.0000000000000901.

Online References

Asthma UK. Personalised asthma action plans. https://www.asthma.org.uk/e75bf921/globalassets/health-advice/resources/children/my-asthma-plan-2021-v5-multi-media-live.pdf

27 | *Surgical Problems in Infancy and Childhood*

ALAN MORTELL and KRIS HUGHES

This chapter will provide you with a complete common-sense understanding of the various presentations of common surgical conditions in infants and children and enable you to assess and understand the indications for referral to a specialist paediatric surgical team.

We propose to go through these sequentially, focusing on modes of presentation, assessment, urgent actions required and management by a specialist paediatric surgical team.

In many respects, paediatric surgery represents a frontier in surgery – it is possibly the most challenging subspecialty in which to conduct research, and yet it is pushing the boundaries of biomedical science to seek innovative, often non-surgical, solutions for intractable problems. This chapter hopes to capture some of these innovations.

Although rare, neonatal gastrointestinal disorders requiring surgical intervention are potentially life-threatening. Despite initial life-saving surgery, they require multidisciplinary management and often have long-term problems.

Neonatal surgical emergencies all require prompt recognition, core investigations to establish the diagnosis, stabilisation, and transfer to a specialist tertiary paediatric surgical service. The main focus will be on prompt recognition and stabilisation with a secondary emphasis on management within a specialist paediatric surgical service.

Thoracic

CONGENITAL DIAPHRAGMATIC HERNIA

Congenital diaphragmatic hernias (CDHs) are developmental defects in the diaphragm that allow herniation of the abdominal contents into the thorax (Fig. 27.1). Through mass-effect, the presence of the abdominal viscera in the chest limits the development of the lungs, resulting in pulmonary hypoplasia and pulmonary artery hypertension. CDH has an incidence of approximately one in 4000 live births. The size and location of the defect can vary with more than over 80 per cent being left-sided. Right-sided CDH tends to have an increased association with congenital heart defects and often have a worse prognosis than left-sided defects, particularly in cases with liver herniation. The two main types of CDH include a Bochdalek hernia and a Morgagni hernia. The Morgagni-type hernia is far less common, is located anteriorly in the diaphragm, and the colon is the most common content of the hernia. These children are usually asymptomatic, and the defect is commonly discovered incidentally on a chest x-ray performed for mild respiratory symptoms. A lateral chest x-ray can be helpful to demonstrate whether it is located anteriorly.

The diagnosis of a Bochdalek-type hernia is most commonly made antenatally, with planned induction of labour being carried out in a tertiary hospital. Before the advent

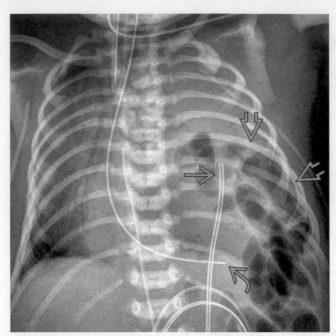

Figure 27.1 Congenital diaphragmatic hernia (CDH). CDH antero-posterior (AP) radiograph in a newborn shows bubbly lucencies (blue arrows) in the left hemithorax, which are typical of bowel in a left CDH. The enteric tube courses into the herniated stomach. There is mass effect with a hypoplastic aerated left lung and mediastinal shift. The umbilical venous catheter (UVC) is malpositioned (blue arrow). (Reproduced with permission from Merrow, A. (2019). *Pediatrics* (2nd ed.). AMIRSYS Publishing.)

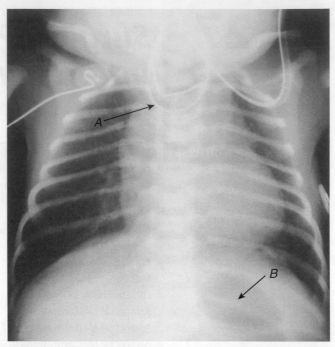

Figure 27.2 Oesophageal atresia with tracheoesophageal fistula. The gastric tube is coiled in the oesophageal pouch (A). Air in the stomach (B) confirms the presence of a fistula between the trachea and the oesophagus. (Reproduced with permission from Verklan, M. T., Walden, M., & Forest, S. (Eds.). (2021). *Core curriculum for neonatal intensive care nursing* (6th ed.). Elsevier Inc.)

of reliable antenatal diagnosis, the typical presentation was of a term newborn unresponsive to adequate resuscitation and intubation who continues to deteriorate with cyanosis and respiratory distress shortly after birth. A scaphoid abdomen may be noted, and the above history points to a diagnosis of CDH, which is confirmed on chest x-ray.

The initial management is airway control, with almost all infants requiring intubation and varying levels of support, including standard mechanical ventilation, high-frequency oscillation, and nitric oxide. It is essential to avoid bag and mask ventilation as any additional air in the intrathoracic stomach and bowel will compromise ventilation and cardiac output. In addition, ventilatory support infants with CDH often require inotropic support to maintain systemic blood pressure. Those who fail to maintain adequate oxygenation and tissue perfusion may need support using extracorporeal membrane oxygenation (ECMO).

The definitive treatment of CDH is surgical repair of the defect. However, surgery is usually delayed until any pulmonary hypertension present is controlled and ventilatory requirements are reduced.

OESOPHAGEAL ATRESIA (OA) AND TRACHEO-OESOPHAGEAL FISTULA (TOF)

Oesophageal atresia refers to a congenital anomaly in which the continuity of the oesophagus is interrupted with or without an associated tracheoesophageal fistula. It is the most common congenital anomaly of the oesophagus, affecting one in 4000 live births. Associated congenital anomalies are present in up to half of all cases, including VACTERL (vertebral defects, anal atresia, cardiac defects, tracheo-oesophageal fistula, renal anomalies, and limb abnormalities) association.

There are five main anatomical subtypes of OA.

Type A: OA without TOF (6 per cent)
Type B: OA with a TOF to the proximal oesophageal segment (5 per cent)
Type C: OA with a TOF to the distal oesophageal segment (84 per cent)
Type D: OA with a TOF to the proximal and distal oesophageal segments (1 per cent)
Type E: A TOF without OA (H-type fistula) (4 per cent)

The diagnosis can occasionally be suspected based on antenatal scans when polyhydramnios and a small stomach are detected. However, it is more common for this anomaly to be detected postnatally during the neonatal period, presenting with failure to tolerate feeds, drooling or foaming, respiratory distress with cyanotic episodes, and an inability to pass a nasogastric tube.

Initial investigations include a chest x-ray, which will often show the nasogastric tube (Replogle tube) arrested in the superior mediastinum (types A to D) (Fig. 27.2). Pure oesophageal atresia (type A) has the additional feature of a gasless abdomen on abdominal radiography.

A preoperative echocardiogram is required to assess for any associated cardiac anomalies and the presence of a right-sided aortic arch that may affect the timing and approach used. Surgical repair is commonly performed via a right-sided thoracotomy, with some surgeons more recently favouring a thoracoscopic approach. Associated long-term problems include gastro-oesophageal reflux disease (GORD), tracheomalacia (with the characteristic brassy TOF cough) and oesophageal dysmotility.

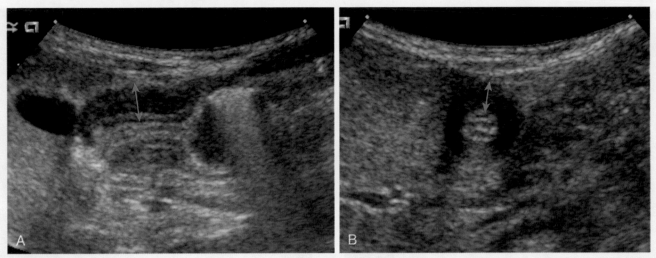

Figure 27.3   Hypertrophic pyloric stenosis (HPS). (A) Longitudinal scan of the pylorus with a single layer of pyloric muscle measuring 4 mm (double-headed arrow). (B) Transverse scan showing the 'donut appearance' of the thick pyloric muscle and central redundant mucosa (double-headed arrow). (Reproduced with permission from McGahan, J. P., Schick, M. A., & Mills, L. (2020). *Fundamentals of emergency ultrasound*. Elsevier Inc.)

Abdomen

INFANTILE HYPERTROPHIC PYLORIC STENOSIS

Infantile hypertrophic pyloric stenosis (IHPS) is a disorder of young infants caused by hypertrophy of the pylorus. It is progressive and can lead to near-total obstruction of the gastric outlet, leading to forceful projectile vomiting. It has an incidence of one to four per 1000 live births, with a male to female ratio of 4:1, with 30 per cent of cases being first-born males. There is a familial predisposition in 7 per cent of cases. Symptoms usually begin between 3 and 5 weeks of age and rarely occur after 12 weeks.

The classical symptom at presentation is forceful, non-bilious vomiting that occurs immediately after feeding, while the infant remains hungry. These symptoms are important differentiating factors that can help rule out gastro-oesophageal reflux. On examination, there may be signs of weight loss and dehydration, and a firm, 'olive-like' mass may be felt in the epigastrium or right upper quadrant of the abdomen (rolling the pyloric mass beneath your fingers on the relaxed abdomen). This examination is facilitated in an awake infant by performing a test-feed, which serves to relax the infant. The typical biochemical changes reported with IHPS are of a hypokalaemic, hypochloraemic metabolic alkalosis and occasional hypoglycaemia. Most often now the typical biochemical pattern outlined above is not seen due to earlier diagnosis because of easier access to ultrasonography. The diagnosis of IHPS is usually confirmed by abdominal ultrasound (Fig. 27.3) and is characterised by a pyloric muscle thickness greater than 3 mm and a pyloric channel length greater than 14 mm.

IHPS is not an acute surgical emergency, and the first aims of treatment are fluid resuscitation and correction of any fluid electrolyte and acid-base abnormalities. The infants should be kept nil by mouth and placed on intravenous fluids with a nasogastric tube sited to decompress the stomach and monitor gastric fluid losses, which should be replaced. Once the patient has normal electrolytes and a normal acid-base balance, surgery can be considered.

The most common procedure performed is an open pyloromyotomy via a supraumbilical incision, although some surgeons favour a laparoscopic approach. Early feeding and discharge are to be expected. There is a small chance of recurrent vomiting, most commonly due to reflux, but rarely is it due to an incomplete myotomy.

DUODENAL ATRESIA

Duodenal atresia (DA) is a congenital abnormality of the upper gastrointestinal tract resulting in the complete obstruction of the lumen of the duodenum and generally results in bilious vomiting in the newborn period. The duodenum is the most common site of neonatal intestinal obstruction, accounting for 75 per cent of cases, and it occurs in approximately one in 3000 live births. Up to 50 per cent of patients with DA will have another congenital abnormality, the most common of which are Trisomy 21, congenital heart defects, annular pancreas, and renal anomalies.

Patients with DA usually present with signs of a proximal (high) intestinal obstruction. Intolerance of feeds and vomiting occurs within the first 24 hours of life. The vomiting may or may not be bilious depending on the level of the duodenal obstruction. If the obstruction is below the level of entry of the bile duct into the second part of the duodenum (ampulla of Vater), then the vomiting will be bilious (85 per cent of cases); an obstruction above this level will cause non-bilious vomiting. They usually pass meconium within the first 24 to 48 hours of life.

The diagnosis can often be suggested based on the findings of antenatal scans, which may show a dilated stomach and duodenum. However, a plain film of the abdomen in suspected cases of DA can often be diagnostic showing a characteristic 'double-bubble' appearance with an absence of gas in the distal bowel (Fig. 27.4). An upper gastrointestinal contrast study can provide a firm radiological diagnosis if there is any doubt. If distal bowel gas is present, a duodenal web with a small central opening may be present, which can lead to a delayed or late diagnosis in some cases.

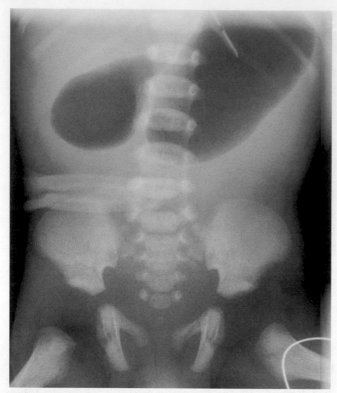

Figure 27.4 Duodenal atresia. Classic double-bubble appearance without distal gas. (Reproduced with permission from Adam, A., Dixon, A. K., Gillard, J. H., & Schaefer-Prokop, C. (2021). *Grainger & Allison's diagnostic radiology: 2-Volume set* (7th ed.). Elsevier Ltd.)

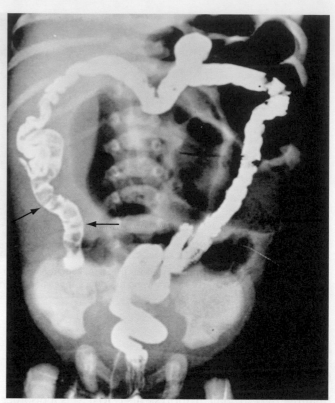

Figure 27.5 Meconium ileus. Film from a barium enema examination in an infant with meconium ileus demonstrating a microcolon and meconium in the distal ileum (arrows). Distended small bowel loops are also noted. (Reproduced with permission from Feldman, M., Friedman, L. S., & Brandt, L. J. (2021). *Sleisenger and Fordtran's gastrointestinal and liver disease—2-Volume set: Pathophysiology, diagnosis, management* (11th ed.). Elsevier Inc.)

Initial management involves holding feeds placement of a nasogastric tube, intravenous fluids, and ideally a preoperative echocardiogram if Trisomy 21 is present. The definitive surgical treatment is a duodenoduodenostomy, effectively bypassing the obstruction.

SMALL BOWEL ATRESIA

Small bowel atresia is the complete obstruction of the lumen of a segment(s) of ileum and/or jejunum. Atresias can occur anywhere along the small bowel; however, the most common sites are proximal jejunum (30 per cent) and distal ileum (30 per cent) with multiple atresias occurring in around 5 per cent of cases. Small bowel atresias have a low (less than 1 per cent) association with other anomalies.

Patients with a small bowel atresia usually present with vomiting, initially with gastric contents followed by bilious vomiting. There can be varying degrees of abdominal distension depending on the level of obstruction; the more distal the obstruction, the greater the distension.

The diagnosis of a small bowel atresia is often made after investigations such as upper and lower gastrointestinal contrast studies, which have ruled out more common causes of obstruction such as DA, Hirschsprung's disease (HD), meconium ileus and colonic atresia.

Initial management involves holding feeds, placement of a nasogastric tube, and intravenous fluids. The surgical treatment is a laparotomy and resection of the atretic segment(s).

MECONIUM ILEUS

Meconium ileus is a small bowel obstruction in the newborn, secondary to inspissation of abnormally viscid meconium, typically at the level of the terminal ileum. Approximately 10 per cent of patients with cystic fibrosis will present with meconium ileus in the newborn period and approximately 90 per cent of infants with meconium ileus will ultimately be diagnosed with cystic fibrosis. In general, newborns with this condition may have abdominal distension at birth.

Meconium ileus can present in two forms. Simple meconium ileus (obstruction without perforation of the bowel) is the most common form, making up two-thirds of cases (Fig. 27.5). The remaining one-third of cases present as complicated meconium ileus, which is obstruction with perforation (early or late).

A plain film of abdomen can show findings suggestive of meconium ileus, usually demonstrating dilated loops of bowel with a 'soap bubble' appearance. Scattered calcifications throughout the abdomen on an abdominal x-ray is usually indicative of prenatal bowel perforation (meconium peritonitis) from complicated meconium ileus. A non-ionic water-soluble contrast enema is usually diagnostic, demonstrating a microcolon and multiple filling defects within the distal ileum.

Once the diagnosis is established the initial management of meconium ileus involves intravenous antibiotic cover, fluid resuscitation, and attempted clearance of the

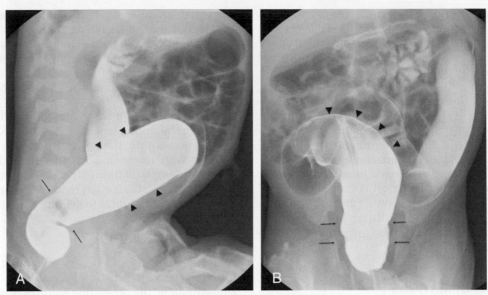

Figure 27.6 Hirschsprung's disease in a neonate with abdominal distention and failure to pass meconium. (A) Left lateral view from a diagnostic contrast enema demonstrates an abnormal rectosigmoid ration. The rectum (small black arrows) is smaller in caliber than the sigmoid colon (black arrowheads). Note the numerous distended small bowel loops throughout the abdomen, suggesting a distal obstructive process. (B) The frontal projection from the contrast enema further demonstrates a mildly serrated appearance to the narrowed rectum (small black arrows). The sigmoid colon (black arrowheads) remains larger in caliber than the rectum. (Reproduced with permission from Donnelly, L. F. (Ed.). (2021). *Fundamentals of pediatric imaging* (3rd ed.). Academic Press.)

inspissated meconium with the use of Gastrografin (hyperosmolar contrast medium) enema. This is generally effective if it can be passed proximal to the obstruction. Given the hypertonic nature of this contrast, infants must be very well pre-hydrated to prevent significant dehydration.

If medical management fails, or in cases of complicated meconium ileus, then surgical intervention may be required via a laparotomy with possible bowel resection and anastomosis, or possibly a temporary stoma.

HIRSCHSPRUNG'S DISEASE

Hirschsprung's disease (HD is caused by a congenital absence of intramural ganglion cells (aganglionosis) in the distal rectum, extending proximally for a variable distance. The extent of disease can affect a very short segment of rectum or can extend to affect the entire colon, and in very rare cases, some or most of the small bowel. However, in the majority of cases (~80 per cent), only the rectum and part of the sigmoid colon is affected. It occurs in approximately one in 5000 births, with males more affected than females, and there is an increased risk of HD associated with Trisomy 21 and some other genetic syndromes.

Presentation is typically within the first few days of life, with a range of symptoms including abdominal distension, delayed passage of meconium, bilious vomiting and explosive gassy bowel movements (either spontaneous or secondary to intervention). Untreated, patients with HD are at risk of developing Hirschsprung-associated enterocolitis (HAEC) due to prolonged faecal stasis and distension resulting in bacterial translocation from the bowel lumen leading to sepsis.

Initial investigation of a suspected case of HD starts with a plain film abdomen (PFA), which may show a distal bowel obstruction; however, the diagnosis is not excluded by a normal appearance. A contrast enema is the most important

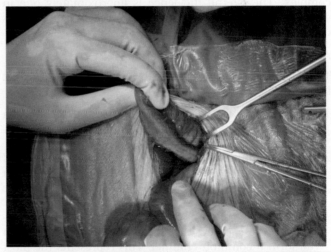

Figure 27.7 Hirschsprung's disease operative findings. Intraoperatively demonstrated sigmoid narrowing which is a typical aganglionic segment in Hirschsprung's disease. (Reproduced with permission from Moenadjat, Y., Panigoro, S. S. (Eds.). (2019). *Bedah Berbasis Kompetensi*. Elsevier.)

imaging study and the presence of a transition zone (calibre change) in the colon is suspicious for HD (Fig. 27.6). The definitive diagnosis of HD is made based on the histological findings after a rectal suction biopsy or an open biopsy in an older child. The classic findings in HD are absent ganglion cells with thickened nerve fibres and an abnormal (absent) Calretinin immunohistochemistry staining pattern.

The definitive treatment of HD is surgical resection (Fig. 27.7) of the aganglionic segment of the bowel with normal ganglionic bowel being brought down and anastomosed to just proximal to the anal canal (pull-through procedure). The level of resection is determined by intraoperative biopsies that are analysed during the procedure to ensure all abnormal bowel is removed while helping to preserve as much normal bowel as possible. Most surgeons prefer to wait until infants are around 4 to 6 months of age prior to performing surgery, as this may be associated with a better outcome. While awaiting the procedure, most infants can be managed at home by their parents with daily transrectal saline irrigation and anal dilatations to empty the colon and prevent faecal stasis. However, some infants (usually those with longer segments of affected bowel) may not respond to irrigation and thus may require the formation of a temporary stoma as a bridge to definitive treatment.

Irregularities in bowel function are common after definitive surgery for HD and tend to increase in proportion to the extent of the initial disease. The most common complications are constipation, incomplete bowel emptying, and faecal incontinence, and patients are still at risk for developing HAEC despite having undergone a technically satisfactory pull-through procedure.

ANORECTAL MALFORMATIONS

Anorectal malformations (ARM) are a spectrum of congenital defects of the lower part of the digestive tract affecting the anus and rectum. They usually manifest as an absent, abnormally placed or narrow (stenotic) anus with an opening (or fistula) occurring outside the anal sphincter muscle complex. The overall incidence is approximately one in 4000. There is significant variation in the clinical features of ARM between males and females.

Anorectal malformations in females

There are three main types of ARM in females, categorised based on the location of the fistula:

1. Rectoperineal fistulas open onto the perineum between the posterior aspect of the vagina and the anal sphincter complex.
2. Rectovestibular fistulas open onto the posterior vaginal wall and can be difficult to identify without a thorough examination. Rectovaginal fistulas can occur but are very rare.
3. Cloacal malformations are with a single perineal opening. In these cases, the urethra, vagina and rectum all form a common channel. This represents the most severe type of ARM.

Anorectal malformations in males

There are three main types of ARM in males, categorised based on the location of the fistula:

1. Rectoperineal fistulas open onto the perineum between the posterior aspect of the scrotum and the anal sphincter complex.
2. Rectobulbar and rectoprostatic urethral fistulas are where the bowel opens into the urethra in one of the two locations.
3. Rectovesical fistula is where the bowel opens into the bladder neck.

The association of ARM with other abnormalities is more likely as the severity of the malformation increases. These defects may fall within the VACTERL association which includes vertebral, anorectal, cardiac, tracheoesophageal, renal and limb abnormalities. Once the diagnosis is made or

suspected, initial evaluation should include investigations to assess for these associated anomalies.

An absent or abnormally placed anus should be identified at the neonatal assessment; however, as some patients have perineal fistulas sufficiently patent to allow the passage of meconium, the diagnosis can sometimes be delayed.

The definitive surgical treatment of ARM is with a posterior sagittal anorectoplasty (PSARP) procedure to create a neo-anus within the sphincter muscle complex. Some patients with lower malformations can be managed initially with simple dilation of the fistula; however, those with higher malformations often require the formation of a temporary stoma as a bridge to definitive treatment.

ACUTE APPENDICITIS

Acute appendicitis is caused by inflammation of the vermiform appendix, which usually results in abdominal pain. Unfortunately, the presenting features of acute appendicitis are similar to many other conditions, making the diagnosis difficult and occasionally delaying treatment.

The classical presentation of appendicitis has the following features after clinical assessment: migratory pain (periumbilical to the right iliac fossa), anorexia, pain on movement, vomiting (following the onset of pain), pyrexia (typically 24 to 48 hours after the onset of pain), and right lower quadrant tenderness (with guarding). While this classical pattern of presentation is typical in older children, it can be difficult to elicit in younger children (<5 years) and those with developmental delay.

The usefulness of laboratory investigations to differentiate appendicitis from other causes of abdominal pain is limited. Nonetheless, they typically form part of the assessment. Common findings associated with acute appendicitis include raised white cell count (WCC) with elevated neutrophils and a C-reactive protein (CRP) level above normal limits. Other tests that can add value to the assessment include urinalysis and urine pregnancy testing in post-menarchal females.

The use of imaging to aid in the diagnosis of acute appendicitis is becoming more common with increased access to ultrasound. However, its value is limited to specific patient groups (Fig. 27.8). It can be helpful in patients with atypical or equivocal clinical findings or in cases where ovarian pathology is suspected as an alternative diagnosis. Computed tomography (CT) is highly sensitive in diagnosing appendicitis; however, it involves a radiation dosage and compliance with lying still, and requires the administration of intravenous and oral contrast to obtain the ideal diagnostic images.

The immediate management of any patient presenting with abdominal pain should include resuscitation with intravenous fluids, baseline blood tests, analgesia and careful clinical examination. It is important to reassess the patient regularly; if there is still suspicion of acute appendicitis after a thorough clinical assessment and repeated physical examination, the patient should be referred to the surgical team. Antibiotics are not typically administered until the diagnosis is made.

There are many differentials to be considered when assessing patients with abdominal pain and these vary in their likelihood with the age and sex of the patient. The main differential diagnoses to consider include:

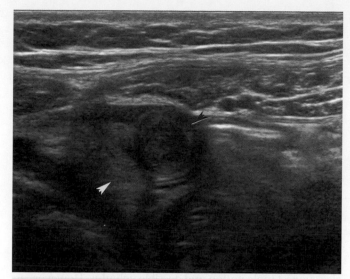

Figure 27.8 Acute appendicitis. B-mode ultrasound to the right lower quadrant shows a dilated rounded structure with debris within it and with wall thickening (red arrow) consistent with acute appendicitis. Note echogenic fat (yellow arrow) seen around the structure consistent with periappendiceal inflammation. (Reproduced with permission from Grajo, J. R., & Lee, L. (2022). *Abdominal imaging: Case review series.* Elsevier Inc.)

Consideration should also be given to the possibility of complex appendicitis (an appendix mass). This is more common in delayed presentations (>3 days) and in younger children (< 5 years) or those with communication difficulties. Delayed diagnosis is associated with a prolonged stay in hospital. The risk of perforation does increase with time and most studies have found an association between pre-hospital delay and the risk of perforation, whereas a large number of studies have not found a negative impact of in-hospital delay of 24 to 36 hours. Despite significant advances in the diagnosis and treatment of appendicitis, perforated appendicitis still occurs in 28 to 29 per cent of cases. In patients felt to have an uncomplicated appendicitis, conservative management with antibiotics alone (and no planned operation) has been utilised with some success. This strategy was particularly helpful during the initial phase of COVID-19 when any surgical intervention was felt to pose a significant risk to staff and patients alike. Patients not improving, with failure of symptom resolution or recurrent symptoms post-discharge, would subsequently undergo a standard appendicectomy (either laparoscopic or open). This strategy is still being employed in certain centres.

MECKEL'S DIVERTICULUM

Meckel's diverticulum is a true diverticulum arising from the antimesenteric border of the ileum. It is the most common congenital abnormality of the gastrointestinal tract and results from incomplete obliteration of the vitello-intestinal duct (omphalomesenteric duct). The 'rule of 2s' has been used to describe its classical features: it affects 2 per cent of the population, it occurs within 2 feet of the ileo-caecal valve, it is two times more likely in males, and it can be approximately 2 inches long.

Meckel's diverticulum is often asymptomatic and the incidental discovery of one is common during abdominal exploration for an unrelated pathology. When symptomatic, Meckel's diverticulum can present with gastrointestinal bleeding or abdominal pain secondary to bowel obstruction, Meckel's diverticulitis, or perforation. A common histological finding in problematic Meckel's diverticulum is ectopic gastric mucosa, which causes bleeding and occasionally perforation.

Meckel's diverticulum is usually not at the top of the list of differential diagnosis when assessing patients with abdominal complaints, but it should be considered in patients with painless lower gastrointestinal bleeding or intussusception (where it can act as a lead point).

The most common imaging modality used to aid in the diagnosis of Meckel's diverticulum is a Technetium-99m radionucleotide scan (or Meckel's scan) (Fig. 27.9), which is used to detect ectopic gastric mucosa.

Symptomatic Meckel's diverticulum should be resected in all patients; however, the management of asymptomatic cases discovered incidentally is controversial and beyond the scope of this text.

MALROTATION AND VOLVULUS

Intestinal malrotation is a congenital anomaly affecting the position and peritoneal attachments of the intestine during foetal development. Malrotation is defined as the incomplete

- acute gastroenteritis (usually vomiting and diarrhoea)
- acute non-specific abdominal pain is a diagnosis of exclusion but is the most common cause of acute abdominal pain
- mesenteric adenitis (enlarged mesenteric lymph nodes possibly due to a recent viral illness)
- constipation
- urinary tract infection (UTI)/acute pyelonephritis (may present with high fever, flank pain, and renal angle tenderness)
- renal colic due to renal calculi is rare in childhood
- sickle cell anaemia with a vaso-occlusive crisis may present with severe abdominal pain
- Crohn's ileitis may present with acute abdominal pain but often gives a more chronic history of bouts of abdominal pain, clubbing, weight loss, chronic diarrhoea and possible perianal disease
- testicular or ovarian torsion (testicular torsion must always be considered as pain can be referred so examination of the groin and scrotum is mandatory. Likewise, ovarian torsion can mimic acute appendicitis)
- right lower lobe pneumonia (may present quite unwell with high fever, tachypnoea and grunting and right-sided abdominal pain)
- Meckel's diverticulum (may closely mimic acute appendicitis)
- intussusception (presents with a classical triad of abdominal colic, pallor and fresh blood per rectum (PR)
- diabetic ketoacidosis (classically presents with Kussmaul respiration and may present with severe abdominal cramps)
- Henoch-Schönlein Purpura (HSP) may cause severe abdominal cramps and tends to precede the classical purpuric rash and arthritis

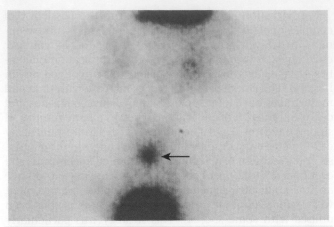

Figure 27.9 Meckel's diverticulum. Technetium-99m pertechnetate scan of a patient with Meckel's diverticulum. Note the blush (arrow) above the bladder. (Reproduced with permission from Holcomb, G. W., Murphy, J. P., & Peter, S. D. (2020). *Ashcraft's pediatric surgery* (7th ed.). Inc.)

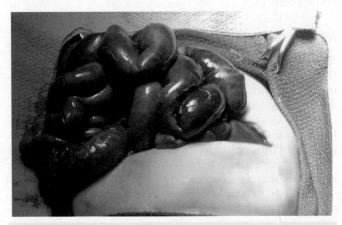

Figure 27.10 Malrotation with midgut volvulus. (Reproduced with permission from Martin, R. J., Fanaroff, A. A., & Walsh, M. C. (2020). *Fanaroff and Martin's neonatal-perinatal medicine, 2-volume set: Diseases of the fetus and infant* (11th ed.). Elsevier Inc.)

or abnormal rotation and attachment of the embryonic midgut around the axis of the superior mesenteric artery. Malrotation occurs in approximately one in 500 births with approximately 75 per cent becoming symptomatic within the first month of life and 90 per cent by 1 year.

Vomiting, which is usually bilious, is the most common presenting symptom of malrotation and volvulus in infancy (Fig. 27.10). It is often associated with abdominal distension and tenderness on examination. As a result of ischaemia secondary to bowel volvulus, hypovolemic shock and metabolic acidosis can develop rapidly with peritonitis on examination, often indicating perforation (Fig. 27.10).

An abdominal x-ray may show a distended stomach with a paucity of gas distally. Unfortunately, there is no single abdominal x-ray finding that is pathognomonic for malrotation and volvulus, and therefore a normal x-ray should not be reassuring. Abdominal ultrasound to examine the orientation of the superior mesenteric artery and vein may also suggest malrotation and possible volvulus. However, an upper gastrointestinal contrast study is the investigation of choice for any child presenting with bilious vomiting (Fig. 27.11). The abnormal findings consistent with malrotation include the duodenum failing to cross the midline and the duodenojejunal flexure lying inferiorly to the duodenal bulb on the right of the spine.

The treatment of patients with confirmed symptomatic malrotation and volvulus should start with appropriate resuscitation with intravenous fluids and nasogastric decompression. Ultimately, an emergency laparotomy and Ladd's procedure is the definitive procedure to prevent major loss of small bowel.

INTUSSUSCEPTION

Intussusception refers to the full-thickness invagination (telescoping) of a part of the intestine into itself. The invagination of proximal bowel into distal bowel causes the mesentery to become compressed, thus compromising the blood supply to the affected portion of the bowel. Any delay in

Figure 27.11 Malrotation and midgut volvulus. (A) Anteroposterior and lateral (B) views from an upper gastrointestinal series demonstrates a 'corkscrew' appearance of the duodenum with the duodenal-jejunal junction to the right of midline (arrow). (CREDIT Reproduced with permission from Fanaroff, A. A., & Fanaroff, J. M. (2022). *Klaus and Fanaroff's care of the high-risk neonate* (7th ed.). Elsevier Inc.)

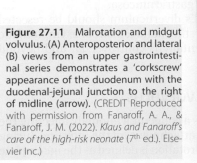

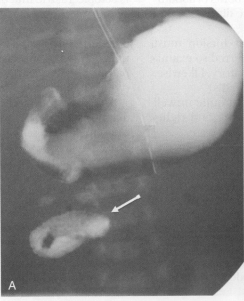

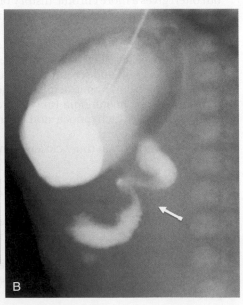

diagnosis can lead to prolonged bowel ischaemia, necrosis, perforation, sepsis and death.

Intussusception is the most common cause of intestinal obstruction in infants between the ages of 6 and 36 months with an overall incidence of 25 to 40 per 100000 live births. The most common type is primary intussusception, which is idiopathic in nature and commonly associated with a preceding viral illness. Primary intussusception is ileocolic and accounts for 90 per cent of all cases. Secondary intussusception is generally associated with an older age group and occurs secondary to a defined pathology, which creates a lead point, such as a Meckel's diverticulum, small bowel lymphoma, or intestinal polyps.

Intussusception typically presents with the sudden onset of intermittent crampy abdominal pain associated with updrawing of the legs and inconsolable crying. Pallor is commonly noted and may be followed by episodes of vomiting and apparent temporary resolution of symptoms before the cycle begins again. Vomiting is initially non-bilious as a reflex response to spasms of pain but then usually becomes bilious in nature as the degree of bowel obstruction evolves. The classical triad of abdominal pain, red-currant jelly stools and a palpable mass are found in less than 20 per cent of cases.

Initial management involves immediate resuscitation with intravenous fluids, the passage of a large-bore nasogastric tube to decompress the stomach, analgesia, and prompt surgical referral. The first line of investigation is ultrasound to confirm the suspected diagnosis followed by non-operative reduction with air enema under fluoroscopic control. This has a success rate of approximately 80 per cent and operative reduction is used in cases in which it fails to reduce the intussusception or where there is evidence of perforation (Fig. 27.12). The recurrence rate for intussusception is 10 per cent with approximately 30 per cent of those recurring within the first 24 hours. With operative intervention and intussusception reduction, the recurrence risk reduces dramatically and falls to almost zero with bowel resection.

BILIARY ATRESIA

Biliary atresia is a progressive, idiopathic fibro-obliterative disease of the extrahepatic biliary tree that presents with biliary obstruction in the neonatal period. It is the most common indication for liver transplants in children. It has an incidence of one in 17000 in Europe with a higher incidence in Asia.

Infants with biliary atresia are typically born at full term with normal birth weight and appear healthy on initial assessment postnatally. Signs of generalised jaundice and scleral icterus usually develop within the first 6 to 8 weeks of life. They may also have pale stools, dark urine and a firm liver.

Laboratory investigations show an elevated conjugated bilirubin (>2mg/dL) with an associated increase in aminotransferases and a significantly raised gamma glutamyl transpeptidase (GGT). In suspected cases of biliary atresia, ultrasound is usually the first imaging modality used to investigate the extrahepatic biliary tree for any abnormalities, particularly dilatation. A radioisotope hepatobiliary scan can also be a useful diagnostic tool (Fig. 27.13); however, a cholangiogram is the definitive imaging modality. Ultimately, the diagnosis of biliary atresia is made with a combination of laboratory investigations, imaging, and histological assessment of a liver biopsy.

While jaundice is a common presenting complaint in infancy, persistent jaundice (more than 2 weeks) should always be evaluated. The critical reason for early investigation in cases of prolonged jaundice is that the success rate of definitive treatment of biliary atresia diminishes with increasing age. Infants who are diagnosed when they are older than 100 days are unlikely to have any success with surgery (Kasai portoenterostomy), resulting in irretrievable cirrhosis, which will usually ultimately require liver transplantation.

Infants with biliary atresia who are jaundiced are at risk for fat-soluble vitamin deficiencies and should be treated with vitamin supplementation. In addition, treatment with ursodeoxycholic acid is recommended both pre- and post-Kasai procedures.

ABDOMINAL WALL DEFECTS

Gastroschisis

Gastroschisis results from a defect in the anterior abdominal wall to the right of the intact umbilical cord. The abdominal contents remain herniated through this small defect in utero and are free floating within the amnion. There is no peritoneal sac covering the bowel (Fig. 27.14), leaving it in direct contact with the amniotic fluid resulting in irritation of the serosal layer of the bowel and formation of a thick peel on its surface. Normal bowel rotation and fixation do not usually occur. The diagnosis is often made antenatally allowing for a planned delivery (vaginal or caesarean) and prompt referral to a tertiary care hospital. Immediate

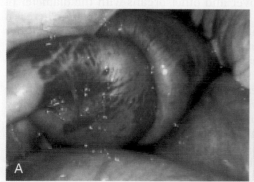
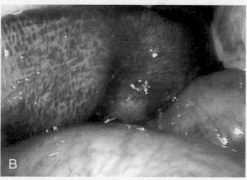

Figure 27.12 Intussusception. (A) The ileoileal intussusception that remained after reduction of the ileum from the colon is seen in this patient with an ileocolic intussusception. (B) The ileoileal portion has been completely reduced. Note the oedema and induration in the wall of the small bowel in both photographs. (Reproduced with permission from Holcomb, G. W., & Rothenberg, S. S. (Eds.). (2022). *Atlas of pediatric laparoscopy and thoracoscopy* (2nd ed.). Elsevier Inc.)

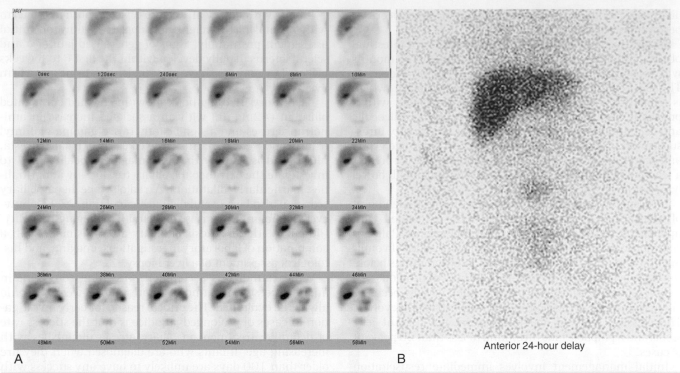

Anterior 24-hour delay

Figure 27.13 Biliary atresia. (A) An anterior image from a normal hepatobiliary iminodiacetic acid (HIDA) scan shows sequential excretion of tracer into small bowel. (B) An anterior image from a hepatobiliary HIDA scan obtained 24 hours after tracer administration in a 3-month-old infant with biliary atresia shows no excretion of tracer into the bowel. (Reproduced with permission from Walters, M. M., & Robertson, R. L. (2021). *Pediatric radiology: The requisites* (4th ed.). Elsevier.)

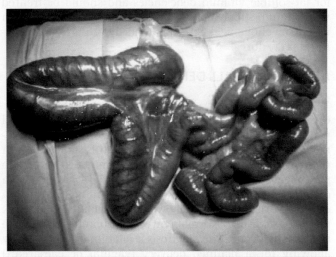

Figure 27.14 Gastroschisis: almost completely eventration of small and large intestines with malrotation. Note the apparent shortening of the mesentery caused by chemical peritonitis. (Reproduced with permission from Schmittenbecher, P. P., (Ed.). (2021). *Pädiatrische Chirurgie: Lehrbuch der Kinderchirurgie – kurz und kompakt* (2 Auflage). Elsevier.)

management post-delivery should involve judicious fluid resuscitation, placement of a nasogastric tube, intravenous broad-spectrum antibiotics and covering the bowel in damp gauze before wrapping the abdomen in clingfilm, while ensuring the small bowel mesentery is not twisted or unduly tractioned. Once transferred to a paediatric surgical unit, management involves either primary closure (if the bowel can be easily reduced into the abdominal cavity) or placement of the herniated bowel into a temporary silicone

covering (known as a 'silo'), allowing for gradual reduction of the bowel into the abdomen over a period of 2 to 3 days so that delayed abdominal closure can be achieved without risking bowel compromise or causing respiratory embarrassment (Fig. 27.15).

Omphalocoele (or Exomphalos)

An omphalocoele is another type of anterior wall defect that results from a central defect of the umbilical ring allowing bowel and other abdominal viscera to herniate. It differs from gastroschisis in that the abdominal contents are covered with a membrane composed of an inner layer of peritoneum fused to an outer layer of amnion (Fig. 27.16). It is common to observe Wharton's jelly inside the sac.

Exomphalos can be grossly classified into two types: minor and major. In an omphalocoele minor, there is protrusion of a small portion of intestine only and the size of the abdominal wall defect is less than 5 cm in diameter. In contrast, in an omphalocoele major, there is protrusion of the intestine, liver and other organs with the diameter of the abdominal wall defect being more than 5 cm. There is a greater association between omphalocoele major and other congenital anomalies, particularly cardiac malformations.

The immediate management is similar to that of gastroschisis but is less time sensitive. It involves fluid resuscitation, placement of a nasogastric tube, intravenous antibiotics, covering the sac in damp gauze before wrapping the abdomen in clingfilm, and prompt referral to a tertiary paediatric surgical centre. Definitive treatment depends on the size of the defect, with some very small omphalocoele minors being closed primarily as an elective procedure once the initial workup has been completed. Echocardiography,

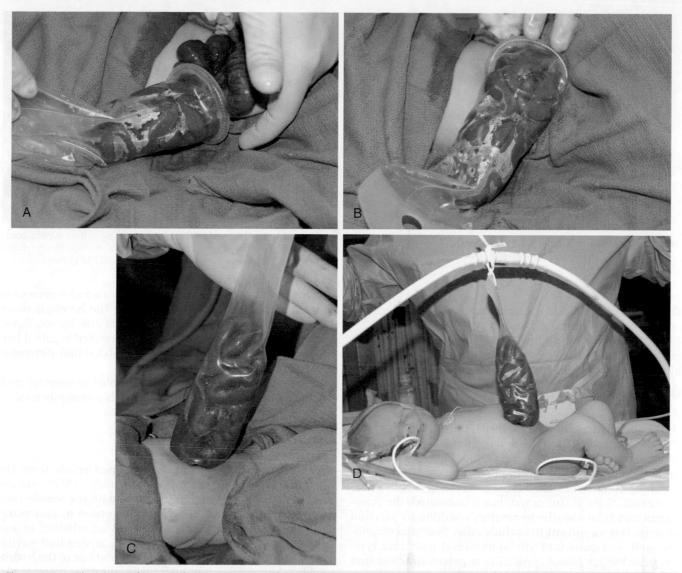

Figure 27.15 Silo. (A) Manufactured silastic silo with a circular spring at its base can be placed at bedside for a newborn with gastroschisis. (B) Bowel loops are gently advanced into the silo, assuring that the mesentery is not twisted. (C) The circular spring at the base of the silo is inserted into the gastroschisis defect and positioned beneath the fascia. (D) The top of the silo is tied to an overhead bar to keep the silo perpendicular to the abdominal wall defect. (Reproduced with permission from Wyllie, R., Hyams, J. S., & Kay, M. (2021). *Pediatric gastrointestinal and liver disease* (6th ed.). Elsevier Inc.)

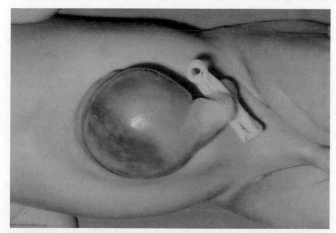

Figure 27.16 Exomphalos. (Reproduced with permission from Quick, C. R. G., Biers, S., & Arulampalam, T. (Eds.). (2020). *Essential surgery: Problems, diagnosis and management* (6th ed.). Elsevier Ltd.)

renal ultrasound, and karyotyping are recommended. The majority of larger omphalocoeles are managed with regular dressings initially using silver sulfadiazine containing a topical agent to encourage epithelialisation of the sac. Surgical closure is delayed until the patient has had time to grow, thereby reducing the size of the defect relative to the patient's abdominal dimensions.

Umbilical Hernia

The incidence of umbilical hernias in Caucasian newborns is 5 to 10 per cent while in African infants it is over 25 per cent. It is also associated with low birth weight, prematurity, Beckwith-Wiedemann syndrome and Trisomies 13, 18 and 21.

Umbilical hernias result from failure of the umbilical ring to close after birth, and are usually asymptomatic. The main complaint is often the cosmetic appearance, with an easily reducible protruding umbilicus (Fig. 27.17). Pain or

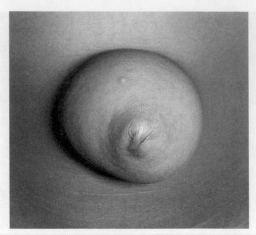

Figure 27.17 Umbilical hernia. (Reproduced with permission from Shiland, B. J. (2020). *Medical terminology & anatomy for coding* (4th ed.). Mosby.)

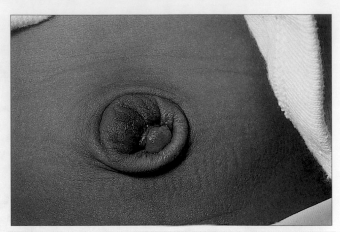

Figure 27.18 This friable red papule at the base of the umbilical cord is a typical umbilical granuloma. (Reproduced with permission from Eichenfield, L. F. (2009). *Dermatología neonatal* (2nd ed.). Elsevier.)

discomfort are rare, and the associated risk of incarceration or obstruction is extremely low.

The majority of umbilical hernias will close spontaneously by the age of 4 to 5 years and surgical repair is usually only considered in cases that persist after this age.

Umbilical Granuloma

An umbilical granuloma is an overgrowth of tissue during the healing process of the umbilicus. It usually presents as a soft, painless, red lump, which is often wet and may leak small amounts of clear or yellow fluid (Fig. 27.18). It can bleed if traumatised by clothing rubbing against it. They are most common in the first few weeks of a baby's life. The exact cause is unknown, but if untreated, the granuloma can take months to resolve, resulting in parental anxiety. It is important to exclude other potential diagnoses such as a persistent vitello-intestinal tract that typically discharges bowel content or a patent urachus that may discharge urine. Either of these aforementioned conditions will require formal resection and closure. Umbilical granulomas are typically managed using topical silver nitrate or steroid cream with some surgeons opting to formally excise them.

Inguinal Region and Scrotum

INGUINAL HERNIA

Hernias and hydrocoeles of the inguinal canal are some of the most common congenital conditions referred to a paediatric surgical service. Inguinal hernias in the paediatric population are typically indirect hernias resulting from persistence of the patent process vaginalis (PPV), which is a peritoneal diverticulum extending through the inguinal canal. They affect both male and female patients and can cause significant morbidity in cases of incarceration and strangulation. They may contain omentum, bowel or an ovary, and they are more commonly found in premature infants.

Inguinal hernias typically present as a painless, intermittent, soft swelling in the groin, which should be easily reduced. They are more often noticed when the patient is crying or straining (Fig. 27.19). They can also present as a painful swelling in instances where the hernia is strangulated due to reduced vascularity of the bowel. Bowel obstruction can also occur with incarcerated inguinal hernias, resulting in bilious vomiting, abdominal distension and acute constipation.

The management of inguinal hernias is surgical with both laparoscopic and open approaches commonly used.

HYDROCOELE

As with inguinal hernias, hydrocoeles result from the persistence of a patent process vaginalis (PPV) and are found to be more common in males, with the female variant being quite rare. They are categorised as communicating or not communicating based on whether or not the process vaginalis is open to the abdominal cavity, allowing peritoneal fluid to move in and out of the hydrocoele. Communicating hydrocoeles tend to have a history of being more prominent during the evening, as the fluid has had a chance to drain by gravity into the PPV throughout the day while the patient is upright and then reducing spontaneously at night as the patient is supine, allowing it to drain back into the abdominal cavity. Non-communicating hydrocoeles present as a persistent swelling in the scrotum or groin, which is less likely to vary in size but may become more prominent if the patient is unwell with a viral-type illness. It is very important to be able to differentiate between a hydrocoele and an inguinal hernia, as the immediate management is different; however, the operative procedure is exactly the same. Differentiation between them can be achieved with a thorough physical examination (Fig. 27.20). The examiner should not be able to 'get above' a hernia on palpation. If bowel is within a hernia, the examiner should not be able to feel a narrow spermatic cord above the scrotum if the swelling is comprised of bowel that has herniated from the abdomen down through the inguinal canal and into the scrotum through a PPV. In the case of a hydrocoele, the examiner should be able to 'get above' the swelling and feel the narrow spermatic cord between their fingers. One exception to this is an encysted hydrocoele of the cord, examination of which may give the impression of it being a hernia.

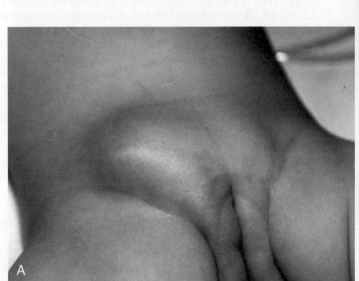

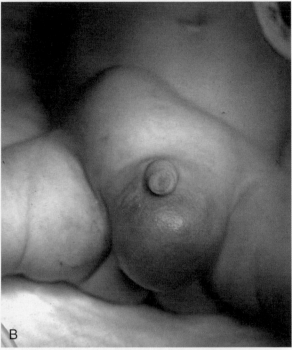

Figure 27.19 Inguinal hernia in an infant. Right inguinal hernias in a female (A) and male (B) infant. Note the asymmetry in the groin area with the prominent bulge indicating the hernia. (Reproduced with permission from Gleason, C. A., & Juul, S. E. (2020). *Avery's diseases of the newborn* (10th ed.). Elsevier Inc.)

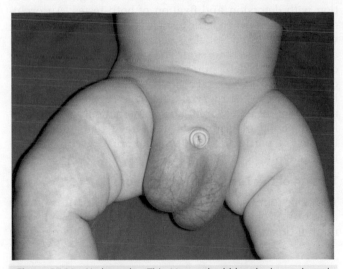

Figure 27.20 Hydrocoeles. This 11-month-old boy had an enlarged scrotum confirmed by transillumination to be the result of hydrocoeles. (Reproduced with permission from Quick, C. R. G., Biers, S., & Arulampalam, T. (Eds.). (2020). *Essential surgery: Problems, diagnosis and management* (6th ed.). Elsevier Ltd.)

Transillumination of a hydrocoele is another often cited finding, where a light is shone through the scrotum illuminating the swelling. Caution should be exercised interpreting this sign in neonates as the bowel wall can be quite thin allowing light to easily pass through, leading to an inadvertent misdiagnosis.

The majority of hydrocoeles will resolve spontaneously by the age of 2 to 4 years and surgical repair is usually only considered in cases that persist after this age or in cases where the hydrocoele is large, thereby causing cosmetic issues or (rarely) impairing mobility.

UNDESCENDED TESTES (CRYPTORCHIDISM)

By definition, cryptorchidism suggests a hidden testis. A testis not within the scrotum at birth that does not descend spontaneously into the scrotum by 3 months of age (or corrected age) is classified as an undescended testis (UDT) (Fig. 27.21). In simple terms, they are classified into palpable and impalpable while under assessment for UDT. A palpable UDT can be felt on physical examination somewhere between the internal ring of the inguinal canal and the scrotum. If the testis is palpable outside of this region, it is further classified as ectopic. An ectopic testis has deviated from the path of normal descent. An impalpable testis cannot be felt on examination and requires a different management strategy, usually involving laparoscopy to determine if the testicle is intraabdominal or atrophic. If atrophic, it can either be removed early or left in situ until the peripubertal period, at which time it may be removed. If desired by the patient, a silicone testicular prosthesis is inserted simultaneously. If the testicle is intra-abdominal, then a laparoscopic first stage orchidopexy (known as a Fowler-Stephens procedure) can be performed by clipping the main testicular blood supply to allow the testis to survive on only the vessels that run along the vas deferens. A delayed procedure up to 6 months later may allow the testis to be brought down into the scrotum on the vasal blood supply with a testicular salvage rate of approximately 85 per cent.

The present evidence indicates that spontaneous descent of a UDT does not occur after 3 months and that germ cell loss is preventable with early surgery. In 2012, the British Association of Paediatric Urologists argued that UDT should be corrected surgically by orchidopexy between 3 and 12 months. The surgical requirement for early operating on these children is tempered by the increased anaesthetic risk with children under 1 year. The main indication for surgical intervention is to facilitate self-examination and reduce the risk of a future missed testicular malignancy. Input should be sought in cases of bilateral impalpable testis and abnormal external genitalia endocrine.

THE ACUTE SCROTUM

Testicular Torsion

Testicular torsion is caused by twisting of the spermatic cord with the subsequent loss of the blood supply to the testicle. This is a surgical emergency for which early diagnosis and treatment are vital to saving the testicle.

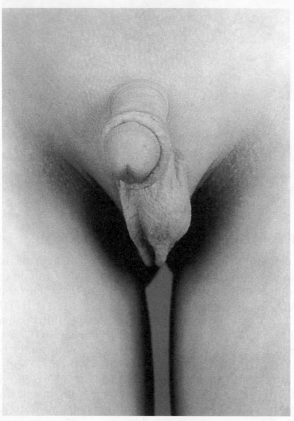

Figure 27.21   Right undescended testis. (Reproduced with permission from South, M. (2012). *Practical paediatrics* (7th ed.). Churchill Livingstone.)

Testicular torsion primarily affects adolescents and newborns and is the most common cause of testicular loss in those age groups (Fig. 27.22). Overall, it occurs in approximately one in 4000 males younger than 25 years old with 65 per cent of cases occurring in boys between the ages of 12 and 18. This increased incidence is thought to be secondary to the increasing weight of the testes during puberty.

Torsion of the testis classically presents with an abrupt onset of severe testicular or scrotal pain, which may radiate to the lower abdomen. It may present with associated inguinal or lower abdominal pain and up to 90 per cent of patients will have associated nausea and vomiting.

Thorough physical examination is key to diagnosing testicular torsion. Testicular tenderness and swelling are the key findings in torsion. The scrotum may be oedematous, indurated, and erythematous if the torsion is longstanding. The testis may lie horizontally, displacing the epididymis from its normal posterolateral position and it may be slightly elevated because of shortening of the spermatic cord from twisting. A reactive hydrocoele may also be present and the cremasteric reflex may be absent.

When clinical findings indicate a high likelihood for testicular torsion, a decision regarding operative exploration, detorsion and fixation needs to be made immediately. Imaging (colour flow doppler) is not routinely done in suspected cases of testicular torsion as it will only serve to delay time-critical surgical intervention.

The treatment for testicular torsion is surgical exploration with detorsion and fixation of both testes. An orchidectomy is performed if the testicle is clearly nonviable. The viability of a torted testicle is dependent upon the duration and completeness of torsion. The typical approximate rates of viability with detorsion within 4 to 6 hours are 100 per cent, 20 per cent after 12 hours and 0 per cent after 24 hours. However, surgery should never be delayed on the assumption of non-viability, as some patients with a prolonged period of symptoms may have had intermittent torsion or a partial torsion (less than 360 degrees), and testicles may still be salvageable.

Torsion of the Testicular Appendages

The appendix testis is a small vestigial structure on the anterosuperior aspect of the testis. It is an embryologic remnant of the Müllerian duct system and typically measures

Figure 27.22 Testicular torsion. Shortly after birth, this newborn was found to have an enlarged and erythematous right hemiscrotum (A). It was unclear whether or not the right hemiscrotum was enlarged at the time of birth. The baby underwent scrotal exploration through a median raphe incision and was found to have an extravaginal testicular torsion (B). The testis is enveloped by the tunica vaginalis and the entire complex has twisted. (Reproduced with permission from Holcomb, G. W., Murphy, J. P., & Peter, S. D. (2020). *Ashcraft's pediatric surgery* (7th ed.). Elsevier Inc.)

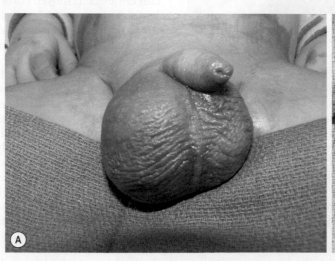
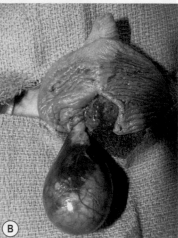

about 0.3 cm. There is also an appendix epididymis, which is a vestigial remnant of the Wolffian duct located at the head of the epididymis. The pedunculated shape of these appendages with a narrow base predisposes them to torsion. Torsion of the appendix testis or appendix epididymis occurs most frequently in boys aged 7 to 12.

The pain of torsion of the appendix testis (or appendix epididymis) is of sudden onset, as is the pain of testicular torsion, and thorough physical examination is required to differentiate between the two as management may differ. In cases of torsion of the appendix testis, physical examination typically demonstrates a non-tender testicle with a tender, palpable, localised mass at the superior pole of the testis. Infarction with necrosis of the appendix testis can be seen as a 'blue dot' sign through the scrotal skin in approximately 21 per cent of cases. A normal cremasteric reflex is usually present and a reactive hydrocoele may be palpated. A normal doppler ultrasound cannot rule out a testicular torsion and scrotal exploration is the only definitive management strategy if there is any concern that a testicular torsion may be present.

Torsion of the appendix testis can initially be treated conservatively using analgesia (non-steroidal anti-inflammatory drugs (NSAIDs), rest and scrotal support to help alleviate swelling. The pain should resolve in 5 to 10 days. Surgical exploration is reserved for equivocal cases and in patients with persistent pain; the contralateral hemiscrotum need not be explored.

Epididymitis

Epididymitis is caused by inflammation of the epididymis and is more common among late adolescents but also occurs in younger boys who deny sexual activity. Several factors may predispose postpubertal boys to develop subacute

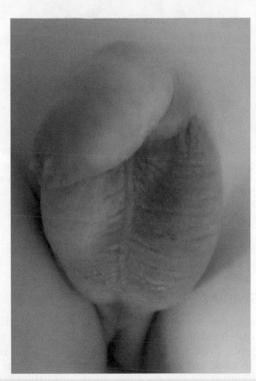

Figure 27.23 Epididymitis on the left. (Reproduced with permission from Fegeler, U., Jäger-Roman, E. (Eds.). (2020). *Praxishandbuch der pädiatrischen Grundversorgung* (2 Auflage). Elsevier.)

epididymitis, including sexual activity, heavy physical exertion and direct trauma (e.g. cycling). Bacterial epididymitis in prepubertal boys is associated with structural anomalies of the urinary tract. Infectious epididymitis in prepubertal boys and adolescents who are not sexually active may be caused by *mycoplasma pneumoniae*, enteroviruses and adenoviruses. Bacterial infection appears to be uncommon in this age group.

Patients with epididymitis may present with acute or subacute onset of pain and swelling isolated to the epididymis. On physical examination, the affected testis has a normal vertical lie. The scrotum may be red and parchment-like and scrotal oedema may be present in 50 per cent of cases (Fig. 27.23). An inflammatory nodule may be felt with an otherwise soft, non-tender epididymis. These patients usually have a normal cremasteric reflex and may experience pain relief with elevation of the testis (Prehn's sign), but this is not a reliable marker for epididymitis.

The diagnosis of epididymitis can be made clinically; however, Doppler ultrasonography may be helpful if the diagnosis is uncertain. This usually demonstrates increased blood flow to the affected epididymis. A urinalysis and urine culture should be obtained in all patients with epididymitis.

Treatment varies according to the severity of the case at presentation and suspected aetiology. The treatment of epididymitis in prepubertal boys depends upon whether they have an associated urinary tract infection or not. Those with pyuria or positive urine cultures should be treated empirically with antibiotics covering coliforms.

Urology

PHIMOSIS

Phimosis is defined as a tight foreskin that cannot be retracted to expose the glans of the penis (Fig. 27.24). In young children, phimosis is normal (physiological), and in older children, infections such as balanitis can cause pathological phimosis. The newborn foreskin is unretractile, and most urologists would recommend not to attempt

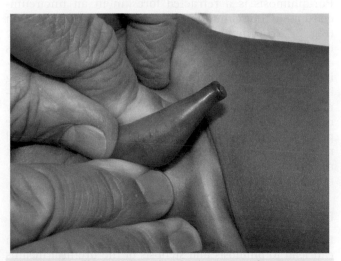

Figure 27.24 Phimosis. (Reproduced with permission from Benoist, G., Bourrillon, A., Delacourt, C., de Billy, B., Liard, A., Collège national des pédiatres universitaires (France)., & Collège national hospitalier et universitaire de chirurgie pédiatrique (France). (2021). *Pédiatrie* (8th ed.). Elsevier Masson.)

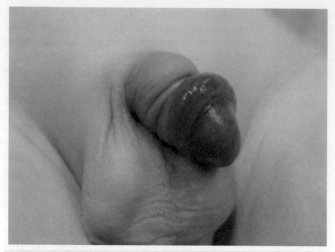

Figure 27.25   Paraphimosis. (Reproduced with permission from Benoist, G., Bourrillon, A., Delacourt, C., de Billy, B., Liard, A., Collège national des pédiatres universitaires (France)., & Collège national hospitalier et universitaire de chirurgie pédiatrique (France). (2021). *Pédiatrie* (8th ed.). Elsevier Masson.)

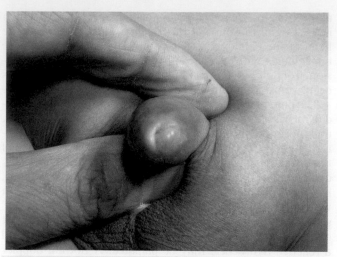

Figure 27.26   Balanitis xerotica obliterans (BXO). (Reproduced with permission from Schmittenbecher, P. P, (Ed.). (2021). *Pädiatrische Chirurgie: Lehrbuch der Kinderchirurgie – kurz und kompakt* (2 Auflage). Elsevier.)

retraction under the age of 6 months. By the age of 1 year, only 10 to 20 per cent of boys will have a retractable foreskin. Up to 90 per cent have a retractable foreskin by school entry. Management of phimosis can be conservative, medical (using topical steroids creams and gentle stretching of the foreskin), or surgical (circumcision or preputioplasty).

While circumcision is one of the most frequently performed surgical procedures worldwide, there is significant variation in the rate between countries. This is due to differing cultural and religious beliefs. At present, the primary surgical indications for circumcision are balanitis xerotica obliterans (BXO) and prophylactic circumcision for recurrent urinary tract infections in boys under 12 months of age with an underlying renal tract anomaly. However, the evidence supporting this is inconsistent.

PARAPHIMOSIS

Paraphimosis is a retracted foreskin in an uncircumcised male that cannot be reduced to its normal position (Fig. 27.25). Impairment of lymphatic and venous flow by the constricting ring of the foreskin causes venous engorgement of the glans with severe, progressive swelling. This can lead to compromised arterial flow resulting in local skin necrosis and even penile necrosis. The primary management of paraphimosis involves the timely reduction of the foreskin back over the glans of the penis. This involves adequate pain control and manual reduction. More invasive techniques such as dorsal slit reduction or urgent circumcision are used if primary management fails.

BALANITIS XEROTICA OBLITERANS

BXO is a chronic, progressive disease of the foreskin, which can lead to phimosis and stenosis of the urethral meatus (Fig. 27.26). In severe cases, it can affect urinary function with spraying and outflow obstruction leading to incomplete bladder emptying. Management with steroid cream is the usual first-line treatment with limited success. Surgical

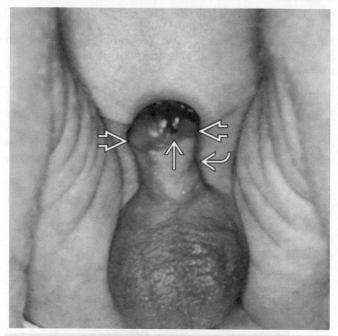

Figure 27.27   Hypospadias. Clinical photograph show that the urethral opening is ventral to the penis tip. Lateral folds of the prepuce and ventral curve of the penile shaft are classic findings of hypospadias. (Reproduced with permission from Woodward, P. J. (2021). *Diagnostic imaging: Obstetrics* (4th ed.). Elsevier Inc.)

treatment with circumcision is frequently necessary and often requires urethral dilatation.

HYPOSPADIAS

Hypospadias is a congenital anomaly characterised by a urethral meatus that opens onto the ventral surface of the penis, proximal to the tip of the glans. The meatus can be located anywhere along the penis from the glans to the scrotum, or in rare cases opens onto the perineum (Fig. 27.27). A ventrally deficient hooded foreskin is typically present and has an unusual cosmetic appearance.

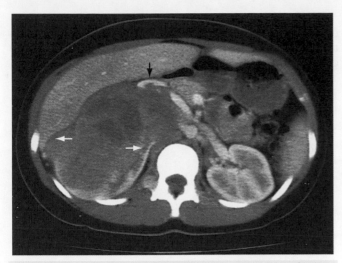

Figure 27.28 Wilms tumour. Computed tomography scan of Wilms tumour. Mass arising out of right kidney (white arrows) displacing the inferior vena cava (black arrow). (Reproduced with permission from Rodgers, A., & Salkind, J. (2019). *Crash course paediatrics* (5th ed.). Elsevier Ltd.)

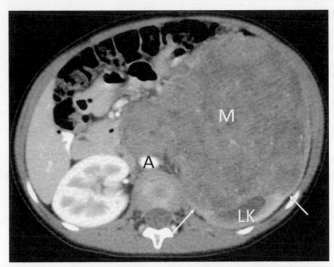

Figure 27.29 Neuroblastoma in a 5-year-old presenting with palpable abdominal mass. Axial contrast-enhanced CT image shows a large mass (M) arising from the left kidney (LK). The parenchyma of the left kidney LK forms a claw sign (arrows), which is helpful in confirming the renal origin of the mass. Note that in contrast to neuroblastoma, Wilms tumour causes displacement of the vessels rather than engulfing them, and when it crosses the midline, the mass passes anterior to the aorta (A) instead of posterior. (Reproduced with permission from Donnelly, L. F. (Ed.). (2021). *Fundamentals of pediatric imaging* (3rd ed.). Academic Press.)

In addition, a chordee, which is a ventral curvature of the penis, has an inconsistent association with hypospadias. They can be classified as glandular, distal or proximal types of hypospadias, depending on the location of the primary urethral opening.

Surgical management depends on the severity of the hypospadias. The more distal types (glandular hypospadias in particular) are considered less severe and do not usually cause any functional impairment; surgical correction may be primarily cosmetic. The proximal types are more complex and surgical correction is often a two-stage procedure requiring grafts of ectopic tissue (foreskin or buccal mucosa) for reconstruction of the urethra. Long-term strictures and urethral fistulae can be problematic.

Neoplasms

WILMS' TUMOUR (WT)

WT is the most common renal malignancy in the paediatric population and is one of the most common cancers in early childhood. Most cases (two-thirds) are diagnosed before 5 years of age. WT can form a component of syndromes such as Beckwith-Wiedemann, wilms tumor, aniridia, genitourinary anomalies, and intellectual disability (WAGR) and Denys-Dash syndrome, with these groups requiring routine screening with serial renal ultrasonography.

Most patients will have a solitary WT, with approximately 5 per cent having bilateral renal involvement. Several gene mutations are associated with WT include p53, WT1, FWT1 and FWT2.

The most common presentation is with a painless, palpable abdominal mass. Occasionally, patients can present with abdominal pain, haematuria or hypertension; however, most are asymptomatic. The diagnosis of WT is prompted by findings of a renal mass on cross-sectional imaging (Fig. 27.28) and confirmed by histology, either by biopsy or based on specimens obtained from surgical excision. Staging is based upon the anatomic extent of the tumour without consideration for genetic, histologic or biomarkers.

The International Society of Paediatric Oncology (SIOP) in Europe stages WTs as follows:

Stage I: tumour limited to the kidney and completely resected
Stage II: tumour extends beyond the kidney but is completely resected
Stage III: invasion beyond capsule, incomplete excision or tumour rupture
Stage IV: distant metastases
Stage V: bilateral renal involvement

Treatment will usually involve preoperative chemotherapy (in patients older than 6 months) followed by a radical nephroureterectomy. The histological staging will determine postoperative chemotherapy and radiotherapy.

NEUROBLASTOMA

Neuroblastomas are tumours of the autonomic nervous system that can develop anywhere along the sympathetic chain. The majority occur in the abdomen, with most arising in the adrenal gland. Neuroblastomas are the most common malignancy in infancy and the most common extracranial solid tumour in children, with 50 per cent of those affected being under 2 years of age.

The presentation of neuroblastoma is variable, and the diagnosis is often made following investigations for complaints such as abdominal pain, Horner syndrome, abdominal/paraspinal mass, and otherwise unexplained secretory diarrhoea.

The definitive diagnosis is made by histologic confirmation or evidence of metastatic disease with an associated rise in urinary catecholamines (homovanillic acid (HVA), vanillylmandelic acid (VMA)). Cross-sectional imaging (Fig. 27.29) should be included when evaluating neuroblastoma imaging. A metaiodobenzylguanidine (MIBG) scan to look for metastatic bone disease is also recommended.

In addition, urinary and serum catecholamine metabolite levels (HVA and VMA) should be measured to assist in the diagnosis and assessment of response to treatment.

Staging of neuroblastoma is planned using the International Neuroblastoma Risk Group Staging System (INRGSS):

L1: localised tumour not involving vital structures and confined to one body compartment

L2: locoregional tumour with the presence of one or more image-defined risk factors

M: distant metastatic disease

MS: metastatic disease in children older than 18 months with metastases confined to skin, liver and/or bone marrow

The treatment plan is typically formulated by an oncology multidisciplinary team (MDT) and involves preoperative chemotherapy, surgical resection and postoperative chemotherapy with radiotherapy.

(Box 27.1)
(Box 27.2)
(Box 27.3)
(Box 27.4)
(Box 27.5)
(Box 27.6)
(Box 27.7)
(Box 27.8)
(Box 27.9)

Box 27.1   Key Points

Failure to pass meconium within the first 48 hours with or without abdominal distension points to a diagnosis of large bowel obstruction.

High up obstruction (duodenal, jejunal or ileal) is associated with bilious vomits or aspirates and the relative absence of abdominal distension.

The standard diagnostic test for Hirschsprung's disease in neonates is rectal suction biopsy while formal full thickness biopsy is preferred in older children. The gold standard curative treatment is a pull through procedure.

Imperforate anus is usually diagnosed on day 1 of life and is an important diagnosis not to miss on newborn examination.

Prior to antenatal diagnosis, the typical presentation of congenital diaphragmatic hernia was of a term newborn infant unresponsive to adequate resuscitation and intubation who continues to deteriorate.

The diagnosis of oesophageal atresia at birth is readily evident in infants when an orogastric tube cannot be inserted further than approximately 10 cm.

Gastroschisis is an open defect of the anterior abdominal wall that results in protrusion of abdominal contents. The defect is mostly on the right side of the umbilicus and the herniating organs are not covered by peritoneum.

Omphalocoele major is associated with other congenital anomalies (in particular cardiac anomalies) in 50 per cent of cases.

In inguinal hernia, the history is of intermittent swelling in the inguinal region and the contents may reach the scrotum.

In terms of undescended testes, reduced fertility, increased risk of testicular torsion and increased risk of seminoma are the key reasons for orchidopexy.

Hypospadias is an abnormal location of urethral meatus on ventral aspect of the penis due to incomplete fusion of paired urogenital folds.

Clinical symptoms of pyloric stenosis include progressive, non-bilious, projectile vomiting that leads to dehydration and weight loss in an infant who is always hungry.

Ileocaecal intussusception is the most common type, and a classical presentation is with episodes of colicky abdominal pain, during which the infant or child draws knees to the abdomen. The infant is pain free between bouts of abdominal colic but remains lethargic.

Surgical indications for circumcision in boys are UTIs with high-grade vesicoureteric reflux or balanitis xerotica obliterans (BXO).

Clinical presentation of acute appendicitis is with initial periumbilical pain, occasionally shifting to right iliac fossa (RIF) and associated nausea, anorexia, vomiting, low-grade fever, occasional diarrhoea and occasional urinary symptoms. If generalised peritonitis develops, the child will look toxic and most unwell.

Acute appendicitis is often difficult to diagnose because of the absence of pathognomonic signs or symptoms, the poor predictive value of laboratory testing, and its varied presentations.

Most cases of Meckel's diverticulum are asymptomatic, but when they do occur, symptoms include painless PR bleeding or acute abdominal pain.

In malrotation, the infant may present in a shocked and collapsed state with bilious vomiting, abdominal tenderness with or without distension, and the passage of dark blood rectally. Presentation is typically under 8 weeks of age.

Late diagnosis of biliary atresia reduces the success of a Kasai portoenterostomy and increases the requirement for liver transplantation.

In testicular torsion, scrotal exploration (ideally **within 4 hours** of the onset of symptoms) with detorsion of the affected side and bilateral testicular fixation should be performed. Emergency surgical exploration is necessary to avoid loss of the testis.

Wilms' tumour or nephroblastoma is one of the most common childhood malignancies with a mean age of diagnosis of 3.5 years. The most common presenting symptom is a large, painless abdominal mass, most likely noted at bath time. Haematuria is unusual in Wilms' tumour.

In neuroblastoma, catecholamine production by the tumour may result in flushing, sweating and irritability. These are quite vague symptoms and thus neuroblastoma can be a very challenging diagnosis to make.

Box 27.2   A Newborn Infant Who Fails to Pass Meconium in the First 24 Hours

A male infant is born by spontaneous vaginal delivery at term and cries at birth. He is breast-fed from birth but his feeding slows after 24 hours. The nursing staff point out that he has not passed meconium and now appears to have mild abdominal distension. His examination is normal apart from abdominal distension and his anus is noted to be patent. An abdominal x-ray is ordered, the infant is transferred to the special care baby unit and placed on an intravenous drip, and a nasogastric tube is inserted. Contact the tertiary paediatric surgical service for advice.

Clinical Pearls

Hirschsprung's disease (HD) is caused by a defect in the cranial–caudal migration of vagal neural-crest cells along the intestine during early embryonic development. The rare long-segment aganglionosis or familial HD (4 to 8 per cent) is of dominant or recessive inheritance with incomplete penetrance. The common, sporadic short-segment HD follows a polygenic inheritance pattern. Differential diagnoses for HD include meconium plug (Fig. 27.30), imperforate anus and meconium ileus.

Interpretation of Investigations

Plain abdominal x-ray shows marked dilatation of the bowel and absence of gas in the rectum. A contrast enema may allow an approximate estimation of the extent of involved bowel by defining a transition zone.

The intraoperative image shows an infant with HD demonstrating distended colon proximal to the affected segment and decompressed small bowel.

Pitfalls to Avoid

Hirschsprung-associated enterocolitis (HAEC), typically manifested by fever, diarrhoea and abdominal distension, is a life-threatening complication In 6 to 60 per cent of HD patients and requires aggressive rectal washouts and systemic antibiotics. It can occur at

any time before or even after a technically satisfactory pull-through operation.

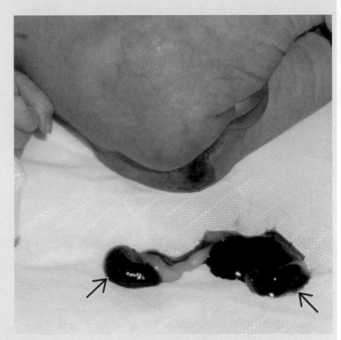

Figure 27.30   Meconium plug. Clinical photograph shows a plug of meconium just passed by a newborn. Meconium is a thick and viscous material that may be aspirated if excreted in utero or during delivery. It causes a chemical pneumonitis, mechanical obstruction of the airways and other problems. (Reproduced with permission from Merrow, A. C., Jr., & Harlharan, S. (Eds.). (2017). *Imaging in pediatrics*, Elsevier.)

Box 27.3   Two-Week-Old With Bilious Vomiting

A 2-week-old infant presents to the emergency department with bilious vomiting. The infant looked well and was passing stool normally. Abdominal examination was essentially normal. While still being observed 4 hours later, the infant deteriorated markedly and developed marked pallor, tachycardia and delayed capillary refill to over 5 seconds. After resuscitation, the infant was taken to theatre where emergency laparotomy revealed intestinal ischaemia from a midgut volvulus.

Clinical Pearls

Bile-stained vomiting in the newborn period is always significant and merits immediate investigation for a surgical cause. Any infant or child with malrotation is at risk of midgut volvulus, which is a surgical emergency. Up to 20 per cent of cases can present after the first year of life and in this group, volvulus is less common. The surgical treatment for malrotation is known as a Ladd's procedure.

Interpretation of Investigations

An abdominal x-ray may not be helpful, whereas an upper gastrointestinal (UGI) contrast study is the definitive investigation of choice to locate the position of the duodenojejunal (DJ) flexure.

In malrotation, you may not see the normal C-shaped loop of the duodenum and the DJ junction is usually lower than the transpyloric plane (L1) and is sited more to the right of the spine (than the normal position to the left of the spine). Small bowel loops will usually be situated mostly on the right side of the abdomen. The caecum can sit higher than usual and to the patients left side and it is often mobile. Doppler ultrasound showing the superior mesenteric vein wrapped in a clockwise direction around the superior mesenteric artery indicating midgut volvulus.

Pitfalls to Avoid

Bilious vomiting should always prompt urgent surgical consultation even in an otherwise well infant. Malrotation is a challenging diagnosis to make. Definitive management is with resuscitation followed by an urgent Ladd's procedure (division of Ladd's bands, widening of the small bowel mesentery, and possible appendectomy) if malrotation and/or volvulus is present.

Recurrent bouts of abdominal pain, irritability and poor weight gain are relatively non-specific symptoms that could indicate malrotation in toddlers and older children.

Box 27.4   A 5-Week-Old Male With Frequent Forceful Vomits

A bottle-fed male infant vomited milk after most feeds, which was worse if he was being moved. Vomiting was forceful and he was hungry afterwards. The infant presented at 6 weeks of age with significant failure to thrive with loose skin folds of the inner thighs and significant pallor.

Clinical Pearls

Hypertrophic pyloric stenosis is an obstructive idiopathic hypertrophy of the pyloric muscle and typically occurs at 1 month, and rarely later than 3 months of age. The curative procedure is division of the circular and longitudinal muscle layers of the pylorus, leaving the mucosa and submucosa intact and this can be done laparoscopically. The open circum-umbilical (Bianchi) approach has a similar cosmetic benefit. Most infants resume feeds and go home 1 to 2 days after the operation. Feeds on demand have become the preferred and most efficient means of postoperative feeding.

Interpretation of Investigations

Ultrasound is accurate, efficient and inexpensive, and has thus become the standard diagnostic test. Protracted vomiting may lead to gastric acid loss and dehydration with renal compensation, creating a hypochloraemic, hypokalaemic metabolic alkalosis, which must be corrected prior to any operative intervention.

Pitfalls to Avoid

The two main complications of pyloromyotomy are an incomplete myotomy (1 per cent of cases) and mucosal perforation (0.5 per cent of cases).

Box 27.5   A Very Pale 4-Month-Old With Blood PR

A 4-month-old male infant presents with a 2-day history of vomiting and loose bowel motions. Four hours post admission, he has an episode of marked pallor and screaming. His examination is unchanged, but he is noted to have tiny amounts of blood in the stool. His pallor settles but he remains unwell.

Clinical Pearls

The classical triad in intussusception is abdominal colic, pallor and blood per rectum. In idiopathic intussusception, the lead point is surmised to be hypertrophy of lymphoid tissue in the distal small bowel wall (Peyer's patches) and in pathological intussusception the lead point can be a Meckel's diverticulum, enlarged mesenteric lymph nodes, a duplication cyst or (more rarely) a lymphoma. The passage of blood PR or red-currant jelly stools is a late sign and occurs in only 15 per cent of cases. A bowel obstruction can develop if the intussusception is not recognised and treated at an early stage.

Interpretation of Investigations

The key investigation is an abdominal ultrasound performed as an emergency. A classical 'doughnut sign' may be seen on ultrasound.

Pitfalls to Avoid

Infants and children with suspected intussusception should only have attempted air enema reduction if on-site paediatric radiological, surgical and anaesthetic expertise is present. Air enema reduction can be successful in up to 90 per cent of cases, but there is a small risk of bowel perforation, which may require immediate needle decompression of abdominal tension prior to definitive laparotomy.

Box 27.6   An 8-Year-Old With Acute Abdominal Pain

An 8-year-old boy attends his family doctor with acute, severe abdominal pain. He is complaining of pain (9 on a scale of 1 to 10 in severity) and nausea. He has no vomiting, diarrhoea or fever. He has no past medical or surgical history and is on no medication. His vital signs are within normal range, though his heart rate is at the upper end of normal.

Clinical Pearls

Abdominal pain is extremely common in children and may reflect a wide variety of conditions. Whenever it lasts for ***more than 4 to 6 hours*** and becomes more intense, or is associated with persistent vomiting or protracted diarrhoea, it must be taken seriously and a surgical cause must be excluded. The diagnosis of appendicitis is made on grounds of history, laboratory findings and repeated clinical examination.

Interpretation of Investigations

The white cell count (WCC) is unable to distinguish between children with or without appendicitis. However, an elevated WCC (neutrophilia) and CRP do increase the likelihood of appendicitis. Diagnostic accuracy is helped by increased use of clinician-performed ultrasound with cross-sectional imaging such as abdominal CT or MRI, which is reserved for cases more difficult to diagnose.

Pitfalls to Avoid

In children with an equivocal diagnosis of acute abdominal pain, active observation is a time-proven and safe management which gives improved diagnostic accuracy. Operative management in acute appendicitis, should only take place *after* resuscitation, rehydration and stabilisation.

Box 27.7 Eight-Week-Old With Prolonged Jaundice

An 8-week-old, breast-fed infant presents with prolonged jaundice and is thought to have breast milk jaundice. His stools are pale and his urine is dark yellow in colour. His sclerae are mildly icteric. He is immediately referred for paediatric assessment. Further testing shows a raised conjugated bilirubin.

Clinical Pearls

Biliary atresia is easy to confuse with breast milk jaundice as most infants with biliary atresia appear well in the first few weeks of life. Main signs of concern are pale stools and dark urine, suggesting obstructive jaundice. Early diagnosis increases the success of the Kasai procedure and may obviate the need for liver transplantation. Biliary atresia is the most common indication for liver transplantation in childhood. The incidence of biliary atresia varies between ethnic groups and is more common in Asian populations.

Interpretation of Investigations

Investigations will show an elevated total and conjugated bilirubin, high alkaline phosphatase and high gamma-glutamyl transferase (GGT). The key initial investigation is the conjugated bilirubin (should be under 20μ mol/L). Ultrasound of the abdomen may show an atretic gallbladder, non-visualisation of the common bile duct with a HIDA scan demonstrating liver uptake, and no excretion of the radio-isotope material into the biliary tree and intestine.

Pitfalls to Avoid

Biliary atresia is often missed due to being misdiagnosed as physiological jaundice or breast milk jaundice. Prolonged jaundice (beyond 14 days in term infants or 21 days in preterms) requires investigation for a pathological cause. If the diagnosis is made late (beyond 100 days of age) then the Kasai procedure is unlikely to be successful. Following the Kasai procedure, clearance of jaundice can be achieved in 60 to 70 per cent of infants, with a 5-year native liver survival of about 50 per cent. Despite a Kasai portoenterostomy, about 30 to 40 per cent of infants will develop end-stage liver disease. Liver transplantation is the only viable treatment option for children who deteriorate after Kasai portoenterostomy. Treating postoperative cholangitis aggressively is an essential element in preventing disease progression.

Box 27.8 A 14-Year-Old With Testicular Pain

A 14-year-old adolescent male presents with a 4-hour history of testicular pain. He has no urinary symptoms. His right testis is swollen and tender to touch. He is immediately referred to the on-call surgical team.

Clinical Pearls

In cases of torsion, testicular pain is of sudden and severe onset. A tender, elevated, transversely located testis with loss of the cremasteric reflex suggests testicular torsion. Torsion can occur at any age but is most commonly seen after puberty. It is an acute surgical emergency and if suspected, surgical exploration should be performed urgently. Key symptoms are testicular pain which may be referred to the abdomen and the affected testis will be swollen and tender. Torsion of the testicular appendages (e.g. the Hydatid of Morgagni) is more likely in the prepubertal age group.

Interpretation of Investigations

A colour-flow doppler study is often unhelpful in the acute setting but may help guide management in cases with symptoms for greater than 24 hours.

Pitfalls to Avoid

All cases of suspected acute testicular torsion should be treated as a surgical emergency. Detorsion and fixation of both testes should take place as soon as possible, even in the non-fasted patient. Pain in testicular torsion may be intermittent or may be a dull ache of gradual onset. The pain may be referred to the abdomen and can be confused with acute appendicitis.

Box 27.9 My Toddler Is Not Quite Right

A 3-year-old girl presented to her family doctor on at least *five occasions* over a 6-month period with vague symptoms of abdominal cramps, bloating, marked irritability and excess sweating. Her mother stated that she was losing weight. She had previously been a cheery and energetic toddler who was very active. She was noted by her mother to be lacking in energy and to be constantly in some discomfort with frequent loose bowel motions. Her mother took her to another GP in the practice and was again reassured. Finally, she brought the toddler to the emergency department to be assessed by the on-duty team.

Her examination showed her to be quite pale and underweight with some degree of abdominal distension without visceromegaly. She was admitted in view of her appearance and her mother's concerns.

She had a full work up, and an abdominal ultrasound showed a large left adrenal mass. Her MRI confirmed this mass and her spot urinary catecholamines were markedly elevated. A diagnosis of neuroblastoma was made, and she subsequently underwent a bone marrow aspirate, a bone scan and metaiodobenzylguanidine (MIBG) scan to assess for metastatic disease.

Clinical Pearls

Neuroblastoma accounts for 10 per cent of all childhood cancers and can be challenging in terms of diagnosis. Some cases regress spontaneously (especially in neonates) while others progress inexorably despite therapy. High rates of survival (over 90 per cent) are achievable if stage 1 or 2 disease is present; however, most children have metastases at the time of diagnosis. Signs and symptoms relating to metastases include bone pain, proptosis and skin lesions. Vasoactive intestinal polypeptide may cause a secretory diarrhoea. There are a variety of neurological symptoms, such as opsoclonus myoclonus (also termed 'dancing eye syndrome'). Overall outcomes are determined by the child's age, histology, and tumour stage.

Interpretation of Investigations

In 90 per cent of cases, catecholamines and their detectable metabolites are found in spot urine samples. Radiological investigations include chest and abdomen x-rays for dystrophic calcification (50 per cent of cases); abdomen ultrasound, CT or MRI for anatomical details of the mass; and metaiodobenzylguanidine (MIBG) scan and technetium bone scanning. Diagnosis is by biopsy and bone marrow aspirate.

Pitfalls to Avoid

Neuroblastoma symptoms are often relatively non-specific and may include irritability, diarrhoea, poor weight gain or weight loss, and excessive flushing or sweating.

Key References

Abdelhafeez, H., & Abib, S. (2020). *IPSO practice guidelines on Wilms tumor.* International Society of Paediatric Surgical Oncology. https://ipso-online.org/guidelines-wt/.

Al-Salem, A. H. (2014). *An illustrated guide to pediatric surgery.* Springer International Publishing.

Benabbas, R., Hanna, M., Shah, J., & Sinert, R. (2017). Diagnostic accuracy of history, physical examination, laboratory tests, and point-of-care ultrasound for pediatric acute appendicitis in the emergency department: A systematic review and meta-analysis. *Academic Emergency Medicine, 24*(5), 523–551.

Bhangu, A., Søreide, K., Di Saverio, S., Assarsson, J. H., & Drake, F. T. (2015). Acute appendicitis: Modern understanding of pathogenesis, diagnosis, and management. [published correction appears in *Lancet, 390*(10104), 1736] *Lancet, 386*(10000), 1278–1287.

Cappendijk, V. C., & Hazebroek, F. W. (2000). The impact of diagnostic delay on the course of acute appendicitis. *Archives of Disease in Childhood, 83*(1), 64–66.

Chan, E., Wayne, C., Nasr, A., & FRCSC for Canadian Association of Pediatric Surgeon Evidence-Based Resource. (2014). Ideal timing of orchiopexy: A systematic review. *Pediatric Surgery International, 30*(1), 87–97.

Di Saverio, S., Podda, M., De Simone, B., Ceresoli, M., Augustin, G., Gori, A., et al. (2020). Diagnosis and treatment of acute appendicitis: 2020 update of the WSES Jerusalem guidelines. *World Journal of Emergency Surgery, 15*(1), 27.

Diamond, D. A., Chan, I. H. Y., Holland, A. J. A., Kurtz, M. P., Nelson, C., Estrada, C. R., Jr., et al. (2017). Advances in paediatric urology. *Lancet, 390*(10099), 1061–1071.

Murphy, F., & Urologist, C. P. (2011). The BAPU consensus statement on the management of undescended testes. http://medi-guide.meditool.cn/ymtpdf/DA7E9AB6-1762-0FA7-E977-E42FC0495970.pdf.

National Health Service. (2015). Commissioning guide: Paediatric orchidopexy for undescended testis. https://www.baus.org.uk/_userfiles/pages/files/Publications/Commissioning%20guide%20for%20orchidopexy%20final%20v7.pdf.

Somani, B. K., Watson, G., & Townell, N. (2010). Testicular torsion. *BMJ, 341*, c3213.

Tam, P. K. H., Chung, P. H. Y., St Peter, S. D., Gayer, C. P., Ford, H. R., Tam, G. C. H., et al. (2017). Advances in paediatric gastroenterology. *Lancet, 390*(10099), 1072–1082.

The Lancet. (2017). Pushing the boundaries in paediatric surgery. *Lancet, 390*(10099), 1006.

Paediatrics in Everyday Practice

28 Common Presentations in Infancy

ALF NICHOLSON and KEVIN DUNNE

For most parents, the first year passes almost in a blur with many sleepless nights, constant worry and wondrous excitement about developmental milestones attained. The first year is a real roller coaster ride for first-time parents in particular, as it is all so new. New parents are also often overwhelmed by a flood of well-meaning advice, which is often conflicting. This leaves new parents uncertain how to proceed or which advice to take. Social media is a further influence, and it can be difficult to sieve through the information overload. The result of all this confusion is that the parents seek medical expert advice.

The great joy of having a newborn baby can be quickly dashed by the reality of excessive crying due to infant colic. In the early days, a baby's head measurements indicating a large or unusually shaped head may be a cause of alarm. Brief, resolved, unexplained events can cause great anxiety, but are just as the name implies. Another common presentation which may be concerning is noisy breathing, whether due to stridor or wheeze, and may require investigation.

In this chapter, we wish to highlight the frequent presentations that cause parents great concern, most of which can be competently managed by their family doctor with back up from a specialist paediatric service as needed.

In the **Clinical Bottom Line** section for each topic, we wish to highlight the key areas to look out for in family practice/primary care and what might be done prior to the child being seen by a paediatrician.

Normal Crying Pattern

Healthy babies signal their need for a response from their caregiver (usually the mother) along a gradient of progressively intense cues, beginning with changed breathing patterns, then increasing movements and vocalisations and finally to a full-blown cry. A newborn infant's cry promotes the secretion of oxytocin in the mother, which in turn promotes responsiveness in her.

Infant Colic

Colic is not serious unless you happen to be the infant's parents!

While it is often difficult to determine when an infant should be considered to have colic, the most widely used definition is the 'rule of threes' proposed by Wessel and colleagues. If an infant cries for more than 3 hours/day for more than 3 days/week for 3 weeks, colic is the diagnosis.

Infantile colic usually begins at about 2 weeks of age and reaches a peak sometime in the second month and then declines to baseline levels at about 4 months of age. The peak of crying may be earlier in formula-fed infants compared to those who are breast-fed. The crying bout may include regurgitation and the passage of gas per rectum. These bouts are resistant to all kinds of soothing attempts, including feeding. In premature infants, the crying pattern is similar, occurring at 6 weeks corrected age.

History

It is important to ask for a detail description of crying pattern, including the timing of the day, duration of each crying bout, the feeding pattern and associated symptoms such as vomiting or an elevated temperature. Infants with a sudden increase in the frequency and duration of inconsolable crying are more likely to have an underlying medical condition.

There are a number of clinical clues that might suggest an alternative diagnosis other than simple colic. These include high-pitched crying with associated back arching with no evening clustering of crying.

Growth parameters such as head circumference should be obtained looking for a rapidly increasing head circumference, which might indicate hydrocephalus.

Urinary tract infection may present with vague symptoms in infancy and therefore one should have a very low threshold for performing urinalysis and urine culture if persistent irritability cannot otherwise be explained.

Differential Diagnoses

INFECTION

Always enquire about a history of recent fever, as the presence of fever in an infant under 3 months old may indicate the possibility of a serious bacterial infection such as urinary tract infection, septicaemia or meningitis.

FEEDING ISSUES

There is an important link between feeding problems and excessive crying. Difficulties with breast-feeding (such as problems of attachment or positioning) may put susceptible infants at risk of increased crying and aversive feeding behaviours. Functional lactose overload occurs when breast-feeds have a low-fat content, resulting in rapid milk transit through the intestine. Undigested lactose ferments in the colon with resulting explosive or frothy stools, excessive crying and a desire to feed very often. You may find the infant gets an associated nappy rash from the acidity of the stools. A few days of lactation support can resolve the issue.

COW'S MILK PROTEIN INTOLERANCE (CMPI)

Some infants with excessive crying have CMPI. A late onset of increased crying in the third month of life or following a switch from breast to formula milk may indicate CMPI.

There is a group of infants with colic that are classified as 'Wessel's plus'. These infants fulfil Wessel's criteria for colic but also show other concerning cues such as clenched fists, flexed legs, back arching, distended abdomens, regurgitation with crying and a pained face when crying. In this 'Wessel's plus' group (especially if associated diarrhoea and/or vomiting), a trial of elimination of cow's milk protein (CMP), either from the mother's diet if breast-feeding or from the infant's diet by changing to a CMP-free formula, may be indicated. The GP Infant Feeding Network (UK) are a useful online resource for the diagnosis and management of all feeding issues in primary care. They have a specific guideline providing help in the diagnosis and management of CMPI including advice on milk selection and the phased re-introduction of CMP.

INCARCERATED HERNIA OR TESTICULAR TORSION

Some infants with an incarcerated hernia or testicular torsion can present with acute onset of crying. An incarcerated hernia may be accompanied by an irreducible groin swelling with abdominal distension. Testicular torsion may be characterised by scrotal swelling, scrotal discolouration and tenderness to palpation. Thus, it is essential to remove the nappy when inspecting the genitalia and hernial orifices to exclude these serious but surgically treatable conditions.

HIRSCHSPRUNG'S DISEASE

Infants with Hirschsprung's disease may present with an abnormal bowel pattern with severe constipation, which causes distress. Symptoms include bilious vomiting, chronic constipation, fever, no meconium passed in first 24 hours of life and poor feeding.

DRUG WITHDRAWAL

Neonatal abstinence syndrome (NAS) is associated with illicit drug use (benzodiazepines, heroin, methadone and opioid analgesics) and is evident soon after birth. These infants may also have symptoms of marked jitteriness, sleeplessness, and tremors. There are a number of international guidelines regarding assessment scores and treatment.

RED FLAG SYMPTOMS

RED FLAG symptoms include bilious or projectile vomiting, fever, lethargy or poor feeding, perinatal risk factors for sepsis (such as prolonged rupture of membranes, presence of Group B streptococcus in the mother, or maternal fever in labour), and pallor with blood in the stool.

MANAGEMENT OF COLIC

It is important to take the problem seriously and to ensure that feeding is adequate and appropriate for the infant. One should conduct a detailed examination of the infant.

Treatment options for breast-fed infants include the probiotic *Lactobacillus reuteri* (strain DSM 17938) and reducing maternal dietary allergen intake. Switching to a hydrolysed formula is an option for formula fed infants.

Parents have historically often used over-the-counter (OTC) treatments to settle their baby. These OTC treatments include gripe water, simethicone drops or lactase drops. There is no convincing evidence that any of these OTC treatments work. Reviewing the infant, checking for normal growth, and–most importantly–listening to the parents and reassuring them that the serious differential diagnoses have been excluded, are all important. The parents need to know that the symptoms will improve with time and should resolve at approximately 4 months of age.

This is an opportune time for the doctor to support the wellbeing of the parents as the impact of being unable to settle your infant can be very tiring and emotionally draining. If necessary, do not hesitate to advise admission to hospital, in order to alleviate a very stressful situation at home. (Box 28.1)

Box 28.1 *Clinical Bottom Line*

Colic is very frequent and causes immense distress to parents. Reassurance and detailed examination of the infant is important to ensure that no 'red flag' symptoms or signs are evident. Avoid frequent milk changes and the use of H2 antagonists or omeprazole. Overall, drug therapy is neither effective nor evidence based. If very severe symptoms of crying with no evening predominance, consider empirical cow's milk protein exclusion on a trial basis for 6 to 8 weeks. Refer directly to hospital if the infant is unwell or feverish or if the parents have reached breaking point.

Infant With a Large Head

The infant with a large head is a very frequent presentation and is most often due to benign familial macrocephaly in families with some first-degree members similarly affected, and which requires no treatment. Classically, the head circumference tracks at or above the 97th centile and developmental progress is normal. Accurate measurement and correct plotting on the centile chart are essential to establish this. Inaccuracies in measurement and charting are avoidable and will lead to unnecessary referral.

Compared to the WHO standard, representative British and Irish heads appear large (median above the 75th centile), but appear to be stable after a rise in the first 6 months of life. The WHO standard extends only to 5 years of age, so the UK 1990 centile chart should be used where head measurement is needed beyond this age.

If the occipitofrontal circumference (OFC) readings are within normal centiles but the head seems large, then consider late intrauterine growth retardation, skeletal dysplasia (such as achondroplasia) or frontal bossing.

Serial measurements of head circumference are very helpful, especially if the head circumference is seen to be crossing centiles upwards, which may be an indicator of raised intracranial pressure (ICP) or hydrocephalus (Fig. 28.1).

HIGH-RISK FACTORS

Look out for any high-risk factors associated with a large head in infancy such as a family history of macrocephaly, preterm birth with history of intraventricular haemorrhages, history of subdural haemorrhages (may be linked to abusive head trauma), neonatal meningitis, history of an open myelomeningocoele or a family history of neurofibromatosis type 1.

SYMPTOMS OF RAISED INTRACRANIAL PRESSURE

The symptoms of raised intracranial pressure (ICP) include irritability, a high-pitched cry, poor feeding, vomiting, seizures, decreased alertness and dilated scalp veins.
(Box 28.2)

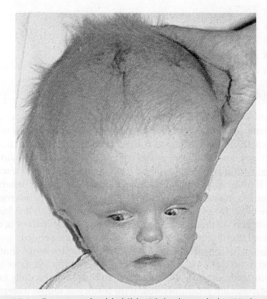

Figure 28.1 Four-month-old child with hydrocephalus. Hydrocephalus is usually caused by obstruction of the flow of cerebrospinal fluid. If hydrocephalus occurs in an infant, the soft bones of the skull push apart as the head increases progressively in size. (Reproduced with permission from Leonard, P. C. (2015). *Building a medical vocabulary: With Spanish translations* (9th ed.). Elsevier.)

Box 28.2 *Clinical Bottom Line*

Regular measurement with referral to appropriate centile charts for head circumference is key. Watch out for a head circumference crossing upwards on repeated measurement. Bear in mind that preterm infants under 37 weeks' gestation require correction on the centile chart to account for their prematurity.

The most common scenario by far is familial macrocephaly, in which the infant's head growth will chart along or just above the 97th centile without any additional symptoms. Checking the head circumference of both parents is helpful in this regard.

Immediate referral is warranted if any features of raised intracranial pressure.

Disorders of head shape

Observation is key for both plagiocephaly and brachycephaly and no active treatment is required. A key differential is craniosynostosis, which may occur along the sagittal, coronal, or lambdoid sutures. Craniosynostosis is a condition in which the head sutures fuse prematurely. This may be noted as a bony ridge or an abnormal head shape. It is important to distinguish this from other causes of abnormal head shape in infancy, as these children require specialist neurosurgical input.

When examining the head from above, the key finding in deformational or positional plagiocephaly is that the ear on the affected side is displaced forward, thereby distinguishing it from lambdoid craniosynostosis where it is displaced backwards. Also, the skull shape in plagiocephaly is like a parallelogram, unlike the trapezoid shape of lambdoid craniosynostosis. Craniosynostosis requires CT scanning for diagnosis and referral to a specialist craniofacial service.
(Box 28.3)

Box 28.3 *Clinical Bottom Line*

The essential finding in deformational or positional plagiocephaly is that the ear on the affected side is displaced forward thereby distinguishing it from lambdoid craniosynostosis. Suspected craniosynostosis requires urgent referral to a specialist craniofacial service.

Brief resolved unexplained events (BRUE)

The key elements of a BRUE are that it only occurs under 12 months of age and includes the occurrence of an episode of pallor or cyanosis and not just colour change. It is a diagnosis of exclusion.

KEY CHARACTERISTICS OF A BRUE

Brief: duration is less than 1 minute
Resolved: the infant returned to their normal state of health after the event with normal observations

Unexplained: the episode is not explained by a medical condition such as gastroesophageal reflux or nasal congestion

Event: at least one of decreased or irregular breathing, marked change in tone or low responsiveness

A low-risk BRUE shows no concerning features on history or examination and ALL of the following criteria are met: being over 2 months of age, being born over 32 weeks' gestation, not requiring cardiopulmonary resuscitation (CPR) by a healthcare professional, an event lasting under 1 minute, and a first event.

Low-risk BRUE do not require investigation and, after a period of observation for 4 to 6 hours, may be discharged home with early medical follow up.

If an infant does not fulfil the criteria for low-risk BRUE, then by definition they fall into the high-risk category. High-risk infants should be admitted to hospital and investigations coordinated based on the history and examination. Investigations include an ECG (to measure the QT interval), a nasopharyngeal aspirate for viruses and *Bordetella pertussis*, a blood glucose and a full blood count.

The key issues are to define level of risk and, if low-risk BRUE, to observe for 4 hours, avoid investigation, and involve parents in agreed management plans.

(Box 28.4)

Box 28.4 *Clinical Bottom Line*

All suspected BRUE episodes should be referred directly to hospital for emergency review. Fortunately, most are low risk and require only observation.

The central issue is to define level of risk. If low-risk BRUE, observe for 4 hours, avoid investigation and involve parents in agreed management plans. Do not be tempted to advise home apnoea monitoring for low-risk BRUE episodes.

Stridor in infancy

Laryngomalacia typically presents with a high-pitched inspiratory stridor with onset usually at 2 to 4 weeks of age. It resolves by 8 to 12 months of age. Stridor is worse during intercurrent upper respiratory tract infections and can be associated with apnoea if laryngomalacia is severe. Severe cases may be accompanied by tracheomalacia which manifests as stridor, coughing with wheeze, and episodes of cyanosis.

Congenital subglottic stenosis usually presents under 3 months with an inspiratory stridor with associated respiratory distress. Acquired subglottic stenosis may develop secondary to prolonged intubation and a cricoid split operation or tracheostomy may be required.

(Box 28.5)

Box 28.5 *Clinical Bottom Line*

A floppy larynx or laryngomalacia is by far the most common reason for stridor in infancy and does cause significant parental concern. It can be very helpful for parents to take an audio or video recording on their smartphone, which can then be sent to your local paediatric specialist service. Watch out for infants with stridor and apparent apnoea (think of tracheomalacia), and stridor with infant haemangiomas in a beard distribution over the chin (may have laryngeal involvement).

If the infant is thriving and if stridor is worse when distressed or during an intercurrent viral illness, then laryngomalacia is very likely. Reassure the parents that the stridor will lessen significantly after 6 to 9 months of age.

Recurrent wheeze in infancy

Recurrent wheezing due to viral infection can subsequently progress to asthma with viral-induced exacerbations.

Initial treatment to manage recurrent wheeze should be with a bronchodilator (either β2-agonist or anticholinergic) and, if symptoms persist, either montelukast or inhaled corticosteroids. There is currently no evidence to support the use of intermittent inhaled corticosteroids for episodic wheeze or as continued prophylaxis.

An infant or child with viral induced wheeze who is well enough to remain at home should not be prescribed oral prednisolone. For those who attend the Emergency Department and who receive bronchodilators, oral corticosteroids may reduce the number of days in hospital.

For multiple trigger wheeze, give a trial of inhaled corticosteroids or montelukast for a defined period (usually 4 to 8 weeks). Consider alternative diagnoses if no response or if troublesome symptoms recur. No treatment has been shown to prevent progression of preschool wheeze to school-age asthma and thus treatment is driven solely by current symptoms.

(Box 28.6)
(Box 28.7)
(Box 28.8)
(Box 28.9)
(Box 28.10)
(Box 28.11)

Box 28.6 *Clinical Bottom Line*

Recurrent wheeze in infancy is very common. The first episode may be due to acute viral bronchiolitis. Enquire about a family history of atopy and whether there is passive smoking at home. The important question is whether or not the wheeze is triggered by intercurrent viral illnesses.

Episodic viral wheeze should be treated depending on a variety of factors. If male and Caucasian with frequent emergency department presentations and a history of atopy, daily inhaled corticosteroids are recommended. However, if female, non-Caucasian, with less frequent and less severe symptoms and no personal or family history of atopy, then intermittent inhaled corticosteroids are recommended.

Persistent wheeze is defined as wheeze episodes more than four times per year, a personal or family history of atopy, episodes lasting more than 24 hours and affecting sleep. In this instance, daily inhaled corticosteroids are recommended. If no history of atopy, intermittent inhaled corticosteroids or daily montelukast are recommended.

Box 28.7   Key Points

An infant should be considered to have colic if they cry for more than 3 hours/day for more than 3 days/week for 3 weeks.

RED FLAG symptoms associated with infant distress include bilious or projectile vomiting, fever, lethargy or poor feeding, perinatal risk factors for sepsis (such as prolonged rupture of membranes, presence of Group B streptococcus in the mother, or maternal fever in labour), and pallor with blood in the stool.

Spend time reassuring the parents when managing infant colic and do not be afraid to advise admission to hospital, if necessary, to alleviate a very stressful situation at home.

The infant with a large head is a very frequent presentation and is most often due to benign familial macrocephaly where some close family members are similarly affected, and which requires no treatment.

Serial measurements of the head circumference are very helpful, especially if the head circumference is seen to be crossing centiles upwards.

The major finding in deformational or positional plagiocephaly is that the ear on the affected side is displaced forward distinguishing it from lambdoid craniosynostosis. Craniosynostosis requires CT scanning for diagnosis and referral to a specialist craniofacial service.

The key elements of a BRUE are that it only occurs under 12 months of age, is only diagnosed when other diagnoses have been excluded and the occurrence of an episode of pallor or cyanosis and not just colour change.

The key issue is to define level of risk and, if low-risk BRUE, to observe for 4 hours, avoid investigation and involve parents in agreed management plans.

Laryngomalacia typically presents with a high-pitched inspiratory stridor with onset usually at 2 to 4 weeks of age. It resolves by 8 to 12 months of age.

An infant or child with viral induced wheeze who is well enough to remain at home should not be prescribed oral prednisolone.

Episodic viral wheeze should be treated with intermittent therapy. Multiple trigger wheeze is defined as wheeze or cough responsive to bronchodilators and breathlessness on most days and a trial of inhaled corticosteroids or montelukast is recommended.

Box 28.8   A Young Infant With Excessive Crying

The parents of a 6-week-old female infant present her to their family doctor with a history of excessive crying and infant distress. She was born by forceps delivery at term and weighed 3.1 kg at birth. She was breast-fed on demand and had an excellent weight gain over the first 6 weeks of age. Her crying was very intense and appeared to be increasing. She tended to cry after feeds and most especially in the evenings. The parents had tried a range of strategies, including swaddling and baby massage, and now were very concerned about her as all strategies had failed to reduce her crying frequency. Her examination is perfectly normal, and she has gained 900 g from birth. A working diagnosis of infant colic is made.

Clinical Pearls

Crying is the young infant's sole way of communicating. All young infant display crying, which peaks at 4 to 6 weeks of age.

Infant colic affects about 30 per cent of young infants and crying tends to cluster during the late afternoon and evening hours. Infants may clench their fists, flex their legs, arch their backs and grimace, giving the impression that they are in pain.

Fussing and crying follows a characteristic crying curve in the first 3 months of life with crying peaking at 6 weeks and then reducing by 3 months of age.

Cow's milk protein intolerance (CMPI) may be a cause of excessive crying. These infants may have 'high-pitched' crying, regularly arch their backs during crying bouts, and their crying pattern does not fit that of evening clustering.

Excessive crying and refusal to feed are not related to silent gastroesophageal reflux (GOR).

In neonatal abstinence syndrome, the crying is high-pitched and inconsolable, usually begins in the first week of life, and may last for over 4 weeks. Exposure to cocaine in utero may cause similar symptoms of excess crying. Lesser degrees of irritability may be evident if the mother is on fluoxetine therapy.

Simethicone and proton pump inhibitors are ineffective for the treatment of colic, and dicyclomine is contraindicated. Evidence does not support chiropractic or osteopathic manipulation, infant massage, swaddling, acupuncture or herbal supplements.

Interpretation of Investigations

Once the history shows the classic features of colic with an evening cluster, no investigations are required. Investigate only if alternative diagnoses are being considered.

Pitfalls to Avoid

Colic is a diagnosis of exclusion after a detailed history and physical examination have ruled out concerning causes.

As doctors, one should never ignore or downplay parental concern about colic and always make sure to regularly monitor the infant with excessive crying.

If the increased crying occurs in the context of a fragile or otherwise challenged family, refer for a specialist paediatric opinion and consider admission to take the heat out of the situation.

Key findings to watch out for on examination include a fever, distended abdomen, full fontanelle or faltering growth and bruising.

Box 28.9   An Infant With a Large or Misshapen Head

A male infant was born by lower (uterine) segment Caesarean section (LSCS) at term with a birth weight of 4 kg and a head circumference at birth of 36 cm. His neonatal course was uneventful and he reached all his developmental milestones. At the 6 weeks check, his head circumference had risen to 39.5 cm and he was noted to have significant head lag. Clinical examination revealed dilated scalp veins and a wide anterior fontanelle. He was referred for urgent paediatric assessment.

Clinical Pearls

Head circumference is measured using a non-stretch tape measure by measuring the occipitofrontal circumference (OFC). The OFC extends from the most prominent part of the glabella to the most prominent posterior area of the occiput of the infant.

Confirm the diagnosis of a large head by plotting the largest of three measurements on the UK-WHO centile chart and checking previous measurements (including OFC at birth) to assess the rate of head growth over time.

The size of the anterior fontanelle varies greatly and if head growth and infant development are both normal, a small or large fontanelle should not cause alarm.

The great majority of head shape abnormalities are positional and the most commonly seen are brachycephaly (flattened occiput) and positional (deformational) plagiocephaly.

The key finding in deformational or positional plagiocephaly is that the ear on the affected side is displaced forward, thus distinguishing it from lambdoid craniosynostosis.

In hydrocephalus, head growth of over 2 cm/week will be seen prior to treatment. Hydrocephalus is usually obstructive in type (postinfectious, posthaemorrhagic or related to Arnold Chiari malformation, aqueduct stenosis or a Dandy Walker cyst of the fourth ventricle). Treatment is by insertion of a ventriculoperitoneal shunt.

Interpretation of Investigations

If raised intracranial pressure (ICP) is suspected, urgent referral for neuroimaging (ultrasound, CT or MRI) is indicated. MRI brain is preferable.

Pitfalls to Avoid

Look for the signs of raised ICP including a bulging anterior fontanelle, splayed sutures, prominent scalp veins, sunsetting of the eyes, a convergent squint of recent onset and a head circumference increasing rapidly and crossing centiles. Cushing's triad of bradycardia, hypertension and a depressed level of consciousness rarely occurs in infancy prior to the closure of the anterior fontanelle. Likewise, papilloedema is rarely seen in infants with raised ICP.

If associated developmental delay, consider neurocutaneous syndromes, particularly neurofibromatosis type 1, and other syndromes such as Soto or Fragile X (molecular testing for FRMI gene of the X chromosome), and confirm by appropriate genetic testing. If coarse physical features or evidence of hepatosplenomegaly with developmental delay, consider mucopolysaccharidoses. Consider Alexander or Canavan syndromes if profound delay is present.

Box 28.10   A Brief Episode of Apparent Apnoea in a Young Infant

A 3-month-old male infant presents with a very brief episode of apnoea requiring stimulation by his parents. He was born at 34 weeks' gestation and spent 4 weeks in the special care baby unit. Apart from feeding issues, there were no major complications and he had received his first immunisations a few days prior to the episode. His parents are both young and were very shocked by the episode, as there is a family history of sudden infant death syndrome (SIDS).

Clinical Pearls

A brief, resolved, unexplained event (BRUE) was previously referred to as an apparent life-threatening event. These episodes are frightening to the observer and are typically characterised by some combination of choking or gagging, apnoea, colour change and marked change in muscle tone.

Low-risk BRUE events occur if the infant is over 60 days of age, the gestational age is above 32 weeks, the first episode did not require cardiopulmonary resuscitation (CPR), there are no concerning features in the history, there is a negative family history of sudden cardiac death, and examination is normal. All other BRUEs are high-risk by definition.

CPR training for low-risk BRUE should be offered to caregivers along with information to further reassure them as to the benign nature of this group. Do not initiate home cardiorespiratory monitoring if BRUE is low risk.

Abnormal vital signs (such as fever, fast respiratory rate or tachycardia) preclude a diagnosis of BRUE.

BRUE infants should be observed for at least 4 hours with pulse oximetry to establish that all observations are stable.

Interpretation of Investigations

For low-risk BRUE, investigations such as chest x-ray, EEG, ECG, echocardiography, and barium swallow are not required. Investigation of high-risk BRUE is less clear cut with little evidence as to how best to proceed.

Low blood glucose measurement can point the clinician in the direction of an occult metabolic disorder such as a fat oxidation defect.

Pitfalls to Avoid

Carefully consider differential diagnoses.

Acute apnoea can occur during intercurrent illnesses such as acute bronchiolitis, pertussis and acute sepsis. Pertussis is a cause of colour change and pauses in breath in young infants but is associated with a paroxysmal cough. A pernasal swab should be requested if this is suspected.

Minor shake injuries in early infancy may be associated with brief periods of apnoea. Ex-preterm infants in car seats may also have apnoea if not given adequate neck support. A history of failure to thrive, an enlarged head circumference, and abnormal breathing all suggest a potential underlying medical condition and thus cannot be classified as BRUE.

Box 28.11 Noisy Breathing in the First Year of Life

An 8-month-old male infant presents with noisy breathing from early infancy and repeated episodes of wheeze brought on by intercurrent viral illnesses. He was born by spontaneous vertex delivery at term and there were no perinatal issues. There is a family history of atopy and asthma. Both parents are smokers. He underwent a number of antibiotic courses with little clinical effect. His examination shows him to be thriving and he has scattered wheezes on auscultation. His chest x-ray is unremarkable. He is referred for specialist opinion.

Clinical Pearls

The key clinical question is whether the infant has stridor (an inspiratory noise) or wheeze with a prolonged expiratory phase of respiration. Parents tend to report noisy breathing and it may be difficult to distinguish one from the other. Smartphone video footage may be helpful in making this distinction. Laryngomalacia is by far the most common cause of inspiratory stridor and noisy respirations in infants.

Wheeze is defined as a high-pitched whistling sound usually in expiration and associated with increased work of breathing and can be divided into either episodic viral wheeze (where the infant only wheezes with an intercurrent viral illness and is otherwise symptom free) or multiple trigger persistent wheeze (where wheeze is brought on by a viral illness and other triggers including exercise, smoke and exposure to allergens).

Therefore, recurrent wheezing in preschool children is common and is frequently triggered by viral respiratory tract infections. Certain phenotypes may respond to treatments differently, depending on the risk factors identified (such as a personal or family history of atopy).

Interpretation of Investigations

Chest x-ray is the key first investigation and may suggest congenital cystic adenomatoid malformation (confirmed by CT), a late-presenting congenital diaphragmatic hernia (usually right sided), or congenital lobar emphysema (also confirmed by CT).

An H-type tracheoesophageal fistula may present with recurrent lower respiratory infections. Diagnosis is by bronchoscopy or OesophagoGastroDuodenoscopy (OGD).

A vascular ring may be suspected on chest x-ray if a right-sided aortic arch is present, on bronchoscopy if extrinsic compression of the trachea is present, and on barium swallow if oesophageal compression is present. MRI or echocardiography are required to diagnose a vascular ring.

Pitfalls to Avoid

If there is no response to treatment, diagnoses to be considered include cystic fibrosis (now detected at neonatal screening in many countries but not universally), a primary immunodeficiency with severe failure to thrive and chronic diarrhoea, and an inhaled foreign body with a sudden episode of choking or primary ciliary dyskinesia (PCD) in which symptoms often date from birth.

In PCD, mean age at diagnosis is 2.6 years in England. Eighty per cent have persistent otitis media with effusion. Half of all children with PCD have situs inversus, and 20 per cent have congenital heart disease.

Vascular rings are very rare and may present with stridor, cough and wheeze.

 Video on the topic The crying infant is available online at Elsevier eBooks+.

References

Bush, A., Grigg, J., & Saglani, S. (2014). Managing wheeze in preschool children. *BMJ Clinical Research Edition, 348*, g15.

Cyriac, J., & Huxstep, K. (2015). Whistles, and wheezes: Don't miss diseases. *Archives of Disease in Childhood Education and Practice Edition, 100*, 132–143.

Drug and Bulletin Therapeutics. (2013). Management of infantile colic. *BMJ (Clinical Research Edition), 347*, f4102.

Fox, A., Lovis, M.-T., & The GP Infant Feeding Network. (October 5, 2019). *The milk allergy in primary care (MAP) guideline 2019*. https://gpifn.org.uk/imap/.

The GP Infant Feeding Network. (n.d.). A website to assist primary care practitioners with best practice in infant feeding. https://gpifn.org.uk/.

Johnson, J. D., Cocker, K., & Chang, E. (2015). Infantile colic: Recognition and treatment. *American Family Physician, 92*(7), 577–582.

McKenzie, S. A. (2013). Fifteen-minute consultation: Troublesome crying in infancy. *Archives of Disease in Childhood Education and Practice Edition, 98*(6), 209–211.

Olsen, A. L., Ammitzbøll, J., Olsen, E. M., & Skovgaard, A. M. (2019). Problems of feeding, sleeping and excessive crying in infancy: A general population study. *Archives of Disease in Childhood Education and Practice Edition, 104*(11), 1034–1041.

Seal A. Fifteen-minute consultation on the infant with a large head. *Archives of Disease in Childhood Education and Practice Edition, 98*(4), 122-125.

Stokes, J. R., & Bacharier, L. B. (2020). Prevention and treatment of recurrent viral-induced wheezing in the preschool child. *Annals of Allergy, Asthma & Immunology, 125*(2), 156–162.

Tate, C., & Sunley, R. (2018). Brief resolved unexplained events (formerly apparent life-threatening events) and evaluation of lower-risk infants. *Archives of Disease in Childhood Education and Practice Edition, 103*(2), 95–98.

Wessel, M.A., Cobb, J.C., el al. Paroxysmal fussing in infancy, sometimes called colic. *Pediatrics.* 1954;14(5):421–435.

Wolke, D. (2019). Persistence of infant crying, sleeping and feeding problems: Need for prevention. *Archives of Disease in Childhood, 104*(11), 1022–1023.

Online References

Joint Trust Guideline for the Management of Neonatal Abstinence Syndrome. file:///C:/Users/kdunne/Downloads/Neonatal-Abstinence-Syndrome-JCG0008-v3.2.pdf.

Neonatal Abstinence Syndrome Advances in Diagnosis and Treatment Elisha M. Wachman, MD1,2; Davida M. Schiff, MD, MSc3; Michael Silverstein, MD,MPH. https://jamanetwork.com/journals/jama/fullarticle/2677452

THE GP INFANT FEEDING NETWORK (UK) A Website to Assist Primary Care Practitioners with Best Practice in Infant Feeding. https://gpifn.org.uk/

29 | *Frequent Flyers in the Toddler Years*

ALF NICHOLSON and KEVIN DUNNE

There was never a child so lovely, but his mother was glad to get him to sleep.

RALPH WALDO EMERSON

The toddler years are indeed challenging for parents. It is a time for the toddler's bold expression of personality often coupled with a battle of wills. Parents and grandparents must set limits for the toddler. Fortunately, parents have a great capacity to forgive and forget the trials and tribulations of the toddler years.

There are a number of frequently presenting issues discussed in some detail in this chapter. These issues include sleep disorders (we all need our sleep), lymphadenopathy (almost universal if you look carefully enough, especially in the posterior neck), delayed speech (the biggest fear relating to autism) and the twenty-first century phenomenon that is constipation.

In the **Clinical Bottom Line** section for each topic, we wish to highlight the key areas to look out for in family practice/primary care and what might be done prior to the child seeing a paediatrician.

Sleep Disorders in Infants and Children

Never underestimate the profound effects sleep disorders can have on children and their families. A child who is often unwilling to go to bed and who frequently wakes up at night will often be tired and irritable during the day. Understandably, this can be highly disruptive to a family. Overall, it is estimated that 20 to 30 per cent of children suffer from sleep disorders, which can affect both their general health and developmental progress. Sleep behaviour varies at different developmental stages. It can be challenging to find a universal definition of a sleep problem as tolerance of sleep behaviours varies between families.

NORMAL SLEEP-WAKE CYCLE

Sleep-wake cycles are governed by a complex group of biological processes. The suprachiasmatic nucleus in the hypothalamus is thought to be responsible for the release of melatonin on a 24-hour cycle in which less melatonin is secreted during exposure to bright light; this is the basis of circadian rhythms. Multiple neurotransmitters are thought to play a role in sleep.

Rapid eye movement (REM) sleep and non-REM (NREM) sleep alternate cyclically through the night. The sleep cycle in infants differs from the sleep cycle in adults. Infants below 6 months spend half of their sleep time in active REM sleep and spend much less time in deep NREM sleep. By 6 months of age, the infant sleep cycle is more similar to that of adults. The child spends the first third of the night mostly in NREM sleep and the last third mostly in REM sleep.

Nighttime sleep gradually becomes consolidated during the first few years of life and most children no longer require daytime napping by the age of 4 years.

COMMON BEHAVIOURAL SLEEP DISTURBANCES

Secondary sleep problems differ according to age group and are much more common than primary sleep disturbances. Waking at night is the most common problem in infants; although toddlers and pre-schoolers can also wake at night, resistance to going to bed is the most frequent sleep disturbance encountered in this age group.

EXCESSIVE NIGHT WAKING AND EARLY MORNING WAKING

By 6 weeks of age, a healthy, well-fed infant should sleep continuously for 5 to 6 hours. An infant waking up excessively during the night may be due to lack of a well-established routine.

DISORDERS OF INITIATING AND MAINTAINING SLEEP

Disorders of initiating and maintaining sleep are by far the most common complaints brought to the attention of a family doctor. The age of onset is generally between 2 and 4 years old with equal gender distribution. It is often very difficult for parents to set limits. Common scenarios include a child delaying bedtime by asking for an extra drink or another story or by searching for their favourite toy. They may have tantrums if their demands are not accommodated. These children become easily hyperexcited and trying to settle them down can be exhausting. Behavioural methods of treatment lead to successful management of these children and seldom require medications. While many parents are now seeking sleep consultants to treat disordered sleep, most children can be treated successfully by their family doctor so long as an effective routine is established.

Another common scenario is frequent nighttime wakening, which is typically intentional and interactional in nature. Management of this problem should also consider the whole family environment and not just the child.

ESTABLISHING A GOOD SLEEP ROUTINE

At bedtime, the child's bedroom should be dark, quiet and at an appropriate temperature. The established bedtime routine should be regularly reinforced.

All environmental stimuli (i.e. noises and light) should be minimised, and children should neither have a large meal before bedtime, nor should they go to bed hungry.

Children should avoid excessive fluid consumption prior to bedtime. Children should also avoid caffeine- and sugar-based drinks such as tea, soft drinks, and fruit juices.

PARASOMNIAS

Parasomnias are classified as disorders of sleep, sleep stages, and partial arousal from sleep. The symptoms appear early in childhood and gradually resolve. The exact aetiology is as yet unknown.

NIGHT TERRORS

A night terror is of sudden onset whereby the child sits up in bed and has intense, inconsolable crying. Although the eyes may be wide open, it is very difficult to wake the child. Signs of autonomic arousal such as tachycardia or tachypnoea during episodes are also seen. The child may even run wildly around the room and bump into furniture with unintelligible vocalisations and have no recollection of it the following morning. Over 30 per cent of toddlers will experience episodes of night terrors, which can last 1 to 10 minutes. Frontal lobe seizures are a differential diagnosis for night terrors but are quite rare.

Night terrors are more likely to occur during times of fatigue or stress. Onset usually occurs between 2 and 4 years of age, has a male predominance, and typically spontaneously resolves by adolescence. Polysomnography shows sudden arousal from slow-wave sleep. In addition to causing the child significant distress, night terrors can also be frightening experiences for parents. Management of night terrors involves waking the child up approximately 1 to 2 hours after going to sleep; this breaks the REM-NREM cycle and significantly reduces night terrors. Medication with diazepam is only necessary in rare circumstances in which both the child and family are highly distressed and is for short-term use only (1 to 2 weeks).

NIGHTMARES

Nightmares are characterised by a frightening dream followed by a period of wakefulness. The child is fully oriented and remembers the event. If the nightmares are recurring and tend to surround the same theme, establish whether there may be an explanation such as a traumatic episode (like a car crash) or a frightening film.

SLEEP WALKING

Sleep walking – or somnambulism – can vary dramatically in its presentation. Activity may range from purposeless automatic behaviours in bed to walking around the house. The child is generally very clumsy and may sustain injury. Verbalisation can also occur (termed somniloquy) with speech usually slurred and garbled. Eyes can be open, but the child cannot be wakened.

Sleepwalking occurs predominantly between the ages of 4 and 8 years and generally resolves by adolescence.

NARCOLEPSY

Narcolepsy is a lifelong neurological disorder of REM sleep in which the hypocretin/orexin axis in the hypothalamus is dysfunctional. It is characterised by sudden onset attacks of daytime sleepiness, sudden loss of muscle control in response to emotional stimuli (termed cataplexy), hypnagogic hallucinations and sleep paralysis.

Children with narcolepsy also suffer from fragmented sleep and find it very difficult to get up in the morning. Understandably, this condition can be highly disruptive for children. They have a characteristically abnormal polysomnogram and sleep latency test and require lifelong treatment and follow-up by a sleep specialist.

(Box 29.1)

Box 29.1 *Clinical Bottom Lines*

Sleep disorders are incredibly common, and the key intervention is to establish a good bedtime routine. Night terrors frequently occur in toddlers; current best advice is to momentarily wake the child up about 2 hours after falling asleep to alter the REM to non-REM sleep cycle.

Lymphadenopathy

Lymphadenopathy is a frequent cause for concern and thus a frequent reason for referral. Parents are often concerned about the possibility of malignancy, especially if the lymphadenopathy is immediately visible (e.g. in the neck region, or, classically, in the posterior triangle).

HISTORY

The sudden onset of unilateral inguinal adenopathy on the same side as a significant cut or graze over the knee suggests infection and is of no concern. On the other hand, progressive enlargement of lymph nodes over the course of weeks or months that is accompanied by systemic symptoms such as pallor, bruising, fever and abdominal distension with joint or bone pain suggest an acute leukaemia. Unexplained fevers, night sweats or weight loss may be presenting symptoms of lymphoma.

Neonatal lymphadenopathy is rare and typically indicates congenital infection such as rubella, syphilis, cytomegalovirus or toxoplasma.

Acute leukaemia is most prevalent in toddlers and young children. Non-Hodgkin's lymphoma tends to occur in school-aged children while Hodgkin's lymphoma is more frequent in adolescence.

Ask about diet (consider toxoplasmosis relating to contact with or consumption of raw or undercooked meat – particularly pork, lamb or venison), ingestion of unpasteurised milk (consequent possible exposure to *Brucella* species and *Mycobacterium bovis*), presence of household pets such as kittens (may cause scratches and transmit *Bartonella henselae* causing cat-scratch disease) or foreign travel (risk of tuberculosis).

Examination for Lymphadenopathy in the Head and Neck

Consider the size (over 1 cm is considered enlarged), texture and tenderness, and the overlying skin of the nodes.

SITES OF REGIONAL LYMPHADENOPATHY AND ASSOCIATED ILLNESSES

Worrying sites of lymphadenopathy include the supraclavicular and bilateral epitrochlear, which may indicate lymphoma. Hilar nodes (picked up on chest x-ray) may indicate sarcoidosis, tuberculosis or lymphoma. Drugs associated

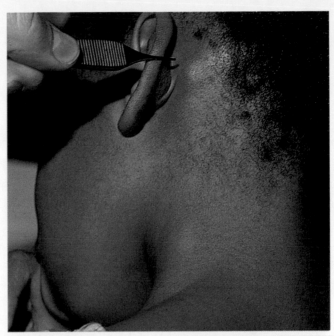

Figure 29.1   Acute postauricular lymphadenitis. This child had folliculotic and crusted scalp lesions and a tender 1.5-cm post-auricular node with overlying erythema. The initial suspicion of bacterial infection was not confirmed. A potassium hydroxide preparation and fungal culture identified tinea capitis as the primary process. (Reproduced with permission from Zitelli, B. J., McIntire, S. C., & Nowalk, A. J. (2017). *Zitelli and Davis' atlas of pediatric physical diagnosis* (7th ed.). Elsevier · Health Sciences Division.)

with generalised lymphadenopathy include allopurinol, captopril, atenolol, carbamazepine, penicillin and tetracyclines.

MANAGEMENT

Enlarged lymph nodes that do not recede after a number of weeks with appropriate antibiotic therapy and without explanation (such as EBV infection) should raise concerns about a potentially malignant cause, especially if systemic symptoms occur.

PATTERNS

Cervical lymphadenopathy is by far the most common pattern and presents with shotty, soft nodes in the anterior and posterior cervical chains due to viral illnesses such as adenovirus, parainfluenza, rhinovirus, influenza, herpes simplex and enteroviruses. This lymphadenopathy can take several weeks to settle and may recur with another viral illness.

Acute Cervical Lymphadenitis

Acute cervical lymphadenitis is due to inflammation of cervical lymph nodes with tender enlargement and is most often due to Group A streptococcus or *Staphylococcus aureus* infection. (Fig. 29.1).

Acute cervical lymphadenitis usually responds well to oral antibiotics, but suppuration and spontaneous drainage can occasionally occur. Acute suppurative lymphadenitis is an indication for ultrasound examination and may require operative incision and drainage (Fig. 29.2). Total excision of the affected gland should take place if atypical mycobacterial infection is suspected.

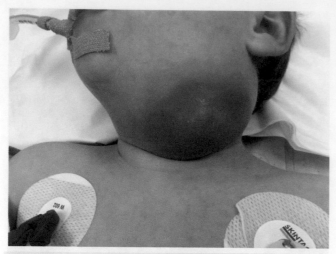

Figure 29.2 Acute cervical lymphadenitis with abscess formation in a child. All the classical signs of acute inflammation are present (i.e. rubor, calor, tumour and dolor). (Reproduced with permission from Cathcart, R. A. (2012). Inflammatory swellings of the head and neck. *Surgery, 30*(11), 597–603.)

Epstein-Barr Virus (EBV) Infection With Lymphadenopathy

Typical symptoms of EBV infection include prolonged pharyngitis with a sore throat, tender and firm cervical lymphadenopathy, malaise, fever, weight loss and anorexia. Splenomegaly is present in over 50 per cent of cases and many are accompanied by mild hepatitis with elevated transaminases. A small minority may have tonsillar lymphoid hyperplasia, which leads to dehydration and possible airway obstruction.

Cat Scratch Disease

This may present as a single enlarged node with no pus (typically in the axilla) several days after a scratch or bite from an infected cat (Figs 29.3 and 29.4).

Atypical Mycobacterial Infection

These infections include *Mycobacterium avium-intracellulare*, *Mycobacterium scrofulaceum*, and *Mycobacterium marinum*.

A typical presentation is an enlarged cervical node in a young child that does not decrease in size after a course of oral antibiotics. The node is often tender and may spontaneously rupture and drain pus. Other glands may be involved (Fig. 29.5).

A tuberculin skin test may be positive, showing 5 to 9 mm of induration. The node should be surgically removed if it drains or continues to enlarge.

Acute Leukaemia and Lymphoma

This is the great fear of parents who present their child with lymphadenopathy. Malignant nodes are usually firm, rubbery, fixed, non-tender, and may be matted together. Typical features include size above 2.5 cm, a steady increase in size over a short period and a supraclavicular location. Systemic symptoms, often non-specific, may be present.

(Box 29.2)

Box 29.2 *Clinical Bottom Lines*

Lymphadenopathy is of great concern to parents but is benign and self-limiting in most cases. If acute fever and cervical lymphadenopathy occur together, think of cervical lymphadenitis, and start oral antibiotics. Beware of firm, rubbery or fixed nodes above 2.5 cm and supraclavicular or epitrochlear nodes. These red flag symptoms require prompt referral to paediatrics to exclude a malignant aetiology.

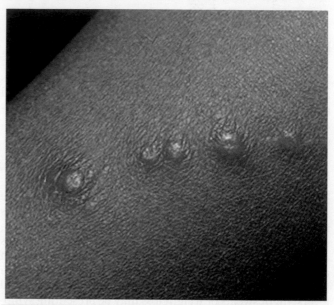

Figure 29.3 Cat scratch disease. A line of papules on the patient's forearm or at the site of a cat scratch. (Reproduced with permission from Fort, G. G. (2021). Cat-scratch disease. In F. F. Ferri (Ed.), *Ferri's clinical advisor 2021* (pp. 323–323). Elsevier.)

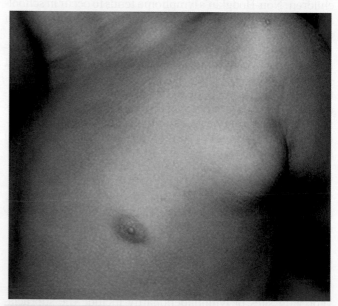

Figure 29.4 Cat scratch disease. Marked enlargement of axillary lymph node. (Reproduced with permission from Fort, G. G. (2021). Cat-scratch disease. In F. F. Ferri (Ed.), *Ferri's clinical advisor 2021* (pp. 323–323). Elsevier.)

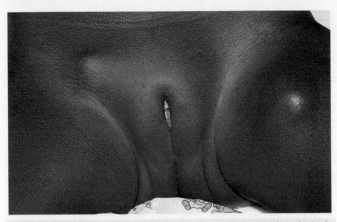

Figure 29.5 Subacute lymphadenitis of a right inguinal node and left femoral node resulted in dramatic swelling in this toddler. Atypical mycobacteria were found to be causative. (Reproduced with permission from Zitelli, B. J., McIntire, S. C., & Nowalk, A. J. (2017). *Zitelli and Davis' atlas of pediatric physical diagnosis* (7th ed.). Elsevier – Health Sciences Division.)

Delayed Speech and Autism

Speech and language issues occur in up to 20 per cent of young children and in some cases may be associated with subsequent learning issues. Although the prevalence of congenital deafness is 1 to 3 per 1000, the rate is much higher in infants who have been in neonatal intensive care (2 to 4 per cent). Universal hearing screening ensures rapid pick up, appropriate investigation and early management (hearing aids or cochlear implants). The goal is to ensure those diagnosed are able to attend mainstream school.

Speech problems may include pronunciation issues, fluency disorders (such as stuttering), or unusual voice quality.

ISOLATED SPEECH DELAY

Most common in boys, these children have difficulty making themselves and their needs understood by parents and other children despite normal intelligence and understanding of language. The outcome is generally excellent despite the emotional difficulties and frustrations these children may endure.

AUTISTIC SPECTRUM DISORDER

Autism spectrum disorders (ASDs) include autism, Asperger syndrome, and pervasive developmental disorder. Regression of skills may occur at between 15 and 24 months of age and can be either gradual or rapid in nature. Regression usually involves the loss of words, gestures and eye contact, and most children plateau in the regressed state rather than regress further. There is a strong preponderance of males (the ratio is 4.5:1) and genetic factors play a significant role.

Diagnostic Criteria for Autism

1. Persistent defects in social communication and social interaction with failure to initiate or respond to social interactions, lack of facial expression and nonverbal communication, and difficulties making friends and sharing imaginative play.

2. Restricted and repetitive patterns of behaviour, insistence on sameness, repetitive motor movements, highly restricted and fixated interests, and an unusual interest in sensory aspects of the environment (apparent pain indifference, excessive smelling and touching of objects and fascination with lights or movement).

3. Symptoms present in the early developmental period, causing significant impairment in social functioning that cannot be better explained by intellectual disability or global developmental delay.

Autism in Preschool Children

ASD usually presents with significant speech delay, and parents are sometimes reluctant to voice concerns about their child's social responsiveness. The Modified Checklist for Autism in Toddlers (MCHAT) is a helpful surveillance instrument, as is the Autism Diagnostic Observation Schedule (ADOS – G).

Autism in School-Age Children

Children in this age group have functional difficulties in the way they use language and may cause their speech to seem robotic. Comorbid conditions such as oppositional defiant disorder, aggressive outbursts and depression are often seen. Other features seen include persistent echolalia, inappropriate attempts at joint play, extreme reactions to any invasion of their personal space, a lack of awareness of classroom norms, a distinct lack of imaginary play activity and an inability to cope with unstructured situations such as school trips or any change to their routine.

Exotic Differential Diagnoses

Landau-Kleffner syndrome occurs in a previously typical child (peak onset 5 to 7 years old) presenting with language regression. There is auditory agnosia, a disappearance of speech, and the child may seem deaf due to impaired cortical processing of sound and language. A marked deterioration in behaviour also takes place. If any seizures occur, they are usually partial and respond well to anticonvulsants. Treatment with corticosteroids somewhat improves the condition, but many will have persisting language and learning issues. Thankfully, Landau-Kleffner syndrome is vanishingly rare.

Medications in ASD

Drugs such as methylphenidate are occasionally used for hyperactivity and melatonin is very useful in treating intractable sleep problems.

(Box 29.3)

Box 29.3 *Clinical Bottom Lines*

Isolated speech delay is especially common in multilingual households. Ensure that a hearing test is ordered and seek speech and language therapy assessment in the community. Parents often fear a diagnosis of autism spectrum disorder, in which poor social interaction and restricted or repetitive patterns of behaviour are also seen in addition to delayed speech. ADOS and MCHAT are useful surveillance tools for autism. Diagnosis of autism requires a full multidisciplinary assessment. Melatonin is very helpful for associated severe sleep issues.

Childhood Constipation

Constipation is very common in both preschool and school-aged children, affecting 5 per cent (over 6 months of symptoms) and 30 per cent (less than 6 months of symptoms) in the UK. The normal range for stool frequency in children is one bowel motion on alternate days to three bowel motions per day.

Diagnostic criteria for functional constipation in children (Rome 3 criteria) must include **at least two** of the following – two or less bowel motions per week, at least one episode of faecal incontinence, painful hard bowel motions, a large faecal mass in the rectum or passage of large stools that may obstruct the toilet.

Most longstanding constipation is secondary to a sedentary lifestyle and inadequate dietary fibre or fluid intake daily. Children with autism spectrum disorder and other neurodevelopmental disorders associated with reduced mobility are at increased risk of developing constipation.

PHYSIOLOGY OF NORMAL DEFAECATION

The trigger for sensing the need to go to the toilet is when the stool reaches the rectum causing it to distend and the internal and external sphincters to relax. The child can then wait to hold onto the stool until they can use the toilet because these sphincters and the pelvic floor puborectalis muscle are under the child's voluntary control. Once these relax, the child can pass stool.

The child can retain stool by not relaxing the external anal sphincter when the internal sphincter is relaxed. If this occurs over a long period, the child cannot keep the external anal sphincter fully contracted and stools leak out of the anal canal. This is how overflow incontinence occurs in chronic constipation.

Anorectal manometry studies have increased our understanding of the pathophysiology of constipation. The most common finding is that the child cannot properly sense a faecal mass in the rectum. Other findings include incomplete relaxation of the internal anal sphincter and paradoxical contraction of the external anal sphincter during attempted defaecation.

KEY POINTS IN THE HISTORY AND EXAMINATION

Most children experience infrequent bowel motions, painful defaecation, retentive posturing or soiling as their presenting symptoms. They may also have urinary incontinence. The Bristol Stool Form chart is helpful in determining the pattern of defaecation.

The age of onset, stool consistency and the presence of associated symptoms help to differentiate functional constipation from secondary causes of constipation. An abnormal growth pattern should always raise concerns about a secondary cause such as hypothyroidism or coeliac disease.

A normal anal wink and cremasteric reflex in males gives reassurance in relation to intact lumbosacral innervation. The perianal area should be inspected for anal tears or fissures. Digital examination of the rectum is generally not recommended beyond infancy in the assessment of constipation.

INVESTIGATIONS

An MRI of the spine is indicated if there are concerns about spinal dysraphism or a tethered cord. Anorectal manometry is occasionally performed to evaluate the integrity of the process of defaecation but is still largely a research tool. Anorectal manometry does have a role as a therapeutic modality in biofeedback therapy for those with chronic indolent constipation and overflow soiling.

DIFFERENTIAL DIAGNOSES

The majority of children will transpire to have functional constipation. The normal passage of meconium after birth and the absence of symptoms before 1 month of age effectively excludes Hirschsprung's disease. Features of Hirschsprung's disease (a rare condition affecting one in 5000 births) include a distended abdomen, failure to thrive and explosive stools on digital rectal examination. Once in a career as a busy general paediatrician, you might be faced with a case of ultra-short segment Hirschsprung's disease masquerading as functional constipation. The definitive diagnosis of Hirschsprung's disease requires a rectal biopsy to confirm the absence of ganglion cells in both Auerbach and Meissner plexuses.

Constipation is a conspicuous feature of anal stenosis, imperforate anus and an open meningomyelocoele, all of which will be obvious in the neonatal period. Medications such as anticonvulsants, opiates, iron preparations and antacids can all be associated with constipation.

TREATMENT OF CONSTIPATION

Constipation can be managed in a primary care setting in the great majority of cases and indeed is a very satisfying condition to treat.

The aims of treatment are to establish normal frequency and consistency of stools, to enable the stools to be passed painlessly and completely, and to resolve rectal bleeding or overflow incontinence. Family education and use of a bowel habit diary are essential.

Polyethylene glycol (PEG 3350) acts by increasing the water content in the large bowel. Stimulant laxatives (such as senna) increase bowel motility whereas rectal suppositories and enemas exert their influence by local stimulation.

DISIMPACTION

Effective disimpaction is a prerequisite for successful maintenance treatment. PEG 3350 is recommended as first-line treatment in an escalating dose regimen for faecal impaction in all age groups. A stimulant laxative (senna, bisacodyl or sodium picosulfate) should be added after 2 weeks if disimpaction is not achieved with PEG 3350. Hospital admission and the use of enemas are now rarely needed for disimpaction thanks to the above medical therapies.

MAINTENANCE

Start and continue maintenance treatment immediately after disimpaction. The dose should be titrated to ideally produce a daily soft stool. It is important to achieve complete rectal evacuation every day or every other day without straining.

After sustained improvement for at least 3 months, gradually reduce the dose of stool softeners over a period of months to maintain stool frequency and consistency and complete rectal evacuation. A major error in management may occur if the treatment is stopped too quickly (usually because of parental concern) and the child relapses. It is useful to pre-empt the anticipated treatment course length at the outset of treatment so that parents are aware that treatment takes time and patience. A period of approximately 6 months is not unusual.

A significant number of trials of treatment in chronic constipation have shown no significant benefits of increased fluid intake, exercise, prebiotics and probiotics, behavioural therapy or other forms of alternative medicine.

(Box 29.4)
(Box 29.5)
(Box 29.6)
(Box 29.7)
(Box 29.8)
(Box 29.9)

Box 29.4 *Clinical Bottom Lines*

Functional constipation is incredibly common and should be managed in family practice/primary care. Be wary of a history of constipation from birth, failure to thrive or abdominal distension. PEG 3350 is the best treatment for both disimpaction and maintenance but must be continued for a lengthy period. Managing constipation is always a marathon and never a sprint! There are useful resources for families provided by eric.org.uk, including stories and cartoon visuals to help children understand what is often a distressing journey. These are particularly useful to support little ones who are retaining stool, encouraging them to relax and overcome the fear to pass stool again.

Box 29.5 **Key Points**

Twenty to 30 per cent of children suffer from sleep disorders, which may affect both their general health and developmental progress.

Disorders of initiating and maintaining sleep are by far the most common sleep complaints brought to the attention of the family doctor.

The most effective way of tackling behavioural sleep disorders is by starting with a correct sleep routine. Ideally, children should learn to fall asleep alone and should sleep in their own bed at all times. Daytime naps should be appropriate for the child's age.

A night terror occurs suddenly, causing the child to sit up in bed with intense, inconsolable crying. They have no recollection of it the following morning. Over 30 per cent of toddlers will experience a night terror.

Nightmares occur during REM sleep and can occur at any age. They are characterised by a frightening dream followed by a period of wakefulness. The child is fully orientated and remembers the event.

Narcolepsy requires lifelong treatment and is characterised by sudden onset attacks of daytime sleepiness, sudden loss of muscle control in response to emotional stimuli (cataplexy), hypnagogic hallucinations and sleep paralysis.

Melatonin is effective for children with autism spectrum disorder (ASD) who suffer with significant sleep issues.

The majority of lymphadenopathy is benign and self-limiting, and confident reassurance is often all that is required. On the other hand, progressive enlargement of lymph nodes over the course of weeks or months accompanied by systemic symptoms weight loss, fevers or night sweats suggests an illness such as lymphoma.

Consider the size (over 1 cm is considered enlarged), texture and tenderness and overlying skin of the nodes. Cervical lymphadenitis should be considered in a child with a fever and a red, tender, warm cervical lymph gland. Oral antibiotics should be started. Lack of improvement warrants an ultrasound scan and consideration should be given to starting intravenous antibiotics.

If non-tender, not red, and soft, consider a viral infection. If firm, hard, rubbery and non-tender, consider malignancy.

Language delay may be receptive or expressive or a combination of both. A formal audiometric assessment and an assessment by a speech and language therapist are required to further assess delayed language.

Autism spectrum disorder (ASD) includes autism, Asperger syndrome and pervasive developmental disorder. Children with ASD have impairment in reciprocal social communication and interaction, circumscribed interests, impairment of imaginary thought and repetitive patterns of behaviour that impede daily functioning.

In ASD, there is a strong preponderance of males (the ratio is 4.5:1) and genetic factors play a significant role. Autism is more common in Down syndrome, tuberous sclerosis, Fragile X and Rett and Angelman syndromes.

Key issues in managing ASD are the use of cognitive behaviour therapy for anxiety, psychoeducational interventions such as applied behavioural analysis (ABA), and therapies focused on communication delivered to small groups of 5 to 6 children.

Constipation is very common and the majority of cases are successfully managed in primary care.

Most have functional constipation and investigations to out rule rare secondary causes are not recommended unless 'red flag' symptoms present, such as delayed meconium passage, failure to thrive or constipation dating from birth.

PEG 3350 is the mainstay of treatment, but prolonged therapy with the dose titrated to stool consistency and frequency may be required. It is a marathon and not a sprint. Stool softeners such as PEG 3350 are perfectly safe for long-term use.

Chronic constipation is debilitating and has a massive impact on both the child and their family, making effective early management both rewarding and important. Few require specialist referral.

Box 29.6   A Toddler Who Just Will Not Sleep

A 2-year-old boy presents to his family doctor with two very distressed parents as he struggles to settle at night and wakes up frequently. He has no relevant past illnesses and is a thriving, well-grown child who has reached all developmental milestones. His examination is quite normal. His parents are quite exhausted and desperate for helpful advice.

Clinical Pearls

The most prevalent sleep problems in toddlers are difficulty falling asleep, difficulty staying asleep, rocking and head-banging, night terrors and nightmares.

The most effective way of tackling behavioural sleep disorders is by starting with a correct sleep routine. Children should learn to fall asleep alone and should sleep in their own bed at all times. Daytime naps should be appropriate for the child's age.

Night terrors occur approximately 90 minutes into sleep during stage 3 or 4 of NREM sleep. Night terrors are usually self-limiting.

Nightmares occur during REM sleep and can occur at any age. They happen in the last third of the night and are remembered in detail by the child.

Rocking and head-banging are more common in boys and are outgrown by 4 to 5 years of age; reassurance is all that is required.

Children with narcolepsy also suffer from fragmented sleep and find it very difficult to get up in the morning.

Interpretation of Investigations

Children with narcolepsy have a characteristic abnormal polysomnogram and multiple sleep latency test and a Cerebrospinal fluid (CSF) hypocretin level under 110 pg/mL.

Frontal lobe seizures may mimic night terrors and are diagnosed on video EEG.

Polysomnography is the gold standard investigation for sleep-disordered breathing.

Pitfalls to Avoid

Always be aware of obstructive sleep apnoea, which affects 3 per cent of children and may be suspected in the presence of nocturnal snoring, poor weight gain, and witnessed episodes of brief apnoea or laboured breathing during sleep.

Children with ADHD or autism spectrum disorder often have great difficulty with either sleep initiation or maintenance and melatonin tends to be an effective treatment.

Sanfilippo syndrome is a very rare condition where symptoms tend to become evident after 2 years of age. Very significant sleep issues and behavioural problems dominate, and the diagnosis is confirmed by elevated urinary glycosylaminoglycans (GAGs).

Box 29.7   Persistent Lymphadenopathy in a Young Child

A 4-year-old girl presents with a history of persistent lymphadenopathy over the past 3 months. She is well-grown, developmentally appropriate, and has no recent history of fevers or systemic upset. Her examination is unremarkable apart from four shotty lymph nodes (each under 1 cm in diameter) located in the posterior triangle of the neck. Her parents are very anxious and concerned about the possibility of malignancy.

Clinical Pearls

Most childhood lymphadenopathy is benign and self-limiting; confident reassurance is all that is required.

Lymphadenopathy that develops rapidly over the course of a few days is more likely to be an infectious process whereas a more indolent presentation may suggest malignant disease.

Toddlers and young children with lymphadenopathy tend to have focal infections that drain into the affected nodal chain or viral illnesses with generalised lymphadenopathy.

If the lymph glands are red, tender, and warm, consider acute bacterial lymphadenitis. If non-tender, not red, and soft, consider a viral infection. If firm, hard, rubbery, and non-tender, consider lymphoma or leukaemia.

Interpretation of Investigations

Acute cervical lymphadenopathy associated with a sore throat in a toddler under 18 months may relate to infection with Group A streptococcus diagnosed by throat swab.

In older children, cervical lymphadenopathy with associated hepatomegaly or splenomegaly should make one consider Epstein-Barr infection (EBV) and prompt a full blood count and EBV titres as investigations.

If cervical lymphadenitis is suspected and oral antibiotics cause no improvement, an ultrasound scan is warranted, and consideration should be given to starting intravenous antibiotics and drainage.

Pitfalls to Avoid

The presence of palpable supraclavicular nodes or bilateral epitrochlear nodes are seen as a red flag for serious illness, including malignancy.

The presentation of atypical mycobacterial infection is with a tender, matted, unilateral enlarged cervical lymph node that may spontaneously rupture and drain. The gold standard diagnostic test is acid-fast staining and culture of the excised node and a positive tuberculin skin test. Excision of the node is advised if the node fails to respond, continues to enlarge or drains spontaneously. This usually solves the problem.

Malignant nodes are usually firm, rubbery, fixed and non-tender, and may be matted. Malignant nodes gradually increase in size. Additional signs suggestive of malignancy are age over 10 years, size over 2.5 cm, glands present for over 6 weeks, and an enlarging and supraclavicular location.

Box 29.8 A 2-Year-Old With Little or No Speech

A male infant is born by lower (uterine) segment Caesarean section (LSCS) at term and weighs 3.5 kg at birth. He has no perinatal issues and has normal developmental milestones apart from speech delay. At 18 months of age, he has not yet started speaking. He lives in a bilingual household and there is no family history of speech delay. His full examination is normal, as is his formal audiometric assessment. His parents are very concerned about the possibility of autism spectrum disorder (ASD).

Clinical Pearls

Speech delay may be due to global developmental delay, hearing impairment, autism spectrum disorder, selective mutism or an isolated disorder of language.

Speech delay may be either receptive or expressive or a combination of both. A formal audiometric assessment and an assessment by a speech and language therapist are required to further assess delayed language.

The majority have isolated speech delay with normal comprehension of language and normal cognitive abilities with an excellent prognosis.

Hearing loss may be acquired in early life (meningitis, significant head trauma or ototoxic drugs) and may also relate to a host of syndromes (including Waardenburg, Alport, Pendred and Lange-Nielsen) with late-onset deafness in neurofibromatosis type 1 and Usher and Hunter syndromes.

Children with autism spectrum disorder (ASD) have impairment in reciprocal social communication and interaction, circumscribed interests, impairment of imaginary thought, and repetitive patterns of behaviour that impair daily functioning.

ASD is relatively common (about one in 100 children).

General warning signs of ASD include a delay or absence of spoken language, not being aware of others, little or no imaginary play, being unresponsive to feelings in others, no purposeful play with peers, inability to share pleasure or to take turn in activities, inability to point at an object, unusual or repetitive hand and finger mannerisms, and heightened reactions to sensory stimuli such as noise or bright lights.

Key issues in managing ASD are the use of cognitive behaviour therapy for anxiety, psychoeducational interventions such as applied behavioural analysis (ABA), and communication-focused therapies delivered to small groups of five to six children.

Interpretation of Investigations

MRI, EEG and metabolic investigations are generally not recommended. Karyotyping via microarray and Fragile X testing are recommended although yield is very low. Whole genome sequencing may be the tool of choice in future investigations of ASD.

Pitfalls to Avoid

Always assess hearing in a child with significant speech delay.

Autism is more common in Down syndrome, tuberous sclerosis, Fragile X and Rett and Angelman syndromes.

Landau-Kleffner syndrome is vanishingly rare and presents in an older child (peak onset 5 to 7 years old) with language regression. Seizures do occur and the EEG in non-REM sleep characteristically shows almost continuous bilateral epileptiform discharges over the temporal lobes of the brain.

Box 29.9 A Toddler With Infrequent Painful Bowel Motions

A 2.5-year-old girl is being toilet trained and has a short gastroenteritis illness lasting 3 days. After recovering from this, she starts to voluntarily withhold stool and has a stool frequency of just one bowel motion every 3 or 4 days. She has experienced great distress on attempted defaecation and one episode of bright red blood. Her past history is unremarkable. She did pass meconium on day 1 of life. She is thriving and developmentally appropriate for her age. Her examination is unremarkable apart from palpable stool in the left side of the abdomen. Inspection of the anal region reveals a small tear.

Clinical Pearls

Constipation is defined as the infrequent passage of hard stools, straining while passing a stool or pain associated with passage of a hard stool.

Well over 90 per cent of constipation seen in childhood is functional and may follow a change in diet, an intercurrent illness, problems with toilet training and major life events.

Encourage children to visit the toilet after each meal for 5 minutes to attempt defaecation. If necessary, they may be supported by a footrest to allow for active straining.

Polyethylene glycol (PEG 3350) is the recommended first-line treatment that promotes disimpaction, improves stool frequency,

reduces pain on defaecation and has fewer side effects than lactulose.

If PEG 3350 is ineffective even in optimal dosage, try combining it with a stimulant laxative such as bisacodyl or sodium picosulfate.

Anal fissures are very troublesome but have a high spontaneous resolution rate with medical treatment. As a result, interventions such as anal stretch, lateral anal sphincterotomy, or injection of botulinum toxin into the sphincters are rarely – if ever – indicated.

Interpretation of Investigations

Routine laboratory evaluation and plain abdominal x-rays are generally not helpful, and investigations are only warranted if there are significant concerns that the constipation is not functional.

Pitfalls to Avoid

Failure to pass meconium within 48 hours of birth suggest Hirschsprung's disease. Other features suggestive of this diagnosis are severe abdominal distension, protracted symptoms dating from birth, a family history, failure to thrive, explosive expulsion of stool after digital examination of the rectum, and narrow ribbon stools.

The spinal and sacral area should be carefully examined for a tuft of hair. A deep dimple or mass in the area should prompt consideration of tethering of the spinal cord.

Key References

Auth, M. K., Vora, R., Farrelly, P., & Baillie, C. (2012). Childhood constipation. *BMJ, 345*, e7309.

Blenner, S., Reddy, A., & Augustyn, M. (2011). Diagnosis and management of autism in childhood. *BMJ (Clinical Research Editon), 343*, d6238.

Bordini, B. J. (2018). Lymphadenopathy and neck masses. In R. M. Kliegman, P. S. Lye, B. Bordini, H. Toth, & D. Basel (Eds.), *Nelson pediatric symptom-based diagnosis* (pp. 647–660). Elsevier.

Friedmann, A. M. (2008). Evaluation and management of lymphadenopathy in children. *Pediatrics in Review, 29*(2), 53–60. https://doi.org/10.1542/pir.29.2.53.

National Institute for Health and Care Excellence. (2010, May 26). Constipation in children and young people: diagnosis and management (NICE guideline cg99). https://www.nice.org.uk/guidance/cg99.

Noe, J. (2018). Constipation. In R. M. Kliegman, P. S. Lye, B. Bordini, H. Toth, & D. Basel (Eds.), *Nelson pediatric symptom-based diagnosis* (pp. 275–282). Elsevier.

O'Donnell, L. J., Virjee, J., & Heaton, K. W. (1990). Detection of pseudo-diarrhoea by simple clinical assessment of intestinal transit rate. *BMJ, 300*(6722), 439–444.

O'Hare, A. (2009). Autism spectrum disorder: Diagnosis and management. *Archives of Disease in Childhood Education and Practice Edition, 94*(6), 161–168.

O'Hare, A., & Bremner, L. (2016). Management of developmental speech and language disorders: Part 1. *Archives of Disease in Childhood, 101*(3), 272–277.

Rosen, D. (2020, September 2). Dyssomnias in children. *BMJ Best Practice.* https://bestpractice.bmj.com/topics/en-gb/781.

Scottish Intercollegiate Guidelines Network. (2016, June). *Assessment, diagnosis and interventions for autism spectrum disorders.* SIGN Publication no. 145. https://www.sign.ac.uk/assets/sign145.pdf.

Simms M. Intellectual and developmental disability. In R. M. Kliegman, P. S. Lye, B. Bordini, H. Toth, & D. Basel (Eds.), *Nelson pediatric symptom-based diagnosis* (pp. 367–392). Elsevier.

The Children's Bowel and Bladder Charity. (n.d.). ERIC. https://www.eric.org.uk/

30 Issues in School-Going Children

ALF NICHOLSON and KEVIN DUNNE

I have never let my schooling interfere with my education
MARK TWAIN, 1907

School's critical role in a child's learning and social development was never more evident than during the period of extended school closures due to the COVID-19 pandemic.

Issues arising during the school-going years include those that interfere with learning, such as attention deficit hyperactivity disorder, developmental coordination disorder, motor tics and the dreaded head lice. Likewise, bed-wetting and obstructive sleep apnoea are evident at night rather than during the school day, but nonetheless interfere with a child's development. All will be explored in this chapter.

In the **Clinical Bottom Line** section for each topic, we wish to highlight the key areas concerning what might be done in family practice/primary care prior to the child seeing a paediatrician.

Attention Deficit Hyperactivity Disorder (ADHD)

ADHD is a neurodevelopmental condition in which affected children (and adults) have problems with attention, impulsivity and hyperactivity.

To make this diagnosis requires the presence of at least six out of nine behavioural features. A diagnosis also requires that these features have been present for at least 6 months with an onset before 7 years of age. They are present in more than one setting and cause significant distress or impairment. The prevalence of ADHD is between 3 and 5 per cent.

INATTENTION FEATURES

These features may include failure to listen to direct conversations, difficulty in maintaining attention, easy distractibility, forgetfulness, a habit of losing possessions, and a lack of organisation.

HYPERACTIVITY AND IMPULSIVITY

Features include being always 'on the go' or always active while seeming unable to rest or stay quiet. This constant movement, walking, running and climbing makes it difficult for caregivers to keep up with them and keep them safe. Affected children tend to find it extremely difficult to wait their turn and may interrupt and talk constantly.

Constant activity may result in poor attention and an inability to finish tasks, which can lead to a perception of laziness or lack of motivation.

The hyperactivity may lessen somewhat over time but may still be an issue in situations where quiet behaviour is expected, such as in the classroom. This often leads to lack of academic progress, particularly in adolescence.

Emotional impulsivity and difficulty controlling emotions may appear in school-aged children as explosive behaviour that also impacts academic progress and causes difficulties with fellow pupils.

Risk-taking behaviour in children (e.g. running out in front of a car) and adolescents (e.g. substance abuse and high-risk sexual activity) pose significant risks to both age groups.

The doctor should not rely on observations made in the clinic, but rather on reports from parents and teachers in particular. There are many differential diagnoses to consider including learning disorders, oppositional defiant behaviour, conduct disorder, anxiety and mood disorders.

TREATMENT OF ADHD

Behavioural parent training helps parents understand their child's troublesome behaviour and make it easier for them to cope.

Stimulant medication can be short-acting or long-acting with the latter favoured as it lasts throughout the day. The most used stimulant medications are methylphenidate and atomoxetine.

Behaviour therapy is recommended for preschool children with ADHD, and school-aged children should receive stimulant medication to dampen down the core symptoms. (Box 30.1)

Box 30.1 *Clinical Bottom Line*

ADHD is very common (one child in every school class) and has many comorbidities. Symptoms of hyperactivity, impulsivity and inattention should be witnessed in more than one setting. Do not rely on behaviour in the practice surgery to determine if ADHD is present. Behaviour therapy is recommended for preschool children with ADHD. Stimulants should only be prescribed by specialists but are very effective in dampening down core symptoms in school-going children.

Developmental Coordination Disorder (DCD)

Developmental coordination disorder is important to identify and treat as it is now recognised as a common condition affecting 5 to 6 per cent of children.

Children presenting with DCD have characteristic features of clumsiness and poor coordination.

They can have issues in everyday self-care such as dressing and tying shoelaces. They often experience difficulties in school such as poor handwriting and may be slower than usual when completing academic assignments or assessments, especially if the task requires motor skills. They often have little interest in sports due to difficulty involving kicking, throwing or catching a ball, and tend to look awkward in the playground or sports field.

Early gross motor milestones in DCD are characteristically within normal limits, but there is a delay in the acquiring new motor skills.

Therefore, DCD is an impairment in motor coordination that significantly interferes with the activities of daily living, leisure, play and academic achievements. A formal occupational therapy assessment is required. The role of this specialist (paediatrician or paediatric neurologist) is to exclude other causes and confirm the diagnosis. DCD may occur in isolation or in association with learning issues or ADHD.

DIAGNOSTIC CRITERIA FOR DCD

These criteria include learning and executing coordinated motor skills below the expected level for the age of the child. The onset is in the early developmental period and the motor skill difficulties are not better explained by cognitive delay, visual impairment or other neurological conditions affecting movement.

Key therapies following diagnosis include regular occupational therapy and school supports (such as use of a laptop for schoolwork) with additional time allowed for examinations. Interventions to boost confidence are essential as self-confidence is a fundamental issue. (Box 30.2)

Box 30.2 *Clinical Bottom Line*

Key features of DCD are poor coordination, poor handwriting and being slow to complete academic tasks. Arrange a formal occupational therapy assessment to make the diagnosis of DCD. Specialist opinion can rule out other causes. Ensure vision testing has taken place. Children with DCD will require support at school such as access to a laptop and additional time for examinations.

Tics

The peak age of tic presentation is 5 to 7 years. Tics are quite common and are described as brief, purposeless, involuntary movements or vocalisations that only occur while awake.

The child with a tic disorder feels the need to perform the tic and a sense of relief when it is over, but their awareness is not altered. Motor tics are simple, sudden, brief movements such as facial grimaces, blinking an eye or shrugging the shoulders. Simple phonic tics include sniffing, making snorting noises, clicking the tongue or clearing the throat. Short utterances, echolalia or coprolalia are complex phonic tics.

Tics are normally benign and do not usually require drug therapy. Disruptive or disabling tics can be treated with clonidine. Common comorbidities associated with tics include ADHD, anxiety and obsessive-compulsive disorder.

Tourette syndrome is diagnosed when a child has a history of multiple motor tics and at least one phonic tic (simple or complex) present for over 12 months. Complex vocal tics in Tourette syndrome include barking and uttering strings of words.

Obstructive Sleep Apnoea (OSA)

OSA may be associated with behavioural problems, failure to thrive, excessive daytime sleepiness and pulmonary

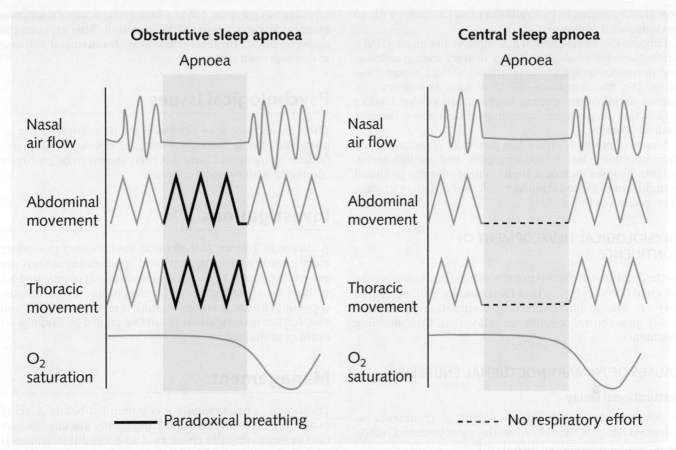

Figure 30.1 Example of polysomnograph results showing the two types of sleep apnoea. Sleep apnoea can be detected by reduced air flow and a delayed desaturation following the apnoea. Normally, the thorax and abdomen move in the same direction; however, the move in opposite directions of each other in obstructive sleep apnoea. This is an abnormal pattern called paradoxical breathing. Conversely, there is neither thoracic nor abdominal movement in central sleep apnoea because the respiratory centre in the brain has stopped instructing the respiratory muscles to move. (Reproduced with permission from Hickin, S. (2013). *Crash course respiratory system* (4th ed.). Mosby.)

hypertension. Behavioural changes such as a depressed mood, emotional outbursts and hyperactivity can all significantly improve following OSA treatment.

SYMPTOMS

Snoring is relatively prevalent in childhood (at least 12 per cent of children snore during sleep), but OSA is characterised by snoring with intermittent episodes of partial or complete upper airway obstruction.

ASSESSMENT

Overnight polysomnography can distinguish between obstructive, central or mixed apnoeic episodes (Fig. 30.1).

SCREENING FOR OSA IN HIGH-RISK GROUPS

In Down syndrome, screen via overnight oximetry annually until 5 years of age. In neuromuscular disease, perform oximetry on all with sleep-related breathing disorders, impaired diaphragm function or a significantly reduced vital capacity.

(Box 30.3)

Box 30.3 *Clinical Bottom Line*

Obstructive sleep apnoea affects one in 30 children with both snoring and upper airway obstruction as key features. Symptoms may include poor weight gain, early morning headaches, or behavioural issues. Smartphone nighttime recordings during deep sleep may be helpful. Some high-risk groups, such as those with Down syndrome, require regular screening. Tonsillectomy and adenoidectomy may be curative.

Nocturnal Enuresis

Nocturnal enuresis (NE) is defined as involuntary voiding of urine occurring at night at an age when the majority of children have achieved continence. Primary enuresis means the child has never been dry, whereas secondary enuresis means the child was previously dry and now has nocturnal wetting or enuresis. Primary enuresis affects approximately 25 per cent of children at age 4 and only 5 to 10 per cent at age seven. By age 10, only 5 per cent will still wet the bed, and the rate of spontaneous resolution is approximately 15 per cent per year throughout the teenage years. It affects boys more than girls and the prevalence appears to be similar in most countries with no obvious racial differences.

Enuresis can be categorised into monosymptomatic (MNE), where there are no daytime lower urinary tract symptoms, and non-monosymptomatic enuresis (NMNE), where these occur. Daytime symptoms of NMNE such as urgency, frequency and daytime wetting imply an underlying bladder dysfunction (organic or functional) and a more complex medical problem.

Monosymptomatic enuresis is generally considered more straightforward but is still complex and multifactorial. Potential causes include a high volume of urine produced at night, small maximal bladder volumes or failing to wake in response to a full bladder.

PHYSIOLOGICAL DEVELOPMENT OF CONTINENCE

As the child grows, there is progressive maturation whereby the child becomes aware that their bladder is filling up and they are able to ignore detrusor contraction signals and finally gain control of sphincter relaxation, thus attaining continence.

CAUSES OF PRIMARY NOCTURNAL ENURESIS

Maturational Delay

A delay in the natural development of continence as described above is thought to be the most common reason for persistent primary nocturnal enuresis.

REDUCED BLADDER CAPACITY

Some children have constitutionally small bladders and thus may end up with a full bladder towards the end of the night, causing the need to void.

Inability to Wake During Sleep in Response to Need to Void

This is a fundamental problem for all children with NE and is believed to be due to a disorder of brainstem arousal that allows us to wake in response to stimuli judged to be of importance.

GENETICS

It is well known that NE is a strongly inherited trait. When one parent has a history of enuresis, the risk in progeny is 44 per cent; this rises to 77 per cent when both parents have a history of NE. There is also a two-fold increase in incidence in monozygotic twins compared with their dizygotic counterparts. There have been a number of gene loci linked with enuresis, including chromosomes 13q, 12q, 5 and 22q11. Unfortunately, this knowledge has not yet led to any new treatments.

Nocturnal Polyuria

Urine production normally falls at night to about 50 per cent of daytime levels. However, in children with NE, there is nocturnal polyuria due to a lack of the normal nocturnal increase in vasopressin (ADH) secretion. This explains the response of two-thirds of children with nocturnal polyuria to desmopressin treatment.

Psychological Issues

These issues have been blamed in the past, but they are far more likely to be associated with the development of secondary enuresis and have not been shown to be positively correlated with primary enuresis.

Investigations

A thorough history and physical examination (including blood pressure measurement and spine examination) are generally enough to elicit a diagnosis of uncomplicated NE without need for extensive investigations. Urine microscopy and culture is an appropriate screening tool. Beyond this, further investigations should be guided by findings on exam or in the history.

Management

Treatment is not typically recommended before 8 years of age. A well-motivated child and family are very important in increasing the chances of a successful outcome. It is vital that the child and family understand that treatment is by no means an exact science and will require lengthy input from all members for a tangible chance at success. Management can be broadly divided into preliminary, non-pharmacological and pharmacological categories.

Preliminary Approach

THE FAMILY

Some children experience significant negative feedback in response to their condition, which may include punishment for accidents. It is crucial to challenge this approach with the family as a whole by explaining the nature of the condition and the impact that such a negative approach can have on the child's self-esteem and on the problem itself. Emphasis must be placed on praise and positive feedback for dry nights and adopting a no-blame approach when accidents do occur. An explanation of the condition should be given to the family and child along with reassurance that the vast majority of cases will resolve in time.

MOTIVATION

The use of a 'star chart' or some form of visual response to a dry night is the method most commonly used. Although there were some early favourable results in studies using this method, no high-quality trial has shown conclusive efficacy using this approach. However, these techniques do serve to highlight the problem to the child and help parents commit to a positive reinforcement approach.

ORAL INTAKE

Children should be encouraged to drink freely during the day with a reduction in fluid intake in the evening, but not so much that the child feels thirsty or punished. Caffeine should be avoided after dinner.

VOIDING

There should be an emphasis on regularly voiding the bladder throughout the day while avoiding overfilling and withholding of urine. Children should void upon waking and regularly throughout the day thereafter. In the evening, they should void after dinner and before bed.

Non-Pharmacological

There is a great deal of research regarding the use of lifting and alarms for the treatment of enuresis; however, it can be confusing and quite contradictory.

LIFTING

This is the process whereby a child is routinely lifted out of bed and brought to the bathroom to void during the night. The idea is that the child will eventually learn to wake themselves and use the bathroom, thus avoiding accidents. The method has been in use for many years. However, there have been no conclusive trials showing supportive results, and its use is fraught with compliance issues from both parents and children alike. While lifting and use of trainers are a pragmatic approaches by parents, they should be discouraged as they do not help the child keep dry because the child is voiding when they have no sensation of the need to void. Trainers reduce the feeling of wetness and are also tend to reduce motivation in the child to improve.

ENURESIS ALARMS

The use of a conditioned treatment with stimulation by alarm after voiding is seen to be a useful method in the management of enuresis. The goal is that the child learns to either finish voiding in the bathroom or to inhibit the voiding reflex through repetitive disturbance by an alarm, which is set to recognise moisture. This technique requires a very well-motivated child and family, as significant disturbance to sleep can be expected initially. In general, the child becomes conditioned to respond more quickly to the alarm, thereby decreasing the frequency of enuresis episodes. An alarm may be used from 8 years of age and upwards. Failure of treatment due to non-compliance has been shown in about 30 per cent of cases. Treatment with an alarm requires nightly commitment and a stable 12- to 16-week period.

Pharmacological Management

DESMOPRESSIN

Desmopressin or DDAVP is a synthetic antidiuretic hormone (ADH) analogue used to artificially induce a

reduction in urine output during the night. ADH is usually released from the posterior pituitary in a circadian pattern, which causes a reduction in urine output overnight by conserving water and concentrating the urine. In young children, this system is immature and prior studies have shown reduced nocturnal levels of ADH in children with enuresis versus normal controls.

Nocturnal polyuria can be treated using desmopressin to reduce the amount of urine throughout the night.

Desmopressin, therefore, does provide effective treatment for the majority of children, with many studies reporting up to 50 per cent cure rates and a 70 per cent improvement in symptoms. However, the relapse rate once treatment is stopped is very high, at 60 to 70 per cent. Due to its immediate effect, it can be used intermittently to help with continence at important times (sleepovers, camping trips). No child with chronic hyponatraemia or a history of hyponatraemia should receive desmopressin as a treatment for enuresis. Desmopressin should also be avoided in children and adolescents with sickle cell anaemia.

Factors that have been identified as predictors of success with desmopressin include a normal bladder capacity, older age (over 8 years old), less severe wetting and one episode of wetting per night.

Dysfunctional Voiding With Daytime Enuresis

This is a commonly seen in young girls and may present with frequent and sometimes continuous leaking and very wet underwear. Daytime wetting occurs after 3.5 years of age combined with either infrequent voiding (under three per day) or urinary frequency (over eight voids per day).

There may also be a history of urgency with holding manoeuvres (e.g. crossing the legs) or, conversely, a need to push in order to urinate.

There may be an interrupted urinary stream or several voids one after the other with possible frequent urinary tract infections. There is also frequently a history of constipation.

If a child has daytime urinary incontinence, it is reasonable to consider oxybutynin or tolterodine twice daily with desmopressin at night, should there be no improvement in enuresis on anticholinergic treatment alone.

If daily symptoms are unresponsive to treatment, always consider a malformation of the kidneys and/or urinary tract (such as an ectopic ureter) or lesions of the spinal cord.

(Box 30.4)

Box 30.4 *Clinical Bottom Line*

Nocturnal enuresis is quite common, often familial and should not be actively treated under 8 years of age. Avoid lifting and the use of trainers. Enuresis alarms and desmopressin are the recommended treatments and can be started prior to referral. Most cases can be managed in the community.

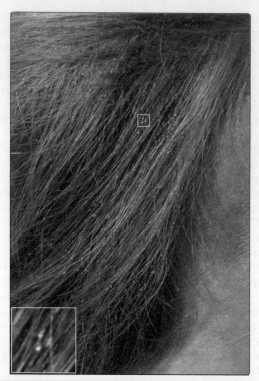

Figure 30.2   Head lice and nits are evident on a hair shaft. Best visualised using a hand lens. (Reproduced with permission from Gawkrodger, D. (2021). *Dermatology: An illustrated colour text* (7th ed.). Elsevier Inc.)

Head Lice in Children

Head lice (*Pediculus humanus capitis*) live exclusively on the human scalp and attach themselves to hair shafts by means of specialised claws (Fig. 30.2). Head lice are wingless insects and thus transmission from host to host can only occur by means of close personal contact as lice cannot fly or jump. Adult lice are about 1 to 3 mm in length and their eggs measure 1 mm and are visible to the naked eye.

SYMPTOMS

Scalp itching is the most common symptom and may be associated with sleep disturbance. Secondary bacterial infection with associated regional lymphadenopathy can complicate the course of infestation with head lice.

DIAGNOSIS

Combing the entire scalp with a fine-tooth comb helps to increase detection rates and this process is enhanced by using hair conditioner in liberal amounts. After each pass, the comb should be inspected for the presence of lice. Eggs should also be detected, with viable eggs being a tan or brown colour and hatched eggs being white or opaque.

TREATMENT

Head lice are found in clothes, bedlinen, and towels, and it seems advisable to change and wash these items regularly during the treatment phase. Washing at temperatures above 50°C is sufficient to decontaminate fabrics. Pediculicide treatment (malathion or permethrin) should be applied on two occasions, 7 days apart. Its mechanism of action is killing nymphs and adult lice. Oral treatment with ivermectin is not recommended.

Eucalyptus, lavender and tea tree oils are natural essential oils, have been tried but have not as yet been evaluated in clinical trials.

WET COMBING OR BUG-BUSTING

This process relies solely on the physical removal of lice and eggs by fine tooth comb with simultaneous use of hair conditioner to facilitate the process.

Electronic combs are enthusiastically marketed but are currently not recommended.

Dimeticone 4% (*Hedrin*) acts by coating the lice and disrupting their ability to manage water, which has a reported cure rate of 70 per cent for head lice following just two clinical trials (caution is urged). It is odourless, non-toxic and generally well-tolerated.

(Box 30.5)

Box 30.5 *Clinical Bottom Line*

Head lice carry an undeserved stigma and are highly prevalent in young children. Wet combing (every 3 days, five times in total) and topical dimethicone 4% are the recommended treatments. Specialist referral is not required, but resistance to treatment is incredibly common.

(Box 30.6)
(Box 30.7)
(Box 30.8)
(Box 30.9)
(Box 30.10)
(Box 30.11)

Box 30.6 Key Points

ADHD is a neurodevelopmental condition in which affected children and adults have problems with attention, impulsivity and hyperactivity.

Diagnosing ADHD requires the presence of at least six out of nine behavioural features that must have been present for at least 6 months, had onset before the age of 7 years, are present in more than one setting and are causing significant distress or impairment. Prevalence of ADHD is between 3 and 5 per cent.

Do not rely on observations made in the outpatients but rather receive reports from parents and teachers in particular.

Stimulant medications are very effective in dampening down the core symptoms of ADHD, and they have an immediate effect.

Behaviour therapy is recommended for preschool children with ADHD whereas school-aged children should receive stimulant medication to dampen down the core symptoms.

Children with DCD have difficulties with daily activities such as dressing, tying shoelaces and grooming. They have difficulties with sports, on the playground and when learning new motor skills, leading to reduced interest in physical activities.

Motor milestones in DCD are characteristically achieved on time but there is a delay in the acquisition of new motor skills.

Tics are quite common and are described as brief, purposeless, involuntary movements or vocalisations that only occur while awake. *Tourette syndrome* is diagnosed when a child has a history of multiple motor tics and at least one phonic tic present for over 12 months.

Sleep-disordered breathing should be considered during routine child consultations. Clinical history taking and overnight oximetry both have limitations in terms of diagnostic precision. Therefore, polysomnography remains the gold standard in the diagnosis of sleep-disordered breathing.

Obstructive sleep apnoea (OSA) is characterised by snoring with intermittent episodes of partial or complete upper airway obstruction.

OSA affects 1 to 3 per cent of all children with increased risk in Down syndrome, neuromuscular disease, craniofacial abnormalities, achondroplasia, Prader–Willi syndrome, mucopolysaccharidoses and in highly obese children.

Nocturnal enuresis is a very common childhood problem. It is a diagnosis of exclusion, and a thorough medical history and physical examination should be conducted to rule out a pathological cause before treatment options are considered.

The natural history of nocturnal enuresis is that it resolves spontaneously in the vast majority of children. Treatment should not be considered until the child is at least 8 years old unless there is significant stigma attached to the condition.

Preliminary methods such as motivational techniques, reducing nighttime fluids and diary keeping will result in improvement in most children and should be tried for at least 3 months before further methods are used.

Alarms require an initiative-taking child and family, and long-term therapy may be required. The risk of relapse is very real.

Head lice infestation is common in childhood, causes considerable distress to children and their families, and may lead to bullying and social stigmatisation.

The prevalence of head lice in school-aged children is approximately 20 per cent in the United Kingdom and various countries in Europe.

It is recommended to carry out wet combing treatment sessions every 3 days for a total of five sessions. Cure rates are reported to be up to 60 per cent as compared to a cure rate of less than 15 per cent with either malathion or permethrin.

Wet combing and topical use of dimeticone are the preferred treatment options as both are acceptable to parents and have few, if any, potential side effects.

Box 30.7 A 9-Year-Old Who Is Always in Trouble at School

A 9-year-old boy is having significant difficulties at school. His class teacher finds him distractable, always 'on the go', never sitting still and usually in trouble. He makes lots of careless mistakes in his schoolwork, blurts out answers before questions are completed and has great difficulty waiting his turn. He has proven to be very disruptive in class. He is frequently in trouble with his peers and has got into a number of fights with his classmates in the school yard.

At home, his parents have noted that he has frequent falls, rarely completes tasks and has great difficulty completing his homework. His past and perinatal history were normal, as were his general and neurological examinations. He has had formal audiometric and visual screening, and both are negative. His parents have asked their family doctor to coordinate a paediatric opinion at outpatients, where he appears quiet and well-behaved.

Clinical Pearls

ADHD has increased prevalence if a positive family history, ex-preterm, acquired brain injury, co-existent conduct disorder, oppositional defiant disorder or mood disorder are present.

Family doctors should not make the diagnosis of ADHD or start stimulant medication without seeking specialist advice.

The revised Conner's Teacher and Parent Rating Scale is a commonly used rating scale in the diagnosis of ADHD and will take the parent or teacher about 15 minutes to answer the questions posed in the scale.

The diagnosis of ADHD is based on meeting DSM-5 or ICD-10 criteria with at least a moderate social and educational impact and evident symptoms occurring in at least two settings.

Hyperactivity and impulsivity are usually readily apparent to family and teachers whereas the manifestations of inattention and distractibility are not as obvious.

Do not advise restrictive diets or the elimination of artificial colourings or additives but rather seek the advice of a paediatric dietitian if any dietary changes are contemplated.

Stimulant medications are very effective in dampening down the core symptoms of ADHD, and they do have an immediate effect.

Methylphenidate is the first-line medication of choice; consider a switch to lisdexamfetamine after a 6-week trial of methylphenidate if not responsive to medication.

While on stimulants, measure the weight of the child or adolescent every 3 months and height every 6 months. Pulse and BP should also be monitored, particularly if dose is adjusted.

If tics occur while on stimulant medication, first consider whether the tics are medication-related and whether the inconvenience of the tics outweighs the benefits of reducing core ADHD symptoms. If required, reduce the dose of stimulants or consider a change to atomoxetine.

Interpretation of Investigations

An ECG is not required before starting stimulant medication.

Pitfalls to Avoid

ADHD rarely exists in isolation and comorbidities are very common.

Common comorbidities include oppositional defiant disorder, conduct disorder, mood and anxiety disorders and learning difficulties.

ADHD should never be diagnosed or excluded based on observation of behaviour in the clinic.

Box 30.8 A 10-Year-Old With Very Poor Handwriting and Last to Be Picked at Football

A 10-year-old is referred for paediatric opinion having had an occupational therapy assessment for suspected DCD. He struggles with his handwriting both in terms of accuracy and speed. He also has trouble with fine motor tasks such as tying his shoelaces. He has poor coordination skills in sports and tends to have little time on the pitch when playing football. His past and perinatal history is normal. His detailed general and neurological examinations are normal.

Clinical Pearls

In DCD, the acquisition of coordinated motor skills is substantially below that expected and interferes with activities of everyday living, academic achievement, leisure and play.

Classical features include clumsiness and poor coordination often with difficulties in handwriting and finishing academic tasks on time. Difficulties with self-care skills such as dressing and tying shoelaces are also common.

DCD affects 5 to 6 per cent of children and has a male predominance. A formal diagnosis under the age of 5 years is made only in cases of severe impairment.

When taking a history, ask about a family history of developmental disorders or muscular dystrophies, a detailed developmental history, measures of academic achievement and any prior or current interventions. Seek formal reports from relevant professionals including the child's teacher, educational psychologist and occupational therapist.

There is an extensive overlap between emotional and behavioural symptoms and DCD with at least 30 per cent having social anxiety.

Training in keyboard and smartphone skills is key for those with poor handwriting.

Active video games may improve overall fitness levels in children with DCD.

Interpretation of Investigations

The Developmental Coordination Disorder Questionnaire, Revised Version (DCDQ-R) questionnaire filled by professionals is useful in diagnosing DCD. The DCD Daily Questionnaire filled in by parents is both valid and dependable in terms of acquisition of motor skills and activities of daily living.

The Handwriting Proficiency Screening Questionnaire is a practical questionnaire developed to detect handwriting difficulties and their impact.

Neuroimaging is <u>not</u> recommended unless alternative diagnoses are suspected.

Pitfalls to Avoid

A comprehensive neurological examination should exclude cerebral palsy or muscular dystrophy.

Comorbidity with conditions such as ADHD occurs frequently.

Box 30.9 A 6-Year-Old With Excessive Snoring and a Drop in School Performance

A 6-year-old boy has been noted by his parents to snore frequently at night. Over the past 2 months, the parents have become concerned that he is tired every morning, and his school performance has dipped according to his class teacher. He has also started to wet the bed despite being previously dry at night. They consequently present to their family doctor for advice. He is the eldest in the family and has no past medical issues. His examination is quite normal. His parents are concerned about possible psychological causes for his current symptoms.

Clinical Pearls

Clinical awareness is key to making the diagnosis of obstructive sleep apnoea (OSA) in otherwise healthy children.

OSA affects <u>1 to 3 per cent</u> of all children with increased risk in Down syndrome, highly obese children and young people, neuromuscular disease, craniofacial abnormalities, achondroplasia, Prader–Willi syndrome and mucopolysaccharidoses.

Common presenting features of OSA are nocturnal snoring and witnessed episodes of brief apnoea or laboured breathing.

OSA can have a significant long-term impact on a child's mental health, quality of life and neurodevelopment.

Children with proven OSA secondary to adenotonsillar hypertrophy should be referred for adenotonsillectomy. In other situations, overnight continuous positive airway pressure (CPAP) is required.

Interpretation of Investigations

Home oximetry is a very helpful screening test in otherwise healthy children. If positive, it is highly predictive (positive predictive value of 97 per cent) of OSA, but a normal or inconclusive study cannot definitively out rule OSA.

Investigations to make the diagnosis include overnight oximetry, transcutaneous CO_2, and the gold standard polysomnography sleep study.

Pitfalls to Avoid

The major issue for family doctors is to be aware of OSA, how common it is and to ask about sleep-disordered breathing in a child who snores.

Children with Down syndrome, muscular disorders, achondroplasia, mucopolysaccharidoses, Prader–Willi syndrome, and craniofacial syndromes should all have regular screening for OSA.

Box 30.10 A 9-Year-Old Boy With Persistent Bedwetting

A 9-year-old boy has never had a dry night since he was born. His parents feel he is too old to still be wetting the bed every night and are upset that it has now affected his school life and his ability to have sleepovers with his friends. His father remembers having a similar problem when he was younger and finding it very distressing. His growth chart shows him to be of above average height and weight. His full examination, including blood pressure measurement and examination of the lower back, is normal.

Clinical Pearls

Neither waking up nor lifting children at night promotes long-term dryness.

Motivational techniques are particularly suited to younger children who respond favourably to reward schemes.

If over 8 years of age, offer a buzzer alarm as first-line treatment to children whose bedwetting has not responded to advice on fluids, toileting or an appropriate reward system.

Box 30.10   A 9-Year-Old Boy With Persistent Bedwetting – cont'd

Offer desmopressin if short-term improvement in bedwetting is the priority. If not completely dry after 1 to 2 weeks of the initial dose of desmopressin, consider doubling the dose.

If accompanied by daytime enuresis, any underlying bladder dysfunction should be identified and treated before initiating specific treatment of bedwetting.

Dysfunctional voiding or 'holding on' behaviour is particularly frequent in young girls and presents with leakage of urine during the day, urgency and frequent episodes of cystitis.

Dysfunctional voiding is managed by increasing fluid intake, avoiding carbonated drinks, regular trips to the toilet (at least six per day), treatment of constipation and, rarely, nighttime antibiotic prophylaxis.

Interpretation of Investigations

Urinalysis is generally the only investigation required.

Pitfalls to Avoid

Consider spinal dysraphism and beware polydipsia secondary to either diabetes mellitus (DM) or diabetes insipidus (DI) as rare differential diagnoses.

The prevalence of enuresis in sickle cell disease is higher than normal and is thought to be due to chronic sickling compromising renal concentration capacity.

Adenotonsillectomy improves enuresis in a significant number of children with obstructive sleep apnoea.

Box 30.11   A Girl With an Itchy Head

A 10-year-old girl is attending primary school and arrives home with a note stating that another child in her class has head lice. A week later she has significant itching of her scalp and a number of head lice are found. She undergoes a few treatments but her head lice infestation persists. Her distraught parents seek advice from their family doctor.

Clinical Pearls

Head lice infestation is common in childhood and causes considerable distress to children and their families and may lead to bullying and social stigmatisation.

The prevalence of head lice in school-aged children is about 20 per cent in the United Kingdom and various countries in Europe.

The female adult louse has a limited life span of 3 to 4 weeks. During that time she will lay 50 to 100 eggs, which are attached to hair shafts in the scalp.

Itching due to head lice infestation is delayed for 2 to 6 weeks during the first infestation but develops after just 1 to 2 days during subsequent episodes.

Wet combing treatment sessions should be carried out every 3 days for a total of five sessions; cure rates are reported to be up to 60 per cent using this method. This compares favourably with a cure rate of less than 15 per cent with either malathion or permethrin.

Wet combing and topical use of 4 per cent dimeticone are viable treatment options as both are acceptable to parents and have few, if any, potential side effects.

Interpretation of Investigations

The diagnosis hinges on the detection of live head lice.

Pitfalls to Avoid

Siblings are frequently also infested with head lice and thus the entire family should be screened; all those affected should be treated simultaneously to break the cycle of reinfestation within the family.

Conventional pediculicides such as malathion, permethrin and phenothrin are increasingly associated with treatment failure due to the emergence of <u>resistance</u> in the parasite population.

▶ **Video on the topic Nocturnal enuresis is available online at Elsevier eBooks+.**

Key References

Blank, R., Barnett, A. L., Cairney, J., Green, D., Kirby, A., Polatajko, H., et al. (2019). International clinical practice recommendations on the definition, diagnosis, assessment, intervention, and psychosocial aspects of developmental coordination disorder. *Developmental Medicine and Child Neurology*, 61(3), 242–285.

Byrne, R., & Kirschner, K. (2018). Unusual behaviors. In R. M. Kliegman, P. S. Lye, B. Bordini, H. Toth, & D. Basel (Eds.), *Nelson pediatric symptom-based diagnosis*. Elsevier.

Gibbons, C., & Nicholson, A. (2008). *Solutions for nocturnal bedwetting in children*. Dublin: ICGP Forum.

Monrad, P. (2018). Paroxysmal disorders. In R. M. Kliegman, P. S. Lye, B. Bordini, H. Toth, & D. Basel (Eds.), *Nelson pediatric symptom-based diagnosis* (pp. 508–542). Elsevier.

National Institute for Health and Care Excellence. (2010, October 27). *Bedwetting in under 19's (NICE guideline [CG111])*. https://www.nice.org.uk/guidance/cg111.

National Institute for Health and Care Excellence. (2018, March 14). *Attention deficit hyperactivity disorder: Diagnosis and management (NICE guideline [NG87])*. www.nice.org.uk/guidance/ng87.

National Institute for Health and Care Excellence. (2020, October 30). *Bedwetting in children and young people overview. NICE Pathways*. https://pathways.nice.org.uk/pathways/bedwetting-in-children-and-young-people.

Nicholson, A., & O'Malley, G. (2016). *When your child is sick: What you can do to help* (2nd ed.). Gill Books.

Pamula, Y., Nixon, G. M., Edwards, E., Teng, A., Verginis, N., Davey, M. J., et al. (2017). Australasian Sleep Association clinical practice guidelines for performing sleep studies in children. *Sleep Medicine 36*(Suppl. 1), S23–S42.

Tebruegge, M., Pantazidou, A., & Curtis, N. (2011). What's bugging you? An update on the treatment of head lice infestation. *Archives of Disease in Childhood Education and Practice Edition*, 96(1), 2–8.

Vande Walle, J., Rittig, S., Tekgül, S., Austin, P., Yang, S. S.-D., Lopez, P.-J., et al. (2017). Enuresis: Practical guidelines for primary care. *British Journal of General Practice: The Journal of the Royal College of General Practitioners*, 67(660), 328–329.

31 *Adolescent Health*

ORLA WALSH

Adolescence

Adolescence is divided into early adolescence (10 to 14 years), late adolescence (15 to 19 years) and young adulthood (20 to 24 years). It is a time of many physical, emotional, social, behavioural and cognitive changes. Each time they look in the mirror, adolescents can see someone different.

For most young people, it is an exciting and enjoyable time filled with new activities and responsibilities. They begin to display autonomy and seek independence from their parents by spending more time with their peers. This can involve experimentation with alcohol, risk-taking behaviours and engaging in romantic relationships. For some, however, this transition can lead to difficulties resulting in significant stress and pressure. Therefore, learning to manage stress is an important life skill adolescents must develop.

Over the past 15 years we have gained a much deeper understanding about how this age group differs from younger and older populations. Significant progress has been made in both the understanding and management of diseases presenting in adolescence such as eating disorders, substance abuse and management of chronic medical illnesses affecting adolescents. Mental health disorders in adolescence are not infrequent and may require psychotropic medications in their treatment.

We now appreciate the importance of a structured transition to adult services for adolescents with chronic illnesses.

We understand the impact that chronic fatigue syndrome can have on a young person's life and can describe assessment and management of this condition in detail. This is one of several conditions occurring in adolescence that will be detailed in this chapter.

In the **Clinical Bottom Line** section for each topic, we wish to highlight key areas to look for in primary care or family practice and what might be done prior to the child being seen by a paediatrician or child and adolescent psychiatrist.

Why Adolescent Health Is Important

Adolescence is a formative time when the foundations for adult life are laid, not least the value of a healthy lifestyle. Substance use, sexually transmitted infections (STIs), mental health issues, obesity and asthma can all impact quality of life into adulthood. For those with chronic medical conditions, an effective transition to adult services may be challenging and needs to be carefully managed. A less than ideal transition process is associated with reduced adherence to treatment and may therefore have long lasting adverse health consequences.

Adolescence is a period where young people learn to develop their independence and life skills such as establishing personal relationships with their peers. We know that young people are uniquely vulnerable to relational, cultural and other environmental factors that contribute to health. Adolescent services in many countries are sadly underdeveloped, and adolescents have in the past been 'a forgotten tribe' in terms of healthcare provision. Considerable skill is required to address their needs which may otherwise go undiagnosed and untreated.

Dealing with adolescent patients is very different from caring for infants, younger children and adults. Adolescence is a unique time for profound brain growth and development. Of all the many changes in adolescence, perhaps the most dramatic are the changes in neuroendocrine function that occur with puberty.

What Makes Adolescents Unique?

BRAIN DEVELOPMENT IN ADOLESCENCE

The frontal lobe of the brain is required for decision making, planning, emotional regulation, and impulse control, and is poorly developed in childhood. Changes of the grey and white matter occur between the ages of 12 and 25 years and are evident on functional MRI studies. Throughout adolescence, increased white matter results in improved integration of memory and experience, both of which are important in decision making.

Selective pruning of grey matter occurs from the back to the front of the brain, resulting in increased cognitive ability. The frontal lobe is the last to show these structural changes, typically occurring in young adulthood. This natural neurodevelopmental sequence may help explain, for example, typical adolescence risk-taking behaviour, decision making and emotional responses.

In adolescence, the limbic system, which consists of deep grey and white matter, develops earlier and quicker than the frontal lobe. This also helps to explain why taking risks is a normal part of adolescent development and is in fact an evolutionary advantage.

PUBERTY

Boys generally experience puberty between 10 and 17 years and girls between 9 and 14 years. The great individual variation in both the onset and completion of pubertal changes can cause significant angst for adolescents who experience either early or late puberty relative to their peers.

Early puberty can be associated with a tendency to join older peer groups and potentially earlier exposure to high-risk behaviours (either sexual experiences or experimentation with drugs). Late puberty can pose different challenges in relation to peer relationships and self-confidence.

Body image becomes more significant during puberty and can lead to unhealthy behaviours including poor eating habits and excessive exercise. Puberty is also a time when sleep patterns begin to change, and many adolescents stay awake late at night and sleep late in the morning. This may relate to later melatonin release in the brain.

Adolescents require 9 to 10 hours of sleep per night and should ideally maintain the same sleep schedules throughout weekdays and weekends. Good sleep hygiene is an important issue in adolescence as sleep deprivation can affect school, social relationships, and both physical and mental health.

RISK-TAKING BEHAVIOURS

For most adolescents, the teenage years are a period of relatively good health, but injuries and suicide account for over three-quarters of all deaths in adolescence. Due to the asynchrony in brain development discussed above, some adolescents feel invincible, resulting in risk-taking behaviours. Examples may include cycling without helmets and alcohol or drug misuse. Sexual risk-taking behaviours can also occur at the risk of unwanted pregnancy and STIs.

Most serious injuries in adolescence relate to motor vehicle collisions. Most of these injuries are preventable by following speed limits, using seat belts, and not driving while under the influence of substances or while using a mobile phone. Late adolescence is a very risky time for road-related injuries and deaths – countries that have adopted a zero tolerance to speeding and drug and alcohol use have shown reductions in both.

PSYCHOLOGICAL ISSUES AND MENTAL ILLNESS

Major psychiatric illness may present in adolescence. Depression, schizophrenia, social anxiety disorder, panic attacks and eating disorders all have a peak of onset during adolescence. Deliberate self-harm is an increasingly common presentation to the emergency department.

Adolescents with mental illness and addictions are more likely to die prematurely than the general population. After accidents, suicide is the second leading cause of death in adolescents and young adults.

SEXUAL HEALTH

Adolescents are least likely to approach adults when they have problems and are more likely to depend on their peers or the internet, both of which can be unreliable sources of information about sexual health. They are also unlikely to talk to their doctor about it for fear of their parents finding out. Therefore, misinformation about contraception and STIs is common, putting many adolescents at risk of becoming engaged in sexual activity without having accurate health information.

SOCIETAL CHANGES

Due to major societal changes including the greater uptake of post-secondary education, there has been a major demographic transition in Europe in recent decades with a consequent delay in leaving home, marriage and childbirth, resulting in a significantly longer adolescent and young adult period (Fig. 31.1).

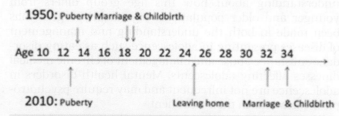

Figure 31.1   Societal changes in puberty, marriage and childbirth in Europe. (Courtesy Prof. Russell Viner.)

Eating Disorders

Eating disorders are clinically diagnosed and classified using one of the two main diagnostic classification systems for mental disorders: ICD-11 (2018) is used by most mental health services in Europe, and the DSM-5 (APA, 2014) is used in North America.

EPIDEMIOLOGY

The three main eating disorders – anorexia nervosa (AN), bulimia nervosa (BN) and binge eating disorder (BED) – have a combined prevalence of 4 per cent. One may also have subclinical eating disorders that are potentially equally disabling in terms of impact on function. A new addition to the DSM-5 classification is avoidant restrictive food intake disorder (ARFID).

Eating disorders occur across the spectrum of socioeconomic class and family income. They have been found to occur in all ethnic groups, cultures and countries. To date, the main body of research has focussed on high-income countries and amongst females.

THE MOST COMMON EATING DISORDERS IN ADOLESCENCE

Anorexia Nervosa (AN)

The main features of AN are a persistent restriction of energy intake with associated weight loss, a great fear of becoming fat, persistent behaviours that interfere with weight gain and a general underappreciation of the seriousness of the situation in terms of low body weight. The peak incidence of onset is 14 to 18 years of age.

Bulimia Nervosa (BN)

Characteristic features of BN include recurrent episodes of binge eating over a discrete period of time and a sense of losing control in terms of how much one is eating. Associated features of BN include self-induced vomiting, laxative or diuretics misuse, fasting and excessive exercise to avoid weight gain. The peak incidence of BN onset is 14 to 22 years.

Binge-Eating Disorder (BED)

Characteristic features of BED include recurrent episodes of binge eating. Patients tend to eat until uncomfortably full (even if not hungry), leading to a consequent feeling of self-disgust. BED most commonly presents in the late teens or early 20s.

Avoidant Restrictive Food Intake Disorder (ARFID):

Characteristic features of ARFID include an inability to meet appropriate nutritional needs leading to significant weight loss or nutritional deficiency. Those with ARFID may require enteral feeding, which leads to significant psychosocial issues. Patients tend to be younger and have a longer duration of illness than those with either AN or BN.

CAUSES OF EATING DISORDERS

Eating disorders have a complex aetiology with biological, environmental and psychosocial factors all coming into play. Contributory factors include pressures around physical appearance and the influence of social media.

Genetic factors are very important and account for 40 to 60 per cent of an individual's likelihood of developing an eating disorder. Top risk factors are female sex, low self-esteem and an anxious or perfection-seeking personality. AN is often linked to the onset of puberty, severe life events or having a medical condition such as diabetes that requires strict dietary control.

PROGNOSIS

The past decade has seen much progress made in the management of eating disorders. Both cognitive behavioural therapy (CBT) and family-based treatment (FBT) have enabled upwards of 40 to 45 per cent of patients to achieve remission, with a further 30 per cent having partial remission.

Adolescents have a better prognosis with early intervention, but a full recovery may take between 2 and 5 years. If left untreated, eating disorders have devastating effects on psychosocial outcomes, educational prospects and engagement in healthy relationships.

MORTALITY

Mortality rates for all eating disorders are high, including a mortality rate in AN that is an astonishing six times that of the general population. Between 5 and 10 per cent of those who present with AN will die prematurely from it within 10 years of onset. The causes of death from AN include cardiac dysfunction resulting from the direct impact of starvation. Suicide risk is higher in patients with eating disorders.

MEDICAL COMPLICATIONS OF EATING DISORDERS

The potential medical complications of eating disorders are extensive. Most are fully reversible with weight restoration; however, potentially irreversible damage to growth, bone health and reproductive health can occur (Table 31.1).

ASSESSMENT

A detailed assessment should include weight and growth patterns, issues around mealtimes, evidence of comorbidity, a family history, a dietetic review and a mental state examination. Baseline physical examination and medical investigations are essential. Family engagement is critical to gather a collateral history and support for the refeeding process.

The indications for hospitalisation for AN are highlighted in Table 31.2.

MANAGEMENT

The goals of management are the stabilisation of vital signs, correction of electrolyte abnormalities, nutritional rehabilitation and motivation to aid recovery. Nutritional rehabilitation includes metabolic recovery, restoration of weight, reversal of medical complications and improved eating behaviours. This requires a multidisciplinary team approach and strong therapeutic alliances with the patient and their family.

Table 31.1   Medical Complications of Eating Disorders

System	Complications
General	Hypothermia
	Nutritional deficiencies: vitamin B_{12}, folate, ferritin, vitamin D
Fluid and electrolytes	Dehydration, hypoglycaemia, hypoalbuminemia, oedema
	Purging: hypochloraemic metabolic alkalosis, low K^+, PO_4, Mg^{2+}, Cl^-, Na^+
	Laxative abuse: hyperchloraemic metabolic acidosis
Head and neck	AN: Dry mucous membranes
	BN: Dental erosions
Cardiovascular	AN: Bradycardia, cardiac arrhythmias, orthostatic hypotension, QTc elongation, mitral valve prolapse, heart failure
	BN: increased risk for cardiomyopathy
Gastrointestinal	AN: Delayed gastric motility and emptying, constipation, superior mesenteric artery syndrome
	BN: Oesophagitis, oesophageal tears (and, rarely, rupture)
	BED: Gastric dilatation, rarely gastric rupture
Pulmonary	BN: Aspiration pneumonia, pneumomediastinum
Renal	Elevated urea and creatinine, decreased glomerular filtration rate (severe fluid restriction/vomiting), renal calculi
Endocrine	Hypothalamic suppression with low gonadotrophic and sex hormones: hypogonadism, amenorrhoea, pubertal delay, low thyroxine, low IGF-1, growth retardation
Haematological	Anaemia, leucopenia, thrombocytopaenia
Musculoskeletal	Muscle wasting, reduced bone mineral density, increased fracture risk
Dermatologic	Acrocyanosis, lanugo hair, hair loss, dry skin
Neurological	Syncope, seizures, structural brain changes, decreased concentration, memory and thinking ability

Table 31.2   Indications for Hospitalisation in Anorexia Nervosa **One or More** of the Following

Severe Malnutrition (Weight <75% Median Body Mass Index for Age and Sex)	Orthostatic Changes in HR (>20 beats/min) or BP (>20 mmHg Systolic/>10 mmHg Diastolic)
Dehydration	Arrested growth and development
Electrolyte disturbance	Failure of outpatient treatment
ECG abnormalities	Acute food refusal
Physiological instability:	Uncontrollable binging and purging
Severe bradycardia (heart rate <50 beats/min daytime, <45 beats/min at night)	Acute medical complications of malnutrition
Hypotension (<90/45 mmHg)	Acute psychiatric emergencies
Hypothermia (<96°F)	Comorbid diagnosis that interferes with the treatment of the eating disorder

Box 31.1   *Clinical Bottom Line on Eating Disorders*

An eating disorder is a diagnosis of exclusion that poses a severe health risk. Differential diagnoses include inflammatory bowel disease, Addison's disease and a hypothalamic tumour. Risk factors include being female, having low self-esteem and a perfectionist personality. There has been a steady rise in prevalence among males. Refer to child and adolescent mental health services (CAHMS) in the community for long-term treatment and refer straight to hospital for medical stabilisation if rapid weight loss (over 1 kg in a week), hypotension, or bradycardia are present, or if the patient is too weak to walk in accordance with *Junior MARSIPAN* guidelines.

Oral feeding is preferred for refeeding. Nasogastric feeds may be required if oral feeding is not working – this may lead to legal and ethical issues if the patient is refusing necessary treatment. Excessive exercise should be discouraged. Desired weight gain may range from 0.5 to 1.0 kg/week, but caution needs to be exercised due to the risk of refeeding syndrome. The key biochemical abnormality of refeeding syndrome is a low phosphate level. Clinical features are a depressed level of consciousness, fluid overload, muscle weakness, diarrhoea and electrolyte derangement.

INTERNATIONAL GUIDELINES

Junior MARSIPAN is the current guideline used in managing those under 18 with anorexia nervosa. It uses both a checklist and traffic-light system to assess risk in a standardised way. It provides guidance on the initial assessment of people with AN, including the exclusion of other conditions associated with rapid weight loss, such as hyperthyroidism.

A detailed treatment plan should be communicated to the patient, family and staff. This international guideline provides a detailed, multi-agency, responsive approach with clear care pathways.

(Box 31.1)

Adolescent Mental Health

During adolescence, mental health issues such as anxiety and depression are prevalent and there is an increased risk of deliberate self-harm and suicidal behaviours. Adolescents require access to user-friendly services specific to their needs. They are more likely to turn to their peers when they experience problems or seek advice.

Doctors need to have a high level of awareness in adolescents with social withdrawal, substance use, poor academic performance, fatigue and somatic complaints. People with mental health problems are more likely to die prematurely than the general population, and suicide is a frequent cause of death for young people aged 18 to 25 years.

ADOLESCENT PSYCHOSIS

Psychosis is characterised by disorganised thinking accompanied by delusions or hallucinations. Primary psychotic symptoms are rarely seen in prepubertal children, meaning that organic causes need to be ruled out in this age group. Many children with psychosis have pre-existing neurodevelopmental or neurocognitive defects. Typical symptoms of psychosis include hallucinations (false sensory perceptions), delusions (fixed false beliefs) and disorganised speech and behaviour. Social withdrawal, flattening of affect and general apathy are often seen.

Table 31.3 Organic Diagnoses to Be Considered in Suspected Psychosis

Symptom/Sign	Possible Organic Cause
Jaundice	Wilson's disease
Rash, arthralgia, myalgia	Systemic lupus erythematosus
Fever	Cerebral malaria, autoimmune encephalitis, thyrotoxicosis, anticholinergic overdose
Previous symptoms associated with fever or high protein diet	Urea cycle defect
Recurrent abdominal pain	Porphyria

Schizophrenia is a severe mental illness that causes psychosis which can first present in late adolescence and young adulthood. It is exceptionally rare under 13 years of age. The differential diagnosis includes delirium, substance abuse, mood disorder and pervasive developmental disorders.

Adolescents with schizophrenia tend to be emotionally unresponsive and show reduced eye contact and body language. They are unable to react appropriately to social cues and often have a depressed mood. Hallucinations are most often auditory and delusions tend to be persecutory. Speech may be disorganised and very difficult to understand. Associated behavioural issues include inappropriate dress, an overall untidy and unkempt appearance and unprovoked aggression.

Clinical assessment requires a meticulous history. Always consider substance abuse, but a wide differential of organic causes must also be considered. The differential diagnoses to be considered in children or adolescents with psychosis are highlighted in Table 31.3.

Investigations for psychosis should include baseline investigations such as ESR, LFTs, TFTs, glucose, electrolytes, a toxicology screen, a brain MRI (looking for focal neurological deficits, features of raised intracranial pressure and history of trauma) and an EEG (looking for non-convulsive status epilepticus).

Second line investigations should include serum copper and caeruloplasmin, serum ammonia, anti NMDA and VGKC antibodies (seen in autoimmune encephalitis) and a urine for porphyria screen.

Consider a primary psychiatric illness if no organic cause is found and refer to a child and adolescent psychiatry team.

(Box 31.2)

Box 31.2 *Clinical Bottom Line on Psychosis*

Adolescents with psychosis have disorganised thinking and hallucinations or delusions. Psychosis is exceedingly rare prior to 13 years of age. Always consider substance abuse or delirium. Prompt referral to CAHMS services is advised.

DEPRESSION

The onset of depression in adolescence is associated with a more severe course of illness and increased risk of poorer academic, occupational, social and psychiatric outcomes. Risk factors include being female, living in poverty, significant family or peer conflict, chronic illness (such as diabetes mellitus), a recent bereavement or a past or family history of depression.

There are multifactorial contributions to depression in adolescents, including structural and functional brain abnormalities and several neurotransmitter systems. Serotonin transporter genes may predispose to depression that runs in families. Numerous cognitive, interpersonal and early developmental theories may also contribute.

Assessment includes an individual interview and collateral information from guardians to assess symptoms and their functional impacts. It is important to assess the severity of the symptoms while keeping in mind how their cultural background may affect the presentation.

General treatment considerations include identifying and addressing stressors and psychiatric comorbidity. Cognitive behavioural therapy (CBT) is one therapeutic option. Medications include selective serotonin reuptake inhibitors (SSRIs) which block the reuptake of serotonin, thereby increasing its concentration in the neurotransmitter systems.

ANXIETY DISORDERS

Unlike anxiety, which is part of normal development, an anxiety disorder occurs when the anxiety is excessive, persistent and interferes with day-to-day functioning. Different categories are based on inborn traits including adaptability, response and sensitivity to situations (e.g. shyness is a risk factor for social anxiety disorder).

Risk factors include environmental factors (life stressors such as parental divorce), adverse events in early childhood, interpersonal stressors and parental factors (overprotection or intrusiveness). Genetic factors are also important with multiple genes involved.

Assessment includes an individual interview and collateral information from guardians to assess symptoms and functional impact. It is important to identify external stressors (such as family conflict), associated physical symptoms, specific worries and thoughts and the level of interference of the anxiety. Psychotherapeutic options for adolescents include cognitive behavioural therapy (CBT) and mindfulness-based therapies. The mainstay of medication management is SSRIs.

DELIBERATE SELF-HARM AND PARACETAMOL POISONING

Common forms of self-harm include cutting the arms or legs with a sharp object, taking an overdose of medication (often paracetamol), or intoxication via alcohol or illicit drug use. Depression is a common comorbidity.

Most cases of paracetamol poisoning in adolescents occur as episodes of self-harm. Post-ingestion of as little as 150 mg/kg within a 24-hour period may result in initial symptoms of nausea and vomiting that usually settle within 24 hours. Persistence of symptoms beyond 24 hours in association with right subcostal pain and tenderness may indicate the development of hepatic necrosis.

Consider giving activated charcoal if a toxic dose has been ingested within the previous hour. Those at risk and who require treatment are identified by a single measurement of the serum paracetamol level taken not less than 4 hours post-ingestion. Using a special nomogram, those whose level is above the treatment line are treated with N-acetylcysteine by intravenous infusion. Adolescents who are malnourished or taking liver enzyme-inducing drugs are at high risk.

Those who have taken a staggered overdose should be treated regardless of the paracetamol level. All require baseline bloods including renal and liver enzymes and INR. Normal liver function tests at 48 hours post-ingestion exclude hepatic damage. ALT levels over 1000 IU/L indicate significant liver injury, and the sequential measurements of the INR offer an important guide to residual liver function.

Adolescents should be admitted to hospital following a significant episode of self-harm. They require formal assessment by a mental health team and a clear follow-up plan prior to discharge. A risk assessment should be performed, exploring the circumstances leading to self-harm and whether there was intent to commit suicide.

SUICIDE AND SUICIDAL BEHAVIOURS

The strongest predictors of reattempts are regret about surviving and high suicidal intent with prior planning. Depression is most strongly associated with suicidal ideation. Psychological traits seen include hopelessness, aggression and impulsiveness. Family and environmental factors include a parental history of suicidal behaviour or mental illness, negative family climate and severe bullying.

Precipitants vary depending on age and can include conflict with parents in young adolescents and conflict with peers or romantic partners in older adolescents.

Protective factors include a positive relationship with a parent, adequate parental supervision, a strong connection to school, reasons for staying alive, and cultural or religious beliefs.

Assessment involves interviewing the adolescent alone (with or without self-reported questionnaire), supplemented by a collateral history including current suicidality, factors that increase distress/reduce inhibition, protective factors, contextual factors and availability of lethal means.

There is conflicting evidence on the use of antidepressants, but epidemiological studies have demonstrated an association between their increased use and reduced rates of suicide in adolescents. Interventions that target family attachment/interaction, mentalisation and substance abuse reduce suicidal ideation and behaviour. (Box 31.3)

Box 31.3 *Clinical Bottom Line on Deliberate Self-Harm*

Deliberate self-harm (DSH) has increased alarmingly in most countries. Many with DSH have comorbid attention-deficit/hyperactivity disorder (ADHD) or conduct disorder. Cutting is the main form of self-harm presenting to family practice and has a low suicide risk but a high risk of recurrence. Deliberate poisoning is the chief presentation of DSH seen in hospital. Risk assessments have been found to be unreliable. Referral to a specialist DSH multidisciplinary team is advised.

Chronic Fatigue Syndrome (CFS)

Chronic fatigue syndrome, as the name suggests, is a long-term illness with a wide range of symptoms including extreme fatigue and general malaise after minimal effort with the result that it becomes very challenging to perform tasks and activities.

In CFS, symptoms cannot be explained by another cause and are present for 4 months in an adult or 3 months in a child or young person. The pattern and severity of symptoms vary greatly and range from mild to severe.

Major symptoms include post-exertional malaise, cognitive dysfunction, sleep disturbance, muscle pain, joint pain, general malaise, headaches, sore throat, dizziness, painful lymph nodes, nausea and palpitations. Younger children have a different set of symptoms with fewer cognitive or sleep problems. Tender lymphadenopathy and dizziness are more likely in preadolescents.

Those with 'mild' symptoms are generally able to carry on everyday activities such as school – however, they may have to give up hobbies to allow extra time for rest. Those with 'moderate' symptoms can usually no longer attend school and sleep a lot during the day. Finally, those with 'severe' symptoms may be house or bedbound, and it takes them a long time to recover from an activity involving extra effort.

CFS is the leading cause of prolonged school absence in adolescence with 1 per cent of secondary school children missing a day a week with only one in 10 having received a diagnosis. About one in 1000 adolescents are so severely affected that they do not attend school at all.

All symptoms experienced (particularly profound fatigue) require assessment in terms of severity, onset and course. A sleep diary should be taken. It is essential to look for a history of chronic illness or similar symptoms in either parent. Twin studies show a moderate genetic risk.

Look for evidence of postural orthostatic tachycardia syndrome during the examination by focusing on blood pressure and heart rate in both standing and lying positions. A detailed neurological examination and palpation for lymphadenopathy or hepatosplenomegaly should also be conducted.

Investigations should incorporate a FBC, CRP, ESR, blood chemistry, creatine kinase (CK), liver function tests (LFTs), thyroid function tests (TFTs), Epstein–Barr virus (EBV) IgM and IgG and urinalysis to exclude alternative causes of fatigue in adolescents.

Referral from primary care to a paediatric or adolescent service is warranted. A paediatrician should be able to make a diagnosis, exclude other causes, treat symptoms, provide advice about sleep and activity, and consider referral to a specialist service if diagnosis is severe. For sleep, advise against oversleeping and to anchor wake up time to avail of the normal cortisol surge in the morning. Prolonged bed rest or complete inactivity should be avoided as physical deconditioning is likely to exacerbate the fatigue.

There is strong evidence for the effectiveness of cognitive behaviour therapy (CBT) especially in younger children and adolescents, in those with significant depression and anxiety, in athletes and others with high levels of pain. If pain is a dominant symptom and simple analgesics and CBT are ineffective, referral to a specialist pain management clinic is warranted. Antidepressant drugs should only be used in those with a severe mood disorder; fluoxetine should be considered as first choice. Be sure to allow adequate time for onset before assessing for a response.

In terms of long-term prognosis, most recover at 6 months with specialist treatment, whereas less than 10 per cent recover without specialist treatment.

(Box 31.4)

Box 31.4 *Clinical Bottom Line on Chronic Fatigue Syndrome*

Chronic fatigue syndrome is the leading cause of prolonged school absence in adolescence. If suspected, advise that the child or adolescent avoid prolonged bed rest or complete physical inactivity. Analgesia for pain and cognitive behaviour therapy are effective, but early referral to a specialised service is advised and improves prognosis.

Transition to Adult Services

Many young people born with complex conditions (e.g. congenital heart disease) now survive well into adult life. For instance, just over 98 per cent of infants born with Fallot's tetralogy now survive into adulthood. Other conditions with greatly improved survival, such as cystic fibrosis, can affect many body systems and aspects of a young person's life and thus transition of their care to adult services requires detailed planning.

The negative consequences of a poorly planned transition from paediatric to adult health services include an increased risk of non-compliance to treatment, patients being lost to follow-up, and psychological distress with a negative impact on both social and educational outcomes.

There is a gap in the current system, which is failing to meet significant health needs of the adolescent population, and we know that such gaps have long-term consequences (Fig. 31.2).

On the other hand, successful transition requires careful collaboration between paediatric and adult services. Rather than occurring as a single event, transition should be a meticulously planned and managed process. A delicate balance must be struck between the young person's need for privacy and confidentiality, and the parents' or caregivers' needs to have sufficient information to provide the ongoing support required. Several models for good transition have emerged with no clear evidence that any one is superior to the others.

Further training is required for healthcare professionals in terms of working with young people, consultation strategies, and multidisciplinary and multiagency teamwork. Professionals working with adolescents in transition should be aware of the evolution of relevant medical conditions (e.g. cystic fibrosis) and their potential consequences in adult life.

As they mature, children should become more involved in decisions relating to their care. This will prepare them for the greater responsibility of managing their own health as young adults. This task is more complicated in a child with chronic illness.

It is important for healthcare professionals to reinforce positive attitudes toward growing up rather than focussing only on medical issues. Support is required for adolescents to care for themselves and to further develop communication and decision-making skills.

Successful transition requires a significant investment in terms of time, resources and commitment. Major keys to success include a recognition of the importance of the process, proper consultation with the professionals and families, flexibility in timing of transition, a period of preparation for the young person and their family, effective information transfer and close monitoring of attendance until the young person is established in the appropriate adult service.

(Box 31.5)
(Box 31.6)
(Box 31.7)
(Box 31.8)

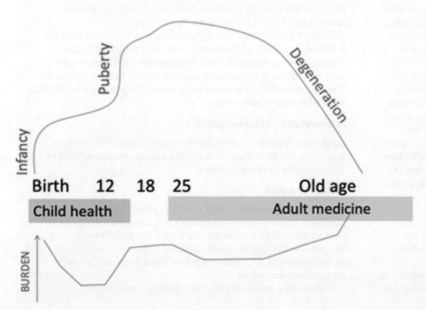

Figure 31.2 Gaps in the health needs of the adolescent population. (Courtesy Prof. Russell Viner.)

Box 31.5   **Key Points**

Adolescence is a time of many physical, emotional, social, behavioural and cognitive changes.

Adolescence is a formative time and when the foundations for adult life are laid, including the value of a healthy lifestyle.

Adolescents are uniquely vulnerable to relational, cultural and other environmental factors that contribute to health.

Responding to the needs of adolescents requires skilled professionals who can engage patients in care and address needs that may otherwise go undiagnosed and untreated.

Adolescents are often simultaneously exploring new experiences and potentially engaging in risky behaviours that can significantly interfere with their health trajectories.

Good sleep hygiene is an important issue in adolescence as sleep deprivation can affect academic performance, social relationships, and both physical and mental health.

The causes of eating disorders are complex and include biological, environmental and psychosocial factors.

The standardised mortality ratio for all eating disorders is three times that of the general population and almost six times higher in AN, which has the highest rate of all mental health disorders.

While most medical complications are fully reversible with weight restoration, potentially irreversible damage to growth, bone and reproductive health can occur.

The goals of management are the stabilisation of vital signs, correction of electrolyte abnormalities, nutritional rehabilitation and motivation to aid recovery.

Adolescence is a time of increased risk of poor mental health with high prevalence of anxiety, depression and amplified risk of deliberate self-harm and suicidal behaviours.

Depression, schizophrenia, social anxiety disorder, panic attacks and eating disorders all have a peak of onset during adolescence.

Common forms of self-harm include cutting the arms or legs with a sharp object, taking an overdose of medication (often paracetamol), or intoxication via alcohol or illicit drug use.

People with mental health problems are more likely to die prematurely than the general population; after accidental death, suicide is the third leading cause of death for young people aged 18 to 25 years.

Chronic fatigue syndrome is a long-term illness with a broad range of symptoms and is a leading cause of prolonged school absence in adolescence.

Prolonged best rest or complete inactivity should be avoided as physical deconditioning is likely to exacerbate the fatigue.

Poorly planned transition from paediatric to adult health services can be associated with an increased risk of non-adherence to treatment and loss to follow-up, resulting in serious consequences.

Transition is a process that should be planned and managed, not a single event.

Box 31.6   **A Non-Compliant Adolescent With Type One Diabetes Mellitus**

You are seeing a 16-year-old male with insulin-dependent diabetes mellitus in clinic following his recent discharge from hospital. He was first diagnosed at the age of 12 after presenting to the emergency room in diabetic ketoacidosis (DKA). Up until a year ago, he had been maintaining excellent glycaemic control. However, in the past 6 months, he has had three admissions for management of DKA. He has also lost weight and has been missing a lot of school. He reports checking his sugars multiple times per day and self-injecting insulin four times per day. He has forgotten his diary today. His review of systems and physical examination are unremarkable.

Obtain further information on history by asking more specific questions. Once you have explained the limits of confidentiality, complete a home, education (i.e. school), activities/employment, drugs, suicidality, and sex (HEeADSSS) screen with him alone.

He lives with his mother and rarely sees his father, who he does not get on with. He and his mother have been fighting a lot recently about his diabetes, so he spends most of his time hanging out with friends. He hangs out with a large group of boys. He is currently struggling in school and wishes to drop out and do an apprenticeship. He is not involved in any extra-curricular activities. He admits to smoking cigarettes and marijuana and drinking alcohol with his friends when they are bored. He is interested in girls but is not sexually active. He describes his mood as somewhat low and says he often feels bored.

Clinical Pearls

The concerning features in this history are his poor relationships with his parents, substance use, low mood and lack of academic engagement, which can all lead to poor compliance with diabetes management.

Assessment of the HbA1c and home glucose monitoring record should take place at each visit to the diabetes specialist clinic. His

ability to recognise and manage occurrences of hypoglycaemia, his injection sites and technique should be assessed. His diet (including carbohydrate counting) requires formal assessment by a specialist dietitian. Dose adjustment of his insulin with intense exercise should be discussed.

Long-term consequences of poor compliance include increased risk of microvascular complications from diabetes (retinopathy, nephropathy, neuropathy), DKA leading to ICU admissions and possibly death, psychosocial, academic and emotional consequences resulting from prolonged admissions, school absences and disrupted relationships.

Firstly, try to provide him with a safe space to discuss how he is feeling. Try to utilise motivational interviewing techniques to enhance his motivation for self-management. With permission, refer him to the diabetes team psychologist to further individual therapy and refer to the team social worker to provide psychosocial support for the whole family.

Interpretation of Investigations

Long-term control is monitored by measuring HbA1c levels and levels less than 7 per cent are associated with lower risks of diabetes-related complications.

Pitfalls to Avoid

There is strong evidence that poorly planned transition from paediatric to adult health services leads to an increased risk of non-adherence to treatment and being lost to follow up. This has adverse consequences in terms of a chronic illness such as diabetes with additional negative impacts on social and educational outcomes.

DKA is still a potentially life-threatening emergency.

Box 31.7 Deliberate Self-Harm

A 13-year-old girl presents with periumbilical abdominal pain ongoing for the past 3 years. It has no known triggers but occurs up to twice per week, with increasing severity over the past 3 months, causing her to be unable to attend school. Her menses are regular, last 5 days and are associated with cramps.

Having explained the limits of confidentiality, complete a HEEADSSS psychosocial assessment with her alone. She lives at home with her mother and younger sister. Her father passed away unexpectedly 3 years ago, and she is not sure of the cause of his death. She has no close friends and does not like any of her teachers. She used to play the piano and go swimming but has stopped in the past year. She has not started dating and is not sure if she is interested in boys or girls. She has never engaged in any sexual activity. She has never tried alcohol, cigarettes or any drugs. She describes her mood as quite low and informs you that she has deliberately cut herself on her inner thighs and forearms with a razor blade on two occasions in the past 3 months following fights with her mother about not wanting to go to school.

On examination, she has well-healed horizontal linear scars on inner thighs and forearms. Her physical examination is otherwise unremarkable.

Clinical Pearls

The loss of her father, lack of engagement with school, loss of interest in participating in activities and confusion regarding her sexuality are all potential contributors to her low mood and deliberate self-harm.

Common forms of deliberate self-harm (DSH) include cutting the arms or legs with a sharp object, taking an overdose of medication (often paracetamol) or intoxication via alcohol or illicit drug use.

Although depression is a common comorbidity, treatment with antidepressants has not been shown to reduce the risk of repetition of DSH in people treated for DSH in hospital. Conduct disorder and attention deficit hyperactivity are common comorbidities in DSH.

Deliberate self-poisoning (over 80 per cent) and self-cutting (10 per cent) are the most common presentations of DSH. For young people with hospital-treated DSH, the key clinical outcomes are rates of suicide and repetition of DSH.

A thorough assessment should be conducted for a young person presenting with DSH by way of discussion with the patient and their family. Specialist DSH multidisciplinary teams enhance both service-user experiences and provide greater support and professional development for clinical staff.

For adolescents, self-motivation to change, positive parenting and healthy sleeping habits all exert a positive effect. Family involvement is critical.

Potential Pitfalls

The main reason for hospital-treated DSH is deliberate self-poisoning, which may be associated with suicidal ideation. Reported repetition rates are approximately 15 per cent at 1 year, and the reported suicide risk is 1 per cent at 1 year.

Self-injury (especially cutting, burning or biting) is the main cause of DSH seen in the community and is equally common among males and females with higher repetition rates and a lower suicide mortality.

Risk assessments have not been demonstrated to reduce repetition of DSH, and there are no widely accepted tools for clinically assessing the subsequent risk of suicide. However, those who present with DSH have a higher relative risk of further DSH and suicide compared with those who have not self-harmed.

Risk categorisation is not a replacement for a thorough clinical assessment. Even if the young person is deemed to be low risk, this should not result in delayed assessment or reduced access to aftercare in the community.

Box 31.8 An Adolescent With an Eating Disorder

A 15-year-old female has always been described by her family as a healthy eater and an active person, but in the last 5 months she has started cutting back on certain foods and is exercising more than usual. She is quite vague when asked about body image. She explains that she initially just wanted to be more healthy and fit, but she now spends a lot of time planning meals and thinking about food, and is terrified of gaining weight. She has never binged or purged or used laxatives or diet pills. She now weighs herself daily. She achieved menarche at age 12 and last menstruated 4 months ago.

A review of systems finds that she is cold all the time, feels tired and becomes dizzy if she stands up too quickly.

Having explained the limits of confidentiality, complete a HEEADSSS psychosocial assessment with her alone.

She lives at home with her mother, father and older sister, with whom she gets on well. She is worried about her end of year exams despite being an excellent student. She is a high achiever with lots of friends and extracurricular activities, including gymnastics three times per week. She has not started dating but is interested in boys. She has never engaged in any sexual activity. She has gone to parties but never tried alcohol, cigarettes or any drugs. She would have previously described herself as very happy, but she has become quite stressed and withdrawn over the past few months. She has never thought of harming herself and there are no safety concerns.

On examination, her height is on the 75th percentile, and her weight is below the 3rd percentile for age. Her vital signs show a postural drop in BP on standing and a heart rate of 40 beats/min and a temperature of 36°C. She is emaciated with sunken eyes and pale skin. She has a delayed peripheral capillary refill of 3 seconds and cool mottled extremities.

Clinical Pearls

The most concerning elements include her decreased energy intake and increased energy expenditure, lack of menstruation and physical symptoms of cold intolerance, fatigue and dizziness. The most likely diagnosis is anorexia nervosa (AN).

Characteristic features of AN include a persistent restriction of energy intake, an intense fear of becoming fat and a persistent lack of recognition of the seriousness of the current low body weight. AN has a peak incidence of onset of 14 to 18 years of age.

The Junior MARSIPAN uses a checklist and traffic-light system to estimate risk assessment of acute medical instability and thereby indicates who needs inpatient care.

A team-based approach focussing on both the medical and psychiatric aspects of the disease is required. Weight restoration is essential to achieve medical stability through frequent monitoring of weight, vitals and electrolytes to monitor for signs of refeeding syndrome.

The gold standard psychiatric treatment for adolescents with eating disorders is family-based therapy once the patient has been medically stabilised.

Interpretation of Investigations

ECG may show sinus bradycardia or a prolonged QTc interval.

Continued

Box 31.8   An Adolescent With an Eating Disorder – cont'd

Electrolytes and renal function: electrolyte abnormalities such as hypokalaemia are common. Liver transaminases may be elevated.

Pitfalls to Avoid

This is a potentially life-threatening condition as the standardised mortality ratio for AN is six times that of the general population and is the highest rate of all mental health disorders in adolescence.

Anorexia nervosa is a diagnosis of exclusion, thus indicating the need to actively consider other diagnoses such as malignancy, inflammatory bowel disease or endocrine disorders, including hyperthyroidism and Addison's disease.

Suggested target weight gain ranges from 0.5 to 1.0 kg/week. Be cautious regarding the risk of refeeding syndrome. The key biochemical abnormality of this is a low phosphate level. Clinical features include a depressed level of consciousness, fluid overload, muscle weakness, diarrhoea and electrolyte derangement.

▶ **Video on the topic Adolescent health is available online at Elsevier eBooks+.**

Key References

Bagnell, A. L. (2011). Approaching the adolescent. In R. Goldbloom (Ed.), *Pediatric clinical skills* (4th ed., pp. 258–264). Saunders.

Carter, G., Page, A., Large, M., Hetrick, S., Milner, A. J., Bendit, N., et al. (2016). Royal Australian and New Zealand College of Psychiatrists clinical practice guideline for the management of deliberate self-harm. *The Australian and New Zealand Journal of Psychiatry, 50*(10), 939–1000.

HSE National Clinical Programme for Eating Disorders. (January 2018). *Eating disorder services.* HSE Model of Care for Ireland (Document Number: CSPD020/2017). National Clinical Strategy and Programmes Division, HSE Mental Health Services. https://www.hse.ie/eng/about/who/cspd/ncps/mental-health/eating-disorders/moc/hse-eating-disorder-services-model-of-care.pdf.

HSE National Clinical Programme for Eating Disorders. (n.d.). *Eating disorders.* National Clinical Strategy and Programmes Division, HSE Mental Health Services. https://www.hse.ie/eng/about/who/cspd/ncps/mental-health/eating-disorders/.

Israni, A. V., Kumar, S., & Hussain, N. (2018). Fifteen-minute consultation: An approach to a child presenting to the emergency department with acute psychotic symptoms. *Archives of Disease in Childhood – Education and Practice, 103*(4), 184–188.

Junior MARSIPAN Working Group. (January 2012). *Management of really sick patients under 18 with anorexia nervosa (College report CR168).* Royal College of Psychiatrists. https://www.rcpsych.ac.uk/docs/default-source/improving-care/better-mh-policy/college-reports/college-report-cr168.pdf.

Katzman, D. K. (2016). *Neinstein's adolescent and young adult health care: A practical guide.* Lippincott Williams & Wilkins.

Lee, L., Upadhya, K. K., Matson, P. A., Adger, H., & Trent, M. E. (2018). The status of adolescent medicine: Building a global adolescent workforce. *International Journal of Adolescent Medicine and Health, 28*(3), 233–243.

National Clinical Programme for Obesity. (2020). *HSE model of care for the management of overweight and obesity.* Royal College of Physicians of Ireland. https://www.hse.ie/eng/about/who/cspd/ncps/obesity/model-of-care/obesity-model-of-care.pdf.

National Clinical Programme for Paediatrics and Neonatology. (2016). *A National model of care for paediatric healthcare services in Ireland.* Clinical Strategy and Programmes Division, Health Service Executive, Royal College of Physicians of Ireland *(Chapter 8): Integrated Care.* https://www.hse.ie/eng/services/publications/clinical-strategy-and-programmes/model-of-care-for-paediatric-healthcare-integrated-care.pdf.

Norrington, A., Stanley, R., Tremlett, M., & Birrell, G. (2012). Medical management of acute severe anorexia nervosa. *Archives of Disease in Childhood – Education and Practice, 97*(2), 48–54.

Patton, G. C., Sawyer, S. M., Santelli, J. S., Ross, D. A., Afifi, R., Allen, N. B., et al. (2016). Our future: A Lancet commission on adolescent health and wellbeing. *Lancet, 387*(10036), 2423–2478.

Shah, R., Hagell, A., & Cheung, R. (February 2019). *International comparisons of health and wellbeing in adolescence and early adulthood.* Association for Young People's Health & Nuffield Trust. https://www.nuffieldtrust.org.uk/files/2019-02/1550657729_nt-ayph-adolescent-health-report-web.pdf.

Society for Adolescent Health and Medicine, Golden, N. H., Katzman, D. K., Sawyer, S. M., Ornstein, R. M., Rome, E. S., et al. (2015). Position paper of the Society for Adolescent Health and Medicine: Medical management of restrictive eating disorders in adolescents and young adults. *The Journal of Adolescent Health: Official Publication of the Society for Adolescent Medicine, 56*(1), 121–125. https://doi.org/10.1016/j.jadohealth.2014.10.259.

The Lancet. (2019). Health and wellbeing in adolescence and early adulthood. *Lancet, 393*(10174), 847.

Walsh, O., & McNicholas, F. (2020). Assessment and management of anorexia nervosa during COVID-19. *Irish Journal of Psychological Medicine, 37*(3), 187–191.

Online References

Young people's mental health. https://www.rcpsych.ac.uk/mental-health/parents-and-young-people.

The Skills Required to Be a Successful Paediatrician

32 Clinical Reasoning and the Clinical Consultation

ALF NICHOLSON and KEVIN DUNNE

I long to accomplish a great and noble task but it is my chief task to accomplish small tasks as if they were great and noble.

HELEN KELLER

There is little doubt that busy clinics and post-take ward rounds can be overwhelming. However, the key role of a senior trainee or consultant is to engage in a positive and energised way when making diagnoses following a consultation. With perhaps three to four clinics per week, it can be significantly challenging to remain empathic and focused, to quickly and efficiently identify common patterns, and to be able to take a closer analytical look when these common patterns do not fit the child or adolescent you are treating either in paediatric clinic (OPD), in ambulatory care, or as an inpatient. This is at the very core of what clinical paediatrics is all about, and these skills require experience and considerable resilience to maintain. The mark of an excellent paediatrician is the ability to quickly identify whether the child requires additional time and thought if the working diagnosis does not appear to fit. This skill is at the core of a successful acute paediatric service and a sustainable and safe clinic service.

As defined by Sir James Spence, an eminent British paediatrician, 'the essential unit of medical practice is the occasion when, in the intimacy of the consulting room or sick room, a person who is ill, or believes himself to be ill, seeks the advice of a doctor whom he trusts. This is a consultation and all else in the practice of medicine derives from it. The purpose of the consultation is that the doctor, having gathered his/her evidence, shall give explanation and advice'.

Consultation in primary care and paediatrics forms the basis of clinical practice. The traditional approach has been that, using a standard format starting with the presenting complaint (as outlined earlier in this book), the doctor goes through a detailed history, systematic examination and the judicious use of investigations to arrive at a diagnosis, and then resolve the problem. The model does not, however, address the issue of how the interview should be conducted or how the doctor-patient relationship should be developed. Most of these soft skills are learned from seniors by simple observation or role modelling. In modern medicine, this traditional model may not be adequate, as doctors now see many complex, life-limiting conditions for which there is no simple cure. Expectations are higher than ever before and the spectre of litigation always looms if a diagnosis is missed

or delayed. Quite often, children and adolescents present with illness without disease (see chapter 34 on illness without disease), in which case a biopsychosocial model of disease is evident.

Modern paediatric consultations do still involve gathering information, a proper clinical examination, and judicious use of investigations; however, detailed planning and explanation in manageable chunks are essential elements and require time. If the explanation and engagement of the child and family is inadequate or rushed, then the family depart dissatisfied, and the problems continue. Shared decision-making is a vital element of the paediatric and adolescent consultation. After a medical consultation, it is important to reflect as a trainee (or even consultant) on how the consultation went and if the time devoted to explanation and planning was adequate. Families can quickly sense a lack of empathy and understanding.

Doctors must capture and shape the attention of the child and family while developing narratives of their experiences and what is actually happening.

The frequent scenario of a paediatrician or family doctor extracting or typing in information on to a computer during a consultation may disrupt the invisible thread between the family and the clinician. Families should feel that the focus is on them and that the doctor has listened, paid attention and shown concern and empathy. This requires expertise in performance and in recognising how the narratives of the doctor and the family intertwine.

Medicine is seen as a science to an undergraduate student, but as a family doctor or paediatrician, the outpatient or ward round consultation should be treated as a performance in certain respects. Families recognise the qualifications and expertise of the doctor conducting the consultation, but what they experience most directly is the performance. Watch how experienced doctors perform and try to emulate their acquired skills with a focus on seeing it all from a family experience perspective. Good eye contact, attentive and empathic listening and taking time to explain are key elements of a successful consultation.

How to Run a Clinic

Most clinics work on a clear start and end time and time allowed for each new and review appointment. Ideally, the ratio of new patient to review patient should be about one to one. This must be managed with lots of advance preparation (definite reasons why appointment at a specialist clinic is required, senior decision making about discharge from the clinic, a robust 'was not brought' policy) and efficient use of nursing and health and social care professionals (HSCPs). New OPD referrals need to be screened, prioritised and divided into urgent (within 1 to 2 weeks), semi-urgent (2 to 12 weeks) and routine (over 12 weeks) categories. Setting these targets requires considerable collaboration and discussion with GP colleagues in the community to ensure that the number of routine referrals is kept to a minimum. This strong relationship with the local GP community with telephone consultations (so-called 'hot lines'), regular continuing professional development (CPD) sessions providing updates and the establishment of health and social care professional (HSCP), or nurse-led clinics are key elements to ensure a manageable stream of patients at the clinic. A population-based view is required whereby the volume of current referrals per week is matched to the clinic slots available, thus ensuring an efficient process of earlier specialist consultation. Particular attention should be given to high volume conditions (such as constipation, enuresis, developmental concerns, feeding issues and faltering growth) to ensure timely consultation, setting clear plans and engaging clinical nurses' specialists and HSCPs to work as part of the clinic team.

The consultant may prepare for the clinic by reviewing the most complex case notes the day before the clinic. On the day, the first key imperative is to arrive ahead of the designated time for the clinic to start. Just turning up at the clinic and working harder and harder to meet the ever-expanding demand is not a viable option. Pre-clinic preparation and efficient use of clinic time slots (usually 3 hours) are essential to a successful general paediatric specialist clinic. All members of the paediatric consultant team must operate the same philosophy, use their experience and areas of particular interest (e.g. food allergy), and work cohesively together and with their GP colleagues to ensure a responsive service geared towards the needs of their local community (Fig. 32.1).

Close collaboration and communication with the primary care team is essential, as are GP support tools such as e-referrals, direct access to diagnostics (simple x-rays and ultrasound), use of virtual clinics (now quite commonplace due to the pandemic), and the increased use of telemedicine. Clinic time slots are precious, and thus every effort should be made to use these time slots efficiently. Work from the Nuffield Trust and others has shown how close collaboration between paediatric specialists and their GP colleagues is the key to a far more effective OPD consultation service.

We should aim to divert routine and review appointment referrals back to the community to free up time for urgent and semi-urgent new referrals to outpatients.

In the outpatients, numerous studies have found that doctors tend to talk too much and listen too little. An excellent tip is to listen attentively without interrupting. The four components of the consultation are its initiation, the gathering of information, explanation and planning and the closing of the consultation.

A consideration of the ideas about the possible causes of the problem **(I)**, concerns **(C)** about the implications of the problem and the family's expectations **(E)** about management and outcome all need to be explored. Explore the family's expectations and concerns. Is the explanation offered understood, does it make sense, and will the treatment plan put forward work for them?

Keeping track of time is incredibly important as most appointments last between 20 and 40 minutes. For the sake of all the other patients arriving that day, it is critical that the clinic runs on time.

CLINIC LETTERS

Clinic letters should be clear, concise, and accurate. The letter should contain all results available or indicate if results are outstanding. Avoid repeating the full history as outlined in the referral letter and giving excessive details of investigations, and never patronise the GP by giving a mini lecture on the topic.

In managing non-attendance (or 'was not brought'), be aware that children are dependent on an adult to bring them to their appointment. Unless there are child protection or safety concern, write to the GP and the parents using a set format stating that they did not attend and that they are being discharged unless fresh concerns have arisen. In

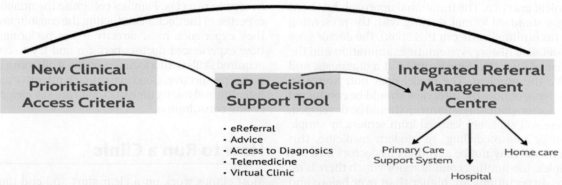

Figure 32.1   Standardised pathways of care. (Courtesy of HSE national OPD group.)

some clinics, the 'was not brought' rate can be as high as 20 per cent, so this element of the clinic needs to be carefully managed.

Pre- and post-clinic meetings are very important to enable the clinic to become a rich learning experience for trainees and students alike. A pre-clinic meeting may highlight what is likely to crop up, and interesting or challenging cases are discussed post-clinic. If required, the evidence base for investigation and treatment is also researched at this time. Making undergraduate students feel like part of the clinic is important; they tend to enjoy it far more when involved in history taking, travelling with the child for investigations (e.g. pulmonary function studies), or to see the clinical nurse specialist.

Becoming a Good Diagnostician

The ability to recognise the rare and obscure presentation and make a diagnosis of a rare condition amid a broad range of common presentations is the defining feature to becoming a successful senior trainee and consultant.

Becoming a good diagnostician should be the goal of every paediatric trainee. The way to develop one's skills is to observe how a senior doctor approaches a clinical problem. The common quality in all good doctors is attention to detail. One needs to know the key symptom and the key clinical sign. Get these correct and everything will usually fall into place.

It is not good enough to state that the child's presenting symptom is a cough. The symptom must be interrogated. How frequent is the cough and what is its duration? Is it present on exercise or at rest? Is it dry or productive? Does the child cough during sleep and have they missed school days? Clearly, a wet cough should immediately alert the doctor to the likelihood that the cough is important.

One must then proceed to find out if the cough is associated with a physical sign. You must know what you are looking for, otherwise you will not find it. If there is air trapping, the chest will be overinflated. The presence of finger clubbing is also a major finding with important diagnostic implications.

When a presumptive diagnosis is made, that is not the end of the matter. One must have a clear understanding about the period during which the child should get better. The diagnosis must be reviewed if improvement does not occur as expected. The ability to stop and change direction when required is the hallmark of a good clinician.

Common sense should always apply. For instance, if parents bring a child back for a second visit, do a careful review. If they come a third time, you need to act and do something else. Either they are overanxious or you have missed something important. The best option is to seek another opinion.

Dealing With Uncertainty

Both doctors and patients find uncertainty to be a very difficult concept and, aside from gaps in current knowledge (and there are many in paediatrics), there is the other issue of whether current medical knowledge applies to the particular sick child. Absolute certainty is unattainable and

thus we must tolerate a degree of uncertainty. In paediatrics, disease progression in acute illness can be quite rapid, so a period of observation or review will reassure a doctor that their initial diagnosis is correct. Dealing with the febrile under 2 years old is a case in point. There are clear discriminators pointing to a viral cause and, if these are present, referral to hospital is not necessary; however, always give the family the option of a review if required.

Clinical experience over time enables the doctor to have seen a vast range of mild illnesses and thereby get a sense of red flag symptoms. Many chapters in this book discuss red flag symptoms, and thus it is essentially about recognising near normality or mild illness and knowing whether the child's condition is deteriorating or atypical. Identify the worst possible outcome and try to assure yourself that it has been effectively ruled out. This technique of reflecting on practice 'in the moment' or reflecting on patients seen over the course of an outpatient session just finished are both valid techniques to obviate errors.

It is never easy, as being overly cautious leads to over investigation and unnecessary referral and a careless approach leads to potential missed diagnoses. At the end of a busy day or clinic, reflect on what you have seen and ask yourself if you are confident about the diagnoses made. Talking to a colleague over a lunch break also helps. This sensitive balance between knowledge based on experience and clinical acumen and a tolerance of an acceptable level of uncertainty is at the core of both general practice and paediatrics.

A Method of Consultation to Reduce Error

An error does not become a mistake until you refuse to correct it.

ORLANDO A BATTISTA

The following principles apply when conducting a consultation (Fig. 32.2).

These five steps do not take a lot of time but are crucial to ensure that you are safely practising what is still an art of medicine. Consider again the illness without disease chapter 34, and the relatively common symptoms of abdominal pain, chest pain or headaches. Consider the worst possible outcome but also consider the overwhelming likelihood that your clinical impression is correct. Paediatrics is both an art and a science after all, and it is both the attention you give to each consultation and this approach to review and documentation that will ensure that you continue to practice well and safely.

Information Overload

By 2022, it is estimated that new technical information will double every 72 hours and that about 50 per cent of what you know in the first year of medical training will be out of date by your third year. Around 5.6 billion internet searches will be done every month and 100 trillion bits per second will travel down one strand of optic fibre.

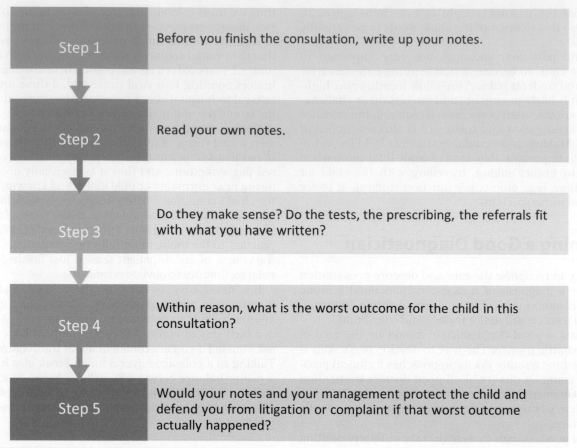

Step 1	Before you finish the consultation, write up your notes.
Step 2	Read your own notes.
Step 3	Do they make sense? Do the tests, the prescribing, the referrals fit with what you have written?
Step 4	Within reason, what is the worst outcome for the child in this consultation?
Step 5	Would your notes and your management protect the child and defend you from litigation or complaint if that worst outcome actually happened?

Figure 32.2　Principles of consultation. (Courtesy of Prof Wayne Cunningham.)

This endless supply of the latest information should not detract from the core essentials to making a clinical diagnosis. Most presentations to the outpatients involve common conditions (such as asthma or constipation) with clearly recognisable patterns of presentation. Making the diagnosis of one of these high-volume common diagnoses involves experience and thereby the ability to recognise the pattern of presentation. What is far more challenging and difficult is a situation in which several classical symptoms are present, but the presentation is atypical, or the child fails to response to treatment. One of the chief responsibilities of a senior decision maker (most often a consultant) is to recognise when the pattern does not fit a common diagnosis. This recognition enables a detailed review of the history, re-examination and comprehensive review of all investigations to date. This clinical skill is key to being a successful consultant because it enables rarer diagnoses to be made. It is all about recognising familiar patterns and then, if the patterns no longer fit, having a detailed re-think involving sub-specialists or referral and investigations to uncover a rare diagnosis. In an average post-take ward round, there may be one such patient (or likewise in an average clinic session) and it is really the responsibility and challenge for the consultant or senior trainee to recognise that patient and to take the time and thought to uncover the diagnosis. As a general paediatrician this ability is the key skill required as the role of a generalist is to effectively manage all the common presentations and to be able to identify rare presentations and seek subspecialist advice if required.

Wellness and Health in Doctors

There is no doubt that being a doctor is both rewarding and demanding, and medicine (in this instance, paediatrics) is challenging both physically and emotionally. There is a balance between wellness and work-related stress in doctors, and we all know colleagues who have lost that balance, allowing work-related stress to dominate. This may happen cumulatively, with too much on-call and overloaded clinics over a sustained period. Stress may dramatically increase following a sentinel adverse event or if an unhappy family is pursuing litigation. Developing coping strategies, having supportive colleagues and engaging in both self-care and reflective practices are all likely to tilt the balance towards wellness and resilience. On the other hand, unrealistic expectations, a perfectionist personality, always wishing to be the 'superhero' and an under-supportive culture at work can tilt the balance firmly towards work-related stress. There is little doubt that a complaint, adverse event or personal illness can all accentuate work-related stress. To promote their own wellness during training, doctors should explore their attitude to work, avoid being a 'superhero', and always be aware of their physical and mental health. Nobody wants to head down the slippery slope of compassion fatigue, burnout, depression, excessive anxiety or disruptive behaviours at work. Physician wellness, on the other hand, has been found to lead to improved system performance and patient outcomes.

In a pressurised health system burdened with administration, altered professional expectations and regulatory policies insufficiently aligned with professional values, the art of medicine can be eroded. Patient-centred health systems, on the other hand, give the doctor a sense of purpose and tend to rehumanise health care.

Burnout is an oft discussed term and contains three dimensions, including emotional exhaustion (always running on a 'flat battery'), depersonalisation (lack of empathy for children and their families) and reduced work satisfaction with decreased feelings of work accomplishment. Burnout and compassion fatigue are both highly counterproductive to excellent patient care. It is now acknowledged that burnout tends to start early during undergraduate education in medicine and, if tackled and addressed, can be prevented later during a long medical career.

The components of wellness, on the other hand, are good physical health, excellent psychological health, self-care, development of resilience and coping strategies and being prepared to engage in reflective practice. Reflective practice is especially important for trainees to be able to reflect on the effects of their experiences and the fact that medicine and paediatrics are inexact sciences. Recognising fallibility and that mistakes do occur are vital learning elements of a successful training programme. Engaging in mindfulness and exercise are particularly useful to promote wellness. Exercise, laughter and meditation have all been shown to increase endorphin levels, which contributes to an overall sense of well-being.

Likewise, many hospitals conduct regular Schwartz Rounds, during which professionals (doctors, nurses, health and social care professionals, or support staff) can recount their experiences of clinical events that have made a significant impact on them. General discussion occurs thereafter in a supportive and confidential atmosphere. We have personally found these Schwartz Rounds to be very helpful.

Therefore, the clinical consultation is at the centre of making a diagnosis. Significant training is required to ensure that consultations are successful and, in relation to ward rounds and clinic sessions, considerable thought should be put in to ensure that high volume does not lead to underperformance. As a career in paediatrics can be stressful and emotionally draining, it is important to develop self-care and wellness strategies, ideally prior to graduation.

The health and wellness of the doctor has a considerable impact on the health of children seen by that doctor. A focus on wellness should commence in the undergraduate years in medical school. Students need adequate coaching and mentoring if they are to successfully develop their own professional identity.

Developing Resilience

Developing resilience is a key skill as a doctor and, if working in a hospital or group GP setting, requires attention to both institutional and individual factors. A strong and supportive institutional culture is fundamental to ensure that the individual can practice with security and confidence.

I cannot overemphasise the importance of a healthy, resilient and well-supported team working within a supportive medical culture – it is this positive working environment that leads to excellent patient care.

(Box 32.1)

Box 32.1 Key Points

Shared decision-making is a vital element of the paediatric and adolescent consultation.

Good eye contact, attentive and empathic listening, and taking time to explain are key elements of a successful consultation.

GP support tools include e-referrals, direct access to diagnostics (simple x-rays and ultrasound), the use of virtual clinics (now quite commonplace due to the pandemic) and increased use of telemedicine.

Clinic letters should be clear, concise and accurate.

Becoming a good diagnostician should be the goal of every paediatric trainee.

The key skill required as a generalist is to effectively manage all the common presentations and to be able to pick out rarer presentations and seek subspecialist advice if required.

Burnout and compassion fatigue are both highly counterproductive to excellent patient care.

Wellness involves good physical health, excellent psychological health, self-care, development of resilience and coping strategies and being prepared to engage in reflective practice.

Recognising fallibility and that mistakes do occur are key learning elements of a successful postgraduate training programme.

Key References

Bhatnagar, G. (2020). Physician burnout. *Lancet, 395*(10221), 333.

Kneebone, R. L. (2017a). Making medicine bespoke. *Lancet, 389*(10064), 19.

Kneebone, R. L. (2017b). Performing magic, performing medicine. *Lancet, 389*(10064), 148–149.

Kneebone, R. L. (2018). Introducing in practice. *Lancet, 391*(10122), 723.

Kneebone, R. L. (2019). Dissecting the consultation. *Lancet, 393*(10183), 1795.

Nuffield Trust. (n.d.). Latest from the Nuffield Trust. https://www.nuffieldtrust.org.uk/.

Rich, A., Viney, R., Needleman, S., Griffin, A., & Woolf, K. (2016). 'You can't be a person and a doctor': The work-life balance of doctors in training-a qualitative study. *BMJ Open, 6*(12). e013897.

The Lancet. (2019). Physician burnout: A global crisis. *Lancet, 394*(10193), 93.

33 Learning From Clinical Events

ALF NICHOLSON and WAYNE CUNNINGHAM

Experience is simply the name we give to our mistakes

OSCAR WILDE

Paediatrics is a wonderful specialty and dealing with children and adolescents is a great pleasure most, if not all, of the time. Societal expectation now is such that mistakes or misadventures are not tolerated, and many countries have very high rates of litigation. As a result, doctors (including GPs and paediatricians) have become most risk-averse and less tolerant of uncertainty. Adverse clinical events do occur relatively frequently, but many do not lead to harm. However, rare sentinel events do happen and can have devastating consequences on the family as well as on the medical and other healthcare professionals involved. One of the great challenges of modern paediatrics is to practise safely without being overcautious or reliant on investigations. Far too often, infants and children are admitted to hospital when a short period of observation (perhaps 4 hours) and input by a senior decision maker would have been sufficient. Our hospital care model needs to move towards an ambulatory model based on prudent use of investigations, the importance of observation over time and empowering both parents and primary care physicians to maintain children in the community and out of hospital.

One might argue that errors in the practice of medicine are ultimately unavoidable, as we all get it wrong at times. However, errors can be minimised using the strategies outlined below.

A New Landscape

The famous painting by *Luke Fildes* from 1891 (Tate Gallery, London) depicts a sick child at home being looked after by the family doctor. The painting highlights the stark differences between past and current paediatric care. In the past, sick children were almost exclusively managed at home by their family doctor. We have now moved to a hospital-focussed model, which accommodates ever-increasing numbers of children admitted to hospital with relatively minor illness, and the upward trend is stark.

341

There have been dramatic changes in disease priorities for child health due to immunisation and improved standards of living. Many 'killer' diseases have disappeared as a result of these changes. Allergic disease, chronic and complex disabilities, and emotional and behavioural problems have all increased in prevalence. In tandem with these are also changes in parental expectation, a desire for faster access to specialist care, and – via the internet – parents are now an 'informed' client group.

Over the past 30 years, there have been many success stories in paediatrics and child health, with a very significant drop in mortality rates for children younger than 5 years in developed countries across the world. Countries that heavily invest in reducing social inequities and supporting families (in particular the Nordic countries and Japan) have the lowest under-5 mortality rates. Conversely, despite being one of the world's wealthiest countries, the United States has a relatively high under-5 mortality rate for a variety of reasons (such as unequal access to health care). Out of 1000 infants born in Sweden and Norway, 997 would be expected to reach their fifth birthday – a stunning achievement.

Sadly, there is still a very high rate of avoidable death in under 5-year-olds in resource-deficient countries, mainly relating to infections, injuries and poor nutrition.

Strategies developed in Ireland and the UK have focussed on patient-centred care, greater cost awareness and accountability, keeping children healthy, using data to plan services, eHealth (never more important than during the COVID-19 pandemic), integrated or joint care, and 'hospitals without walls'. Safe high-quality care can be delivered now and into the future by empowering parents and supporting primary care doctors.

Safe Practice

One of the significant challenges is supporting doctors in primary care in this ever-developing, fast changing world of modern paediatrics. Most have received just a few weeks of undergraduate training and 4 to 6 months in hospital-based paediatrics thereafter.

Responding to Errors

Response when an error has occurred is indeed very challenging and the doctor involved often becomes the 'second victim'. A sentinel event while in a training programme can have a devastating psychological effect on a trainee and the whole multidisciplinary team. Errors are inevitable and the secret is to learn from them, to share that learning, and to establish a 'safety net' to catch errors and thus avoid or lessen any potential harm to the child.

What those affected want or need when an error has occurred is shown in Fig. 33.1.

These are reasonable expectations and, in many ways, how you respond when an error has occurred defines you. It is not an easy process, but both the doctor and patient (and the family) proceed on a shared journey with both determined that every effort will be made to avoid a similar error in the future.

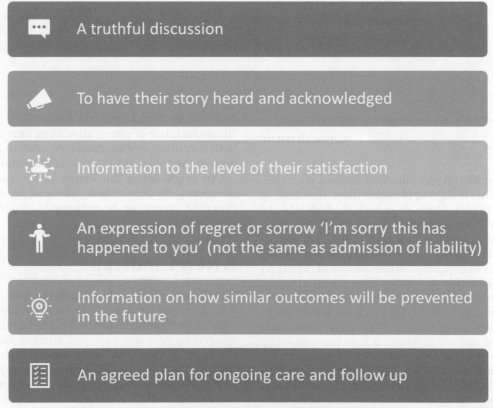

A truthful discussion

To have their story heard and acknowledged

Information to the level of their satisfaction

An expression of regret or sorrow 'I'm sorry this has happened to you' (not the same as admission of liability)

Information on how similar outcomes will be prevented in the future

An agreed plan for ongoing care and follow up

Figure 33.1 Strategy when dealing with errors.

The Medical Protection Society recommends the ASSIST method as an approach to deal with a complaint or when an error has happened (Fig. 33.2).

There are a number of golden rules to follow after a complaint and when legal action is likely or already in process (Fig. 33.3).

Safe HealthCare in Hospitals

Hospital-based paediatrics is also very challenging, but there are helpful rules in place to ensure high-quality care. These again focus on documentation, excellent communication between healthcare professionals, learning from near misses, proper and formalised efficient handover, and a commitment both at an individual and corporate level to quality improvement. These principles need to be enshrined during undergraduate education and are a major component of outcome-based postgraduate training curricula in paediatrics. As a consultant, it is critical to listen carefully to junior members of the team, all other team members and to parental concerns. As a trainee, you must be confident enough to speak up on call or on a ward round and voice your concerns. Do not be deferential to your superiors but remain respectful of their expertise and experience. Assert yourself. The quality improvement process is now firmly established in hospital practice with paediatricians such as Dr Don Berwick having been international leaders in the field of quality in health care.

The **five** key elements for quality health care for children are as follows:

PATIENT PARTNERSHIP

The purpose of all health services is to provide for patient needs in a manner that serves patient preference. This requires a new relationship between patients and providers that recognises this and balances it with other demands such as cost,

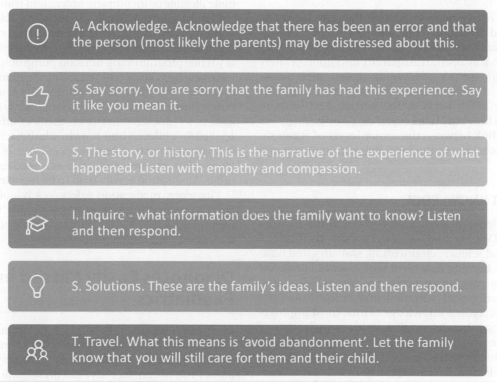

A. Acknowledge. Acknowledge that there has been an error and that the person (most likely the parents) may be distressed about this.

S. Say sorry. You are sorry that the family has had this experience. Say it like you mean it.

S. The story, or history. This is the narrative of the experience of what happened. Listen with empathy and compassion.

I. Inquire - what information does the family want to know? Listen and then respond.

S. Solutions. These are the family's ideas. Listen and then respond.

T. Travel. What this means is 'avoid abandonment'. Let the family know that you will still care for them and their child.

Figure 33.2 ASSIST method when medical error has occurred.

Contact your medico-legal indemnifier immediately	After a complaint, doctors enter a legal world of which they have no experience and even less control. This is the world of lawyers. You are not a lawyer, so do not try to be one.
Follow their advice	Always follow their advice. Do nothing without checking with your medico-legal advisor: never write letters, attend hearings, give statements without checking. Never ever go to the public domain be that the press or social media.

Figure 33.3 Golden rules after a complaint.

staff availability, location and the wishes of other patients. Focussing on the outcomes that matter to patients and their experience within the health system is important and can only be developed in partnership. Getting real patient input requires the development of training and support for patients and families who wish to become more involved.

CLINICAL LEADERSHIP

The role of leaders is to promote, articulate and share a vision of quality for the real world. Leaders shape a culture and help create the conditions that enable staff to deliver quality care. Primary attributes of professional health leaders are their credibility and their understanding of the complexity of the healthcare system. Clinical leaders should act to the values of their organisation as well as the values that speak to them. Leadership must be sought, nurtured, coached and developed.

INTEGRATED GOVERNANCE

Integrated governance helps to provide the structures and agreed rules and standards that enable complex healthcare systems to achieve quality. Governance also provides accountability that is open, transparent and appropriately responsive. The integration of governance structures across traditional lines (clinical, operational, finance) accepts the interdependency of all parts of the system and leads to improvements in how they work together. Good governance serves as a vital link between the senior levels of organisations and those working in the front line with children and their families.

IMPROVEMENT KNOWLEDGE

Improvement science has emerged both from the theories of W. Edwards Deming and experience from the fields of psychology, social science, engineering, statistics and business know-how. Deming described four essential areas for improvement: the psychology of change, an understanding of systems, measurement variation and various methods of building improvement knowledge. Thus, most improvement methodology has its origins in the application of Deming's theories, including the Model for Improvement. Regardless of which method is applied, the value of using proven methods is now well accepted in health care. Leading principles include the importance of standardisation and ensuring that all activity benefits the patient. All methods highlight the need to access the unique knowledge and experience that frontline staff possess and to involve them in any change process. Everybody working in health care should have a basic understanding of quality improvement methods recognising that it is a shared responsibility. Some may require advanced training to support implementation and quality improvement efforts.

DATA

The need for measurement and data is central for all quality improvement initiatives. It is impossible to show evidence of improvement without data. For clinicians, this requires a new understanding about the application of data that differs from that used in medical research. Understanding the value of using small amounts of data over time, and the importance of how that data is presented to influence behaviour, is critical. Better use of information technology to assist with data collection and analysis helps support the implementation of national models of care.

SAFE PRESCRIBING AND AVOIDANCE OF MEDICATION ERRORS

Safe prescribing is a key area as medication errors can occur at any point in the medication process, including prescribing, transcribing, dispensing or the administration of medications.

Children are uniquely vulnerable to medication errors due to weight-based dosing, the need for dilution to administer small amounts of medication, immature hepatic and renal mechanisms of drug metabolism in children, and the inability of young children to self-administer medications or to communicate side effects. Computerised prescription order entry (CPOE) is now used in many hospitals and helps to eliminate illegible or incomplete orders and transcription errors.

Clinical pharmacists in the inpatient setting also play an important role in reducing medication errors. SMART pumps are infusion delivery systems that decrease reliance on memory while programming infusion pump doses and rates. They have also been shown to reduce medication errors.

Medication safety in the community is also an issue, and publications such as *Medicines for Children* in the UK provide leaflets to educate parents on medications commonly prescribed for children and how to administer them.

Medication errors tend to occur out of hours and most often related to misreading or not reading the medication order. Medication errors tend to be reported by nurses.

Therefore, medication safety is a major priority – strategies to reduce the risk of error include CPOE, barcoding technology with SMART pumps, mobile application devices and workflow management systems.

Diagnoses Easily Missed in Paediatrics

In essence, we are reflecting on potential errors in different situations that will hopefully help you on your journey to safer practice. Experience is incredibly important and allows you to consider atypical presentations and gives you a 'sixth sense' that a diagnosis may need to be reviewed. As experienced paediatricians, we wish to highlight situations in which you must be aware of potential diagnoses that are essential not to miss:

The Newborn Examination

These examinations are most often performed in high volume under time pressure by junior residents or senior house officers (SHOs). The examination takes about 5 to 6 minutes at most and involves taking a brief history. What we are always careful about not missing are an absent red reflex (indicating a potential cataract), a submucous cleft palate, developmental dysplasia of the hip (DDH), imperforate anus and absent femoral pulses. All these can easily be missed at the newborn check, as can central cyanosis due to cyanotic congenital heart disease (hence all newborns have pulse oximetry prior to hospital discharge). All have major consequences if not diagnosed; thus, picking up all of the above requires superior clinical technique. The reader should also refer to Chapter 4 (the newborn and 6-week examination) for further discussion.

RED REFLEX ABSENT

Examination of the red reflex requires experience and patience. A delayed diagnosis of cataract will affect visual outcome, so prompt referral to a paediatric ophthalmologist is required. Absence of the red reflex is also seen in retinoblastoma.

SUBMUCOUS CLEFT PALATE

Submucous cleft palate is also easily missed and may present subsequently with a history of feeding issues including milk coming down the nose.

DEVELOPMENTAL DYSPLASIA OF THE HIP (DDH)

Picking up an unstable or dislocated hip requires proficient technique in both Barlow and Ortolani testing and ultrasound screening for high-risk infants. Despite this, DDH can still be missed with the later requirement for operative intervention.

IMPERFORATE ANUS

Always check for anal patency and ensure that meconium has been passed.

REDUCED VOLUME OF FEMORAL PULSES

Femoral pulses are difficult to palpate and the ductus arteriosus remains open for a number of days leading to weak rather than absent femoral pulses. Coarctation of the aorta is the most frequently missed congenital heart disease. These infants present subsequently with poor feeding, poor weight gain, and evidence of heart failure with fast respirations, a big liver and occasionally cardiogenic shock.

The 6-Week Check

These examinations are generally performed in primary care. To maintain clinical skills, we recommend that a small number of GPs in a practice develop expertise via a high volume of examinations. Again, the examination is an opportunity to pick up on conditions that may not have been noted on the newborn examination, such as a congenital cataract, DDH or a cardiac murmur.

A NEW MURMUR

The murmur of a ventricular septal defect may not be obvious until the 6-week check. At this examination, the murmur may be loud, pansystolic and heard all over the preacordium. Some may have associated poor feeding, sweating during feeds and poor weight gain due to congestive heart failure.

CENTILES

At the 6-week check, we focus on issues related to feeding and weight gain, assessment of head growth and plotting on a centile chart, and also ensuring that both testes are descended.

JAUNDICE THAT IS NOT CLEARING AFTER 2 WEEKS

If jaundice is present or slow to clear, the main questions to ask are related to stool and urine colour. Pale stools and dark urine associated with prolonged jaundice require a blood test to assess for a raised conjugated bilirubin level and to investigate for biliary atresia.

Infancy

MY BABY IS 'NOT RIGHT'

The assertion by a mother that 'my baby is not right' should always raise concerns as it reflects maternal instinct, which always deserves ultimate respect. It has a myriad of potential causes, but alarm bells should always ring, especially in the under 8-week age group.

In the setting of fever, a concern about lethargy (and thereby an affected feeding schedule) should point to sepsis. The 'traffic light' system is helpful in this instance. Bacterial sepsis is now quite rare due to vaccination, so you are less likely to see invasive meningococcal disease during your paediatric training, which may make it more difficult to recognise when encountered for the first time. Significant clinical clues are pallor, cold peripheries, a petechial rash (not always present) and an infant who is 'just not right'. Meningococcal disease and viral illness are relatively indistinguishable in their early stages. Therefore, you should always seek to review the infant, or observe the infant in hospital for a longer period to investigate for an elevated heart rate, as tachycardia is the cardinal sign of septic shock in infancy. Always check for a non-blanching rash. Always listen to the mother; if she is concerned, you should be too.

NIGHTMARE COLIC

Colic is another relatively frequent symptom that should not be underplayed (see chapter 28). It is common, usually peaks at 6 to 8 weeks of age and predominantly occurs during the evening. Consider intolerance to cow's milk protein if very severe and if no evening predominance. Exclusion of milk protein may transform the infant and offer immense relief to the parents. Be very aware that an infant who is constantly crying is a great source of stress in the household. Parents can find it all 'too much', and hospital referral is advised if you suspect that either or both parents has had enough. Abusive head trauma is far more common in infants with colic and needs to be considered and prevented if possible.

TREMULOUS JERKS

Infantile spasms tend to occur in clusters and may be confused with tremulousness. The clustering and slowed acquisition of developmental milestones are characteristic and infantile spasms require prompt investigation (EEG showing hypsarrhythmia) and treatment.

EARLY HAND PREFERENCE BEFORE 18 MONTHS OF AGE

Developmental limit ages are described in the chapter 3 on systems and development, but the chief issue is that urgent neurology referral is needed if an infant is developmentally regressing or has lost acquired skills. An early hand preference (before 18 months of age), inability to sit alone by 9 months of age and absence of parachute reflexes all point to a possible diagnosis of cerebral palsy.

CONSTIPATION FROM BIRTH

Delayed diagnosis of Hirschsprung's disease is common. The greatest clue is failure to pass meconium within 24 hours of birth but presentation with enterocolitis at 2 or 3 months of age is possible. Infants with enterocolitis associated with Hirschsprung's disease present with diarrhoea, shock, fever and abdominal distension, and require prompt hospitalisation.

BILIOUS VOMITS

Bilious vomits (grass green) in an infant are always significant and should prompt urgent surgical consultation to exclude obstruction (e.g. malrotation with a midgut volvulus).

Toddlers

HEAD TILT

Head tilt or torticollis is relatively common and usually benign. However, if associated with vomiting and a new squint due to a sixth nerve palsy and ataxia, a posterior fossa brain tumour should be considered.

FUNNY BREATHING AT NIGHT

Snoring is also relatively common; however, in about 3 per cent of toddlers, it may be associated with episodes of apnoea with or without cyanosis. If evident during deep sleep, this indicates obstructive sleep apnoea. Adenotonsillectomy is curative but keep in mind that obstructive sleep apnoea is far more common in craniofacial disorders, severe obesity and in Down syndrome than in the general population.

AN ACUTE LIMP

Transient synovitis (usually of the hip) and minor trauma are very common in toddlers. A toddler refusing to walk or bear weight is likely to have either of these two conditions. However, septic arthritis needs to be considered if there is a high fever, if the affected joint is held in a position of comfort and if the toddler refuses to walk. Never discharge a toddler with a limp until the limp has disappeared or a diagnosis has been made. A fever above 38.5°C, refusal to bear weight, an ESR above 40 mm/h, and a white cell count above 12.0×10^9 are four Kocher criteria that help distinguish septic arthritis from transient synovitis.

PROLONGED FEVER

Kawasaki's disease is both an exotic condition and a cause of a prolonged fever in young children. It needs to be distinguished from conditions such as adenovirus infection, measles, parvovirus B19 and Group A streptococcal infections. Fever must be evident for 5 days or more and other criteria need to be met. The key intervention is intravenous immunoglobulin, which reduces the incidence of coronary artery aneurysms from over 25 per cent to under 5 per cent if given within 10 days of fever onset. Irritability is a dominant feature in Kawasaki's disease.

WORRISOME BRUISING

Bruising is relatively frequent in toddlers and is generally over the anterior tibial surfaces. Unusual patterns of bruising, delayed presentation or other concerns should point to a possible diagnosis of non-accidental injury, and an in-depth review by a hospital paediatric team and social work team is now mandated. Both coagulopathy (Von Willebrand's disease, immune thrombocytopaenic purpura (ITP)) and Mongolian blue spots may present as apparent bruising with concerns of physical abuse. Coagulation screening is essential as is a skeletal survey. It is impossible to age bruising in children.

PERSISTENT COUGHING

Choking episodes are common in toddlers as they often place objects in their mouths. A witnessed choking event is by far the most important factor in pinpointing an early diagnosis of foreign body inhalation. If the event goes unnoticed, the child may then present with a dry, persistent cough. Peanuts, carrots and raisins are frequent offenders. A chest x-ray may show air trapping or atelectasis, but bronchoscopy is the main investigation. Therefore, a persistent cough following a choking episode (however brief) should always raise concern about possible foreign body inhalation.

CALL TO THE SURGICAL WARD

Abdominal pain 8 weeks post-appendicectomy with or without distension may indicate possible obstruction due to adhesions. Post-tonsillectomy bleeding may indicate infection in the tonsillar bed.

School-Going Children

NEW ONSET BED WETTING

About 30 per cent of children with newly diagnosed diabetes mellitus have at least one related medical visit to their GP prior to the diagnosis, causing some to evolve into diabetic ketoacidosis. Consider diabetes in all children who have secondary nocturnal enuresis (dry at night before but now wet), polyuria, polydipsia (especially if nocturnal) and weight loss. A single capillary blood glucose above

11.1 mmol/L indicates diabetes. Diabetes is usually type 1 (95 per cent) and its prevalence has increased steadily across Europe and North America. A high blood sugar level should prompt same-day referral to hospital.

HEADACHES

Headaches are very common in healthy school-going children and are usually due to tension or migraine. A crescendo pattern of headaches, early morning headaches relieved by vomiting or a new squint should always prompt consideration of a brain tumour with raised intracranial pressure.

DAYDREAMING

Daydreaming is very common in schoolchildren but must be distinguished from childhood absence epilepsy. Childhood absence seizures begin with a sudden impairment of consciousness, where the child stares blankly and is unresponsive, and usually last between 8 and 15 seconds (always less than 30 seconds). There is no recollection of the event and no postictal phase. Some patients may be aware of a 'lapse' in concentration or losing track of a conversation (those in the child's company may report the same). Seizures typically occur on a daily basis with tens of seizures occurring each day. All of the history is important in determining whether or not the episodes are seizures.

SYNCOPE

Simple faints or vasovagal syncope are most commonly triggered by a warm environment, prolonged standing, painful stimuli (a blood test) or insufficient intake. Be aware of long QT syndrome as a differential for either an apparent faint or seizure; the best way to pick this up is to order an ECG. Exertional syncope should always be of concern, so an accurate history is of the utmost importance. Refer to Chapter 11 (congenital heart disease) for more information.

Adolescence

A full and detailed adolescent history is vital, as is taking time to discuss issues with the adolescent alone in addition to discussing parental concerns. Risk-taking behaviour and cyberbullying are current issues of increasing prevalence.

SUICIDE RISK

Deliberate self-harm is increasingly prevalent and always requires input from the Child and Adolescent Psychiatry team either in hospital or in the community. Risk assessment for suicide following an episode of deliberate self-harm is quite challenging.

WEIGHT LOSS

Extreme weight loss with amenorrhoea in girls and associated altered body image are characteristic of anorexia nervosa. Anorexia nervosa is a critical diagnosis for which the Junior MARSIPAN criteria for hospitalisation are very helpful. Beware of differentials of anorexia, including craniopharyngioma, Addison's disease and Crohn's disease.

HIP OR KNEE PAIN

Slipped capital femoral epiphysis occurs during periods of rapid growth in adolescence when shear forces, especially if obese, lead to epiphysis displacement. A chronic slip is the most common presentation, with symptoms often present for weeks or months as the slip progresses. Pain is often referred to the knee, which can be very misleading. The key physical sign is loss of internal rotation of the leg in flexion with pain at extreme movement. Anteroposterior and lateral x-rays of both hips are required to diagnose the condition. The adolescent is admitted to hospital and placed on bed rest to avoid acute displacement of a chronic slip. Surgery is required to stabilise a displaced capital femoral epiphysis. Avascular necrosis and chondrolysis are the complications of slipped capital femoral epiphysis that we are trying to avoid, and both are markedly reduced post screw fixation (less than 1.5 per cent).

TESTICULAR PAIN

Many boys experience testicular pain, which most often relates to viral epididymo-orchitis. However, a sudden onset of testicular pain (with sometimes misleading severe abdominal pain, mimicking appendicitis) with a tender, elevated, transversely located testis and loss of the cremasteric reflex suggests testicular torsion. This is a surgical emergency requiring prompt surgical treatment and detorsion. (Box 33.1)

Box 33.1   **Key Points**

Adverse clinical events occur relatively frequently, but many do not lead to harm. Sentinel events are devastating for both the family and the professionals involved.

A sentinel event while in a training programme can have a devastating psychological effect on a trainee and the whole multidisciplinary team.

The Medical Protection Society recommends the ASSIST method (Fig. 33.2) as the correct strategy to handle a complaint or when an error has occurred.

For safer care in hospitals, focus on documentation, excellent communication between healthcare professionals, learning from near misses, formalised efficient handover and a commitment both at an individual and corporate level to quality improvement.

Factors that make children uniquely vulnerable to medication errors include weight-based dosing, dilution to administer small amounts of medication, immature hepatic and renal mechanisms of drug metabolism in children, and the inability of young children to self-administer medications or communicate side effects.

Experience is incredibly important and allows you to consider atypical presentations and gives you a 'sixth sense' that the diagnosis may need to be reviewed.

Key References

Abrams, D. J., Perkin, M. A., & Skinner, J. R. (2010). Long QT syndrome [published correction appears in *BMJ, 340*, c366]. *BMJ, 340*, b4815.

Berwick, D. M., Blanton Godfrey, A., & Roessner, J. (2002). *Curing health care: New strategies for quality improvement*. Jossey-Bass.

Clarke, N. M., & Kendrick, T. (2009). Slipped capital femoral epiphysis. *BMJ, 339*, b4457.

Deming, W. E. (2012). In J. Orsini, & D. D. Cahill (Eds.), *The essential deming: Leadership principles from the father of quality*. McGraw-Hill Education.

Hill, I. D. (2020). Using QI to break bad habits. *Journal of Pediatrics, 225*, 1–2.

Institute for Health Improvement. (n.d.). *Improving Health and Health Care Worldwide*. www.ihi.org.

Kahn, S., & Abramson, E. L. (2019). What is new in paediatric medication safety? *Archives of Disease in Childhood, 104*(6), 596–599.

Medicines for Children. (n.d.). *We provide practical and reliable advice about giving medicines to your child*. https://www.medicinesforchildren.org.uk/.

National Clinical Programme for Paediatrics and Neonatology. (n.d.). *A National Model of Care for Paediatric Healthcare Services in Ireland*. https://www.hse.ie/eng/services/publications/clinical-strategy-and-programmes/model-of-care-for-paediatric-healthcare-executive-summary.pdf.

Nicholson, A. (2021). Further reflections on the report of the Mother and Baby Homes Commission. *Irish Medical Journal, 114*(3), 303.

34 Illness Without Disease

WAYNE CUNNINGHAM

The paediatrician's mission is to relieve anxiety – and all our knowledge, research, diagnosis and treatments are only means to that end

DR HARRY H. GORDON

Care of a patient who has illness without disease (also termed somatisation) can be a significant challenge for doctors in every clinical field of medicine, and paediatric practice is no exception. Fortunately, although somatisation can feel frustrating for doctors and families, caring for children with somatisation can be one of the most rewarding types of clinical work. Somatisation, or more correctly, care of the somatising patient, is an important part of medical practice, and the purpose of this chapter is to outline how doctors might better understand the condition, its diagnosis and help restore their patient to good health.

Here we present a method for diagnosing somatisation, offer advice about how to recognise 'red flags', and appropriately investigate common paediatric presentations where somatisation is common, but serious physical pathology must not be missed.

Somatisation

What, then, is somatisation? Our way of explaining somatisation (from the Greek 'soma' or 'body') to families is as the process through which children and young people have bodily symptoms caused by some form of unresolved psychological stress. The key word is 'unresolved'. Everyone, including children, suffers from stress. Most stress is eventually resolved in some way, and we carry on with our lives and do not become unwell. However, stress is sometimes unable to be resolved, causing us to suffer bodily symptoms that can range from being a mere nuisance to being quite disabling. Regardless of the form that it takes and what part of the body it affects, somatisation is always characterised by a lack of demonstrable underlying pathology. For example, there are no brain tumours causing the child's headache, no sign of inflammatory bowel disease causing abdominal pain or bloating, and no ECG abnormality to account for palpitations or syncope.

The concept of stress is mostly familiar to children and their parents, but a further concept is worth exploring – that the mind and the body are, in fact, connected. This link is at the heart of somatisation.

The explanation is as follows: we are all the things that collectively make us a person – our bodies, minds, relationships, spirituality, history, perceived futures, schoolwork, aspirations, cultures, values, beliefs and so on. Unresolved stress in any of these areas may lead to psychological distress and the experience of bodily symptoms thereby termed somatisation. Helping patients to arrive at an understanding that somatisation is not 'made up' or 'fake' or 'just in their heads' is the starting point for healing.

Somatisation is a legitimate, real, and entirely acceptable diagnosis. However, somatisation is a challenge to the conventional way that doctors think about the cause and effect of disease. Consider the following ideas. Children present to their doctor because they are suffering and need help. They will usually have discoverable pathology such as acute asthma or appendicitis that appropriately fits conventional medical history taking, examination, investigation and intervention, all of which lead to a successful outcome. However, somatisation does not usually 'seem' to fit, and sometimes two undesirable things happen. The first is that children with somatisation are often over-investigated, which carries cost and risk to patients and healthcare systems. The approach of 'diagnosis by exclusion' wastes time and resources. It is a search for a pathology that does not exist. It also risks patients developing 'somatic fixation' with an over-emphasis on physical symptoms and investigations while avoiding questions about personal and psychological stressors. The second adverse outcome is that doctors lose confidence, thus becoming unwilling or unable to consider the possibility of somatisation, thereby persisting with a purely biomedical model of practice which fails the child and family.

In 2013, Drs Mann and Wilson helpfully suggested several key questions that may help to diagnose somatisation. Firstly, ask what was going on in the child's and family's life when the symptoms started, and then ask whether the symptoms ever relate to pressures at home or in school. Enquire further whether there are times when symptoms get better or disappear and whether there are times when symptoms are always, or very likely, to be present.

Carefully exploring the above questions allows identification of possible stressors. Often, there is a clear temporal relationship to the patient's symptoms, especially where there has been a marked change in a child who was quite well who now has new, emergent symptoms.

Once diagnosed, or even suspected, empathy towards the child and normalisation of the diagnosis are required. At some time in life, just about everyone experiences bodily symptoms in relation to stress, ranging from a dull headache after an overly busy day at work, or the 'butterflies' of anxiety before sitting an important examination, to the often debilitating symptoms of irritable bowel syndrome. It is essential to show empathy to the child and family and ensure them that you understand their suffering is real. Normalisation means carefully explaining how common and, in fact, normal it is to suffer bodily symptoms at times of stress. In our experience, normalisation of the somatisation experience is extremely powerful and therapeutic. Families need to hear that they are not making this up and that they are not alone in their experiences.

In terms of providing support after making a diagnosis of somatisation, much depends on how receptive or accepting the patient and their family indicate themselves to be. Be aware that a family may have a particular health belief system shaped by prior experiences or interactions with the healthcare system. A family may be deeply entrenched in biomedicine and insist that there is a physical cause for their symptoms that must be uncovered by further investigations or obtaining further opinions. This can be very challenging and unsettling for doctors, and takes confidence and fortitude to resist these requests. Sometimes it is best to obtain specialist assistance from psychologist colleagues. Another challenge for doctors is realising that, unlike acute asthma or appendicitis, the unresolved stress may not be easily 'fixable'. Family discord and poverty or other stressors can all manifest as somatisation, and none can be fixed with a simple intervention. Our approach is to individualise the management in open discussion with the child and their parents to plan a path forward.

Even though a child may present with what appears to be classical somatisation, be alert to atypical or red flag features that should alert you to organic pathology. Always be willing to revisit the diagnosis if symptoms change or if the child is not improving. Under various headings, we will now explore some characteristics of somatisation presentations in children, and some of the red flags that should alert the doctor to serious underlying pathology.

Functional Abdominal Pain (FAP)

This concept was originally described in 1958 by Apley and Naish. They reported that, in a sample of 1000 healthy school children, just over 10 per cent reported recurrent abdominal pain. Their three observations are still pertinent to this day: '*First*, the high incidence of recurrent abdominal pains, especially at certain ages and particularly in girls. *Second*, the high incidence of abdominal pain and other complaints in the families of affected children. *Third*, the lack of evidence of any physical cause, and the positive association of frequent emotional disturbance'.

Several differentials (Crohn's disease, coeliac disease and peptic ulcer disease) need to be considered, but investigations should be kept to a minimum and should be reserved for red flag symptoms as described below.

Obtain a detailed history exploring stressors at home and at school. There may well be a family history of somatisation symptoms or irritable bowel syndrome. Explore ideas linking unresolved stress to bodily symptoms with sensitivity, as parental acceptance of this approach will have a very positive impact. A full physical examination is essential, including plotting growth on a centile chart.

It is important to note that children with functional abdominal pain do experience real pain, and it is not in their imagination, nor are they faking it. It is quite tempting to repeatedly request unnecessary diagnostic tests, thereby promoting a cycle of anxiety around symptoms and further health-seeking behaviour.

In addition to FAP, there are other identified subgroups of recurrent abdominal pain. These include abdominal migraine (intermittent episodes of often severe pain with headache, photophobia, nausea, vomiting and pallor in a child with a first-degree relative with migraine), functional dyspepsia (the abdominal pain normally occurs in the epigastric region), and irritable bowel syndrome (the abdominal pain is associated with altered bowel habit and symptoms of bloating).

The key question relates to the site of pain in the periumbilical region as most likely to be functional abdominal pain. The more lateral the pain, the more likely that the pain has an organic cause and requires investigation.

Eosinophilic oesophagitis should be considered if episodic abdominal pain is associated with dysphagia or a history of food impaction.

Treatment Approach

Although clinically challenging, this is a very rewarding condition to manage as a family doctor or paediatrician. The primary objective is to detect any stressors (physical or psychological) or environmental factors that may be causing the pain or allowing it to continue. It is crucial that the child attends school every day, even if the abdominal pain is still present. Parents and the school must work together to support the child. The aim is that the child returns to normal school, social and sports activities to lead as normal a life as possible.

It is vital that the child (where age-appropriate) and the family accept the biopsychosocial model both in terms of explaining the condition and acting as a path to recovery. This model works on the premise that the child's personality can be affected by triggers (psychological or physical) and can be affected by feedback from family or peer group. Recognition by the family and dealing with such triggers are vital for recovery.

Investigations should be limited to a 'one-stop' approach (blood tests and faecal calprotectin). This is important as further investigations are highly likely to have a low yield in the absence of 'red flag' symptoms as outlined in Table 34.1.

Table 34.1 Red flags pointing to alternate diagnoses

- pain localised away from the umbilicus
- anorexia and weight loss with consequent faltering growth
- gastrointestinal (GI) bleeding (haematemesis, melaena or bloody diarrhoea)
- profuse diarrhoea
- extraintestinal symptoms such as fevers rashes or recurrent aphthous ulcers
- a family history of coeliac disease
- abnormal biochemistry (elevated bilirubin or transaminases, low albumin)
- a high faecal calprotectin level
- iron deficiency anaemia or an elevated C-reactive protein (CRP) or erythrocyte sedimentation rate.

Other Symptoms Due to Somatisation

PRIMARY HEADACHES

Primary headaches are benign, not caused by underlying disease, and can be diagnosed through history and physical examination. Examples include tension headaches and migraines.

Tension headaches often start slowly in the morning and worsen as the day progresses. The pain is often described as a band around the head; a continuous pressure pain that is not throbbing. Sensitivity to light or sound is rarely seen. Tension headaches can disrupt normal living with loss of school attendance and is often associated with persistent use of analgesics without relief.

Childhood migraines are much like those experienced by adults. The attacks tend to be shorter and less often compared to adult migraines and respond better to treatment. A family history of an affected first-degree relative with migraine is the rule and various triggers, especially foods, may be present. Gastrointestinal symptoms are common in childhood migraines, including abdominal pain, nausea and vomiting. For more information, see chapter 18 (the child with headaches).

CHEST PAIN

Chest pain is relatively common in childhood and adolescence. Most are idiopathic, psychogenic or musculoskeletal. In the absence of known congenital heart disease, only a small minority have a cardiac cause. Chest pain lasting several seconds or up to 2 minutes is likely to originate from the chest wall.

In adolescents, other cardiac somatic symptoms such as transient chest pains with or without hyperventilation, a feeling of breathlessness, syncope or near-syncope, and palpitations may coexist with anxiety and depression. For more information, see chapter 11 (congenital heart disease).

VASOVAGAL SYNCOPE

Vasovagal syncopal episodes (simple faints) are very common, occurring in almost a quarter of school-age children. Episodes are often preceded by feeling light-headed, nauseous or sweaty. Recognised triggers include hot environments while standing such as school assembly, hunger or the sight of blood. Exertional chest pain or syncope may have a cardiac cause. Be concerned if there is a family history of sudden cardiac death. For more information, see Chapter 11.

(Box 34.1)
(Box 34.2)

Box 34.1 **Key Points**

Somatisation is when children and young people have bodily symptoms caused by some form of unresolved psychological stress.

Somatisation is a legitimate, real and entirely acceptable diagnosis. Once diagnosed, or even suspected, good management by the doctor is based on empathy and normalisation.

In a consultation where somatisation is possible, undertake detailed exploration of the symptom pattern paying special attention to the temporal relationships between life events and the patient's symptoms.

Then, explore the symptoms in terms of their impact both on the child and the family considering life events, current stressors in the family (marital discord, financial pressures or bereavement) and secondary gain (perhaps not going to school) in the child.

Thereafter, explore past medical history and family history of somatisation, and undertake a detailed system review.

A detailed physical examination of the child, including plotting growth centiles, is of paramount importance and should not be glossed over regardless of a working clinical diagnosis.

Investigate judiciously as one should not get on the 'investigation train' and struggle to jump off.

Use empathy and normalisation as your consultation tools.

While the initial consultation may take longer by the above approach, there will be considerable savings in terms of avoiding unnecessary investigations and specialist appointments if this approach is followed.

Functional abdominal pain is very common, and the localisation of pain to the periumbilical region makes it most likely to be functional abdominal pain.

Red flag symptoms include recent weight loss, pain away from the periumbilical area, nocturnal pain causing awakening or alteration of the bowel habit.

In the absence of red flags, the one-stop approach to investigations includes a full blood count, coeliac screen and blood inflammatory markers (CRP), and stool for calprotectin appears sensible with a pickup rate between 5 and 10 per cent.

Acceptance of the biopsychosocial model (whereby a physical or psychological trigger is affected by the child's developing personality and influenced by parental and peer feedback) is the key to understanding the condition and to recovery.

Tension headaches often begin gradually and escalate throughout the day. The pain is constant, squeezing, non-pulsatile and band-like.

Most chest pain in childhood is idiopathic, psychogenic or musculoskeletal.

Vasovagal syncope may be recurrent and is precipitated by well-known triggers such as the sight of blood, heat, hunger or prolonged upright position.

Box 34.2   11-Year-Old Girl With Recurrent Abdominal Pain

A bright, high-achieving 11-year-old girl presents with recurrent bouts of dull, crampy periumbilical abdominal pain. She is the eldest child in her family and all her grades in school have been excellent. The episodes of pain are more common on school days and she must rest with each. Her family are extremely concerned and attend for advice. Both parents are professionals, and her father travels frequently with his work. Both are convinced of a serious underlying cause for their daughter's symptoms.

Clinical Pearls

The key aspects of this scenario are the recurrent episodes of pain, the fact that it is always periumbilical and that most episodes are seen at school. Regular school attendance is important and should be encouraged despite ongoing pain episodes.

Functional abdominal pain (FAP) is defined as episodic or continuous abdominal pain which, after appropriate evaluation, cannot be fully explained by another medical condition, and as where a loss of daily function is present.

Children with FAP with higher levels of functional impairment tend to be both anxious and perfectionistic. It is postulated that visceral hypersensitivity may play a significant role in the aetiology of FAP.

In FAP, there is insufficient data to recommend either mebeverine or antidepressants. Short trials of peppermint oil or antispasmodics may be considered. Food exclusions (such as dairy or gluten) should be limited, and early reintroduction should be attempted to ascertain efficacy.

Hypnotherapy has some beneficial effects in reducing short-term pain. Neither cognitive behaviour therapy nor yoga therapy have proven efficacy in FAP.

Acceptance of the biopsychosocial model is the key to understanding the condition and indeed to recovery.

Role of Investigations

In the absence of red flags, the 'one-stop' approach to investigations includes a full blood count, coeliac screen, blood inflammatory markers (CRP) and stool for calprotectin appears sensible with a pick-up rate between 5 and 10 per cent.

Potential Pitfalls

The most common pitfall is to over-investigate and set off on a journey whereby more and more investigations are performed with little to no resolution of symptoms.

Red flag symptoms include pain not in the periumbilical region, nocturnal pain causing awakening, weight loss, diarrhoea or blood in the stools. Red flag symptoms should prompt further assessment and investigation.

 Video on the topic Recurrent abdominal pain is available online at Elsevier eBooks+.

Key References

Andrews, E. T., Beattie, R. M., & Tighe, M. P. (2020). Functional abdominal pain: What clinicians need to know. *Archives of Disease in Childhood, 0*, 1–7.

Apley, J., & Naish, N. (1958). Recurrent abdominal pains: A field survey of 1,000 school children. *Archives of Disease in Childhood, 33*(168), 165–170.

Crushell, E., Rowland, M., Doherty, M., Gormally, S., Harty, S., Bourke, B., et al. (2003). Importance of parental conceptual model of illness in severe recurrent abdominal pain. *Pediatrics, 112*(6 Pt 1), 1368–1372.

Korterink, J. J., Diederen, K., Benninga, M. A., & Tabbers, M. M. (2015). Epidemiology of pediatric functional abdominal pain disorders: A meta-analysis. *PLoS One, 10*(5), e0126982.

Lauck, S., & Gage, S. (2018). Headaches. In R. M. Kliegman, P. S. Lye, B. Bordini, H. Toth, & D. Basel (Eds.), *Nelson pediatric symptom-based diagnosis* (pp. 439–454). Elsevier.

Mann, B., & Wilson, H. (2013). Diagnosing somatisation in adults in the first consultation: Moving beyond diagnosis by exclusion. *British Jounral of General Practice, 63*, 607–608.

Miranda, A. Abdominal Pain. In R. M. Kliegman, P. S. Lye, B. Bordini, H. Toth, D. Basel (Eds.), *Nelson pediatric symptom-based diagnosis* (pp. 161–181). Elsevier.

35 Professionalism, Advocacy and Ethics in Child Health

FIONNUALA GOUGH, DAVID MISSELBROOK, SHAISTA SALMAN and MARTIN WHITE

'There is no keener revelation of a society's soul than the way it treats its children'

NELSON MANDELA

Dealing with sick children and their families demands the highest of professional standards. In many ways, how you respond to difficult and challenging situations defines you.

By virtue of their role in treating children, child health professionals should assume an advocacy role and should speak out on issues of concern. Currently, these issues may relate to immunisation, prevention of obesity, avoidance of physical punishment, road safety and caring for homeless or refugee children. However, these issues vary between countries and even between different sections of society.

Professionalism

Professionalism is realised through a partnership between patient and doctor; one based on mutual respect, individual responsibility and appropriate accountability.

Graduating doctors should commit to setting the highest professional standards, being an effective communicator, scholar, leader in their field, team player and global practitioner with transferrable skills.

These commitments form the basis of a social contract between the medical profession and society. The development of your professional identity begins during your time as a medical student and should be nurtured. You will see examples of good professional behaviour in your teachers, and you should try to emulate this behaviour. Professionalism is a key pillar in medical training that students should display in their attendance and punctuality, and in courteous and appropriate behaviour during clinical interactions with patients and families. Students should also demonstrate professional behaviour in terms of student selected research projects, continuous assessment and taking examinations.

These commitments evolve into a quest for excellence, formation of professional identity and the assumption of leadership roles. Professional values (or virtues) exist within the three key areas of *professional expertise, integrity* and *compassion*. Professional expertise includes professional training, a sound knowledge base, an ability to analyse and use evidence, and a commitment to lifelong learning.

Integrity denotes a focus on vocation and altruism, diligence in attending to duties, respect for colleagues and patients alike, truthfulness, accountability and self-regulation. It is critical to develop a sense of compassion and maintain a focus on empathy while taking a thoughtful patient-centred approach.

We should all aim to link individual clinical expertise to the most recent evidence available with the aim of being a reflective and thoughtful doctor. The dictum of Socrates states that 'to know thyself is the beginning of wisdom'. Willingness to learn from your mistakes is an essential characteristic of a reflective professional. Competence and performance must be continually verified during training and throughout your career. These reflective personal traits are just as important as proficiency in knowledge and technical skills.

Trainee education and training curricula explore the knowledge, competencies and values needed to obtain specialist qualification. Nowadays, greater emphases are placed on being an effective collaborator and seeking feedback from colleagues about your performance, and on the ability to effectively communicate with families in difficult situations, including end-of-life care and breaking bad news.

An Advocacy Role for Child Health Professionals

These early years (starting in the womb) have lifelong effects on many aspects of health and well-being – from obesity, heart disease and mental health to educational achievement and economic status

MARMOT (2010)

It has long since been established that a child's early experiences have a major impact on their lifelong health.

Children require safe and secure housing, adequate and nutritious food, access to medical care, secure relationships with adult caregivers, nurturing and responsive parenting, and high-quality learning opportunities at home, in child-care settings and at school.

ADVERSITY AND POOR ADULT OUTCOMES

Children and young people thrive if they can live in a safe and supportive environment that provides them with the right conditions and opportunities to reach their full emotional and developmental potential.

In a recent Danish study (DANLIFE), early childhood adversity was found to be associated with a fourfold increase in mortality before the age of 35 years, with the most common causes of death being accidental injury, suicide and cancer.

This study provides a striking picture of links between adversity and early mortality in a country (Denmark) with high social equality and a globally renowned social security system to support vulnerable families.

Poor-quality housing and living in overcrowded conditions are associated with an increased risk of childhood home injuries including domestic fires. Lack of access to a healthy diet negatively impacts school attendance and learning.

SLAPPING

Compelling international evidence continues to emerge highlighting the long-term effects of slapping children. If a child is under 18 months, it has been found that slapping has a wholly negative effect on the parent-child relationship. Slapping increases both aggression and oppositional defiant behaviour in both preschool and school–aged children. Slapping has a deleterious longer-term impact leading to increased suicide rates, moderate to heavy drinking and adult substance abuse. Parents should use positive reinforcement of appropriate behaviours and set limits.

HOMELESSNESS

Homelessness and poor housing conditions are both linked to poverty and have a deleterious effect on children's health. Preterm birth is more likely if the mother is homeless or living in temporary accommodation during pregnancy.

REFUGEE CHILDREN

In 2018, the worldwide number of people forcibly displaced from their homes due to conflict, persecution, natural disasters and famine reached the staggering total of 68.7 million – over half of whom are children. Child refugees and asylum seekers are more vulnerable to physical and mental health issues than children in the host population. Apart from a long and often complex legal immigration process following arrival in a new country, refugee children have to learn a new language and adapt to a new culture. They face challenges with integration in the host country and difficulties navigating the healthcare system, are often housed in sub-standard and overcrowded accommodations, and experience loneliness, isolation and often a delay in access to education. Sadly, they may also experience racism and discrimination. Refugee children and their families should be supported in navigating the healthcare system. Access to interpreters and allowing additional time for appointments are essential.

Paediatricians may also receive requests for age determination in asylum seeking children and adolescents. The age of asylum seekers may be uncertain as they often flee without documentation. All methods of radiological age estimation (both dental and skeletal using bone age) can provide an estimation of age. Unfortunately, this estimation is largely inaccurate, especially in older children and adolescents.

Child refugees and asylum seekers are a very resilient group with a great capacity to survive and flourish. Addressing their health needs should be a priority across Europe.

Key Ethical Principles in Child Health

Doctors should not only concentrate on the view of parents but also consider the interests of the child in accordance with Article I of the Rights of the Child from the United Nations Convention. Thus, it is important to seek active involvement of children in decisions about their own health.

Contentious ethical issues are frequently encountered in both neonatology and paediatrics. Some of the most challenging of these relate to issues around consent – particularly the age of consent, how best to seek the views of the child or young person, and in seeking consent for research relating to children or genetic testing. Confidentiality is of the utmost importance in all instances but is especially so in conversations with adolescents.

To empower families to make an informed decision, they should receive detailed information about proposed investigations or procedures in language they can understand. Children should also be informed of proposed plans using language they too can understand. Consent is all about informed choices made freely without any hint of coercion. If a child who is too young to give consent expresses an opinion, this should be taken into consideration – this is termed assent.

The relationship with both the child and family should be built on a spirit of partnership and mutual respect. In essence, consent should be viewed as a continuing process. Active engagement of the child and family in decisions has been shown to improve compliance with treatment. Rarely, legal advice is needed to resolve difficult issues in situations where conflict has arisen and, most importantly, to protect the weak and vulnerable.

Families should have sufficient time to reflect on information received and then make an informed choice. The risks and benefits of the proposed treatment should be clearly outlined.

Avoid an overly paternalistic approach and give enough detail to enable the family to make an informed decision. A faster decision by the parents may be needed in an emergency. If verbal consent has been given, then write an account of the information imparted to obtain consent.

END-OF-LIFE CARE

This poses significant challenges as the views of fellow colleagues (including nursing and health and social care professionals) and those of the family may not always align but nevertheless must be respected. This requires considerable training, a proper allocation of time and excellent communication skills. One also needs to be culturally sensitive as different religious cultures have quite diverse views on end-of-life care. In these situations, always provide comfort and try to reduce any potential pain or suffering.

However, respecting the values and beliefs of a family does not mean advocating life-sustaining treatments if the benefits are clearly outweighed by significant burdens to the child.

PAEDIATRIC PALLIATIVE CARE

Paediatric palliative care (PPC) has a clear focus on relieving the child's suffering through the control of pain and other distressing symptoms. The key aims of PPC are to enable the infant or child to have as active and full a life as possible. PPC supports families and helps them cope with significant added burdens. PPC is appropriate in children with life-limiting conditions when premature death is inevitable, in conditions for which there is no known cure, and when there is severe disability with likely premature death.

Palliative care services always aim to improve quality of life, and its introduction should <u>not</u> be left until a decision is made to withdraw or withhold life-sustaining treatment. The team should help the family live in the knowledge of an uncertain future. There is a delicate balance between 'care' and 'cure' for an individual child, and families should receive continued support even if active treatment has stopped. All decisions reached in consultation with the family should be recorded and details of supportive care should be set out. Decisions may need to be reviewed after further discussion and can result in a change of plan.

END-OF-LIFE CARE AMONG DIFFERENT CULTURES

Both Western and Islamic traditions agree that there is no moral, legal or religious duty to attempt resuscitation where such an attempt would be futile and would not benefit the patient. Unfortunately, some families may not fully understand this issue and thereby confuse not for resuscitation orders with a failure to provide all proper medical help to their child.

Doctors must therefore do their best to communicate realistic options with patients and families, and what they understand to be in the best interests of the patient.

DEALING WITH CONFLICT

In difficult and emotionally draining circumstances, it is not surprising that conflict between families and health care professionals may develop. Asking spiritual leaders (e.g. an Imam for Muslim families) or senior family members may help calm the situation.

Conflict may also arise within the team and generally relates to differing views about the child's prognosis, and an external opinion may be required. If a second opinion has been sought, it is best if the family first meet the designated clinician prior to them seeing the child. Legal opinion is always a last resort. When resolving conflict with the family, always give the family additional time to reflect on the advice given. These are certainly difficult, emotional times for the family and the healthcare professionals involved. When conflict develops, an already difficult situation becomes far more stressful. Always seek to avoid any escalation to conflict within the team or with the family. Family needs and wishes must be respected despite the best interest of the child being paramount.

Continued support of families is essential even if there is a breakdown of trust between the family and the professionals involved. The goal should always be to provide pain relief, relieve suffering, and to allow infants and children to die with dignity. Appropriate religious, cultural and counselling support should be offered.

(Box 35.1)
(Box 35.2)
(Box 35.3)
(Box 35.4)
(Box 35.5)

Box 35.1 Key Points

Good doctors combine individual clinical expertise and best available external evidence to try to become thoughtful, evidence-based practitioners who continue to show empathy in the care of their patients.

Contentious ethical issues are frequently encountered in both neonatology and paediatrics. Chief amongst these relate to issues of consent with particular reference to the age of consent, seeking the views of the child or young person, consent for research relating to children and consent for genetic testing. Confidentiality is imperative in all instances but especially so in conversations with adolescents.

End-of-life care requires considerable training, time and excellent communication skills. One also needs to be culturally sensitive as different religious cultures have quite diverse but important views on end-of-life care.

Families wish to be treated with dignity, respect and honesty. Children, especially if over 10 years of age, need to have potential medical decisions explained to them, and their feedback should be sought. Consent in terms of medical treatment, the conduct of research, the performance of genetic testing and in extreme situations is a key issue.

Box 35.2   Refusal of Treatment

A 14-year-old is admitted to hospital with anorexia nervosa and a 2-kg weight loss over the past week. She is under the combined care of a general paediatrician and a child and adolescent psychiatrist. In hospital, she continues to struggle and has now lost more weight and has electrolyte disturbances. The issue of nasogastric feeding is raised, but the patient herself is not eager to have a nasogastric tube. The team should request a meeting with the family to discuss further management and treatment options.

Pearls of Wisdom

When treatment is refused, the key legal principle is that one should follow what is in the best interest of the child or young person.

Young people from 14 to 18 years are widely regarded as being able to give their own consent to treatment. This is sometimes referred to as a Gillick competence. In broad terms, the young person should demonstrate an understanding of their illness, the proposed treatment and the consequences if treatment is unsuccessful.

Issues With Potential for Controversy

Doctors should establish that there is a threat to the child's life or a significant risk to their physical or mental health if the treatment is withheld. Written support from a colleague should be sought and all the steps to obtain consent taken. The most frequently cited example is the refusal of a Jehovah's Witness family to allow a newborn infant to receive a blood transfusion that is necessary for survival.

Young people with mental illness may refuse proposed treatment. Most disputes can be resolved with sufficient time and energy to discussions with the young person and the family. If resolution proves elusive, the appropriate legal steps should be taken.

Box 35.3   Consent for Research in Children

You are a developmental paediatrician, and, in your region, you look after a number of children with complex disability and intractable seizures. Parents are seeking your advice on the use of medicinal cannabis and you have been approached by colleagues to be part of a clinical trial assessing effectiveness of this form of treatment.

Pearls of Wisdom

All research proposals should have a formal evaluation by a research ethics committee prior to commencement.

The key question for this committee is whether the research proposed is likely to answer a valid scientific question. Written consent is also significant, and the family need to be reassured that they may withdraw their consent at any time without adversely affecting the care received.

Issues With Potential for Controversy

An individual clinician should never attempt to coerce a family to partake in a clinical trial involving their child. It is good practice to seek assent from the child to be involved in research when the parents have given formal consent.

The main issues in this example are the somewhat unproven use of medicinal cannabis for this purpose, the size of the trial, the vulnerability of affected families and the need to ensure that the proposed trial is able to answer the questions asked , see Chapter 38 (Critical Appraisal).

Box 35.4   Ethical Issues Surrounding Genetic Testing in Childhood

A 35-year-old father of three children has just been diagnosed as having Huntington's disease, and the family have requested that the children be tested to exclude the condition. The children are 5, 7 and 10 years of age.

Pearls of Wisdom

It is quite appropriate for genetic testing of minors to be performed if the problem in question can be rectified, treated or prevented (e.g. cystic fibrosis as per American College of Medical Genetics guidelines in 2018).

Issues With Potential for Controversy

From a legal perspective, one should not be willing to permit testing as the evidence suggests that being diagnosed with a genetic condition (in this case, Huntington's disease) may lead to stigmatisation and intense anxiety about the future.

There is near-universal agreement that testing should not be performed in adult-onset diseases where there is no treatment, such as Huntington's disease.

Genes that confer susceptibility to obesity, diabetes and coronary artery disease are increasingly being discovered. It is inappropriate to offer any testing for these genes until a clear intervention is available.

Testing a child for carrier status requires a paediatrician or geneticist to discuss the pros and cons of testing to enable a fully informed decision to be reached. The family should receive follow-up support and counselling.

In summary, it is not appropriate to test for untreatable adult-onset diseases (as in our case, Huntington's disease). Formal genetic testing should wait until the young person is old enough (over 18 years of age) to request testing for themselves.

Box 35.5   Controversies and Challenges Around End-of-Life Care

You are a neonatologist working in a regional neonatal intensive care unit. An ex 24-week gestation infant with a birth weight of 520 g has had a stormy perinatal course with fulminant necrotising enterocolitis and grade 4 intraventricular haemorrhages with post-haemorrhagic hydrocephalous requiring placement of a ventriculoperitoneal shunt. He is now over 6 months old and is on continuous oxygen due to chronic lung disease. He has had an MRI brain scan showing major ischaemic changes in addition to hydrocephalous. He has markedly reduced vision due to retinopathy of prematurity. His family are devout Muslims. You ask to speak to the parents and grandparents as part of a multidisciplinary team discussion.

Pearls of Wisdom

This clearly is a very challenging scenario for the family and all staff involved. In certain clinical situations active treatment may not be commenced, may be limited or may be withdrawn. Infants born with anencephaly or under 22 weeks' gestation may not be resuscitated following discussions with the parents, and artificial ventilation may be withdrawn in cases of severe birth asphyxia where profound brain damage is anticipated.

In relation to issues surrounding Charlie Gard and other high-profile cases, we may need to consider a lower threshold for innovative but as yet untested treatments when there are no other options. Cost and the perennial issue of limited resources need to be considered and disputes of this kind should ideally be resolved without resorting to the legal process.

Conflicts between parents and doctors that end up in court lead to long delays in both a final decision and the timely introduction of potential life-saving treatments. Going to court should therefore be seen as an absolute last resort in these difficult situations.

As always, the essential question to consider is whether the anticipated suffering is likely to exceed any future prospects that can be envisaged for the infant or child.

Issues With Potential for Controversy (and There Are Many!)

A multidisciplinary team approach involving the family enables better communication and allows differences in opinion to be respectfully aired.

In order to minimise conflict with parents and families, general advice supports the early use of palliative care. There should be a recognition that parents are under extreme stress and that they should be offered appropriate pastoral support. Also be cognisant that staff are under significant stress. It is best to have a designated lead clinician to provide continuity of clear information to the family and to seek second opinions or external advice (both ethical and legal) as required. Also consider the earlier involvement of mediation services if conflict is anticipated or becoming evident.

Generally speaking, try to resolve disputes by discussion, consultation and consensus. It is important to acknowledge that discussions about limiting care are taking place while the family are under enormous stress.

Key References

Bengtsson, J., Dich, N., Rieckmann, A., & Rod, N. H. (2019). Cohort profile: The Danish LIFE course (DANLIFE) cohort, a prospective register-based cohort of all children born in Denmark since 1980. *BMJ Open, 9*(9), e027217.

De Lourdes Levy, M., Larcher, V., Kurz, R., & Ethics working group of the Confederation of European Specialists in Paediatrics (CESP), (2003). Informed consent/assent in children. Statement of the ethics working group of the Confederation of European specialists in Paediatrics (CESP). *European Journal of Pediatrics, 162*(9), 629–633.

Dunne, M., & Meinck, F. (2020). Childhood adversity and death of young adults in an affluent society. *Lancet, 396*, 449–450.

Fryer, A. (1997). The genetic testing of children. *Journal of the Royal Society of Medicine, 90*(8), 419–421.

Fryer, A. (2000). Inappropriate genetic testing of children. *Archives of Disease in Childhood, 83*(4), 283–285.

Lagercrantz, H. Observations on the case of Charlie Gard. *Archives of Disease in Childhood, 103*, 409–410.

Larcher, V., Craig, F., Bhogal, K., Wilkinson, D., Brierley, J., & Royal College of Paediatrics and Child Health (2015). Making decisions to limit treatment in life-limiting and life-threatening conditions in children: A framework for practice. *Archives of Disease in Childhood, 100*(Suppl.1(2)), s1–s23.

Linney, M., Hain, R. D. W., Wilkinson, D., Fortune, P.-M., Barclay, S., Larcher, V., et al. (2019). Achieving consensus advice for paediatricians and other health professionals: On prevention, recognition and management of conflict in paediatric practice. *Archives of Disease in Childhood, 104*, 413–416.

Puntis, J. W. (2021). COVID-19: Children on the front line. *Archives of Disease in Childhood, 106*(7), e28. https://doi.org/10.1136/archdischild-2020-319671.

Richards, S., Aziz, N., Bale, S., et al. (2015). Standards and guidelines for the interpretation of sequence variants: a joint consensus recommendation of the American College of Medical Genetics and Genomics and the Association for Molecular Pathology. *Genetics in Medicine, 17*(5), 405–424.

Rod, N. H., Bengtsson, J., Budtz-Jørgensen, E., Clipet-Jensen, C., Taylor-Robinson, D., Andersen, A.-M. N., et al. (2020). Trajectories of childhood adversity and mortality in early adulthood: A population-based cohort study. *Lancet, 396*(10249), 489–497.

Sauer, P. J., Nicholson, A., & Neubauer, D. (2016). Advocacy and ethics group of the European Academy of Paediatrics. Age determination in asylum seekers: Physicians should not be implicated. *European Journal of Pediatrics, 175*(3), 299–303.

Smith, R. (2006). Medical professionalism: Out with the old and in with the new. *Journal of the Royal Society of Medicine, 99*(2), 48–50.

Stevens, A. J. (2020). How can we meet the health needs of child refugees, asylum seekers and undocumented migrants? *Archives of Disease in Childhood, 105*, 191–196.

Takahashi, R., Kruja, K., Puthoopparambil, S. J., & Severoni, S. (2019). Refugee and migrant health in the European Region. *Lancet, 393*, 2300–2301.

Wilkinson, D., & Savulescu, J. (September 4, 2018). *Ethics, conflict and medical treatment for children: From disagreement to dissensus.* [Internet]. Elsevier.

Online References

EAPC Abstracts. (2019). *Palliative Medicine, 33*(1), 118–589. https://doi.org/10.1177/0269216319844405.

Faculties of Public Health Medicine and Paediatrics. (November 2019). *The impact of homelessness and inadequate housing on children's health.* Royal College of Physicians of Ireland. https://rcpi-live-cdn.s3.amazonaws.com/wp-content/uploads/2019/11/Impact-of-Homelessness-full-position-paper-final.pdf.

NSPCC Learning. (2020, June 10). *Gillick competency and Fraser guidelines.* National Society for the Prevention of Cruelty to Children. https://learning.nspcc.org.uk/child-protection-system/gillick-competence-fraser-guidelines.

The Marmot Review. (2010, February). *Fair society healthy lives – strategic review of health inequities in England post-2010.* http://www.instituteofhealthequity.org/resources-reports/fair-society-healthy-lives-the-marmot-review.

United Nations Human Rights Office of the High Commissioner. (1990, September 2). *Convention on the rights of the child. Adopted and opened for signature, ratification and accession by General Assembly resolution 44/25 of 20 November 1989 entry into force 2 September 1990, in accordance with article 49.* https://www.ohchr.org/EN/ProfessionalInterest/Pages/CRC.aspx.

36 Interpretation of Laboratory Results

ALF NICHOLSON and MICHAEL RIORDAN

Technology is a useful servant but a dangerous master
CHRISTIAN LOUS LANGE

We aim to ensure both helpful and necessary laboratory testing in children and to avoid extensive testing if possible. Before you order an investigation, it is important to justify it and to be able to interpret the result in the clinical context.

In this chapter, we look at relatively frequently performed blood investigations in infants and children including the full blood count, coagulation screen, electrolytes, thyroid function tests, liver function tests, calcium, phosphate, and alkaline phosphatase, cerebrospinal fluid, and their interpretation in the clinical context.

(Box 36.1)
(Box 36.2)
(Box 36.3)
(Box 36.4)
(Box 36.5)
(Box 36.6)
(Box 36.7)
(Box 36.8)
(Box 36.9)
(Box 36.10)
(Box 36.11)
(Box 36.12)
(Box 36.13)

Box 36.1 A Child With a Swollen Knee and Widespread Bruising

A 3 year old boy is seen in the emergency department with a swollen knee after a simple fall. The child has multiple large bruises in the arms and legs and is reported to have bled after a religious circumcision. Blood tests include full blood count and clotting screen.

Clinical Pearls

In taking the history from the parents, enquire about evidence of widespread bruising, epistaxis lasting more than 20 minutes, and evidence of haematomas. Haemophilia should be considered if there is a history of bleeding following a circumcision early in infancy. Bleeding from the umbilical stump is linked to factor XIII deficiency. Haemophilia (the diagnosis in this case) can be subdivided into factor VIII deficiency (haemophilia A) or factor IX deficiency (haemophilia B) and can present with a bleeding frenulum (Fig. 36.1), or haemarthroses or intramuscular haematoma following trauma or intramuscular injection.

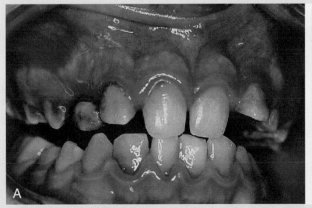
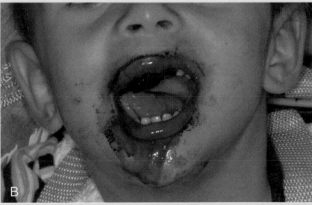

Figure 36.1 (A) Gingival haemorrhage around an exfoliating maxillary right primary canine in a child with haemophilia B. Normally, exfoliation of primary teeth is not of major concern and bleeding is locally controllable. (B) A boy with haemophilia presenting following minor trauma to the labial frenum. Note the poorly formed clot in the mouth and continued oozing after several days. (Reproduced with permission from Widmer, R. P., & Cameron, A. C. (Eds.). (2022). *Handbook of pediatric dentistry* (5th ed.). Elsevier Ltd.)

Continued

Box 36.1   A Child With a Swollen Knee and Widespread Bruising – cont'd

Bleeding may become evident as the child starts to mobilise around 18 to 24 months of age. The child may then develop spontaneous haemarthroses, typically seen in weight-bearing joints such as the hip, knee or ankle joints.

Severity depends on the level of factor VIII or IX levels and if the factor activity is less than one per cent, then it is by definition severe. Bleeding complications can also occur in female carriers.

In mild haemophilia, desmopressin is recommended to treat bleeds, for dental procedures, and prior to minor surgical procedures. Recombinant factor replacement therapy is the mainstay of treatment in both moderate and severe haemophilia.

Recombinant factor VIII or IX concentrate is the mainstay of treatment, but inhibitors to clotting factor replacements develop in a minority of cases.

Key findings in examining a child with a possible coagulopathy may be chronic arthropathy in weight-bearing joints (haemophilia), joint laxity (Ehlers–Danlos syndrome), thumb anomalies (Fanconi anaemia or thrombocytopaenia in absent radius syndrome), the presence of hepatosplenomegaly (acute lymphocytic leukaemia (ALL)) and examination of the skin (petechiae or ecchymoses).

The classical presenting features of acute immune thrombocytopaenia (ITP) are an acute onset of petechiae and purpura in association with nosebleeds or bleeding gums and an otherwise well-looking child.

Von Willebrand disease is associated with the delayed formation of platelet plugs and is generally inherited in an autosomal dominant fashion with desmopressin (DDAVP) being the treatment of choice.

Primary platelet disorders such as Glanzmann thrombasthenia or Bernard–Soulier syndrome cause relatively mild mucocutaneous bleeding.

Life-threatening illnesses such as sepsis may be associated with disseminated intravascular coagulation (DIC) with a consequent generalised consumption of clotting factors, anticoagulant proteins and platelets. DIC is managed in an intensive care setting by platelet transfusion, fresh frozen plasma, and fibrinogen concentrate and possibly anticoagulants if major vessel thrombosis.

Vitamin K deficiency is seen in breast-fed newborns, children with cholestatic liver disease and rarely post accidental ingestion of rat poison and is treated with intravenous vitamin K.

Interpretation of Investigations

Firstly, request a full blood count and platelet count looking for anaemia and thrombocytopaenia.

The prothrombin time (PT) is prolonged either by deficiency of a clotting factor or if an inhibitor is present. The PT measures both the extrinsic and common coagulation pathways.

The partial thromboplastin time (APTT) is prolonged if there are deficiencies of factors VIII, IX and XI. Factor XII deficiency may cause a prolonged APTT in an otherwise asymptomatic child. The APTT measures both the intrinsic and common pathways.

The bleeding time will be prolonged in platelet function abnormalities, thrombocytopaenia and von Willebrand disease.

Features seen in DIC include the prolongation of both PT and APTT, low fibrinogen levels, a low platelet count and elevated D-dimer levels

Pitfalls to Avoid

Be aware that up to one-third of children with factor VIII deficiency will not exhibit a family history if due to a new genetic mutation.

ITP is a diagnosis of exclusion with a normal blood film apart from thrombocytopaenia. Request a bone marrow examination if either leukaemia or marrow hypoplasia is suspected.

If thrombocytopaenia in an adolescent or pre-adolescent girl, consider systemic lupus erythematosus and perform an antinuclear antibody test. If thrombocytopaenia in a boy with eczema and recurrent infections, consider Wiskott–Aldrich syndrome.

Menorrhagia is another frequent symptom in von Willebrand disease (VWD) and the observation that improvement occurs after starting oral contraceptives is insufficient to rule out VWD.

Parents who are reluctant to allow administration of Vitamin K to their newborn infant (especially if breast-fed) need to be made aware of the risk of catastrophic haemorrhage due to vitamin K deficiency in a condition called haemorrhagic disease of the newborn.

Box 36.2   A Very Ill 2-Year-Old With Suspected Sepsis and Acidosis.

A 2-year-old child is admitted with a short history of high fever, headache, lethargy and poor skin perfusion. Sepsis is suspected and bloods taken include blood gas analysis and lactate levels. Blood gas analysis shows a marked metabolic acidosis.

Clinical Pearls

A pH less than 7.35 is defined as acidosis and is respiratory in origin if the pCO_2 is high and metabolic if a change in bicarbonate concentration. Metabolic acidosis results in tachypnoea in an attempt to blow off CO_2 to compensate with characteristic deep and rapid breaths (Kussmaul respiration).

Causes of metabolic acidosis with a normal anion gap include marked diarrhoea (the most frequent reason) and types 1 and 2 renal tubular acidosis. Type 1 relates to an inability to secrete hydrogen ions in the distal tubules and type 2 is due to impaired bicarbonate resorption in the proximal tubule.

The normal anion gap is 10 to 18 mmol/L. Metabolic acidosis with an increased anion gap is seen in diabetic ketoacidosis (DKA). Severe acidosis in DKA is reversed by fluid and insulin replacement.

Interpretation of Investigations

An unwell infant or child with likely sepsis and an increased anion gap metabolic acidosis may have a high lactate as the cause.

Pitfalls to Avoid

Poisonings can also be associated with increased anion gap metabolic acidosis and include salicylate, ethylene glycol and carbon monoxide poisoning.

Organic acidaemias can present with increased anion gap metabolic acidosis often in the neonatal period.

Box 36.3 A 6-Week-Old Male With Forceful Vomits

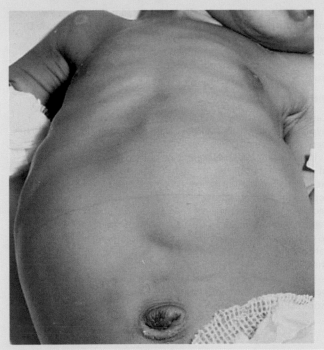

Figure 36.2 Pyloric stenosis may cause epigastric distension by the obstructed stomach. This patient also exhibits a visible wave of peristalsis, which moves from left to right. (Reproduced with permission from Zitelli, B. J., McIntire, S. C., & Nowalk, A. J. (2017). *Zitelli and Davis' atlas of pediatric physical diagnosis* (7th ed.). Elsevier.)

A 6-week-old male infant is admitted with a 1-week history of projectile milk vomits, irritability, and weight loss. Blood tests include blood gas analysis, which shows a marked metabolic alkalosis.

Clinical Pearls

The diagnosis in this instance is hypertrophic pyloric stenosis.
Visible peristalsis may be present (Fig. 36.2).
The loss of gastric fluid by persistent vomiting leads to a metabolic alkalosis linked to protracted vomiting. Loss of potassium and chloride ions leads to a hypochloraemic hypokalaemic metabolic acidosis.

Interpretation of Investigations

If metabolic alkalosis with a low urinary chloride (under 15 mEq/L), the main causes relate to excessive vomiting (pyloric stenosis in infancy, bulimia in teenagers) and chronic use of diuretics.
If metabolic alkalosis with a high urinary chloride (over 15 mEq/L), the main causes include Bartter and Gitelman syndromes.

Pitfalls to avoid

Both Bartter and Gitelman syndromes are autosomal recessive in inheritance. Bartter syndrome is characterised by marked hypokalaemia, metabolic alkalosis with a low chloride and increased levels of renin and aldosterone.
Neonatal Barrter syndrome is associated with failure to thrive and dehydration due to both polyuria and polydipsia and is a differential diagnosis for late presenting pyloric stenosis. Gitelman syndrome is milder and associated with hypomagnesemia.
Cystic fibrosis may present with pseudo-Barrter syndrome with marked hypochloraemic metabolic alkalosis

Box 36.4 A 2-Year-Old With Severe Gastroenteritis and an Abnormal Serum Sodium

A 2-year-old child is admitted with a 3-day history of vomiting, poor oral intake and very frequent loose stools. The child is clinically dehydrated (Fig. 36.3), and her electrolytes are tested with a serum sodium of 154 mEq/L.

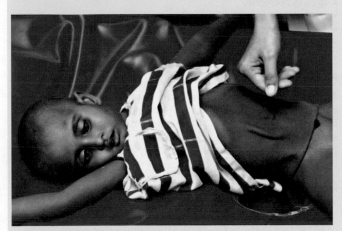

Figure 36.3 A child, lying on a cholera cot, showing typical signs of severe dehydration from cholera. The patient has sunken eyes, lethargic appearance and poor skin turgor but within 2 hours he was sitting up, alert and eating normally. (Reproduced with permission from Sack, D.A., Sack, R. B., Nair, G. B., & Siddique, A. K. (2004). Cholera. *Lancet, 363,* 223–233.)

Clinical Pearls

The kidney relies primarily on the energy dependent movement of sodium to regulate water homeostasis. Sodium concentrations are dependent on both the amount of sodium present in the plasma and the amount of water. Both sodium and water status need to be considered when assessing electrolyte measurements. Clinical assessment by history and examination is essential to allow the correct interpretation of electrolyte measurements with a focus in taking the history on both fluid intake and fluid losses. Fluid losses may be in stool, vomits or urine.
The focus of clinical examination should be an assessment of the child's volume status looking for pulse rate, blood pressure, dryness of mucous membranes, and capillary refill time.
By far the most seen cause of hyponatraemia is salt depletion due to either excessive loss or inadequate intake. Salt depletion is associated with clinical signs of dehydration.
Salt depletion most often relates to acute gastroenteritis in children, but excessive sodium losses may also be renal (tubular immaturity in preterms, diuretic therapy, osmotic diuresis in DKA, and the recovery phase of acute tubular necrosis), endocrine (hypoaldosteronism or congenital adrenal hypoplasia) or cutaneous (cystic fibrosis, prematurity, burns).
Hyponatraemia caused by dilution is very rare and is associated with excess water retention. In children with CNS malignancies, the cause most often relates to the syndrome of inappropriate antidiuretic hormone secretion (SIADH) in which the urine osmolality will be inappropriately high in the context

Continued

Box 36.4   A 2-Year-Old With Severe Gastroenteritis and an Abnormal Serum Sodium – cont'd

of a low serum sodium. Clinical signs of dehydration are absent in SIADH.

Hypernatraemia (a plasma sodium greater than 145 mEq/L) is usually prevented by thirst and renal concentrating mechanisms. A water deficit is by far the most common cause of hypernatraemia and is due to inadequate water intake or excessive water loss associated with severe gastroenteritis (as above). Breast-fed neonates can develop severe hypernatraemic dehydration associated with difficulties in the initial establishment of breast-feeding.

Excessive salt intake can cause hypernatraemia (examples include the inadvertent administration of hypertonic feeds, iatrogenic administration of excess sodium or deliberate salt poisoning).

Interpretation of Investigations

Hyponatraemia arises from either water retention or sodium losses.

Hyponatraemia and highly concentrated urine are normal findings in a child with dehydration where appropriate ADH secretion tries to correct dehydration by making the kidney retain water. Urine sodium concentration in this scenario will be low and clinical history and signs of dehydration will usually be obvious.

Excessive water loss can also occur as a consequence of impaired renal water retention due to diabetes insipidus (either central or nephrogenic) or an osmotic diuresis associated with glycosuria or hypercalcaemia.

Infants and children with diabetes insipidus (DI) have a low urinary osmolality. A fluid deprivation test is used to diagnose DI where a 4-hour fluid fast leads to an elevated serum osmolality but unchanged urinary osmolality. Administration of injectable vasopressin helps distinguish central (where there is a response) from nephrogenic DI.

Pitfalls to Avoid

Care should be taken to avoid an excessively rapid correction of hyponatraemia (>10 mmol/day), particularly if the abnormality has been longstanding.

In managing hypernatraemia, be guided by your assessment of whether or not the child is dehydrated. In the initial phase of treatment, normal (0.9 per cent) saline should be used to slowly replace the fluid deficit over 48 to 72 hours. Isotonic fluids are not recommended to reduce the risk of an overly rapid correction in serum sodium, which can cause cerebral oedema, thereby leading to central pontine demyelinosis. Close monitoring is essential and a rate of fall in plasma sodium of no more than 1 mEq/L/h should be the target.

Hypernatraemic dehydration has been misinterpreted as salt poisoning in the past and great care is needed in making this extremely rare diagnosis.

Box 36.5   A 6-Month-Old With Hypoglycaemia

A 6-month-old is seen in the emergency department with a 1-day history of fever and increasing lethargy and unresponsiveness. A bedside glucose level is 1.2 mmol/L and a blood glucose confirms this result.

Clinical Pearls

Hypoglycaemia, although rare beyond the neonatal period, is an acute emergency that may result in seizures, permanent brain damage and even death.

The brain solely relies on glucose as a primary source of energy. The brain also uses ketones as an alternative source of energy during periods of starvation.

The symptoms of hypoglycaemia are many and varied but include sweating, anxiety, hunger, weakness, pallor, lethargy, headache, irritability and – although rare – lost consciousness.

Hypoglycaemia in newborns is very common and associated with prematurity, small for gestational age infants, infants of diabetic mothers, transient hyperinsulinism, Rhesus incompatibility, neonatal sepsis and Beckwith–Wiedemann syndrome.

Persistent hypoglycaemia in infancy may be due to hyperinsulinism (either congenital hyperinsulinism or insulinoma) with characteristically very high glucose infusion rates required to prevent hypoglycaemia. Another cause is hypopituitarism, which predisposes to fasting hypoglycaemia. Microphallus is a useful clinical sign in males with hypopituitarism.

Due to glucose-6-phosphatase deficiency, fasting hypoglycaemia is also a feature of Addison's disease and glycogen storage disease types 1a and 1b.

Infants and children with medium chain acyl-coenzyme A dehydrogenase deficiency, see Chapter 19 (Inborn Errors of

Metabolism) (mercifully shortened to MCADD) have hypoketotic hypoglycaemia usually brought on by fasting stresses.

Interpretation of Investigations

The key investigation is the critical sample at the time of hypoglycaemia (blood sugar less than 2.6 mmol/L), testing for:
- blood glucose
- insulin and C-peptide
- growth hormone
- cortisol
- beta-hydroxybutyrate and free fatty acids
- acylcarnitine profile of the urine
- urine for organic acids

Pitfalls to Avoid

Always check the blood glucose in an infant or child with a seizure or impaired level of consciousness. If the blood glucose is low (under 2.6 mmol/L), check the urine for ketones and take a critical sample as above. Absence of ketones in the urine should prompt consideration of hyperinsulinism or a fatty acid oxidation disorder (such as MCADD).

Be wary of the sick infant or child with congenital adrenal hyperplasia during an intercurrent illness, when they may develop adrenal crisis with hypoglycaemia.

For the emergency treatment of hypoglycaemia, give a bolus of 10 per cent dextrose rapidly and thereafter a continuous infusion. Glucagon may be used to treat hypoglycaemia if the hypoglycaemia occurs in a known diabetic or if hereditary hyperinsulinism.

Box 36.6   A 6-Year-Old With Diarrhoea and Associated Hypokalaemia

A 6-year-old child is admitted with a 2-day history of fever, vomiting and diarrhoea. The child is noted to have at least six to eight bowel motions of watery consistency per day. Bloods confirm a potassium of 3.0 mEq/L.

Clinical Pearls

Potassium is a major intracellular cation with the kidneys playing a major role in eliminating potassium from the body.

Hypokalaemia in the context of an acidosis should prompt consideration of a possible renal tubular acidosis. If hypokalaemia is associated with normal blood pressure, consider significant vomiting and diarrhoea (by far the most common reason), diabetic ketoacidosis, renal tubular acidosis, and Bartter and Gitelman syndromes.

If hypokalaemia is associated with elevated blood pressure, consider primary hyperaldosteronism, Cushing's syndrome or 11 beta hydroxylase deficiency.

Severe hypokalaemia may be associated with symptoms such as muscle weakness, paralytic ileus and gastric dilatation. The treatment of hypokalaemia is by potassium administration, ideally by mouth.

Hyperkalaemia is linked to a reduction in urinary potassium excretion and either the release or redistribution of intracellular potassium.

Interpretation of Investigations

The normal serum concentration of potassium is 3.5 to 5.5 mEq/L. Hypokalaemia is seen in acute gastroenteritis (as in the example above), and hyperkalaemia is a feature of acute kidney injury (AKI).

Pitfalls to Avoid

Moderate or severe hyperkalaemia requires prompt treatment. The major risk with hyperkalaemia is cardiac arrhythmias. The characteristic ECG changes are tall, peaked T waves.

In tumour lysis syndrome, a significant release of potassium may cause severe hyperkalaemia.

Treating hyperkalaemia involves cardiac membrane stabilisation (achieved with calcium gluconate), shifting potassium into the intracellular compartment (using beta 2 agents such as salbutamol, dextrose infusions or sodium bicarbonate administration to correct an associated acidosis), and eliminating excess potassium (by stopping parenteral potassium administration or total parenteral nutrition (TPN), the administration of loop diuretics and, if necessary, using acute dialysis).

Box 36.7   A Jaundiced Girl With a History of Recent Foreign Travel

A 12-year-old girl is seen in the emergency department with a 1-day history of yellow discolouration of the eyes and skin. She was recently abroad and had a fever with loose stools 10 days ago. Blood tests performed include liver function tests and a hepatitis screen. Hepatitis serology confirmed the diagnosis of hepatitis A.

Clinical Pearls

Children under 5 years old with hepatitis A are often asymptomatic and anicteric.

After an incubation period (which may last between 15 and 40 days), symptoms of malaise, fever, right hypochondrial pain and anorexia are followed 2 to 7 days later by jaundice. Recovery within 2 weeks is expected.

Hepatitis A is transmitted via the faeco-oral route with the greatest faecal excretion of the virus occurring prior to the onset of jaundice.

Infection in contacts can be prevented by giving intramuscular immunoglobulin within 2 weeks of exposure. Hepatitis A vaccine confers long-term protection.

There are many extrahepatic causes of raised transaminases including coeliac disease, thyroid disease, adrenal insufficiency, muscular dystrophy, or viral myositis, and both immune and non-immune red cell haemolysis.

With mild and isolated elevation of the transaminases without any symptoms in the child, the best strategy is to repeat 6 to 8 weeks later and, if back to normal, the child can safely be discharged.

Mild elevation of transaminases in an obese child may be due to non-alcoholic fatty liver disease.

Interpretation of Investigations

The key investigations are aspartate aminotransferases (AST), Alanine aminotransferases (ALT), serum bilirubin, gamma glutamyl transferase (GGT), alkaline phosphatase, serum albumin, international normalised ratio (INR) and prothrombin time.

Aminotransferase levels of 10 to 100 times normal are found in hepatitis A and diagnosis is confirmed by hepatitis A IgM.

Both ALT and AST are good biomarkers of the natural history of viral hepatitis where high levels fall as the child recovers. The degree of elevation of both ALT and AST is not a good marker of hepatocellular damage.

Persistently elevated transaminases after 8 weeks require investigation. Differentials to consider include congenital infections, Alagille syndrome, choledochal cyst, cystic fibrosis, liver-based inborn errors and viral hepatitis (in infants). In older children, consider viral hepatitis, Wilson disease and autoimmune liver disease.

Liver ultrasound is a very useful investigation if transaminases are persistently raised and may show benign hamartomas or hepatoblastoma, non-alcoholic fatty liver disease, choledochal cyst, biliary atresia and (rarely) portal vein thrombosis.

Pitfalls to Avoid

Rarely fulminant hepatitis may follow hepatitis A infection.

In acute liver failure, the single most important investigations are the prothrombin time (PT) and INR. If the INR is prolonged, then vitamin K should be given intravenously and then the INR repeated. If the INR remains prolonged, this suggests impaired hepatic synthesis and requires urgent referral to a liver unit.

Box 36.8   An 8-Year-Old With an Incidental Raised Bilirubin

An 8-year-old is seen in outpatients with vague symptoms of tiredness and a recent viral illness. A serum bilirubin is checked and found to be mildly elevated.

Clinical Pearls

An isolated rise of a mild degree in unconjugated bilirubin is seen in Gilbert syndrome, which affects over 5 per cent of the population.

Gilbert syndrome is benign, and a mild elevation of unconjugated bilirubin occurs with fatigue, exercise, fasting and febrile illness. The diagnosis is invariably a clinical one.

Crigler–Najjar syndrome, by contrast, is associated with marked unconjugated hyperbilirubinaemia in newborns with a consequent risk of kernicterus. It is treated by exchange transfusion followed by liver transplantation.

Interpretation of Investigations

The key investigations include both direct and indirect bilirubin, aminotransferase levels and INR.

A mild elevation of unconjugated bilirubin is seen in Gilbert syndrome and all other laboratory investigations are normal.

A two- or threefold rise in unconjugated bilirubin will be seen following a 24-hour fast but, unsurprisingly, few families volunteer for this confirmation.

Both conjugated bilirubin and alkaline phosphatase will rise if biliary obstruction or cholestasis are evident.

An older child presenting with conjugated hyperbilirubinaemia, high transaminases, and normal albumin and INR is likely to have either autoimmune hepatitis or Wilson disease. Wilson disease is important to diagnose, and tests include urine copper and liver copper estimation via liver biopsy.

Pitfalls to Avoid

A mild rise in unconjugated bilirubin in a well child usually indicates Gilbert syndrome.

However, a 4-week-old well infant with jaundice, pale stools, dark urine and raised conjugated bilirubin needs prompt investigation to rule out biliary atresia and alpha 1 antitrypsin deficiency. In unwell infants of this age group with conjugated hyperbilirubinaemia, consider sepsis, disseminated herpes simplex infection or neonatal haemochromatosis. On the other hand, a 4-week breast-fed infant with unconjugated hyperbilirubinaemia most likely has breastmilk jaundice.

Box 36.9   A 7-Day-Old With an Abnormal Thyroid Screen

A 7-day-old infant is referred with an abnormal thyroid screen result on heel prick testing. The baby is asymptomatic, bottle-fed and thriving. Thyroid function tests are taken.

Clinical Pearls

Hypothyroidism may be congenital or acquired. The congenital form (as above) is picked up on newborn screening.

Acquired hypothyroidism in childhood is usually due to autoimmune thyroiditis. Children with Turner syndrome, Klinefelter syndrome, Down syndrome, coeliac disease or diabetes mellitus are at increased risk of autoimmune thyroiditis. There are often few complaints in acquired hypothyroidism apart from slow growth, weight gain or a goitre. The examination may show a goitre, growth deceleration, dry hair and delayed return of ankle jerk reflexes.

Acquired central hypothyroidism (low T4 and low TSH) is due to central nervous system tumours affecting the hypothalamous (hamartoma) or anterior pituitary gland, cranial irradiation or head trauma.

The treatment of hypothyroidism is L-thyroxine with normalisation of the TSH and free T4 levels, indicating adequate dosage.

Interpretation of Investigations

Congenital hypothyroidism is picked up by an elevated TSH level on the newborn Guthrie card test.

With an elevated TSH in the newborn screen, thyroid function tests are coordinated, and a thyroid scan will diagnose an absent or lingual thyroid gland or, more commonly, a normal or enlarged thyroid gland which is not functioning properly (dyshormonogenesis).

Investigations in autoimmune hypothyroidism show a low or low-normal thyroxine (T4), a high level of thyroid stimulating hormone (TSH), and positive anti-thyroperoxidase and anti-thyroglobulin antibodies.

Pitfalls to Avoid

In hypopituitarism, an elevated TSH will not be seen on the newborn screen; hypothyroidism may be missed as a result.

If the TSH fails to fall on L-thyroxine treatment, always first consider non-compliance with treatment. However, be aware that drugs (such as rifampicin and carbamazepine), the timing of giving L-thyroxine (not during or immediately after meals) and malabsorption conditions of the small intestine (where it is absorbed) may all interfere with delivery of L-thyroxine.

Box 36.10   A 2-Year-Old With Delayed Walking and Swollen Wrists

A 2-year-old child with Indian parents is referred because of delayed walking. The child is noted to be short, have swollen wrists (Fig. 36.4), a rachitic rosary on chest inspection and marked bowing of the legs (Fig. 36.5). Bloods tests are taken.

Clinical Pearls

Rickets is due to deficient mineralisation of the osteoid matrix of bone, resulting in softening and weakening of the bones. Clinical features of rickets include softening of the cranial bones (craniotabes), a rachitic rosary along the costochondral junctions, wrist swelling and bowing of the tibiae.

Rickets may be seen in preterm infants (rickets of prematurity), X-linked hypophosphataemic rickets (with striking tibial bowing), Vitamin D deficiency and chronic renal failure.

Rickets is most often due to vitamin D deficiency and those children especially at risk are of dark skin pigmentation with limited sun exposure, especially if breast-fed.

Interpretation of Investigations

Diagnosis of rickets is most often made by x-ray (Fig. 36.6). Blood investigations show low calcium and phosphate, elevated alkaline

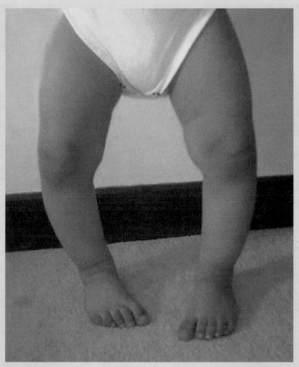

Figure 36.5 Softening of the growth plates of a child's bones causes the bowed legs and the thickened ankles seen in rickets. (Reproduced with permission from Cifu. D. X. (2021). *Braddom's physical medicine and rehabilitation* (6th ed.). Elsevier Inc.)

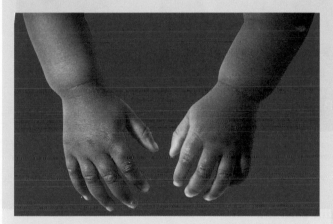

Figure 36.4 Hands and forearms of a young child with rickets show prominence above the wrist, resulting from flaring and poor mineralisation of the lower end of the radius and ulna. (Reproduced with permission from Bullough, P. G. (2009). *Orthopaedic pathology* (5th ed., pp. XX). Mosby.)

phosphatase and high parathyroid hormone (PTH) levels. The 1,25-dihydroxyvitamin D level may initially rise in response to PTH but subsequently drops due to limited 25-hydroxyvitamin D, which is the main circulating form of Vitamin D and has a long half-life. It is the best indicator of Vitamin D status and is not susceptible to fluctuations.

Pitfalls to Avoid

Tibial bowing is a striking feature of X-linked hypophosphataemic rickets. Always consider rickets in a child with delayed walking, especially if in a high-risk group.

Continued

Box 36.10   A 2-Year-Old With Delayed Walking and Swollen Wrists – cont'd

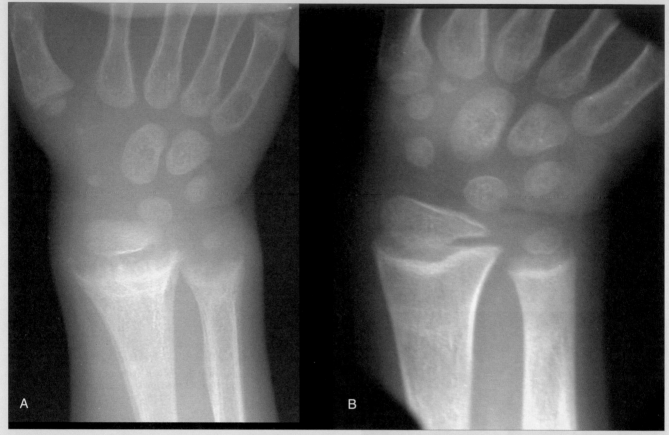

Figure 36.6   Rickets. A 1-year-old baby presented with swollen wrists. **(A)** X-ray shows widening and fraying of the distal end of the metaphysis of both the radius and ulna consistent with rickets. **(B)** After 5 months treatment with Vit D, growth has resumed and fraying of the distal radial and ulnar metaphyses has resolved. (Courtesy Prof. Stephanie Ryan.)

Box 36.11   A 3-Day-Old With Jitteriness and a Low Serum Calcium

A 3-day-old male infant is admitted with excessive tremors and jitteriness of the face, arms, and legs, and possible seizure activity. Blood glucose is normal and a blood calcium and magnesium are taken.

Clinical Pearls

Parathyroid hormone (PTH) and 1,25-dihydroxyvitamin D both regulate serum calcium levels. Hypocalcaemia is relatively common within 72 h of birth and is seen most often in infants of diabetic mothers, preterms and those with birth asphyxia.

Hypocalcaemia after 72 hours may be due to congenital hypoparathyroidism, maternal hyperparathyroidism and vitamin D deficiency.

In DiGeorge syndrome (22q11), there is hypoplasia of the parathyroid glands with associated congenital hypoparathyroidism.

Children with mild hypocalcaemia are often asymptomatic. Paraesthesiae, muscle cramps, laryngospasm, tetany and seizures are seen in severe hypocalcaemia. Chvostek and Trousseau's signs should be checked.

Hypocalcaemia may present with seizures that tend to be multifocal in neonates and generalised tonic clonic in older children. Some newborns may also have stridor or apnoea.

Children with mild hypercalcaemia are often asymptomatic but if severe they can have symptoms such as drowsiness, irritability and a depressed level of consciousness. Other symptoms include thirst, anorexia, confusion and depression.

Interpretation of Investigations

The normal range for serum calcium is 2.2 to 2.6 mmol/L. Hypocalcaemia may occur in very ill children with sepsis but, if the child is well, the key investigation is measurement of the parathyroid hormone (PTH).

A low-serum calcium with a low PTH level is seen in DiGeorge syndrome, familial hypoparathyroidism and maternal hyperparathyroidism in pregnancy.

A low-serum calcium with an elevated PTH is seen with vitamin D deficiency, malabsorption, use of anticonvulsants and pseudohypoparathyroidism.

An ECG is helpful in hypocalcaemia and may show a prolonged QT interval.

An elevated parathyroid hormone (PTH) level is seen in primary hyperparathyroidism following renal transplantation and, if ectopic, PTH production due to malignancy. Low phosphate levels are typical in primary hyperparathyroidism.

Familial benign hypercalcaemia is of autosomal dominant in inheritance with typical hypercalcaemia with a normal calcium to creatinine clearance ratio (under 0.01) and rarely causes symptoms.

Pitfalls to Avoid

Hypercalcaemia with a normal PTH is seen in Williams syndrome and usually disappears by 12 months of age. Williams syndrome is diagnosed by fluorescent in situ hybridization (FISH) analysis.

Hypercalcaemia with a low PTH is seen in hypervitaminosis A or D, sarcoidosis, thiazide diuretics or relating to immobilisation.

Box 36.12   A Febrile and Irritable Infant

An 8-month-old infant presents with a 1-day history of fever, irritability and vomiting. A lumbar puncture is performed and a turbid sample is obtained.

Clinical Pearls

Immunisation has been outstandingly successful in reducing the burden of meningitis across the world. *Defeating Meningitis by 2030* hopes to prevent epidemics caused by *Neisseria meningitidis*, substantially reduce neonatal deaths from *group B Streptococcus* infections, and decrease growing antimicrobial resistance. As always, prevention is the key to reduce morbidity and mortality from meningitis across the world.

Interpretation of cerebrospinal fluid (CSF) begins with inspection of the colour of the sample obtained. Normal CSF is clear and colourless. In meningitis, the fluid is turbid and often under pressure.

In traumatic taps (very common in paediatrics) or intracerebral haemorrhage, the fluid is blood-stained. Obtaining the red blood cell (RBC) count in tubes one and three is helpful as the RBC count is unchanged in central nervous system (CNS) haemorrhage but may decline in a traumatic tap.

Interpretation of Investigations

CSF should be sent for microscopy (total and differential cell counts), biochemistry (CSF glucose and protein) and bacteriology (Gram stain and culture and sensitivity). If antibiotics have been given prior to the lumbar puncture (LP), then DNA-PCR testing for specific agents should be performed.

In bacterial meningitis, there is characteristically an increase in white cells often above 1000/mm³ typically neutrophils, but meningitis can occur with an excess of lymphocytes or even a mixed picture. The CSF glucose level is lowered due to the bacterial consumption of glucose and is less than two-thirds of the blood glucose.

In bacterial meningitis, CSF protein is raised above 50 mg/dL, but interpretation may be difficult in a traumatic tap as blood cells also falsely raise protein levels. Gram stain may be positive for bacteria, but all CSF samples must be sent for culture and sensitivity if meningitis is suspected (even if negative).

The characteristic CSF picture in viral meningitis is lymphocytosis with normal protein and glucose and a negative Gram stain. In contrast tuberculosis (TB) meningitis typically shows raised white cells (classically lymphocytes) with an elevated protein, low glucose and a negative Gram stain. Acid-fast testing and TB culture both have a low level of sensitivity.

In herpes simplex encephalitis, cerebrospinal fluid (CSF) examination shows an increased number of white cells and red cells and an elevated CSF protein. MRI brain scan and EEG may show a temporal lobe focus. Polymerase chain reaction (PCR) of CSF for herpes simplex DNA provides a specific diagnosis.

Pitfalls to Avoid

Despite immunisation, meningitis is still seen and requires a high index of suspicion in the pyrexial infant. Timing of the lumbar puncture is key. Be aware of contraindications to LP, including fulminant sepsis and raised intracranial pressure.

Correct technique is also important. Here the key to success is correct positioning with an experienced helper. Use topical anaesthetic cream on the skin at the site of the LP.

The three key elements to obtaining a satisfactory CSF sample are good preparation, good nursing assistance and good technique. HHV6 infection can be associated with a bulging or full fontanelle and febrile seizures.

Blood glucose should be measured at the same time as performing a lumbar puncture. The normal ratio of CSF to blood glucose is 2:3.

Box 36.13   Key Points

It is important to justify an investigation before you order it and then be able to interpret the result in the clinical context.

The child with haemophilia will often have no problems until they start to mobilise around 18 to 24 months, when 'pea-sized' lumpy bruises are commonly seen. The classical presentation of spontaneous haemarthrosis is expected in weight-bearing joints such as the hip, knee or ankle joints.

For moderate to severe haemophilia, recombinant factor replacement therapy is the mainstay of treatment.

Diarrhoea is the most common cause of metabolic acidosis with a normal anion gap.

The diagnosis of lactic acidosis should be considered in all severely ill infant with sepsis or hypotension, and children with an increased anion gap metabolic acidosis. The diagnosis can be confirmed by measurement of the serum lactate level.

If metabolic alkalosis with a low urinary chloride (under 15 mEq/L), the main causes relate to excessive vomiting (pyloric stenosis in infancy, bulimia in teenagers) and chronic use of diuretics.

Sodium concentrations are dependent on both the amount of sodium present in the plasma and the amount of water.

Salt depletion is associated with clinical signs of dehydration.

A water deficit is by far the most common cause of hypernatraemia and occurs due to inadequate water intake or excessive water loss associated with severe gastroenteritis.

Excessive water losses can also occur as a consequence of impaired renal water retention due to diabetes insipidus (either central or nephrogenic) or an osmotic diuresis associated with glycosuria or hypercalcaemia.

For hypoglycaemia (blood glucose under 2.6 mmol/L), the absence of ketones in the urine should prompt consideration of hyperinsulinism or a fatty acid oxidation disorder (such as MCADD).

In tumour lysis syndrome, massive amounts of potassium are released from the intracellular compartment and severe hyperkalaemia can ensue if any associated renal impairment.

The major risk with hyperkalaemia is cardiac arrythmias. The characteristic ECG changes are tall, peaked T waves.

With mild and isolated elevation of the transaminases without any symptoms in the child, the best strategy is to repeat 6 to 8 weeks later and if back to normal, the child can safely be discharged.

In acute liver failure, the single most important investigations are the prothrombin time (PT) and international normalised ratio (INR).

An isolated rise of a mild degree in unconjugated bilirubin is seen in Gilbert syndrome, which affects over 5 per cent of the population.

Acquired hypothyroidism in childhood is usually due to autoimmune thyroiditis. Children with Turner syndrome,

Continued

Box 36.13   Key Points—cont'd

Klinefelter syndrome, Down syndrome, coeliac disease or diabetes mellitus are at increased risk of autoimmune thyroiditis.

Clinical features of rickets include softening of the cranial bones (craniotabes), a rachitic rosary along the costochondral junctions, wrist swelling and bowing of the tibiae.

Diagnosis of rickets is most often made by x-ray. Blood tests show decreased calcium and phosphate, increased alkaline phosphatase, increased 1,25 hydroxy vitamin D levels, and increased parathyroid hormone levels.

Children with mild hypocalcaemia usually have no symptoms. In severe hypocalcaemia, symptoms such as paraes-

thesiae, muscle cramps or spasm, laryngospasm, tetany and seizures may occur. Chvostek and Trousseau's signs should be checked.

CSF should be sent for microscopy (total and differential cell counts), biochemistry (CSF glucose and protein) and bacteriology (Gram stain and culture and sensitivity). If antibiotics have been given prior to the lumbar puncture, then DNA-PCR testing for specific agents should be performed.

The <u>three</u> key elements to obtaining a satisfactory CSF sample are good preparation, good nursing assistance and good technique.

Key References

Assadi, F. (2008). *Clinical decisions in pediatric nephrology A problem-solving approach to clinical cases.* Springer Nature.

Bhatnagar, N., & Hall, G. W. (2018). Major bleeding disorders: Diagnosis, classification, management and recent developments in haemophilia. *Archives of Disease in Childhood, 103*(5), 509–513.

Chaker, L., Bianco, A. C., Jonklaas, J., & Peeters, R. P. (2017). Hypothyroidism. *Lancet, 390*(10101), 1550–1562.

Flood, V. H., & Scott, J. P. (2018). Bleeding and thrombosis. In R. M. Kliegman, P. S. Lye, B. Bordini, H. Toth, & D. Basel (Eds.), *Nelson pediatric symptom-based diagnosis* (pp. 682–700). Elsevier.

Nadar, R., & Shaw, N. (2020). Investigation and management of hypocalcaemia. *Archives of Disease in Childhood, 105*(4), 399–405.

The Lancet. (2020). A new roadmap for meningitis. *Lancet, 395*(10232), 1230.

Online References

Meningitis Research Foundation. (n.d.). *Defeating meningitis.* https://www.meningitis.org/our-work/action-and-support/meningitis-2030.

37 ECG Interpretation

WILLIAM EVANS

This chapter focusses on electrocardiogram (ECG) interpretation with the aim of improving your ability to distinguish normal from abnormal ECGs and to identify specific abnormalities.

Paediatric trainees often struggle with the ECG interpretation. This chapter will look in detail at the interpretation of an ECG, the common normal variants and ECG changes that require recognition and appropriate referral.

A recent study from the United States shows that education of paediatric residents on ECG interpretation – focussing specifically on distinguishing normal from abnormal and identifying specific ECG findings – significantly improves their ability to interpret ECG abnormalities (Fig. 37.1). Sinus arrhythmia and Wolff–Parkinson–White syndrome were among the most frequently misinterpreted ECG findings for paediatric trainees. Normal variant ECGs seemed to provide the greatest difficulty for residents.

ECG Interpretation and Cardiac Arrhythmias

The four-step approach for ECG interpretation outlined in this chapter enables a trainee, family doctor or consultant to differentiate a normal tracing from an abnormal one.

The ECG leads need to be correctly placed (Fig. 37.2).

It is important to note that in infants and children, the normal ranges of heart rate, BP and respiratory rate vary significantly with age.

The *essential differences* in infants and children are:

Firstly, the normal heart rate is much higher, with a normal heart rate of 110 to 160 per minute under 12 months of age.

There is often sinus arrythmia, whereby the heart rate varies quite considerably with respiration.

The cardiac axis is deviated to the right in newborns, and T wave inversion is normal in leads V1 to V3, and Q waves are normal in the inferior leads (aVF, II and III) and V5 and V6.

The QRS axis is +110 degrees in neonates, +70 degrees from 1 month to 3 months of age and +60 degrees from 3 months to 16 years of age.

The corrected QT interval is less than 0.49 seconds under 6 months of age and less than 0.44 seconds over 6 months of age.

Step One: Determine the Rate and Rhythm

Using lead II, calculate the approximate heart rate by counting the number of large boxes between two QRS complexes where the heart rate = 300 ÷ number of large boxes between two QRS complexes (Fig. 37.3].

RHYTHM

For sinus rhythm, there should be a P wave before each QRS complex with a regular PR interval (Fig. 37.4). The P waves should be upright in 1, aVF and negative in aVR.

Commonly seen sinus rhythms include:

Sinus arrhythmia is a normal variation in sinus rhythm that occurs with respiration. The heart rate rises and falls with inspiration and expiration (Fig. 37.5). The variation is more pronounced in young children and less pronounced in infants and adolescents.

Sinus bradycardia is a slow sinus rhythm seen normally in aerobically trained individuals, but also occasionally in hypothyroidism and long QTc. The heart rate is under 60 beats per minute (Fig. 37.6).

Sinus tachycardia is a fast sinus rhythm consistent with anxiety, crying, fever, sepsis and occasionally hyperthyroidism (Fig. 37.7).

The heart rate is over 140 to 160 beats per minute.

Each P wave is normally followed by a QRS with a constant PR interval. If some or all P waves are not followed by a QRS or the PR intervals vary, then atrioventricular (AV) block is present (Fig. 37.8).

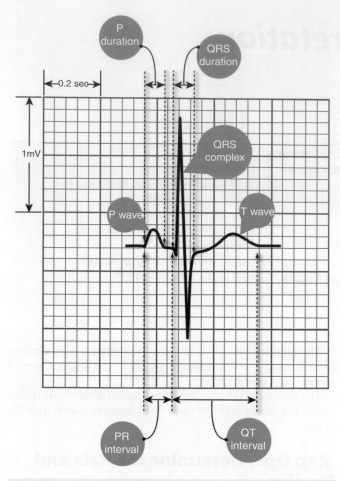

Figure 37.1   Evaluating an ECG.

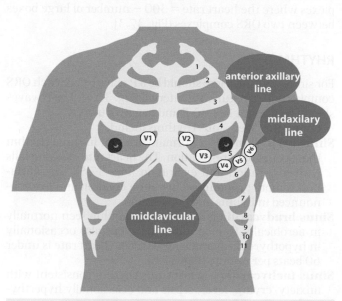

Figure 37.2   Praecordial leads placement.

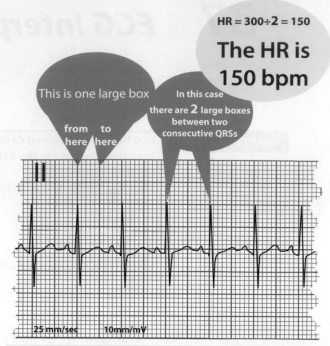

Figure 37.3   Evaluating heart rate.

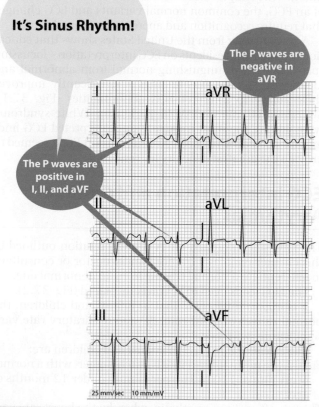

Figure 37.4   Sinus rhythm.

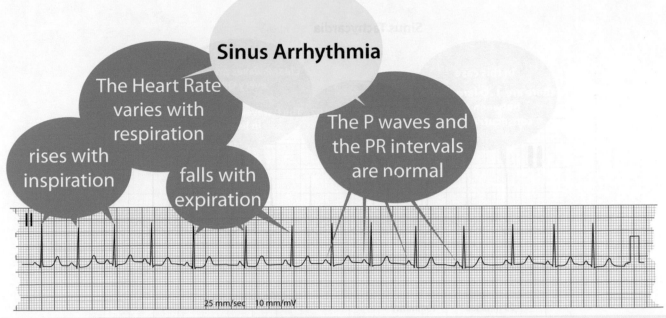

Figure 37.5   Sinus arrythmia.

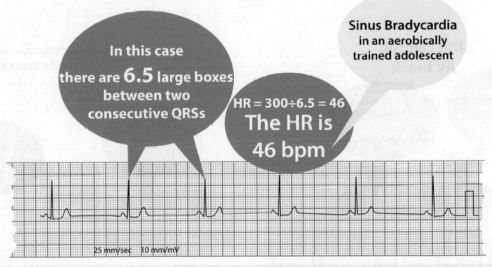

Figure 37.6   Sinus bradycardia.

Step Two: Evaluate the PR, QRS and QT Intervals

Using lead II, inspect the PR, QRS and QT intervals. Measured values can be expressed either as seconds or milliseconds. For example, one small box is 0.04 seconds (40 msec), and one big box is 0.2 seconds (200 msec) (Fig. 37.9).

PR intervals and QT intervals are often expressed in seconds.

PR INTERVAL

The normal PR interval is 0.12 to 0.2 seconds (Fig. 37.10). At any age, a PR interval of 0.2 seconds (200 msec or one big box) is long and consistent with first-degree AV block (Fig. 37.11).

In infants and young children, however, a PR interval of 0.16 (160 msec or four small boxes) is long and consistent with first-degree AV block. A prolonged PR interval is seen in myocarditis, rheumatic fever, hypothermia and Duchenne muscular dystrophy. In complete heart block, the atria and ventricles beat independently of each other, the QRS is normal and the ventricular rate is regular but slow (30 to 40 beats per minute). Congenital complete heart block is most often seen in infants born to mothers with connective tissue disorders with anti-Ro and anti-La antibodies (most commonly systemic lupus erythematosus).

A short PR interval can adjoin the QRS and may be normal if the QRS is narrow or it may be abnormal and consistent with pre-excitation if the QRS base is wide. In a condition known as Wolff–Parkinson–White syndrome, the ECG appearance is of a short PR interval associated with a widened QRS (Fig. 37.12). The widened QRS pattern consists

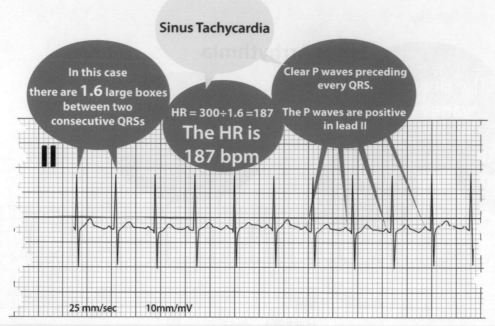

Figure 37.7 Sinus tachycardia.

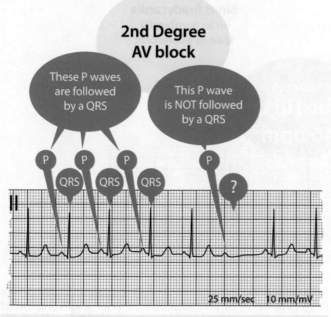

Figure 37.8 Second degree AV block.

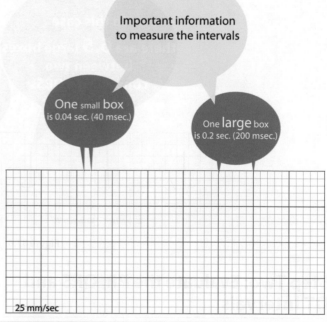

Figure 37.9 Measure the intervals.

of a characteristic upstroke or downstroke (depending on the lead) forming a delta wave on the proximal portion of the QRS. The ECG appearance of pre-excitation is caused by an early excitation of the ventricles via congenital bypass tracts. Pre-excitation is associated with SVT and most children and adolescents with pre-excitation and SVT should undergo electrophysiology studies with pathway ablation.

QRS

A normal QRS is usually only about one small box wide (.04 seconds or 40 msec). A wide QRS is usually two small boxes

or more (0.08 seconds or 80 msec). A wide QRS is seen in ventricular hypertrophy, bundle branch block, WPW, ventricular arrythmias or with a pacemaker.

QT AND T WAVES

The most important interval is the QTc interval and lead II or V5 should be used. A QTc interval > 0.45 seconds (> 450 msec) warrants further attention. A markedly prolonged QTc interval (>480 msec) can place a person at risk of life-threatening ventricular arrhythmia. Therefore, the QTc

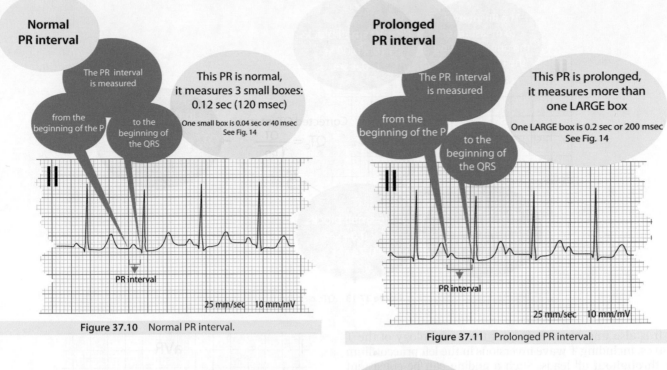

Figure 37.10   Normal PR interval.

Figure 37.11   Prolonged PR interval.

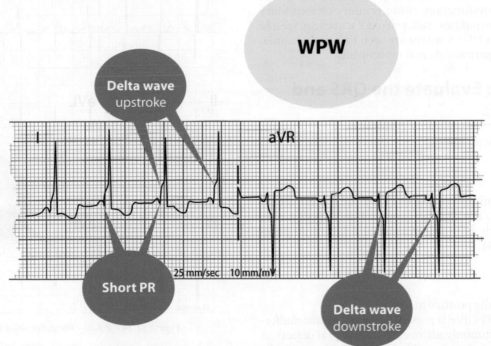

Figure 37.12   Wolff–Parkinson–White (WPW) syndrome.

must be checked closely in *every* ECG. The most accurate way of measuring the QTc is known as the tangent method: the end of the T wave is defined as the point where the tangent on the steepest point of the terminal limb of the T wave intersects with the isoelectric baseline. The preceding R-R interval before the measured T wave is the reference heart rate (Fig. 37.13).

Long QT syndromes are usually inherited in an autosomal dominant fashion and thus there may be a family history of sudden death. Romano–Ward syndrome is inherited in an autosomal dominant fashion and Jervell and Lange-Nelson syndrome has associated deafness and is inherited in an autosomal recessive fashion. Most pathogenic variants for prolonged QT interval involve a sodium or potassium channel. Long QT syndromes may present with syncope, seizures, palpitations or presyncope. Acquired prolongation of the QT interval may arise due to hyperkalaemia, hypocalcaemia or hypomagnesaemia, secondary to myocarditis, or with a variety of medications including amiodarone, quinidine, sotalol, erythromycin, procainamide, methadone and haloperidol.

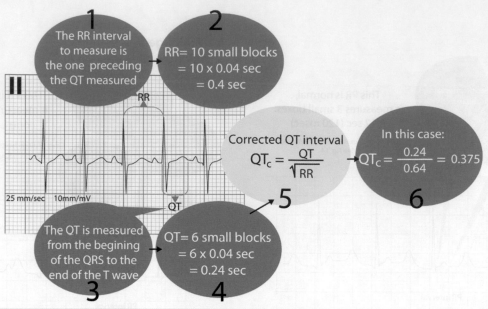

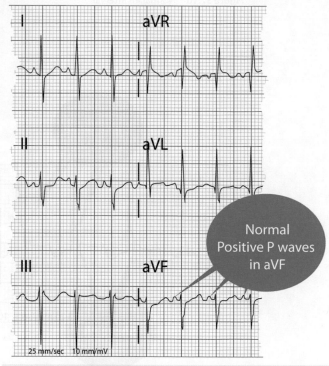

Figure 37.13   QTc calculation.

It is also important to inspect the morphology of the T waves, including T wave inversions in the left praecordium or throughout all leads. Such a finding can be consistent with myocardial dysfunction, either primary or secondary to metabolic abnormalities. Tall, peaked T waves are seen in hyperkalaemia and flat T waves are seen in hypokalaemia, hypothyroidism, pericarditis and myocarditis.

Step Three: Evaluate the QRS and P Wave Axis

Use aVF for this evaluation.

P AXIS

The P wave is normally positive in aVF. If the P wave is negative in aVF, then the electrical conduction direction may be abnormal, such as in a low atrial or a left atrial pacemaker (Fig. 37.14).

QRS AXIS

The QRS is normally positive in aVF.

A negative QRS in aVF is present in some cardiac malformations, most commonly atrioventricular septal defects. A superior axis is seen in tricuspid atresia, Ebstein anomaly, and atrioventricular septal defects (Fig. 37.15).

Step Four: Evaluate for Right and Left Ventricular Hypertrophy

First, always check for the standardisation marks on the ECG, which are usually seen in multiple leads and are two big boxes tall for normal, full standard. For consistency, ECGs should always be performed using full-standard settings.

Figure 37.14   P Axis – normal positive P waves.

RIGHT VENTRICULAR HYPERTROPHY

To determine the presence or absence of right ventricular hypertrophy (RVH), use only lead V1.

There are **three** rules for RVH (Fig. 37.16):
1. Upright T waves in V1 after about 7 days of age. The T waves in V1 are inverted after 7 days and remain so until adolescence, after which time the T wave in V1 becomes upright.
2. An RSR' pattern in V1 in which the R' is taller than the R.
3. A pure R wave in V1 after about 6 months of age.

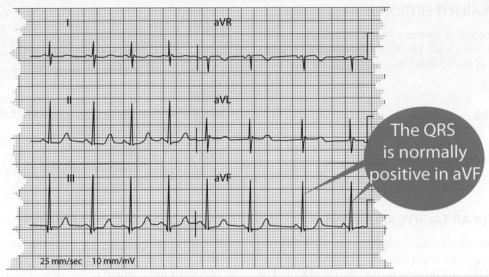

Figure 37.15 Normal QRS axis.

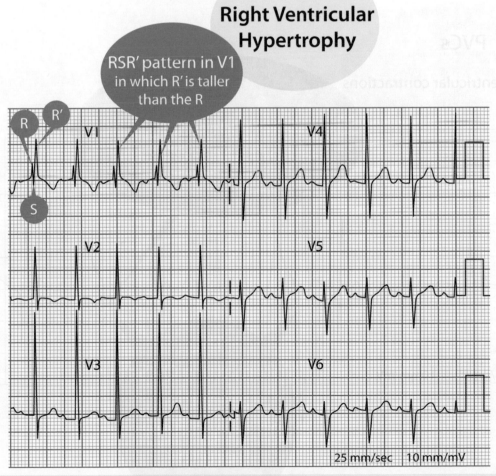

Figure 37.16 Right ventricular hypertrophy (RVH).

LEFT VENTRICULAR HYPERTROPHY

To determine presence or absence of left ventricular hypertrophy (LVH), use only lead V6. If the R wave in V6 intersects the baseline of the lead V5 in a standard 12 lead ECG, there is LVH.

Arrhythmias

Premature atrial and ventricular contractions are seen quite often and are regarded as normal variants (Figs 37.17 and 37.18).

SUPRAVENTRICULAR TACHYCARDIA (SVT)

SVT is a narrow complex tachycardia that occasionally can be difficult to differentiate from sinus tachycardia and a re-entrant mechanism is the most common cause of SVT. The P wave is buried in the T wave of the preceding cycle. The heart rate in SVT is over 180 (in children) and over 220 (in infants). Non-specific presenting symptoms include pallor, irritability and chest pain, and they may have features of heart failure (such as tachypnoea and hepatomegaly). SVT is distinguished from sinus tachycardia by its sudden onset, absence of rate variation, unresponsiveness to a fluid bolus and no P waves being visualised on ECG (Fig. 37.19).

Management of SVT involves ice immersion in infants and a Valsalva manoeuvre in children (ask the child to blow into an empty 10 mL syringe).

In those who are acutely compromised or in whom initial vagal manoeuvres were not successful, adenosine should be given intravenously, or direct current (DC) cardioversion may be required.

VENTRICULAR TACHYCARDIA (VT)

VT is a broad complex tachycardia and usually presents with a very compromised, ill, hypotensive child who may progress to full cardiac arrest (Fig. 37.20). If not in shock, amiodarone is recommended and, if shock is evident, DC cardioversion is required. It is possible, however, to have short runs of VT and be asymptomatic.

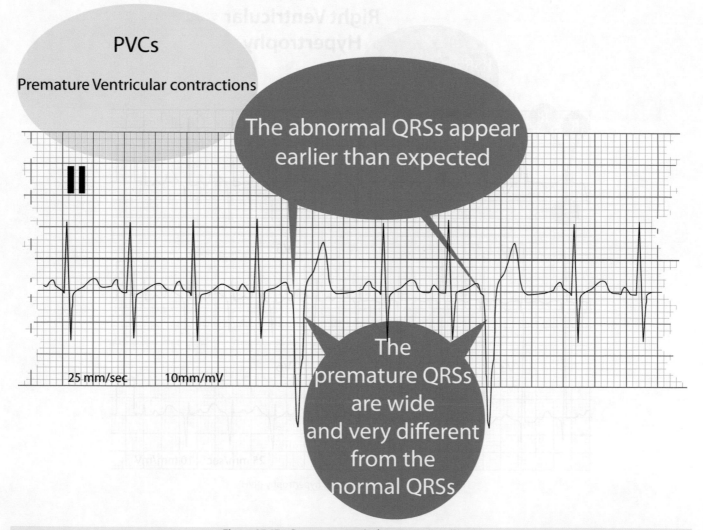

Figure 37.17   Premature ventricular contractions (PVCs).

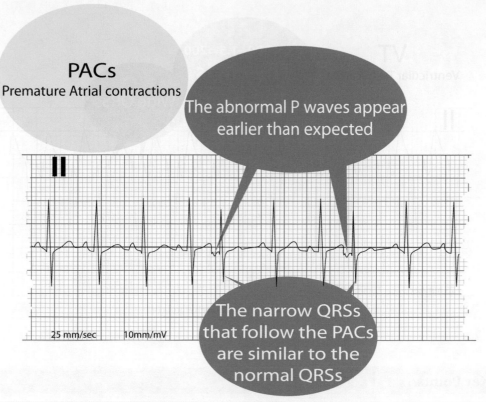

Figure 37.18 Premature atrial contractions (PACs).

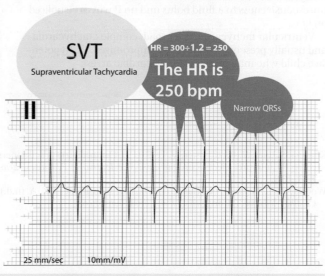

Figure 37.19 Supraventricular tachycardia (SVT).

DC cardioversion with 0.5 to 2.0 J/kg is appropriate for unstable patients or those with wide-QRS tachycardias, as wide-QRS SVT is difficult to distinguish from ventricular tachycardia. The cardioverter/defibrillator needs infant or paediatric paddles. Firstly, synchronise the equipment with the QRS, as unsynchronised defibrillation may cause ventricular fibrillation requiring immediate repeat cardioversion. Infants and children require deep sedation for electrical cardioversion. Trained anaesthetic personnel should administer deep sedation.

(Box 37.1)

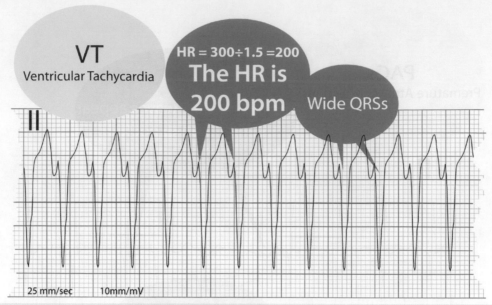

Figure 37.20   Ventricular tachycardia (VT).

Box 37.1   Key Points

The four-step approach for ECG interpretation outlined in this chapter enables a trainee, family doctor or consultant to differentiate a normal tracing from an abnormal one.

Step one is to evaluate the rate and rhythm; step two to evaluate the PR, QRS and QT intervals; step three to evaluate the QRS axis; and step four to evaluate for left or right ventricular hypertrophy.

The QRS axis is +110 degrees in neonates, +70 degrees from 1 month to 3 months of age and +60 degrees from 3 months to 16 years of age.

A markedly prolonged QTc interval (>480 msec) can place a person at risk of life-threatening ventricular ar-

rhythmia. Therefore, the QTc must be closely checked in *every* ECG.

Premature atrial and ventricular contractions are seen quite often and are regarded as normal variants.

Supraventricular tachycardia is distinguished from sinus tachycardia by its sudden onset, absence of rate variation, unresponsiveness to a fluid bolus and no P waves visualised on ECG.

Ventricular tachycardia is a broad, complex tachycardia and usually presents with a very compromised, ill, hypotensive child who may progress to full cardiac arrest.

References

Evans, W. N., Acherman, R. J., Mayman, G. A., Rollins, R. C., & Kip, K. T. (2010). Simplified pediatric electrocardiogram interpretation. *Clinical Pediatrics, 49*(4), 363–372.

Khanna, S., Iyer, V. R., & Vetter, V. L. (2019). Can pediatric practitioners correctly interpret electrocardiograms? *The Journal of Pediatrics, 206,* 113–118.

Woosley, R. L., Heise, C. W., Gallo, T., Woosley, D., & Romero, K. A. (n.d.). *CredibleMeds.org.* QT drugs list. www.crediblemeds.org.

38 *Critical Appraisal of the Literature*

CONOR HENSEY and STEPHEN ATKIN

Evidence-based medicine is the conscientious, explicit and judicious use of current best evidence in making decisions about the care of individual patients. The patient should be at the centre of this quest, and it is the task of the doctor to provide the information to facilitate the patient's or family's choice. Therefore, evidence-based practice provides a systematic approach to enable clinicians to use the best available evidence to help them solve a clinical problem. In paediatrics, it is fair to say that high quality evidence underpinning clinical practice is evident, especially in oncology and neonatology. Virtually all children with cancer are enrolled in multicentre clinical trials to identify which treatment gives the very best results. Clinical decisions elsewhere in paediatrics are quite complex and the evidence base is often incomplete and tends to inform rather than determine clinical decisions.

The **five** key steps to ensure the practice of evidence-based medicine are:
1. **Ask** patient-centred, focussed questions about the care of individuals, communities or populations. The PICO (PICO stands for **P**opulation, **I**ntervention, **C**omparison and **O**utcome) helps to ask pertinent questions in assessing the current medical literature.
2. **Acquire** the best available evidence relevant to your question.
3. **Appraise** the evidence for validity and applicability to the problem at hand.
4. **Apply** the evidence by engaging in collaborative decision-making with individual patients and/or groups.
5. **Assess** the outcomes and evaluate your new or amended practice.

Keeping Up To Date With the Medical Literature

It can be very challenging to separate the important literature, which should inform our clinical practice, from the large volume of irrelevant or poor-quality studies.

It is important to develop a system which makes this easier and helps you engage with colleagues and the latest evidence. Social media and modern technology make this easier, and with the continued development of FOAMed (Free Open Access Medical Education), there is a growing community focussed on evidence-based practice and knowledge translation.

Twitter is a great resource to direct you towards new, relevant evidence and information. Following important paediatric medical journals and key people who share an interest in paediatric FOAMed will provide a gateway to information and a way to connect with likeminded individuals. Another way to stay up to date is to subscribe to eTOC for important journals relevant to your speciality.

Some additional paediatric specific online resources which are very helpful include:

Don't Forget the Bubbles – https://dontforgetthebubbles.com/

This is a paediatric blog providing online medical education for paediatric medical professionals including 'The Bubble Wrap', which provides a short summary and review of selected articles.

Cochrane Child Health – https://childhealth.cochrane.org/

This website provides news, updates and links to Cochrane Reviews in Child Health and other paediatric evidence-based content.

Evidence Alerts – https://www.evidencealerts.com/ and www.nhs.uk/news/

This free service notifies physicians and researchers about newly published clinical studies from high quality journals. Notifications can be refined by speciality and clinical importance.

These tools will keep you updated on important medical literature; however, without skills in critical appraisal, you will not be able to evaluate the relevance and validity of results presented and apply the evidence in practice.

Critical Appraisal

Critical appraisal is a detailed look at relevant research papers to assess their validity, reliability, importance and applicability to clinical practice.

Location and Selection of Studies

TACKLING BIAS

It is important to be aware of bias. An example of publication bias is that studies with positive results are more likely to be published. Most major journals are written in English and are thus more likely to be referenced by study authors – this is termed citation bias.

Study Design

There are a few study design types with which you should be familiar, including (Fig. 38.1):

QUALITATIVE STUDIES

Qualitative studies seek to explore patient attitudes, beliefs, and experiences, and their interactions with healthcare professionals.

QUANTITATIVE STUDIES

The research career of a student or junior doctor often begins with a case report (we all have to start somewhere!) which may progress to a case series, therein reflecting a group of patients with the same condition and often a literature review of that condition.

Moving upwards, a case control study looks at patients and controls and studies relevant exposures and their links to outcome. A cohort study studies two separate groups with just one receiving an exposure of interest.

A cross-sectional study is the observation of a defined population at a single point in time or a defined period wherein exposure and outcome are simultaneously determined.

Randomised Controlled Trials

A randomised controlled trial (RCT) is the gold standard in determining whether an intervention is effective. Bias is minimised by blinding and randomisation. Participants

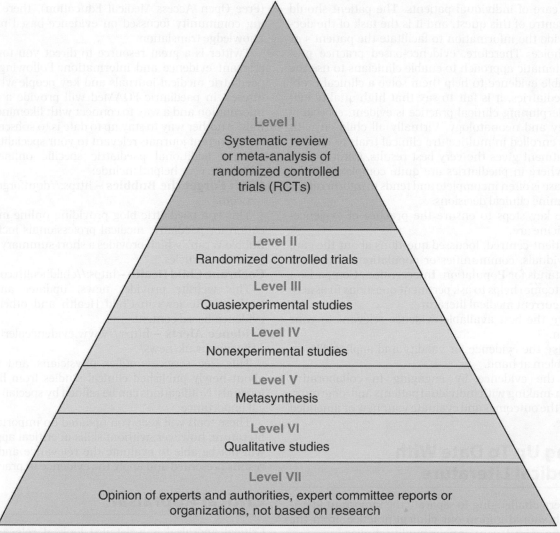

Figure 38.1 Levels of evidence. Evidence hierarchy for rating levels of evidence associated with a study's design. Evidence is assessed at a level according to its source. (Reproduced with permission from Lobiondo-Wood, G., & Haber, J. (2022). *Nursing research – binder ready: Methods and critical appraisal for evidence-based practice* (10th ed.). Elsevier.)

should be randomly allocated to either a treatment or control group.

In a single-blinded trial, the participants are not aware whether they have received the treatment or not. In a double-blinded trial, neither the participants nor those giving the intervention are aware who has received the treatment. Therefore, RCTs enable the rigorous assessment of a single variable and they can be pooled for meta-analysis. They are expensive to run and may last a long time. RCTs may at times be ethically problematic, as a trial may have to be stopped early if dramatic effects are seen. RCTs are less effective for interventions that require operator training (e.g., catheterisation) and for trials of complex interventions (e.g. multidisciplinary team interventions).

The so-called consolidated standards of reporting trials (CONSORT) flowsheet is a tool that allows a detailed assessment when reporting an RCT. Firstly, assess the allocation looking at the randomisation process, stratification and whether there are potential confounders. Look for the power calculation and how sample size was worked out. All participants should be followed up and reasons for those dropping out should be displayed. The presentation of results should be clear and precise.

A DEEPER DIVE INTO THE STATISTICAL CONCEPTS IN RCTS

The so-called baseline characteristics of the intervention and control groups should be broadly similar.

When establishing a trial, there should be a sample size large enough to have a high chance of detecting a worthwhile effect (if one exists). Before commencing the trial, calculate the sample size needed to detect a true difference between the control and intervention groups. The expected standard power is 80 per cent. It is important to study all the results, including participants who complete and those who withdraw from the trial.

The null hypothesis assumes there is no statistical significance between the two variables. If accepted, this means that there is no difference in clinical efficacy between two treatments.

The P-value measures whether a particular outcome may have arisen by chance if the null hypothesis were true. A P-value of less than one in 20 ($p < 0.05$) is deemed statistically significant and will allow the researcher to reject the null hypothesis.

Confidence intervals are increasingly used, with a 95 per cent confidence interval meaning that there is a 95 per cent chance that the true size of effect will lie within this range.

The concept of an odds ratio is important, with higher-odds ratios indicating more effective interventions. An ineffective intervention will have an odds ratio under one and, conversely, the odds ratio will be over one if the outcome is positive. The number needed to treat (NNT) reflects how many children need to receive the intervention to prevent an unwanted outcome. The ideal NNT is one; the higher the NNT, the less effective the intervention. As an example, the NNT for therapeutic cooling in cases of neonatal encephalopathy is seven.

Critical Appraisal of Different Study Designs

In the critical appraisal process of a journal article, there are a few initial questions that are worth considering before detailed critical analysis.

1. Does this study ask a clearly focussed question?
2. Have valid methods been used to address this question?
3. Are the results important?
4. Can I apply the results to my patients or the local population?

If the answer to any of these four questions is a clear no, perhaps you should proceed no further. If an article warrants detailed critical appraisal, you should always start by looking at the research methodology used in the study.

INTERPRETING NEGATIVE CLINICAL TRIALS

If the clinical trial did not show a treatment effect, could this be because the sample size was not big enough to have a reasonable chance of finding one? The smaller the trial, the less chance it has of showing a treatment effect, even if there is one. In addition, the smaller the treatment effect of practical importance, the bigger the trial required need to identify it.

CLINICAL AND STATISTICAL SIGNIFICANCE

If a study is clinically significant, the treatment must produce a worthwhile effect in terms of the patient's health. For example, a drug that lowers cholesterol by less than 1 per cent is of no clinical use. If a study is statistically significant, then the treatment benefit must be such that an occurrence by chance is unlikely.

Systematic Reviews

Systematic reviews have increasingly become more relevant and seek to combine valid studies following a clear methodological approach with meta-analyses, proving very helpful in summarising the results. Systematic reviews give a panoramic overview of all primary studies on a topic.

Avoiding bias is key – a systematic review should therefore follow an explicit and reproducible methodology. First, identify all primary studies (not just in the English language) and only select the best studies for further analysis. It is helpful to include a meta-analysis of the results from selected studies and graphically represent these results for greater clarity using a Forest plot.

The Forest plot is a display reflecting the participants in both intervention and control groups with outcomes expressed as relative risk. Confidence intervals are displayed for each study and for the overall pooled results (Fig. 38.2). A Forest plot reflects the level of heterogeneity seen and what influence each individual study has had on the overall result when they are pooled together. In essence, a picture paints a thousand words!

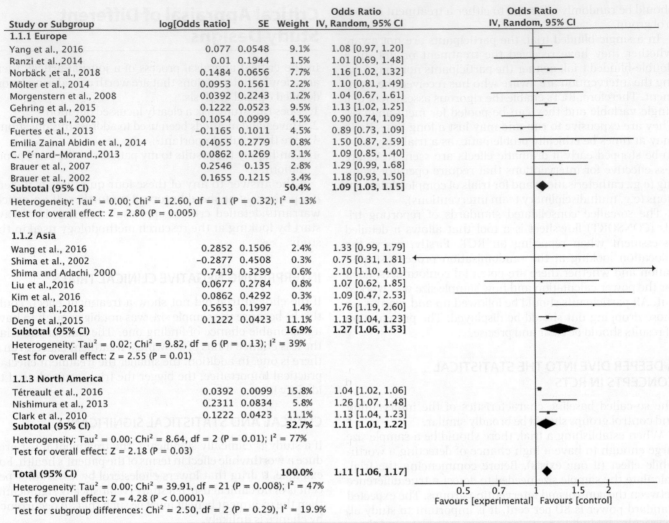

Figure 38.2   Forest plot of the association between traffic-related benzene and the development of asthma in children. (Reproduced with permission from Han, K., Ran, Z., Wang, X., Wu, Q., Zhan, N., Yi, Z., et al. (2021). Traffic-related organic and inorganic air pollution and risk of development of childhood asthma: A meta-analysis. *Environmental Research*, 194(110493), 110493.) CI = confidence interval.

ADVANTAGES AND DISADVANTAGES OF SYSTEMATIC REVIEWS

A major advantage of a systematic review is that it enables the pooling of results from a number of studies. They may increase overall confidence from small studies and may be updated if new evidence becomes available. They tend to have the final word on a clinical query and help identify areas where more research is needed.

Disadvantages of systematic reviews are that they are quite expensive and time-consuming. There may be publication bias where a test called the funnel plot is a useful barometer. They help summarise the evidence dating back 2 years, as it often takes this length of time to conduct a systematic review, which needs to be updated on an ongoing basis.

CRITICAL APPRAISAL OF SYSTEMATIC REVIEWS

In your assessment of a systematic review, assess whether the literature search included published and unpublished materials and studies not written in English. Ensure only high-quality studies are included using a scoring system to rate studies and ensure that at least two experts perform the analysis. Ensure that the results are clearly and precisely presented and that they might apply to a local population. Comprehensive assessment tools include the very detailed QUOROM (quality of reporting of meta-analyses) statement, but perhaps both AMSTAR and CASP checklists are easier to navigate for busy clinicians.

(Box 38.1)

Box 38.1   Key Points

Evidence-based medicine is the conscientious, explicit and judicious use of current best evidence in making decisions about the care of individual patients.

In a randomised controlled trial (RCT), participants are randomly allocated to a test treatment and a control group.

The RCT is the gold standard to test the effectiveness of an intervention by which bias is reduced through randomisation and blinding.

A meta-analysis is a systematic review that uses quantitative methods to summarise the results.

The term number needed to treat (NNT) refers to the number of patients receiving the intervention to prevent one person having the unwanted outcome.

Systematic reviews allow for the pooling of results and may be expanded if new evidence becomes available. They are rightly regarded as having the final say about a clinical question.

Resources including online for further information, support, and training:

Critical Appraisal in General

Leen, B., Bell, M., & McQuillian, P. (2014). The Evidence-Based Practice (EBP) Group South East. *Evidence-Based Practice: A Practice Manual.* Health Service Executive. https://www.drugsandalcohol.ie/21949/1/EBPManual.pdf.

Saaiq, M., & Ashraf, B. (2017). Modifying "Pico" question into "Picos" model for more robust and reproducible presentation of the methodology employed in a scientific study. *World Journal of Plastic Surgery, 6*(3), 390–392.

UCL Great Ormond Street Institute of Child Health. (2017, March). *Critical appraisal of a journal article.* University College London. https://www.ucl.ac.uk/child-health/sites/child-health/files/library_critical_appraisal_handout.pdf.

van Loveren, C., & Aartman, I. H. (2007). The PICO (patient-intervention-comparison-outcome) question. *Nederlands Tijdschrift voor Tandheelkunde, 114,* 172–178.

Young, J. M., & Solomon, M. J. (2009). How to critically appraise an article. *Nature Clinical Practice Gastroenterology & Hepatology, 6*(2), 82–91. https://doi.org/10.1038/ncpgasthep1331.

Critical Appraisal of Certain Kinds of Study

Jansen, M., & Ellerton, P. (2018). How to read an ethics paper. *Journal of Medical Ethics, 44*(12), 810–813.

Moher, D., Cook, D. J., Eastwood, S., Olkin, I., Rennie, D., & Stroup, D. F. (1999). Improving the quality of reports of meta-analyses of randomised controlled trials: The QUOROM statement. Quality of Reporting of Meta-analyses. *Lancet, 354*(9193), 1896–1900.

Moralejo, D., Ogunremi, T., & Dunn, K. (2017). Critical Appraisal Toolkit (CAT) for assessing multiple types of evidence. *Canada Communicable Disease Report, 43*(9), 176–181.

Critical Appraisal Tool Collections

AMSTAR (n.d.). *Checklist.* Assessing the methodological quality of systematic reviews. https://amstar.ca/Amstar_Checklist.php.

Appraisal of Guidelines for Research and Evaluation (AGREE). (n.d.). *Advancing the science of practice guidelines.* http://www.agreetrust.org/.

Cadogan, M. (2019, May 2). *FOAM • LITFL • FOAMed resources.* Life in the Fast Lane • LITFL. https://litfl.com/foam/.

CONSORT. (2010). *The CONSORT Flow Diagram.* http://www.consort-statement.org/consort-statement/flow-diagram.

Critical Appraisal Skills Programme (CASP). (n.d.). http://www.casp-uk.net/.

Dawes, M., Summerskill, W., Glasziou, P., Cartabellotta, A., Martin, J., Hopayian, K. et al. (2005). Sicily statement on evidence-based practice. *BMC Medical Education, 5*(1), 1.

JBI. (n.d.) *Critical Appraisal Tools.* Faculty of Health and Medical Sciences, The University of Adelaide. https://jbi.global/critical-appraisal-tools.

McVeigh, J. (1998). How to read a paper. *Physiotherapy, 84*(12), 623–624. https://doi.org/10.1016/s0031-9406(05)66166-4.

Resources for Critical Appraisal – http://www.londonlinks.nhs.uk/groups/clinical-librarians-information-skills-trainers-group/trainers-toolkit/resources-for-critical-appraisal.

SIGN – The guideline developer's handbook by the Scottish Intercollegiate Guidelines Network is a useful source of guidelines. https://www.sign.ac.uk/.

The Centre for Evidence-Based Medicine. (n.d.). *Critical appraisal tools.* University of Oxford. https://www.cebm.ox.ac.uk/resources/ebm-tools/critical-appraisal-tools.

The Centre for Evidence Based Medicine has a broad range of resources to help navigate critical appraisal.

The Centre for Evidence-Based Medicine. (n.d.). Nuffield Department of Primary Care Health Sciences. http://www.cebm.net.

The Critical Appraisal Skills Programme (CASP) allows access to critical appraisal checklists enabling assessment of different types of study.

39 Practical Procedures in Neonatology and Paediatrics

EUGENE DEMPSEY and JOHN MURPHY

Introduction

Practical procedures in newborns and infants can be daunting for the doctor new to paediatrics. Newborn care is a procedure-driven speciality. Infants as young as 22- or 23-weeks' gestation are now surviving. It is no longer acceptable that trainees perform procedures without first undergoing adequate training in a simulated environment where learning should occur in a safe environment. Historically, most procedural training has occurred in the inpatient setting. However, the learner is the priority in the simulation environment. A reduction in exposure to procedures, changes in training curricula and changes in clinical practice mean that opportunities to perform procedures are reduced. Thus, it is essential that when trainees are performing their first procedure in the neonatal unit, they have had the necessary exposure in the simulation area in advance. Simulation is best defined as an instructional strategy 'used to replace or amplify real experiences with guided experiences that evoke or replicate substantial aspects of the real world in a fully interactive manner'. These facilities do not need to be high fidelity and every centre should strive to ensure access to neonatal mannequins and the necessary essential equipment to replicate the real-world scenario.

Some key aspects of simulation based medical education (SBME) include feedback, deliberate practice, curriculum integration, outcome measurement, skills acquisition and maintenance. Feedback can be from a facilitator or a peer. The session can be video recorded and reviewed afterwards by a group of peers for this purpose. There are many elements of deliberate practice including focused repetitive practice that leads to precise measurements that yield informative feedback where trainees also monitor their progress. Curriculum integration is seen as an essential component of SBME, where it complements clinical education. Outcome measurement is critical to the success of simulation training and the establishment of reliable metrics is essential. A metric should be clear, concise, unambiguous, and have high intra- and inter-rater reliability. It should allow a quantitative distinction between the performance of novices and experts and permit the quantitative definition of proficiency. Metric units of task execution are the units of performance that are associated with the optimal performance of that skill. A metric unit should include steps within which the procedure is performed, the instruments used and how they should be used, and, crucially, should also include what should not be done (i.e. errors). Competence is achieved through the vehicles highlighted above in the simulation environment. With competence comes confidence, and confidence is the key to success.

Preparation Prior to the Procedure: General Principles

The importance of adequate preparation cannot be overstated. 'Fail to prepare, prepare to fail' holds true for any of the procedures outlined below, whether it is the placement of a peripheral cannula through to the emergency insertion of a pigtail catheter or an emergency intubation. It is essential that one is familiar with the equipment being used, optimises the position of the patient in advance, calculates necessary measurements, is aware of the potential complications and how to deal with these, and that an experienced assistant is present for the procedure. Analgesia is important for a number of these procedures from sedation and muscle relation for a newborn intubation to the use of sucrose for venous cannulation. The procedures outlined below include umbilical catheterisation, peripherally

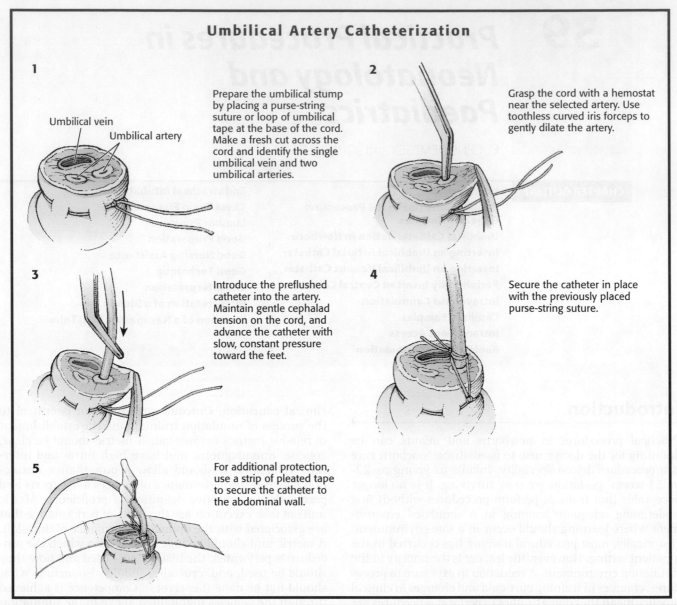

Umbilical Artery Catheterization

1

Umbilical vein
Umbilical artery

Prepare the umbilical stump by placing a purse-string suture or loop of umbilical tape at the base of the cord. Make a fresh cut across the cord and identify the single umbilical vein and two umbilical arteries.

2

Grasp the cord with a hemostat near the selected artery. Use toothless curved iris forceps to gently dilate the artery.

3

Introduce the preflushed catheter into the artery. Maintain gentle cephalad tension on the cord, and advance the catheter with slow, constant pressure toward the feet.

4

Secure the catheter in place with the previously placed purse-string suture.

5

For additional protection, use a strip of pleated tape to secure the catheter to the abdominal wall.

Figure 39.1   Umbilical artery catheterisation. (Reproduced with perfrom Roberts, J. R. (2018). Roberts and Hedges' clinical procedures in emergency medicine and acute care (7th ed.). Elsevier Inc.)

inserted central catheters, newborn intubation, radial line insertion, peripheral venous cannulation, lumbar puncture, chest drain insertion, and nasogastric tube placement.

Umbilical Catheterisation in Newborns

Newborn infants (both term and preterm) have easily accessible umbilical vessels with two arteries and one vein present in the umbilical cord. Measurements should be performed in advance to determine how far one needs to place the umbilical venous and arterial catheter. There are various nomograms in use; please refer to your own institutional guideline to determine the appropriate insertion length. Ensure that you are adhering to a sterile technique and wearing the appropriate gown, hat, mask and double gloves for the procedure. Always ensure equipment is placed to the dominant hand side (e.g. right side for right-handed person) for ease

of access. We would generally recommend placement of the arterial catheter first as this can be the more difficult procedure and may require further cut downs on the cord.

Inserting an Umbilical Arterial Catheter

Decide the distance for insertion using the formula (weight in kg × 3) + 9 cm or defer to your own institutional guidelines for measurements. Flush the catheter with 0.9 per cent saline. Wrap a tie loosely around the base and cut the cord down to 3 cm. Stabilise the artery by holding the adjacent cord with forceps and gently locate the arterial opening using fine-toothed forceps. Encourage it open with a dilator. Do not force the dilator. Gently ease the umbilical arterial catheter into the artery. Carefully advance the catheter (Fig. 39.1). Significant resistance is sometimes felt. Do

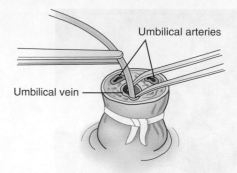

Figure 39.2   Inserting the catheter into the umbilical vein. (Reproduced with permission from Cameron, P., Browne, G. J., Mitra, B., Dalziel, S., & Craig, S. (Eds.) (2019). Textbook of paediatric emergency medicine (3rd ed.). Elsevier Ltd.)

not try to advance as it may be entering a false tract. As the catheter enters the vessel further, gently pull the cord superiorly to aid passage into the iliac artery. Secure the line and check its position with a chest and abdominal x-ray. Trainees are encouraged to practise in the simulation setting, ideally with fresh umbilical cord.

Inserting an Umbilical Venous Catheter

Flush the lumen of the umbilical venous catheter with 0.9 per cent saline. Clean the umbilical cord and place a tie lightly around the base. Cut the cord to about 3 cm in length from the umbilicus. The umbilical vein is large and may ooze blood when the cord is cut. Using a sterile technique, identify the vein (single, large, patulous oozing vessel compared to the two arteries) and insert the umbilical venous catheter about 5 cms (Fig. 39.2). Withdraw to ensure blood return and then insert the umbilical venous catheter to the predetermined length. The most common problem encountered is 'bouncing' at approximately 5 to 6 cm, which may reflect the fact that the catheter is attempting to enter the left portal vein. Carefully advance the catheter and do not force it. Check the position with both a chest and abdominal x-ray when both lines are placed. Again, trainees are encouraged to practise in the simulation setting, ideally with fresh umbilical cord.

Peripherally Inserted Central Catheter

Peripherally inserted central catheters (PICCs) are used in the care of preterm and critically ill term neonates and children (Fig. 39.3). This form of central venous access allows the provision of fluids, medications and concentrated nutritional solutions. PICC insertion is challenging and has a wide array of potential complications. Insertion success rates vary and enhancing PICC insertion skills is important to reduce potential complications and ensure patient safety. Simulation models exist that mimic the clinical conditions for PICC insertion. Choosing the correct vein is the most important element. Typically, the upper limb brachiocephalic vein is the most ideal. The

long saphenous is also an excellent site but involves a longer distance to achieve optimal placement and will occasionally enter the lumbar plexus. Critical to success are familiarity with equipment, optimal positioning of the patient when the insertion site is chosen and careful meticulous sterile procedure to avoid any subsequent central line infections. Position is verified with contrast injected as the x-ray is performed. It is essential that the catheter is positioned outside of the heart.

Intravenous Cannulation

Commonly used sites for venous blood sampling and cannulation include the dorsum of the hand or foot or the anterior cubital fossa. Wiping with an alcohol swab will make the vein more visible.

Introduce a cannula at an angle of 45 degrees through the skin and into the vein. Once in the vein, a flashback of blood will occur, and then reduce the angle to go a short distance along the vein. While holding the needle still, advance the cannula over the needle and into the vein with blood flowing up the cannula. Remove the needle and dispose of it carefully into the sharps container. Take a sample of blood with a syringe and then attach a T-piece connector and flush with 0.9 per cent sodium chloride. Firmly secure the cannula. Seal the end with a bung and connect an infusion.

Capillary Samples

Firstly, make sure the heel is warm. In newborns, use the sides of the heels (Fig. 39.4). Clean the area with an alcohol swab and use a sterile lancet to create a puncture about 2 mm deep. A second puncture may sometimes be required. A spring-loaded automatic lancing device is more convenient and also ensures consistency in penetration depths. Collect the blood sample into a capillary tube.

Intraosseous Access

This is an emergency procedure in which venous access is not possible. It is rarely performed in newborn infants but more typical in infants and children with sepsis presenting to the emergency department. Intraosseous needle insertion is the fastest way to give fluid resuscitation in a peripherally shut down infant or child. The site used is the flat anterior surface of the tibia, a finger breadth below and medial to the tibial tuberosity (Fig. 39.5). The anteromedial tibia is the first choice and presents a flat, stable surface. The anterolateral femur is the next most commonly selected site. Clean with an alcohol swab. Firmly insert the intraosseous needle at 90 degrees to the skin surface using a turning or boring motion. This may be done manually or with a drill. There is a sudden 'give' when the needle enters the bone marrow. After ensuring the needle is stable, remove the stylet and flush with saline. Attach a syringe and aspirate bone marrow if possible. Secure the intraosseous needle with an adhesive dressing and attach a pre-primed intravenous extension set and flush with

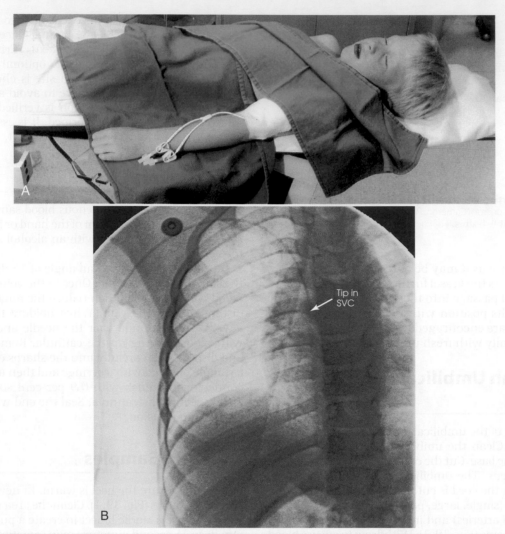

Tip in SVC

Figure 39.3   (A) Postinsertion image of a double-lumen PICC line in a 7-year-old boy (shown in the interventional suite). Conscious sedation was used for this procedure. (B) Digital image of PICC line showing the distal tip of the catheter positioned in superior vena cava (SVC). (Reproduced with permission from Frank, E. D., Long, B. W., & Smith, B. J. (2011). *Merrill's atlas of radiographic positioning & procedures* (12th ed.). Mosby.)

normal saline, ensuring that there is no extravasation. Replace with a more secure intravenous access when possible. Intraosseous samples should never be run in a blood gas machine.

Radial Artery Cannulation

Support the wrist slightly extended. Find the radial pulse (just medial to the radial styloid) and insert the cannula towards it at a shallower angle (30 degrees) than for venous cannulation. A light source is often helpful for transillumination of the underlying vessel in newborns, particularly in preterm infants. The flashback will be pulsatile. Advance the cannula and remove the needle. While removing the needle, make sure that appropriate pressure is applied to the cannula to prevent blood loss. Connect to lockable bungs or connectors and flush with 0.9 per cent saline. When taking arterial blood samples from the line, do so slowly so as to prolong the lifespan of the radial

line. Remove the radial line if there are any signs of digital ischaemia.

Endotracheal Intubation

All trainees should have completed the Neonatal Resuscitation Programme (NRP) training prior to being on call for neonatology and should avail of training using mannequins. Endotracheal intubation is a difficult skill to learn, and every effort should be made to ensure appropriate time is given to trainees to acquire this skill. Mannequins of different sizes (term and preterm) are an essential element of any newborn training program me. It is essential that trainees be familiar with the equipment and have practised in the simulation lab. Requirements in terms of equipment include non-sterile gloves, suction, a bag valve mask linked to an oxygen supply, a laryngoscope with a bright light and different sized blades, an endotracheal tube of suitable size, a means of securing the tube once the newborn is intubated, and a stethoscope to aid in determining appropriate positioning.

Term infants require a 3.5 mm size endotracheal tube and preterm infants need a size 3.0 or 2.5 mm. Pre-medication is now routinely given prior to intubation using the FAST pneumonic (Fentanyl-Atropine-Suxamethonium-Tube) as pre-medication makes intubation easier and less traumatic for the infant. Various other agents are used; please defer to institutional practice.

Position the head of the newborn infant in a neutral position, preoxygenate with bag valve mask ventilation via Neopuff device, T piece, or flow-inflating bag attached to a manometer. Avoid hyperextension of the neck. As a general rule, the aim is to avoid overinflation of the chest. For preterm infants, set pressure at 25 cm H_2O and PEEP of 5 cm H_2O on the Neopuff device. Following insertion of blade, apply gentle pressure on the cricoid cartilage using the little finger of the left hand to bring the cords into view (Fig. 39.6). An assistant can also perform this task. Gently suction out secretions. Insert the endotracheal tube past the vocal cords and position at the vocal cord line on the ETT. Do not insert the tube if the vocal cords cannot be seen. Listen for air entry; louder sounds on the right indicate that the tube may be in the right main bronchus–if so, pull the tube back slightly and listen again. Secure the endotracheal tube and confirm its position (Figs 39.4 and 39.5).

A trainee undertaking an intubation should recite the following steps as the laryngoscope blade is being advanced:

I am now placing the blade on the tongue – I can now see the uvula – next I can see the posterior pharyngeal wall – next I will push the blade forwards and identify the epiglottis – I will lift up the epiglottis and the cords come into view in front of it – then I insert the tube through the cords.

A CO_2 detector should be used to confirm that the tube is in the trachea. The detector changes from purple to yellow when the tube is correctly placed. If there is no colour change, the tube is most likely in the oesophagus and must be removed and a further attempt made. Other ways to confirm correct placement include equal air entry heard bilaterally and 'misting' of the endotracheal tube. Straight

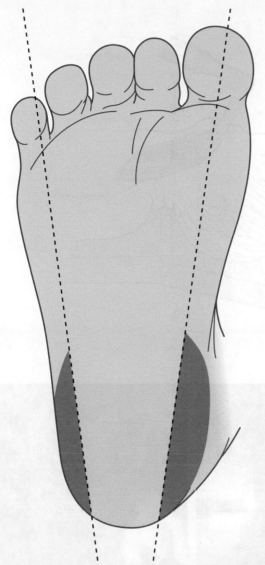

Figure 39.4 The shaded areas indicate the lateral and medial aspects of the heel, which are suitable for heel-pricks. (Reproduced with permission from Rennie, J. M. (2012). *Rennie & Roberton's textbook of neonatology* (5th ed.). Saunders.)

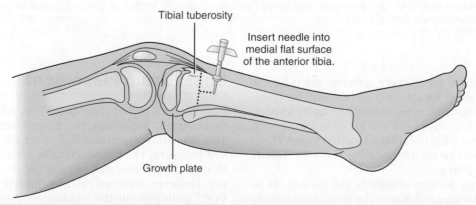

Tibial tuberosity

Insert needle into medial flat surface of the anterior tibia.

Growth plate

Figure 39.5 Insertion of the intraosseous needle into the anterior tibia. (Reproduced with permission from Zimmerman, J.J., & Rotta, A.T. (2022). Fig. 14.2: Insertion of the intraosseous needle into the anterior tibia. *Fuhrman & Zimmerman's pediatric critical care* (6th ed., p. 95). Elsevier Inc.)

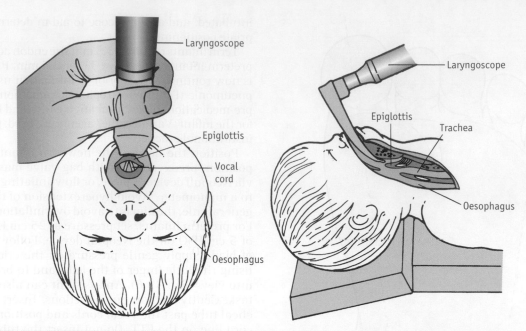

Figure 39.6   Neonatal intubation. (Reproduced with permission from Henderson, C., & Macdonald, S. (2004). *Mayes' midwifery – a textbook for midwives* (13th ed.). Bailliere Tindall.)

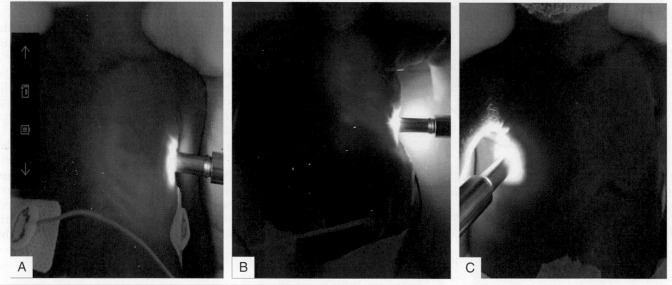

Figure 39.7   High-intensity fibre optic light demonstrating increased transillumination on left half of chest suggestive of left side pneumothorax (A and B) compared to normal right chest (C). (Reproduced with permission from Rajiv, P. K., Lakshminrusimha S., & Vidyasagar, D. (Eds.). (2019). *Essentials of neonatal ventilation* (1st ed.). Elsevier.)

blades are used (size 00 for the very preterm, size 0 for the moderate preterm, size 1 for the term infant), and the endotracheal tube is made easier to manipulate by using a stylet. The tube is inserted 6 cms plus 1 cm for each kg (i.e. in a term infant weighing 3 kg, the tube is inserted 9 cm). However, the tube should be no further than 6 cm for infants weighing less than 750 g.

Videolaryngoscopy is increasingly being used so as to visualise what the trainee is doing so the consultant trainer may give guidance; this significantly increases the intubation success rate.

Chest Drain Placement

Insertion of a pigtail chest-drain is one of the less common (but critically important) procedures seen in newborn care. This is often a procedural skill of which trainees have limited exposure. The introduction of surfactant and advances in ventilation have reduced the incidence of pneumothorax. However, reported rates in the recent COIN and SUPPORT trials indicate the incidence of pneumothorax is now between 3 per cent and 9 per cent in very preterm newborns. Transillumination may help identify a pneumothorax

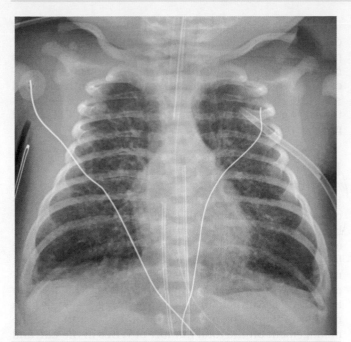

Figure 39.8 Anterior–posterior radiograph of a 1-day-old full-term male with meconium aspiration syndrome (MAS). The lungs are hyperinflated (flattened diaphragms and 10–11 rib lung expansion) with patchy, rope-like opacities projecting from the hilum to the periphery. A 'high'-lying umbilical arterial catheter is seen at T6 and a malpositioned umbilical venous catheter is seen close to the right atrium. The percutaneous chest tube present on the left was placed to drain a large pneumothorax, a common complication in severe MAS. (Reproduced with permission from Goldsmith, J. P., Karotkin, E. H., Suresh, G., & Keszler, M. (2017). *Assisted ventilation of the neonate: An evidence-based approach to newborn respiratory care* (6th ed.). Elsevier Inc.)

(Fig. 39.7). It is no longer acceptable that trainees insert catheters without proper preparation, training and skills acquisition in a simulation environment. Pigtail catheters are dependable, safe and effective, have few complications, are associated with less discomfort, and possibly less trauma than the previously used trocars. Ideal placement is the fourth intercostal space, midaxillary line. Two types of catheters exist: one for direct placement and the second utilising a Seldinger technique. This procedure requires a skilled assistant. Sucrose should be given and consideration should be given to local anaesthetic prior to the procedure. Gentle but firm pressure is applied for the direct placement applying pressure until a 'give' is felt. The needle should not be inserted more than 1 cm. The needle is withdrawn as the catheter is advanced. A needle and syringe are used initially in the Seldinger technique. The needle is advanced to 1 cm through the skin and the syringe is aspirated as the needle advanced. When air is aspirated, remove the syringe and place the guidewire through the needle, then remove the needle, leaving the guidewire in situ. A dilator is advanced over the guidewire to ensure an appropriate size tract for the catheter. The dilator is removed and the pigtail is passed over the guidewire and advanced approximately 5 cm into the chest. The guidewire is removed and the catheter secured. A three-way tap is applied to the catheter. Confirm resolution of the pneumothorax and catheter position with a chest x-ray (Fig. 39.8).

Lumbar Puncture

A lumbar puncture (LP) is a procedure in which an aspiration needle is inserted into the sub-arachnoid space of the spinal cord, usually in the interspace between L4 and L5. The main indications for an LP in newborns and infants are to diagnose bacterial and viral meningitis, herpes and candida infection, and metabolic disorders such as hyperglycinaemia.

The key to success is correct positioning with an experienced helper. Use topical anaesthetic cream on the skin at the site of the LP. When performing an LP in a newborn, the aim is to obtain a 'champagne' (clear) tap rather than 'coke' (blood-stained) tap. A traumatic LP is defined as a CSF specimen with over 500 RBCs/mm³. The procedure can be technically challenging. The LP success rate in newborns is 50 to 60 per cent compared with 80 to 90 per cent in older children.

The **three** key elements to obtain a satisfactory CSF sample are good preparation, good nursing assistance, and good technique.

Good Preparation

A 25-gauge short bevel needle with a stylet is most commonly used. The other items are an antiseptic solution (chlorhexidine), masks, gloves, and gowns. The infant's oxygen saturation and heart rate should be monitored during the procedure. Free flow oxygen and suctioning should be readily available if required. Sucrose should be administered just prior to the attempt.

Three CSF tubes marked 1, 2, 3 are required. Tube 1 is for culture and Gram stain, Tube 2 is for glucose and protein, and Tube 3 is for cell count and polymerase chain reaction (PCR).

Good Nursing Assistance

The nurse places the infant on their side at right angles to the hard surface. One hand is placed behind the knees and the legs are held at right angles to the hips. The other hand is placed behind the infant's shoulders. The neck must not be flexed; it is best to keep the head in a neutral position (Fig. 39.9). Some flexion of the lower spine opens up the lumbar spaces, but the nurse should only do this right before the needle is inserted. If available, a second nurse can collect the CSF samples in the marked tubes.

Good Technique

The doctor should sit at eye level to the infant's spine. The infant's head is on the doctor's left. The end of the spinal cord in a term infant lies at L2–L3 and thus, in newborns, the preferred space for needle insertion is between L4–L5. Identify the L3–L4 space by drawing an imaginary line along the tops of the iliac crests. Then identify the L4 spinous process and locate the L4–L5 space. It can be

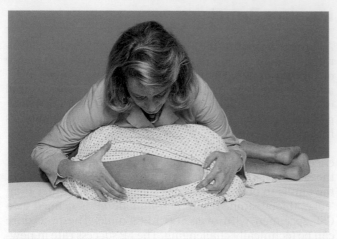

Figure 39.9 Side-lying position for lumbar puncture. (Reproduced with permission from Hockenberry, M. J. & Wilson, D. (2018). *Wong's Nursing care of infants and children* (11th ed.). Mosby.)

helpful to place the thumb and index finger around the L4 spinous process.

The LP needle is inserted into the L4–L5 aiming towards the umbilicus. Once the skin has been entered, stop and wait for the infant to settle. Many recommend that the stylet be removed at this point. The advantage of early removal of the stylet is that it reduces the chances of the needle going beyond the CSF space and entering the venous plexus and resulting in a bloody tap. The needle is advanced slowly until CSF flow is obtained. The usual length of needle insertion is 0.5 cm.

Ten drops of CSF should be collected in each of the three tubes.

The needle is withdrawn and a pressure dressing is applied to prevent CSF leak followed by a Band-Aid. The samples are then promptly sent to the laboratory.

CSF Interpretation

The cerebrospinal fluid (CSF) is examined for red blood cells (RBC), white blood cells (WBC), CSF glucose and protein, Gram stain and culture, and PCR for certain microorganisms. Normal CSF is clear and colourless, and blood in the CSF usually indicates a bloody tap with a decreased number of RBCs in bottle 3 compared to bottle 1. It takes 300 to 400 WBCs to turn CSF turbid.

In normal CSF, the glucose concentration is two-thirds that of the serum glucose concentration. The normal CSF protein is less than 0.45 g/dL in infants over 2 months of age but is higher (under 1.0 g/dL) in term infants in the neonatal period and slightly higher (under 1.15 g/dL) in preterms in the neonatal period. The CSF protein is elevated in the great majority of infants and young children with bacterial meningitis. CSF changes

in bacterial meningitis include 100 to 10, 000 white cells (polymorphs predominate) with an elevated CSF protein over 0.5 g/dL and a decreased CSF glucose. The normal newborn CSF values are neutrophils 0, lymphocytes $<20\times10^9$/L in infants less than 1 month old, and $<10\times10^9$/L in infants over 1 month old with protein less than 1.0 g/L, glucose above 2.5 mmol/L, or a CSF/blood glucose ratio above 0.6.

Interpretation of a Bloody Tap

If there is a traumatic tap, the question is whether one can correct the number of WBCs to compensate for the blood in the CSF. The formula varies from 1 WBC for every 500 to 1000 RBCs in the sample. In practice, these formulae have not proven to be dependable in ruling out meningitis, as adjusting the WBC in the CSF reduces false-positives while increasing false-negatives. The formula is particularly unhelpful when evaluating a sample in a newborn infant. The message is that it is best to base the management on the total number of WBCs in the CSF and ignore the RBCs. Using various calculations to reduce the number of WBCs in the CSF is risky and may lead to a delay in the treatment of a meningitis case. In the case of a bloody tap in a newborn, always start intravenous antibiotics pending the culture report and microbiology guidance.

Insertion of a Nasogastric (NG) Tube

Nasogastric tubes are frequently used in neonates. The main indications for NG tube insertion are feeding the preterm infant and gastric drainage for the relief of bowel obstruction. Older infants with feeding or swallowing problems may also require NG feeds.

Prior to NG insertion, one should wash hands and put on gloves and an apron. Estimate the length of tube by measuring from the tip of the infant's nose and passing the tragus of the ear on to the xiphisternum (Fig. 39.10). Lubricate the end of the NG tube using plenty of lubricant. Local anaesthetic spray may be applied to the back of a child's throat to lessen discomfort.

Gently slide the tube along the floor of the nasal cavity, initially aiming towards the occiput. There will be slight resistance as the NG tube passes into the oesophagus. Advance the NG to the predetermined distance. Attempt to aspirate gastric fluid into the syringe and check on a pH strip (pH should be under 5.5) and attach the tube to a drainage system or spigot. Check the position of the NG tube by performing an x-ray where a correctly placed NG tube should be seen passing below the diaphragm.

(Box 39.1)

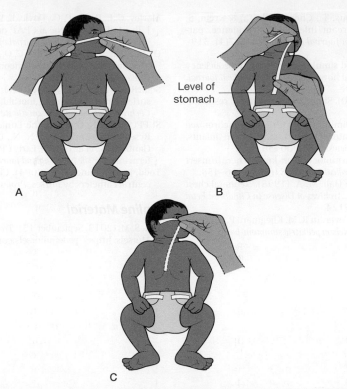

Level of
stomach

A

B

C

Figure 39.10   Measuring the length of the nasogastric tube prior to insertion: measure from ear to nose, then from nose to xiphisternum, noting the distance markers on the tubing. (Reproduced with permission from Johnson, R., & Taylor, W. (2006). *Skills for midwifery practice* (2nd ed.). Elsevier.)

Box 39.1   **Key Points**

Competence in practical procedures is achieved through demonstration, observation and practice. With competence comes confidence, and confidence is the key to success. Simulation-based education programmes place the learner first.

Commonly used sites for venous blood sampling and cannulation include the dorsum of the hand or foot or the anterior cubital fossa.

Intraosseous needle insertion is the fastest way to give fluid resuscitation in a peripherally shut down infant or child.

The **three** key elements to obtaining a satisfactory CSF sample are good preparation, good nursing assistance and good technique. The lumbar puncture (LP) needle is inserted into the L4–L5 aiming towards the umbilicus.

For intubation, preoxygenate with bag valve mask ventilation and position the infant's head in a neutral position, thus avoiding hyperextension of the neck. Gentle pressure on the cricoid cartilage using the little finger of the left hand brings the cords into view.

Check the position of the NG tube by performing an x-ray where a correctly placed NG tube should be seen passing below the diaphragm.

Key References

American Academy of Pediatrics, & American Heart Association. (2021). In G. M. Weiner (Ed.), *Textbook of neonatal resuscitation* (8th ed.). *American Academy of Pediatrics.*

Aziz, K., Lee, H. C., Escobedo, M. B., Hoover, A. V., Kamath-Rayne, B. D., Kapadia, V. S., et al. (2020). Part 5: Neonatal resuscitation: 2020 American Heart Association guidelines for cardiopulmonary resuscitation and emergency cardiovascular care. *Circulation, 142*(16, Suppl. 2), S524–S550. https://doi.org/10.1161/CIR.0000000000000902.

The S.T.A.B.L.E. Program. (n.d.). *Neonatal Education.* https://stableprogram.org/.

Additional Reading Material

Ang, H., Veldman, A., Lewis, A., Carse, E., & Wong, F. Y. (2012). Procedural training opportunities for basic pediatric trainees during a 6-month rotation in a level III perinatal centre in Australia. *The Journal of Maternal-Fetal & Neonatal Medicine, 25*(11), 2428–2431.

Bourgeois, F. C., Lamagna, P., & Chiang, V. W. (2011). Peripherally inserted central catheters. *Pediatric Emergency Care, 27*(6), 556–561, quiz 62–63.

Cates, L. A. (2009). Pigtail catheters used in the treatment of pneumothoraces in the neonate. *Advances in Neonatal Care, 9*(1), 7–16.

Chopra, V., Ratz, D., Kuhn, L., Lopus, T., Chenoweth, C., & Krein, S. (2014). PICC-associated bloodstream infections: Prevalence, patterns and predictors. *The American Journal of Medicine, 127*(4), 319–328.

Gallagher, A. G. (2012). Metric-based simulation training to proficiency in medical education: What it is and how to do it. *Ulster Medical Journal, 81*(3), 107–113.

Garvey, A. A., & Dempsey, E. M. (2020). Simulation in neonatal resuscitation. *Frontiers in Pediatrics, 8*, 59.

Greenough, A., Milner, A. D., & Dimitriou, G. (2004). Synchronized mechanical ventilation for respiratory support in newborn infants. *Cochrane Database of Systematic Reviews, 4*, CD000456.

Griffiths, J. R., & Roberts, N. (2005). Do junior doctors know where to insert chest drains safely? *Postgraduate Medical Journal, 81*(957), 456–458.

Hourihane, J. O., Crawshaw, P. A., & Hall, M. A. (1995). Neonatal chest drain insertion—an animal model. *Archives of Disease in Childhood Fetal and Neonatal Edition, 72*(2), F123–F124.

Lye, P. S., & Densmore, E. M. (2018). Fever. In R. M. Kliegman, P. S. Lye, B. Bordini, H. Toth, & D. Basel (Eds.), *Nelson pediatric symptom-based diagnosts* (pp. 701–725). Elsevier.

Morley, C. J., Davis, P. G., Doyle, L. W., Brion, L. P., Hascoet, J. M., Carlin, J. B., et al. (2008). Nasal CPAP or intubation at birth for very preterm infants. *The New England Journal of Medicine, 358*(7), 700–708.

O'Shea, J. E., Thio, M., Kamlin, C. O., McGrory, L., Wong, C., et al. (2015). Videolaryngoscopy to teach neonatal intubation: A randomized trial. *Pediatrics, 136*(5), 912–919.

Soll, R. F., & Morley, C. J. (2001). Prophylactic versus selective use of surfactant in preventing morbidity and mortality in preterm infants. *Cochrane Database of Systematic Reviews, 2*, CD000510.

SUPPORT Study Group of the Eunice Kennedy Shriver NICHD Neonatal Research Network, Finer, N. N., Carlo, W. A., Walsh, M. C., Rich, W., Gantz, M. G., et al. (2010). Early CPAP versus surfactant in extremely preterm infants. *The New England Journal of Medicine, 362*(21), 1970–1979.

Todd, J., & Hammond, P. (2004). Choice and use of peripherally inserted central catheters by nurses. *Professional Nurse, 19*(9), 493–497.

Online Material

Fox, S. M. (2013, September 13). *Traumatic Lumbar Puncture*. Pediatric EM Morsels. https://pedemmorsels.com/traumatic-lumbar-puncture/.

Index

Note: Page numbers followed by "f" indicate figures, "t" indicate tables and "b" indicate boxes.